GASTROENTEROLOGY

PATHOPHYSIOLOGY AND CLINICAL APPLICATIONS

Harvey J. Dworken, M.D.
Associate Professor in Medicine,
Case Western Reserve University;
Director, Division of Gastroenterology,
University Hospitals,
Cleveland, Ohio

BUTTERWORTHS
Boston · London

Contents

Preface

While the objectives of this work remain essentially unchanged from those of its predecessor volume, *The Alimentary Tract,* usage of the original version has suggested a number of conceptual alterations. The text has been rewritten almost completely, and summarizes much of the mass of new information which has become available during the past seven years. The scope has also been increased greatly in order to make the book more useful to house officers and to practising physicians. The bibliography has been expanded and, since there is much to be learned from past medical experiences, brief historical notes have been added liberally throughout the text, usually at the ends of chapters. The rule for these is that no eponymic terms be applied without there being at least a laconic notation of the persons involved, their dates, their fields and locations of work, and their patrimony. One thus learns quickly that the edifice of modern gastroenterology stands on a foundation which owes no particular allegiance to any one place or any one time. The major thrust of the work remains unchanged. The text is designed to be read first, and then summarized if desired with illustrated lectures and demonstrations. Content may then be firmly fixed in memory by discussion in small groups of the problems and clinical conferences placed at the end of each chapter.

Though it may appear to be an act of hubris for a single author to attempt to write a complete text on alimentary disease in these days of burgeoning research and increasing specialization, it is my hope that certain advantages may be realized. Among these are a fairly uniform approach to the material with a minimum of unplanned repetition, treatment of each topic which is less detailed than in a work by subspecialists but which is nonetheless broad enough in scope to fill the needs of students and physicians, and the opportunity to inject the personal reactions of a single physician who has had the good fortune to live through a period of great change in his field of major professional interest. The text itself, while indubitably greater in length and breadth than its predecessor, will certainly weigh less heavily than multiauthored books and should, with luck, be readable through with a minimal amount of literary sedation.

Throughout the book, I have striven to achieve a logical development of each topic, citing appropriate references, and indicating where more information is needed, all with the interests of the readers and their patients clearly in mind. Should it succeed, the mighty effort required will have been worth the while.

Harvey J. Dworken

Cleveland, 1981

Acknowledgments

Many friends and colleagues have helped me during the course of my research and writing of this text. I owe great thanks to Case Western Reserve University and to Dr. Charles C.J. Carpenter, Chairman of the Department of Medicine, for granting me a sabbatical leave of six months to get this project under way. The entire staff of the Allen Memorial Library, Cleveland, was inordinately helpful and patient in providing me with an office and in complying with many requests, large and small. Most supportive were Lydia Holian, Associate Librarian, and Glen Jenkins of the Howard Dittrick Museum of Historical Medicine. For reading portions of the text and offering useful suggestions, thanks should go to colleagues Donald D. Anthony, James M. Boyle, Lansing C. Hoskins, John B. Marshall, Mary Petrelli, and Anthony S. Tavill, as well as to two anonymous referees solicited by my publishers, and to many students. Dr. Yao Shi Fu, of the Department of Pathology, deserves double recognition for both his editorial guidance and his preparation of the numerous photomicrographs which illustrate this volume. Typing chores were ably performed by Eleanor Anthony and Laraine Crosen, and much help and useful commentary has been provided by Patricia J. Sheehan, Editor, and Elizabeth O'Neill, Associate Editor at Butterworths.

HJD

Chapter 1

History Taking in Gastrointestinal Disease, and Evaluation of Abdominal Pain

In this book we intend to undertake a thorough examination of the digestive tract, its diseases and their treatment, and to delineate their pathophysiology to the extent that that is possible in these waning years of the twentieth century. At first, we focus briefly on the individual patient with a digestive disorder, with the aim of developing a logical approach to the diagnosis of our patient's problem in the most direct fashion and with the least discomfort and expense. We commence by suggesting an approach to history taking, and follow with a plan for evaluating abdominal pain by both physical diagnosis and by ancillary diagnostic procedures which will be described more fully later.

HISTORY TAKING

Derangements of normal physiology eventually approach the level of perception and manifest themselves to patients as symptoms. All too often, such symptoms do not appear until disease has become well established, and even then they might be nonspecific and may define the disease process imperfectly. Despite this inexactitude, a careful physician can often delineate the progress of a disorder and deduce the mechanisms involved. Success in these efforts is limited by the experience of the physician, the adequacy of the approach to the patient, and by the patient's own ability to describe the difficulty intelligibly. Taking the time to talk with patients and caring enough to employ an orderly and complete approach often makes the task more simple. Gastrointestinal complaints can be grouped under a number of headings, each of which should be investigated thoroughly. It is the purpose of this section to suggest such an approach.

Pain

Type. Cramplike pain usually suggests hyperperistalsis of the type associated with inflammation or obstruction of the small intestine or colon. It is also encountered frequently with psychogenic or functional alimentary disorders. A steady pain suggests a localized disorder. Sharp pains are most often due to spasm of intestinal musculature or acute inflammation of the viscera or peritoneum, whereas dull pains suggest visceral distention associated with partial obstruction or chronic inflammation. Patients with peptic ulcer or esophagitis often describe their discomfort as burning.

Severity. The patient's own description of the discomfort is extremely helpful, even when one discounts for hyperbole. The pain of acute peritonitis is often so excruciating that the patient cannot tolerate movement of the abdomen, or even deep breathing, as in acute pancreatitis or perforated peptic ulcer. Such pain is usually sudden in onset, though it may have been preceded by less intense pain for hours or days. The pain of an inflamed gall bladder or appendix progresses more slowly and usually does not reach such extreme intensities. Cancer may be painless until it causes visceral obstruction or spreads to surrounding tissues. Under this circumstance, pain gradually becomes more severe, prolonged, and relentless.

Location. Location is a very important determinant, the general location of pain often suggesting the organ involved. Biliary tract, pancreatic, and duodenal disorders commonly produce pain in the right upper abdomen; cecal, appendiceal, and lower ileal diseases, in the right lower section; and descending colonic or sigmoidal disorders, in the left lower abdomen. Supraumbilical pain relates mainly to organs above the jejunum, including gall bladder, liver, pancreas, duodenum, and stomach. Usually, the more sharply localized the pain, the more likely is the parietal peritoneum to be involved. Infraumbilical pain suggests small intestinal or colonic disorders. Vague, diffuse lower abdominal discomfort often accompanies inflammatory or psychogenic intestinal disease. One must always be mindful of the fact that not all abdominal pain stems from the alimentary tract—primary diseases of the urogenital system and the large abdominal arteries also cause abdominal pain!

Radiation. Patterns of pain radiation often suggest disease loci. Thus, right upper abdominal pain which radiates posteriorly and upward to a point between the shoulder blades suggests inflammation in the gall bladder or biliary tree. Pain in a similar part of the abdomen referred as well to the right scapuloclavicular junction suggests inflammation of the diaphragm, such as occurs with a subphrenic abscess. The pain of a penetrating peptic ulcer or of retroperitoneal disorders such as pancreatitis, cancer of the pancreas, or aneurysms of the abdominal aorta are often most severe in lower dorsal or upper lumbar levels of the back. A psoas abscess may produce pain that radiates downward into the groin and thigh.

Relationships. Knowledge of what relieves or aggravates pain is frequently a helpful indication of disease. Immediate aggravation by meals suggests that the disease somehow interferes with normal postprandial hyperperistaltic reflexes, a situation encountered in partial intestinal obstructions, intestinal inflammations, or in psychogenic disorders. Pain that appears some hours after a large meal suggests interference with normal gall bladder emptying or pancreatic secretion, as in cholelithiasis or pancreatitis. The pain of peptic ulcer or esophagitis is often promptly relieved by eating, whereas the patient with alcoholic gastritis may experience partial, transient relief from a drink of spirits.

Vomiting often relieves the pain of gastric retention or intestinal obstruction, whereas it usually does not affect, or worsens, symptoms of cholecystitis or pancreatitis. Passage of stool or flatus commonly improves the discomfort of inflammatory or obstructive lower bowel disorders.

Borborygmi (audible bowel sounds) related to abdominal cramps suggest the sort of hyperperistalsis that may accompany obstructive or inflammatory disease or some disorders or intestinal motility, such as the irritable bowel syndrome. A previous history of abdominal surgery might implicate postoperative adhesions as a cause of the obstruction. Chills and fever with abdominal pain suggest abscess formation or extensive inflammation. A recent abdominal injury prior to the onset of pain draws one's attention to the possibility of intra-abdominal hemorrhage or visceral perforation.

Anorexia and Weight Loss

Many patients are endowed with very frail appetites, and anorexia in such individuals may accompany any feeling of unease and be of little diagnostic value. However, significant and documentable loss of weight is always an important symptom, whether accompanied by anorexia or not.

Anorexia associated with fever suggests inflammatory disease or abscess. The resultant loss of weight is caused by both decreased caloric intake and increased metabolic demands. Malignant neoplasms also lead to prodigious losses of weight because of the increased metabolic requirements of the malignant tissue. Anorexia may also be caused by certain drugs, such as digitalis, or by a fear of the patient that eating will aggravate the abdominal pain.

In patients in whom weight falls despite a good or increased appetite, one must think of hypermetabolic states, such as hyperthyroidism, or conditions wherein normal metabolic pathways are interrupted by disease, such as uncontrolled diabetes mellitus, or disorders of intestinal absorption. Food faddists, such as vegetarians, commonly lose weight because of simple caloric inadequacy and protein malnutrition. More tragic cases of weight loss despite a good appetite exist in our society among those persons who are either too poor or too old, or both, to obtain the food necessary to maintain nutritional parity. Misdirected appetites for alcohol or drugs also frequently lead to weight loss stemming from caloric inadequacy.

Regurgitation and Heartburn (Pyrosis)

Regurgitation is a passive symptom in which esophageal, gastric or duodenal contents appear in the mouth without being preceded by retching or vomiting. If the contents merely taste like previously swallowed material, the chances are good that they have never entered the stomach and are regurgitated because they were sequestered in a diverticulum or were unable to traverse the full length of the esophagus because of obstruction or muscular dysfunction of that organ.

Regurgitation of sour and partially digested contents suggests that the reflux arose in the stomach and passed too readily retrograde into the esophagus. This symptom implies decreased competence of the sphincteric mechanism at the lower end of the esophagus, and the possible presence of a hiatal hernia. Bitter regurgitant fluid, particularly if it is bile stained, represents reflux of duodenal contents. This is encountered commonly in patients with previous partial gastric resections who also suffer from decreased competence of the gastroesophageal sphincter, and in many patients with gastritis or gastric ulcer.

Heartburn is a burning distress usually felt beneath the sternum, and commonly aggravated by large meals and by lying down. It results from irritation of the esophageal mucosa by acid or bilious gastric contents, and its occurrence correlates well with gross or microscopic findings of esophagitis in the lower esophagus. Assuming a recumbent position facilitates flow from stomach to esophagus and aggravates heartburn. Ingestion of antacids generally brings prompt relief.

Dysphagia

The patient who complains of difficulty in swallowing almost invariably has a disorder that can be precisely diagnosed. Dysphagia should be clearly distinguished by history from the feeling of a lump in the throat that does not interfere with swallowing and is usually psychogenic in origin.

Most disorders compromising the lumen of the esophagus (e.g., stricture, cancer or an obtruding mediastinal mass) gradually lead to a progressive form of swallowing difficulty, wherein the patient first experiences trouble with solid, then with liquid foods. Achalasia is the outstanding exception, patients usually experiencing equal difficulty from the start with solids and liquids, or even having more trouble with the latter.

Relationships. A history of heavy smoking in a patient with dysphagia makes one suspect a carcinoma of the esophagus. Nasogastric intubation in the recent past or a history of ingestion of caustic agents favors a diagnosis of stricture of the esophagus. Raynaud phenomenon or thickening of the skin is often found with scleroderma of the esophagus. Although loss of weight occurs with almost all forms of dysphagia, its absence favors a diagnosis of diffuse esophageal spasm. Previous heartburn or sour regurgitation suggests that dysphagia results from esophagitis and stricture, whereas pain with dysphagia (odynophagia) supports the impression of an esophageal ulcer, ulcerated neoplasm, or *Candida* or herpetic esophagitis.

Nausea and Vomiting

As an isolated symptom, nausea is often functional in origin, commonly accompanying the constipation and flatulence frequently associated with the irritable colon syndrome. However, since nausea may also be an early sign of disorders, such as digitalis intoxication, pregnancy, or hepatitis, its significance should never be minimized without fuller investigation. A careful history of drug ingestion, disease exposure, and menstrual activity should be obtained. Nausea, especially in the morning, may be an early symptom of alcohol withdrawal. Its relief by a drink of spirits is diagnostic.

A single episode of vomiting, while especially significant in an adult, might merely be an accompaniment to an infection or fever and have no specific import in relation to alimentary disease. Repeated vomiting, however, is another matter, and is often critically important.

Type of vomiting. Repeated vomiting of recently ingested gastric contents is commonly encountered in gastritis, peptic ulcer, alcoholism, and pancreatitis, and is occasionally seen in certain types of drug intoxication (e.g., digitalis) or in metabolic disorders, such as uremia.

Retention vomiting is usually the result of obstructions from ulcer or neoplasm. It is typified by vomitus, usually voluminous, containing food eaten many hours or several days before. The absence of bile staining indicates that duodenal contents are not able to reflux into the stomach.

Hematemesis implies that bleeding has arisen from above the ligament of Treitz (duodenal-jejunal junction). Coffee-grounds vomitus has the same significance, but indicates that blood has been in contact with acid gastric contents long enough to convert hemoglobin to acid hematin. Vomiting of blood-free contents once or twice prior to hematemesis suggests that retching may have produced tears of the gastroesophageal junctional mucosa (Mallory-Weiss syndrome).

Fecal vomiting, wherein gastric contents smell and taste fecal in character, is a rare, though highly significant, symptom of lower small intestinal or colonic obstruction.

Relationships. A history of ulcer pain, often for months or years, frequently precedes the onset of ulcer bleeding. Prior history of regular alcohol intake suggests erosive gastritis or bleeding esophageal varices as a cause of hematemesis. Multiple bleeding erosions may also be caused by salicylate ingestion. The use of anticoagulants may also precede upper gastrointestinal bleeding in patients with an ulcer history.

Patients with repeated or retentive vomiting often have a prior history of ulcer, whereas patients with fecal vomiting from chronic intestinal obstruction usually have had abdominal cramps, constipation, or loss of weight.

Distention of the Abdomen

This, like nausea, is often a functional symptom associated with the irritable colon syndrome, especially if it comes and goes over a long period of time and is unassociated with any more ominous symptoms such as loss of weight or blood in the stool. However, the symptom always demands further investigation.

Lower abdominal distention, recent in onset, occurring before and relieved by a bowel movement, suggests partial lower bowel obstruction, even when unaccompanied by pain or bleeding. Such obstructions may be seen in patients with colonic neoplasms, diverticulitis, or endometriosis. Thus, menstrual history, bowel regularity, and changes in weight must be investigated.

A middle-aged or older man with obstruction of the neck or the urinary bladder may complain of lower midabdominal distention without being particularly concerned, or even aware, that he is not urinating freely. In a woman such progressive distention may be coming from an enlarging ovarian cyst, a fibromyoma of the uterus, or even an unsuspected pregnancy.

Patients with partially obstructed loops of bowel due to adhesions, rotations, inflammatory disease, or neoplasm, or with disordered bowel motility, such as occurs in diabetic enteropathy, scleroderma, or intestinal pseudoobstruction, may note areas of distention in the abdomen from time to time. At times distention of these bowel loops is accompanied by severe cramps and borborygmi. These patients often lose weight from fasting because of awareness that eating leads to an aggravation of cramps and distention.

Diffuse distention of the abdomen, progressive and unrelenting, is commonly associated with the presence of free fluid in the peritoneal cavity (ascites). Since ascites is commonly seen in chronic liver disease, a history of alcoholism or jaundice is often confirmatory. The ascites of tuberculous peritonitis is commonly accompanied by fever and loss of weight, as is the ascites seen in malignant neoplasms that have metastasized to the peritoneal cavity.

Jaundice

Primary considerations. Jaundice may appear with or without the presence of amber-colored bilirubin in the urine, and with or without brown bile pigment in the stool. For reasons described in Chapter 8, the first few minutes of an interview with a jaundiced patient can reveal much about the pathophysiology of the disease. Normally colored urine and stool in an icteric patient defines hemolysis as the major cause of jaundice. Amber urine with normally colored stool indicates primary disease of liver parenchyma; amber urine with clay colored or lightly pigmented stool suggests an obstructive element to the jaundice, either in the liver itself or in the extrahepatic biliary tree.

Associated Symptoms. When jaundice is preceded by a period of malaise, frequently associated with fever and nausea, or when arthritis or urticaria have been part of the prodromata, viral hepatitis becomes strongly suspect. Itching suggests biliary tract obstruction. A preceding period of constant upper abdominal pain, often radiating into the back, suggests extrahepatic obstruction from neoplasms in or around the extrahepatic biliary ductal system. Intermittent previous attacks of upper abdominal pain, previous knowledge of gallstones, or both indicate that biliary calculi may have entered and blocked the common bile duct. High fever and hematuria may precede the jaundice of leptospirosis. Disorientation and irrational behavior indicate extensive hepatic necrosis.

Interrelationships. Since certain types of jaundice are familial, information regarding the possibility of similar difficulties in blood relatives should be obtained. Some other types of jaundice are contagious. Thus, in attempting to validate an impression of viral hepatitis, one should determine whether any personal or sexual contacts have recently had the disease, if the patient has had any injections recently, if injectable drugs from unsterile syringes have been used, if any transfusions of blood or blood products have been received, if a cut with an instrument possibly contaminated with someone else's blood has been sustained, or any raw or partially cooked food that may have been in contact with infected sewage has been ingested. Further types of jaundice are drug or chemical related, necessitating a full report from patients or drugs used, of occupational exposures to possible hepatotoxins, or of exposures to possibly toxic agents in other ways (such as a halothane anesthesia for surgery). Finally, since alcohol is a ubiquitous and common cause of liver disease, a careful history of its use should be taken in every case.

Bowel Action, Character of Stools, and Gastrointestinal Bleeding

Constipation. Chronic constipation is a troublesome symptom in our society, particularly where diets tend to be low in bulky foods with indigestible residues. A careful history of eating habits and a food inventory should be taken in all patients with this complaint. Questions should also be asked about anal discomfort, hemorrhoids, and bleeding, which often accompany this disorder. Since patients also experience constipation in response to emotional strain, social history is usually important in evaluating the complaint.

Acute constipation, or constipation of recent onset, carries more ominous implications, since it may indicate the onset of partial intestinal obstruction, particularly by an enlarging colonic cancer. Relevant associated symptoms such as loss of weight, crampy abdominal pain, and blood in the stools should be questioned. It is also well to bear in mind that certain drugs, such as anticholinergics, aluminum- or calcium-containing antacids, and anodynes, such as codeine, may also be constipating.

Diarrhea. Acute diarrhea may be a symptom of a variety of intestinal infections ranging from viral to protozoan. Thus, a careful history of exposure (travel through an endemic area, possible outbreak of viral or bacterial diarrhea, and food poisoning), should be taken. More and more fresh water supplies are becoming infected with *Giardia*, *Campylobacter*, and *Yersinia*, so any changes in the source of drinking water should be noted. Certain antibiotics, such as clindomycin, often cause diarrhea. The presence of blood in the stool suggests active colonic mucosal friability such as is seen in ulcerative colitis or cancer of the colon. A previous history of pelvic irradiation suggests radiation colitis. Chills and fever may accompany colitis, diverticulitis, or typhoidlike infections. Secretory diarrheas continue even when patients abstain from eating, whereas osmotic diarrheas improve with fasting.

Some chronic diarrhea, especially if it alternates with periods of constipation and is accompanied by little or no loss of weight, suggests the irritable colon syndrome. Sustained diarrhea with loss of weight may accompany chronic Crohn disease, ulcerative colitis, or one of the malabsorption syndromes. In such patients, arthritis or skin eruptions, such as erythema nodosum or pyoderma gangrenosum, may also be present.

Character of Stools. Patients with constipation frequently have small, hard, round (scybalous) stools. If the patient also notes mucus on the stool, the diagnosis of irritable colon is suggested. Occasionally, collections of mucus may appear grossly to resemble flatworm segments.

Watery stools may typify any of the acute diarrheas, a secretory diarrhea due to vasoactive intestinal polypeptide, an osmotic diarrhea due to ingestion of laxatives, or the diarrhea caused by unconjugated bile acids or dihydroxy fatty acids. A soft, pasty stool, particularly if it has a strong odor, suggests malabsorption. Ribbonlike stools, although often described as suggestive of rectal cancer, are much more commonly noted by patients with irritable colons. Fibrotic rectal strictures, such as occur in chronic ulcerative colitis, lymphogranuloma venerum, or radiation proctitis may also narrow the diameter of stools.

Heed carefully the man who states that he passes air or stool with his urine, or the woman who passes gas or stool vaginally while defecating. These complaints are diagnostic of fistulas from the rectum or sigmoid to the urinary bladder or vagina, and may complicate cases of Crohn disease, colonic diverticulitis, or, rarely, cancer.

Gastrointestinal Bleeding. Blood in the stool may come from one of many sources. Hemorrhoidal blood often streaks the surface of an otherwise normal stool. Occasionally a prolapsing internal hemorrhoid will bleed profusely at stool, the blood being shed in large 10- to 15-ml spurts, unaccompanied by stool and appearing essentially odorless. It is surprising to find that some patients will allow this condition to continue for months unchecked, occasionally suffering the secondary effects of blood-loss anemia as a consequence of their procrastination in seeking medical care.

Bleeding may also accompany fissures, but such bleeding is invariably accompanied by anal pain at stool and is not likely to be nearly so voluminous as the bleeding from internal hemorrhoids. Thrombosed external hemorrhoids are usually also quite painful, but rarely do they bleed.

The character of bloody bowel movements resulting from colonic lesions above the anus depends on the extent and nature of the disorder and the rapidity of the bleeding. Thus, when ulcerative colitis is mild and limited to the rectum, stools may be formed or soft and contain variable proportions of blood and mucus. This combination may be exactly the same in patients with carcinomas of the distal colon and rectum. When colitis is more extensive and ulcerations deep, stools become looser and bleeding greater, reaching at times the level of exsanguinating hemorrhage. In such cases bowel movements also tend to have a highly offensive odor, owing to the partially digested blood protein and necrotic tissue in the stool.

On the other hand, patients with a localized arterial rupture from a colonic diverticulum or from colonic angiodysplasia have profusely bloody bowel movements that are only slightly odorous. A similar set of complaints occurs in patients with sudden mucosal necrosis produced by mesenteric vascular lesions resulting in acute ischemia.

The usually liquid red- or plum-colored stools seen in massive upper gastrointestinal bleeding are among the most malodorous of all blood-containing stools. Here blood is shed heavily in the esophagus, stomach, or upper intestine, is partially digested by intestinal proteolytic enzymes, and possibly because of its sheer volume, progresses very rapidly through the distal intestine before the red heme pigment has lost all its usual color.

More typically, when blood in amounts greater than 30 to 40 ml is lost into the upper alimentary tract, the resulting stool is formed or soft, depending on the amount of blood lost, and is either reddish black or jet black in color with a shining or tarry quality to the surface. This is true melena and should be carefully distinguished from the dull gray–black or black color imparted to stools by orally ingested iron or bismuth. The ingenuous should also learn to distinguish the bluish black color of berry residues in stool from melena.

In using the presence of melena to approximate the level in the gastrointestinal tract at which bleeding occurred, it is safe to assume that lesions below the ileocecal junction rarely cause melena. As indicated above, however, the converse of this statement is not true—bloody stools may originate from lesions at any level of the tract. In a patient beyond infancy, hematemesis accompanying melena or bloody stools indicates bleeding above the ligament of Treitz.

One final consideration in regard to gastrointestinal bleeding is detecting from history, insofar as possible, the possible cause(s) of the hemorrhage. Thus, a patient with a previous history of peptic ulcer is a likely candidate for hemorrhage from a recurrence of that lesion. A patient with cirrhosis of the liver may well be bleeding from esophageal varices. The use of anticoagulants may facilitate bleeding from an ulcer, while salicylates and alcohol cause diffuse hemorrhagic gastritis. Patients with consumptive coagulopathies or thrombopenia frequently bleed from the intestinal tract. One or more of the curious telangiectases of the Oster-Weber-Rendu syndrome or von Willebrand disease may lead to intestinal bleeding, whereas others may be visible on the lips or buccal mucosa. The incidence of peptic ulcer, and thus gastrointestinal bleeding, is increased in patients with chronic obstructive lung disease, rheumatoid arthritis, and hyperparathyroidism. Major lower bowel hemorrhage may arise from a bleeding colonic diverticulum in patients with chronic constipation, from colonic ischemia in patients with congestive heart failure, or from uremic colitis in chronic renal disease. Although such observations cannot be considered to be anything other than tentative on the basis of history alone, they are extremely useful as a guide for further diagnostic studies.

Anorectal Symptoms

Pain and Discharge. Confined anal pain is aggravated by defecation and is almost invariably associated with anal inflammation, such as a mucocutaneous fissure, a thrombosed external hemorrhoid, or a perianal abscess. Pain radiating toward the anus from within the pelvis and occurring in spasms lasting for several minutes or more (proctalgia fugax) is occasionally experienced by patients with the irritable colon syndrome. Rectal cancer causes no pain until the process has extended into the perirectal tissues, at which time a boring, continuous discomfort occurs. Such pain frequently radiates toward the sacrum.

Tenesmus is a distressing feeling of rectal urgency that may be present in any acute diarrheal disorder and is often painful. It is associated with spasm of the anal and rectal muscles and may also be experienced by patients with perirectal inflammations such as prostatitis.

Anal discharge varies from clear mucus to frank pus. The former is commonly seen in irritable colon syndrome but may also be encountered in patients with bacterial colitis, rectal cancer, or mild degrees of ulcerative colitis. Prolapsed internal hemorrhoids and anal fissures often become inflamed, and mucus is secreted from the overlying or surrounding mucosa. Pus is commonly associated with ulcerative colitis or with spontaneous drainage of a perirectal abscess.

Prolapsing of Tissue and Perianal Mass. Internal hemorrhoids are the most common cause of tissue prolapsing through the anal ring. The patient may note that although the prolapse may be reduced by digital pressure against the mass, the process is likely to recur later either at stool or in association with walking or exercising. Prolapsing of tissue, especially in elderly persons, may also be the first symptom of eversion or prolapse of the rectum. It is less common, but not exceedingly rare, for a pedunculated rectal or sigmoidal polyp to prolapse repeatedly through the anus.

Perianal masses are most commonly folds of redundant skin associated with stretching by internal hemorrhoids. If the mass is quite painful, however, it is more likely to be due either to a thrombosed internal hemorrhoid or to a perianal abscess.

Pruritus. Perianal itching frequently accompanies hemorrhoids or long-standing diarrhea. It is also at times a consequence of sustained perianal moisture and poor hygiene, especially when tight undergarments are worn in hot weather. Prolonged anal pruritus, especially if it is also a complaint among other members of the household, suggests infection with pinworms (*Enterobius vermicularis*).

Emotional Background

Since many gastrointestinal disorders, such as irritable colon, peptic ulcer, ulcerative colitis, and Crohn disease are adversely influenced by emotional stresses, obtaining a precise notion of a patient's psychological status is an essential element in planning treatment. Numerous occasions arise where friendly personal discussion and counseling will do more for the patient's physical status than will any amount of medication.

To counsel patients one must know something about them, and there is no better way to know than to ask. It is important to learn whether they are nervous, compulsive, or depressed, and to discover something about their fears, concerns, and angers. Problems are usually personal, not global. One is more likely to worry oneself into an ulcer or a relapse of colitis from concerns about domestic, financial, occupational, or sexual problems than from anxiety over world peace, environmental pollution, and honesty in Washington. Once the nature of the concerns is clarified, counseling can begin.

Family History

Certain gastrointestinal disorders show a clear genetic inheritance and are potentially lethal, but treatable if diagnosed early. Among these are familial polyposis of the colon and Gardner syndrome, which frequently lead to intestinal cancer, Wilson disease, which can lead to progressive liver and brain damage, hemochromatosis, and multiple endocrine adenomatosis. Once this type of diagnosis is made in the proband, other family members should be so informed, and then evaluated.

Other disorders, such as Crohn disease, sprue, and peptic ulcer, are familial, though not clearly hereditary. This knowledge is useful in making tentative diagnostic deductions that can, at times, be helpful and timesaving. For example, the appearance of an anal fistula in a patient whose sibling is known to suffer from Crohn disease might lead one to order more extensive X rays of the intestinal tract than otherwise, and so arrive at a more prompt diagnosis. Similarly, upper abdominal pain in a patient with an immediate blood relative with known peptic ulcer should cause a physician to consider the likelihood of an ulcer, even though the pain pattern itself is atypical.

Occupational History

Some occupations are more continuously stressful than others and may predispose to peptic ulceration. One study has shown that ulcer incidence is higher among factory supervisors and transportation and unskilled workers than it is in the general population, while the incidence is very low among agricultural workers. Irritable colon symptoms are also common among patients in stressful occupations. When inquiring about occupational stresses, it is well to know something about certain practices in United States industry. Production-line workers whose output is lower than average may be penalized by their fellow workers whose productivity and income must of necessity be geared to that of the slowest worker on the line.

Workers in the steel industry must change shifts weekly and commonly have trouble readjusting sleep and leisure activities so often. Urban transit workers are expected to collect fares, struggle with heavy vehicular traffic, and adhere to fixed schedules, and they are liable to penalties whenever their performance falls short. Prolonged strikes may also place serious financial and emotional stresses on the worker whose financial reserves are not adequate to withstand lengthy periods of greatly reduced or no income.

In contrast with the important effects that occupational stresses may have on the gastrointestinal tract, exposures to potential occupational toxins are limited. Among these are carbon tetrachloride, a potent hepatotoxin, and lead, a neurotoxin that may cause severe abdominal cramps as an early symptom. Responsible industry carefully monitors exposures to these agents, but irresponsibility is frequent, especially when previously unimplicated toxic agents are involved.

Habits

Diet. Many Americans subsist on a low residue "hamburger, fried potato, and ice cream" diet. Many Americans are also constipated and overweight and suffer the long-term complications of that diet—hemorrhoids, diverticulosis of the colon, and diverticulitis. It is not uncommon, on the other hand, to encounter the careless vegetarian suffering from both diarrhea and malnutrition. One cannot treat these disorders without having knowledge of dietary habits and making efforts to help the patient realize the need for correcting them.

Drugs and Treatments. The incidence of medication taking in this country, whether it is obtained over the counter or through a prescription, is so great that it is distinctly unusual to encounter a patient who is not taking one or several drugs. Aspirin, acetaminophen, cold preparations, vitamins, and contraceptives are among the most common. All are potentially toxic. This chapter has already suggested some of the gastrointestinal symptoms and disorders that may be drug or treatment induced. Later chapters, especially Chapters 6 and 7, refer to others. At this point it is essential only to note that no history is complete without reference to a catalog of drugs taken either currently or in the past, with special note taken of treatments, such as radiation therapy or blood transfusions. Specific inquiries should also be made about certain drugs, such as aspirin and contraceptives, because their very ubiquity makes many people fail to realize that they are potentially disabling medicaments.

Alcohol. No treatise on gastrointestinal history taking can be considered complete without special mention of ethyl alcohol, for here is a popular, possibly addicting chemical that, operating alone, can severely damage the stomach, injure the small bowel, and destroy the liver and pancreas. Its abuse is the cause for expenditure of untold millions of dollars for medical care and service in the United States annually. The volume of alcoholic intake is generally underestimated by most consumers, at least when one compares the intake admitted by a patient with the amount attested to by the observant spouse. Most physicians are well aware of these discrepancies and often automatically multiply a patient's acknowledged consumption by a factor of four or five to arrive at the probable intake. Often they are doubtless correct, but occasionally a patient is misjudged and the start of proper treatment is delayed. When doubt about the fact or the amount of alcoholic intake exists, collateral history from family or friends can often clarify the matter.

EVALUATING ABDOMINAL PAIN

A physician's record in medical diagnosis is punctuated by successes and failures. With time, it is governed increasingly by remembrances formed from previous experiences. When confronted by a symptomatic patient, the physician remembers to ask questions whose answers tend to exclude certain diagnoses, while making others more likely. When the limits of the history-taking process are reached, physical examination, radiological and laboratory tests, and occasionally even exploratory surgery are employed to arrive at a precise, single diagnosis. We have just reviewed the history-taking process as it applies to the diagnosis of digestive diseases, and come now to consider physical and ancillary methods of diagnosis.

The location of abdominal pain brings certain diagnostic possibilities to mind. In this section, specific remembrances of disorders commonly causing abdominal pain are outlined, and ways to confirm or exclude them by physical and ancillary diagnosis are suggested. Appendicitis, diverticulitis, splenic subcapsular hemorrhage, and inflammatory disorders of the biliary tree are used as models of painful disorders in each quadrant of the abdomen.

The Lower Right Quadrant

Appendicitis is suggested by the recent onset of localized pain in the lower right quadrant of the abdomen. The pain is often preceded by several hours of a less intense, less sharply localized periumbilical discomfort frequently associated with nausea, vomiting, and slight fever. The shift of pain to the lower right quadrant (LRQ) signals the onset of parietal peritonitis. Chills and high fever are distinctly unusual in uncomplicated appendicitis and suggest perforation with formation of an abscess, or even a wholly different disease, such as typhoid fever or the acute megacolon of ulcerative colitis. Diarrhea preceding or contemporaneous with the pain is also foreign to one's remembrance of uncomplicated appendicitis and suggests instead acute Crohn disease or, if the patient has been taking antibiotics, a drug-induced enterocolitis. Recent constipation is compatible with acute appendicitis. Prolonged constipation associated with scybalous, often mucoid, stool or episodes of abdominal bloating leads to the suspicion of an irritable colon as the cause of the pain. The presence of fever, however, excludes that diagnosis. Acute constipation with the inability to pass gas, suggests the presence of an intestinal obstruction. Here the pain tends to be crampy rather than steady, as it would be with appendicitis, and the cramps are often associated with borborygmi and sometimes localized distention of the abdomen. History of blood in the stool erases all remembrance of appendicitis and leads instead to the thought of colitis or colonic neoplasm. One of the major concerns of surgeons treating younger patients with symptoms suggesting appendicitis is the problem of mesenteric adenitis. This diagnosis is suggested by concurrent or slightly previous symptoms of an upper respiratory infection with the abdominal discomfort.

Disease in organ systems other than the gastrointestinal tract must also be considered in patients with either LRQ or lower left quadrant pain. Chief among these are ruptured or twisted ovarian cysts, tubal pregnancies, endometriosis, pelvic inflammatory disease, and acute ureteral obstructions. Appearance of pain between menses suggests the possibility of a ruptured cyst or a tubal pregnancy, while the pain of endometriosis usually occurs with menstruation. Ureteral or renal pelvic pain often has an associated component of back as well as lower quadrant abdominal discomfort, and the pain tends to radiate to the groin or pelvic area. Furthermore, the patient often has a history of urinary tract infections, acute hematuria, or disorders such as gout or chronic diarrhea that predispose to the precipitation of ureteral calculi.

The pain of appendicitis may be mild or atypically located in patients with a retrocecal appendix, or in older patients. Complications, such as perforation and abscess, appear to be higher than usual in both groups. With a retrocecal appendix the pain may not shift, and localization may be in the back or the right flank. While older patients may have little or no pain and complain only of a bloating discomfort in the LRQ and fever, their symptoms may also be identical to those in younger persons.

Abdominal examination in uncomplicated appendicitis usually reveals moderate spasm of the musculature of the lower right abdominal wall. Palpation must be gentle. The examiner should be comfortably seated, and thus not forced to employ the hand for support and diagnosis simultaneously. Slightly deeper pressure in the area of spasm usually elicits tenderness and should also be done with great concern for the comfort of the patient. The elicitation of rebound tenderness is usually not helpful as an additional means of demonstrating parietal peritonitis. Psoas and obturator signs are frequently positive in patients with inflammation of a retrocecal appendix.

A palpable mass in the LRQ suggests an appendiceal abscess, Crohn disease, a neoplasm, or an ovarian cyst. Its presence speaks against uncomplicated appendicitis. Bowel sounds are generally reduced or normal in acute appendicitis. Their total absence suggests fairly extensive peritonitis or ileus and may indicate an appendiceal or cecal perforation, or the ileus of a toxic megacolon. Peristaltic rushes are associated with obstructing lesions but may also be seen with certain types of acute enterocolitis, such as bacillary, amebic, or antibiotic-induced forms. Rectal and pelvic examinations should always be done in patients suspected of having appendicitis, the former to confirm point tenderness in the LRQ and to localize abdominal masses, the latter to identify painful gynecological disorders.

Laboratory work is straightforward. Polymorphonuclear leukocytosis with a total count between 10,000 and 15,000 per ml supports the diagnosis of appendicitis. A higher count suggests an abscess or purulent peritonitis. A lower white count is strong evidence against appendicitis, and a count below 5,000 suggests lymphadenitis or typhoid infection. Stools should be negative for occult blood. Microscopic examination of the freshly passed stool for *Endamoeba histolytica* or *Giardia*, and stool cultures, are clearly indicated in patients with abdominal pain, diarrhea, and fever. Significant anemia favors colitis or even neoplasm as the underlying cause of pain. Abdominal X rays or computed tomograms are often helpful to rule out bowel obstruction and LRQ masses. If all evidence points to appendicitis, a barium enema should not be performed. It is a good screening procedure, however, in those patients with suggestive pain when other studies tend to exclude appendicitis.

The Lower Left Quadrant

Diverticulitis is a common cause of pain in the lower left quadrant (LLQ). Save for its left-sided location, symptoms and signs are much like those of appendicitis. Remembrance of diverticulitis is stirred most clearly when an older patient, often one with long-term constipation, complains of a new cramping or steady pain associated with fever. There is usually some derangement of bowel activity, most often diarrhea with or without tenesmus, but occasionally constipation and bloating. Small amounts of blood and mucus may be noted in the stool. Free perforation of a diverticulum into the peritoneal cavity is suspected when the pain spreads upward and to the right, while becoming increasingly intense. As with appendicitis, chills and spiking fever suggest localized perforation with formation of an abscess.

Lower urinary tract symptoms, such as dysuria and frequency, are commonly observed. These result from direct extension of the sigmoidal inflammatory process to the urinary bladder, and are more common in men. With advance spread of the inflammation, a spontaneous fistula may develop between colon and bladder, leading to pneumaturia. At times, pneumaturia is the sole symptom of chronic diverticulitis.

There are no symptoms of diverticulitis that cannot be produced as well by an obstructing carcinoma of the descending or sigmoid colon, and the two conditions occasionally coexist. Patients with cancer may have noted a period of bleeding at stool before the onset of pain, while patients with diverticulitis frequently offer a lengthy history of prior bowel irregularity. However, these symptoms are not truly diagnostic. In Crohn disease of the colon, characterized by inflammatory obstructing lesions of the rectum and sigmoid, or in radiation colitis, a similar set of symptoms may appear. At times, patients with Crohn disease have had a previous history of cramps and diarrhea without bleeding, while patients with ulcerative colitis more usually note considerable blood in their stools and may have suffered bleeding for some time prior to the onset of abdominal pain.

The acute onset of left flank and lower left quadrant pain with bloody diarrhea and fever and without a preceding history of bowel disease should call to mind the possibility of a distal bowel infarction, especially in patients with evidence of vascular disease or a hypovolemic state. Such symptoms also suggest infectious types of colitis, ranging from amebiasis to bacterial infection, the former being most commonly associated with bleeding. A history of the recent use of broad-spectrum antibiotics, especially clindomycin, suggests the possibility of a drug-induced colitis. The absence of fever and bloody stools in patients with moderate to severe left lower quadrant pain excludes none of the disorders discussed above and adds the need to consider the possibility of an irritable colon. This common disorder occurs in all age groups, may be associated with excruciating discomfort, and is often preceded by a history of mucoid, frequent stools alternating with constipation. The diarrhea is almost never associated with watery stools. Endometriosis and pelvic inflammatory disease are among the most common urogenital disorders causing LLQ pain.

On examination of the patient with LLQ pain, tenderness can be elicited in all of the conditions mentioned. The presence of a palpable loop of lower bowel is also common. An extremely tender or fixed mass, or both, suggests inflamed bowel, abscess, or neoplasm. Peritoneal signs, such as muscular rigidity and ileus, indicate the presence of pericolitis, and may occur with severe colitis or diverticulitis. Marked tympany with distention of the abdomen raises the specter of bowel perforation, especially where percussion over the liver shows that the usual area of dullness is absent.

Pelvic and rectal examinations should always be performed in patients with LLQ pain, followed by proctosigmoidoscopy if signs do not point to a bowel perforation. Stools should be examined for pus cells and parasites, and blood and stool cultures should be performed where infection is suspected. Plain abdominal X rays are useful in revealing such concomitants of abdominal pain as megacolon, ileus, or free perforations of the bowel, and may also demonstrate colonic obstruction or a feces-filled colon. Barium enema is usually indicated once perforation or a condition prone to perforation, such as severe colitis or massive infarction, have been ruled out. Although colonoscopy is at times very useful in diagnosis, its use should be reserved for those instances in which the cause of the pain has not been clearly defined by the studies suggested above.

The Upper Left Quadrant

Splenic subcapsular hemorrhage is a signal cause of upper left quadrant (ULQ) pain. The discomfort is often mild at onset and tends to worsen in time. The pain is steady, and often aggravated by deep breathing if the underside of the left diaphragm is involved by the associated inflammation of the splenic capsule. Pain may be referred to the left shoulder. Since splenic hemorrhage generally follows trauma, the patient should be questioned about athletic or automobile injuries within the previous four to six weeks. In persons taking anticoagulants or suffering from a spontaneous disorder of blood clotting, the trauma may have been very mild indeed, or may have even passed unnoticed.

The pain of splenic infarction is usually sharp and sudden in onset. It is most likely to occur in a patient who has a possible source of emboli in the left side of the heart. The pain of hemorrhage, on the other hand, is of more gradual onset, although much more ominous. In time, as bleeding continues, the pain of the subcapsular hemorrhage may become agonizing. If the splenic capsule ruptures and blood enters the peritoneal cavity freely, a catastrophic spreading form of pain appears, and the patient is likely to pass suddenly into shock. A carefully taken history and precipient observation usually prevents the physician from withholding an essential operation until this dreadful complication occurs.

A pseudocyst or abscess in the body or tail of the pancreas often causes steady ULQ pain, which has a tendency to radiate into the back. An enlarging aneurysm of the abdominal aorta or the splenic artery may do the same. Distinguishing these pains from that of splenic affections may be very difficult. Left epigastric pain arising from a peptic ulcer, however, is usually relieved promptly by eating, at least during the early days of the disease. If the pain is steady, low in intensity, and aggravated by meals, the possibility of a gastric cancer arises. The relief of ULQ pain by defecation or the passage of flatus suggests distention of the splenic flexure by gas, a frequent concomitant of the irritable colon syndrome. Jejunal obstruction may also cause ULQ pains, but these are usually crampy, and often associated with vomiting or borborygmi.

Physical examination may disclose a spleen enlarged to percussion or palpation in patient with subcapsular hemorrhage. The patient may appear pale. Pancreatic pseudocysts and vascular aneurysms are often palpable and slightly tender, and lie medial to the splenic area. Bruits are often audible over aneurysms or when the aorta is compressed by a pancreatic neoplasm or pseudocyst. There may be signs of an effusion at the base of the left lung and decreased movement of the diaphragm if subdiaphragmatic peritonitis is present.

Anemia in the absence of occult or gross blood in the stool should recall the possibility of a subcapsular hematoma of the spleen in a patient with ULQ complaints, especially if bizarre forms of red blood cells are found. An elevated ratio of serum amylase or urinary amylase to creatinine supports the impression of pancreatitis or pseudocyst. Plain films of the abdomen usually demonstrate splenomegaly and some aneurysms. An upper gastrointestinal series may show an ulcer or cancer of the stomach, as well as rightward displacement of the fundus by an enlarged spleen or anterior displacement of the body by a retroperitoneal mass such as a pseudocyst, neoplasm, or aneurysm. An enlarged spleen will often cause downward displacement of the splenic flexure of the colon after a barium enema. Abdominal ultrasonography and computed tomography are very useful in demonstrating fluid-filled tumors, such as aneurysms and cysts, and solid masses; celiac arteriography is effective in demonstrating solid masses, such as carcinomas of the pancreas and splenic hematomas.

The Upper Right Quadrant

Inflammatory disorders of the biliary tree are among the prime causes of upper right quadrant (URQ) pain. When stones impact in the outlet of the gall bladder, the resultant edema and inflammation of that organ lead to a steady pain that frequently radiates to the back and the right scapular area. The pain usually lasts for hours and may be associated with, though unrelieved by, vomiting. Chills and fever in addition to the pain suggest empyema of the gall bladder, while associated jaundice or dark urine indicates cholangitis from calculous obstruction of the common bile duct. Crampy URQ pain, especially if it is associated with bloating, belching, and nausea, is more likely the result of functional bowel disease. Sudden sharp and severe URQ pain in a young black patient suggests the possibility of a hepatic infarction associated with sickle cell anemia.

Other types of URQ pain tend to be less severe though more persistent. Sudden distention of the liver in a patient with right heart failure may lead to both URQ discomfort and shortness of breath. Patients with acute hepatitis will often have URQ pain as a chief complaint, but this symptom is generally associated with constitutional symptoms, such as lassitude, nausea, and fever. Patients with primary or metastatic hepatic neoplasms often complain of a feeling of heaviness or dull pain in the URQ.

Pains caused by pancreatitis and acute cholecystitis are often difficult to distinguish from each other. There is a tendency for pancreatic pain to localize somewhat closer to the midline, and to radiate directly into the back instead of to the scapula, but these are frail reeds on which to rest a diagnosis. A preceding history of alcoholism, recent abdominal trauma, or mumps supports the possibility of pancreatitis. Peptic ulcer pain, too, is usually more in the midline, but when the pain penetrates into the back, it may resemble biliary tract discomfort. Usually, there is a history of previous relief of pain by food. A subhepatic abscess is commonly associated with rigors, fever, and dull URQ pain. So also is the pain caused by abscesses in the substance of the liver. Patients with this disorder often have a preceding history of pelvic inflammatory disease or concomitant amebic colitis. Where an abscess is located in the subphrenic area, the URQ pain is often aggravated by inspiration.

Physical examination in patients with inflammatory disorders of the biliary tree commonly demonstrates spasm of the abdominal musculature in the URQ. An enlarged, tender gall bladder, which can usually be felt with light palpation, suggests empyema or hydrops of that organ. The presence of a sharp, tender liver edge suggests either hepatitis or hepatic congestion. Enlargement of the liver by one or more nodules of malignant tumor is usually made readily apparent by the hard consistency of the liver. In peptic ulcer disease, the tenderness tends to be more toward the midline, but this location is variable. If the patient has a free perforation of an ulcer into the peritoneal cavity, the musculature of the abdominal wall becomes extremely rigid, and peristaltic sounds are usually absent. When a large amount of free air is present in the peritoneal cavity, percussion dullness over the liver disappears.

A white blood count is essential for the evaluation of patients with URQ pain. Leukocytosis suggests abscess or inflammation of the gall bladder or pancreas, and tends to rule out an uncomplicated peptic ulcer. Elevated serum amylases are not specific, but tend to support an impression of pancreatitis. Obstruction of the biliary tree by calculi or enlargement of the head of the pancreas by inflammation or pseudocyst may cause obstructive jaundice and elevation of the serum bilirubin. The presence of hypotension, elevated hematocrit, or methhemalbumin in the blood supports the impression of hemorrhagic pancreatitis in a patient with severe URQ pain. Where the hematocrit is low, especially if the patient has been taking anticoagulants and shows no evidence of occult blood in the stool, the physician should recall the possibility of intramural hemorrhage into the intestine or mesentery.

Plain abdominal X rays are employed to demonstrate the presence of free air in the peritoneal cavity from a perforation, opaque biliary calculi, calcifications in the substance of the pancreas, or localized areas of ileus in the jejunum or colon. Presence of the last sign suggests the diagnosis of pancreatitis with regional peritonitis. Further evaluation includes the use of the upper gastrointestinal series to demonstrate intrinisic disease of the stomach, duodenum, or jejunum and the possibility of displacements associated with enlargement of the gall bladder or pancreas. Where this study is negative, one may wait for the subsidence of pain before ordering X rays of the gall bladder and biliary tree. Upper gastrointestinal endoscopy will occasionally reveal the presence of ulcers not detected by X ray, and the use of endoscopic retrograde contrast studies or the pancreatic duct and biliary tree is likely to detect abnormalities in these areas that cannot be demonstrated by any other technique. Ultrasonography and computed tomography are also indicated, often as the first diagnostic procedures in patients with unexplained URQ pain because enlargements of the gall bladder or pancreas, calculi in the gall bladder, and masses in the liver are commonly detected easily by these procedures.

CONCLUSION

This discussion suggests an orderly approach for evaluating pain appearing in any quadrant of the abdomen. The approach requires an adequate knowledge of the major disorders which may occur in the abdomen, their usual presenting and associated symptoms, and the physical findings that may be anticipated. Each diagnostic procedures should be employed to answer a specific question, and those which are least costly and least troublesome for the patient should be used first. The willy-nilly use of any and all diagnostic procedures tends to add much to the patient's discomfort and little to the solution of the clinical problem.

The physician of the 1980s is at considerable risk of suffering from an abundance of riches when the full range of diagnostic procedures currently available is critically analyzed. Not only have conventional radiological procedures been improved, but entirely new techniques, such as ultrasonography and computed tomographic scanning, have been shown to be capable of duplicating, supplementing, or even replacing the older modalities. While not attempting to denigrate these new procedures, for they are indeed remarkable, it is important to point out that many of the conditions which they demonstrate so well were, in the past, demonstrated also by other procedures, although not always so well or so easily.

The central physician, the adviser who was first consulted by the patient, must remain central during the diagnostic and therapeutic process, lest the better interests of the patient become subverted amid a welter of duplicative diagnostic procedures. Physicians must choose carefully among the variety of available tests, in order to delineate an appropriate program for each patient, the one which is the most accurate, the least uncomfortable and risky, and the least expensive. Unless the central physician, with the full knowledge and agreement of the patient, has remained in control of the diagnostic program, there is danger that it might, like the horseman of Stephen Butler Leacock, have "rode madly off in all directions."* One must carefully consider the possible benefits and disadvantages of each procedure before advising that it be undertaken.

There has as yet been nothing better devised to furnish the basis and rationale for the supplemental diagnostic workup than the complete history and physical examination. It is unlikely that there ever will be. For not only

*From *Gertrude the Governess* (1911).

do physicians acquaint themselves with the setting of the patient's illness while taking a history, but so also do they get to know the patient at the same time, and to provide a feeling of assurance and sympathy. No history recorded on a questionnaire or obtained by a third party is likely to replace the direct interview between a patient and an informed physician in the quiet of a consulting or hospital room.

It is the purpose of this text to inform physicians and students about digestive disorders, their pathophysiology, their symptoms, and their physical findings; it has been the purpose of this first chapter to suggest ways of framing the interview and diagnostic program of patients with these disorders. I hope that the effort will, to a significant degree, prove successful.

CHAPTER 2

A Survey of Gastrointestinal Hormonology

In the past twenty years, technological advances have permitted protein chemists to purify, characterize, and in many instances, synthesize an increasing number of gastrointestinal hormones. Immunochemical techniques have facilitated the identification of cellular sites in which these hormones are stored and perhaps produced. Radioimmunoassay has provided the mechanism for the measurement of these hormones in body fluids. The upper gastrointestinal tract has proved to harbor the largest, if not the most important, endocrine gland system in the body. Because many of the hormones produced in this system have effects on more than a single component of an organ, and indeed on more than one organ, it is worthwhile to obtain an overview of their actions prior to considering the physiology and pathophysiology of the organs individually.

Most of the gastrointestinal hormones appear to have effects that are localized to the gut. A few, such as enteroglucagon and somatostatin, have systemic effects as well. Of the multiple effects which they have been demonstrated to exert on the gastrointestinal tract in human beings and other animals, it is not clear in every case which are truly physiologic and which are merely incidental effects of pharmacologic doses. Thus, the exact importance in maintaining homeostasis, particularly of the candidate hormones, has not been established.

Each of the gastrointestinal hormones is a polypeptide whose effects depend on its molecular structure (Tables 2–1 and 2–2). Gastrin and cholecystokinin (CCK), for example, possess identical four-amino residues at the carboxyl terminal of the polypeptide chain and have similar stimulant effects on the stomach, gall bladder, and pancreas. This residue alone is cap-

---

I wish to thank Dr. James M. Boyle for his help in preparing this chapter.

Table 2-1. Gastrin-Cholecystokinin Family

Human big gastrin (G 34, mol wt 3,839)

1 2 3 4 5 6 7 8 9 10 11 12 13 14 15 16 17 18
Pyro-Leu-Gly-Pro-Gln-Gly-His-Pro-Ser-Leu-Val-Ala-Asp-Pro-Ser-Lys-Lys-Gln

19 20 21 22 23 24 25 26 27 28 29 30 31 32 33 34
-Gly-Pro-Trp-Leu-Glu-Glu-Glu-Glu-Glu-Ala-Tyr-Gly-Trp-Met-Asp-Phe-NH_2
|
R

Porcine cholecystokinin—variant (39 amino acids, mol wt 4,678)

1 2 3 4 5 6 7 8 9 10 11 12 13 14 15 16 17 18 19 20
Tyr-Ile-Gln-Gln-Ala-Arg-Lys-Ala-Pro-Ser-Gly-Arg-Val-Ser-Met-Ile-Lys-Asn-Leu-Gln

21 22 23 24 25 26 27 28 29 30 31 32 33 34 35 36 37 38 39
-Ser-Leu-Asp-Pro-Ser-His-Arg-Ile-Ser-Asp-Arg-Asp-Tyr-Met-Gly-Trp-Met-Asp-Phe-NH_2
|
R

Cerulein (10 amino acids, mol wt 1,352)

SO_3H
|
Glp[a]-Gln-Asp-Tyr-Thr-Gly-Trp-Met-Asp-Phe-NH_2

Human little gastrin (G 17, mol wt 2,098) is 18-34 of G 34
Human minigastrin (G 13, mol wt 1,647) is 22-34 of G 34
Porcine cholecystokinin (33 amino acids, mol wt 3,918) is 7-39 of cholecystokinin variant
Gastrin I, R = H
Gastrin II and CCK R = SO_3H

Source: Go VLW, Owyang C. Radioimmunoassay of gastrointestinal hormones. In: Glass GB, ed. *Progress in Gastroenterology*, vol 3. New York: Grune and Stratton, 1977:155. Reprinted by permission.
[a]GLP = pyroglutamyl.

able of producing the effects of the full molecule, although not to the same degree. Similarly, the effect of CCK on the oxyntic (acid-secreting) cells of the stomach is not nearly as strong as the effects of equal amounts of gastrin, even though it appears to have a stronger affinity for surface receptors on these cells. Because of this, equimolecular doses of CCK inhibit the full effect of gastrin in the secretion of acid. While hormones of the secretin family also have structural and functional similarities, the entire molecule is required to induce the key physiologic responses. These hormones include secretin itself, vasoactive intestinal polypeptide (VIP), gastric inhibitory polypeptide (GIP), and glucagon.

Table 2–2. The Secretin-Glucagon Family

Secretin (27 amino acids, mol wt 3,055)
His-Ser-Asp-Gly-Thr-Phe-Thr-Ser-Glu-Leu-Ser-Arg-Lev-Arg-Asp-Ser-Ala-Arg-Leu-Gln-Arg-Leu-Leu-Gln-Gly-Leu-Val-NH_2

Glucagon (29 amino acids, mol wt 3,484)
His-Ser-Gln-Gln-Thr-Phe-Thr-Ser-Asp-Tyr-Ser-Lys-Tyr-Leu-Asp-Ser-Arg-Arg-Ala-Gln-Asp-Phe-Val-Gln-Trp-Leu-Met-Asp-Thr

Vasoactive intestinal peptide (28 amino acids, mol wt 3,326)
His-Ser-Asp-Ala-Val-Phe-Thr-Asp-Asn-Tyr-Thr-Arg-Leu-Arg-Lys-Gln-Met-Ala-Val-Lys-Lys-Tyr-Leu-Asn-Ser-Ile-Leu-Asn-NH_2

Gastric inhibitory polypeptide (43 amino acids, mol wt 5,104)
Tyr-Ala-Glu-Gly-Thr-Phe-Ile-Ser-Asp-Tyr-Ser-Ile-Ala-Met-Asp-Lys-Ile-Arg-Gln-Gln-Asp-Phe-Val-Asn-Trp-Leu-Leu-Ala-Gln-Gln-Lys-Gly-Lys-Lys-Ser-Asp-Trp-Lys-His-Asn-Ile-Thr-Gln

Other Gastrointestinal Peptides

Motilin (22 amino acids, mol wt 2,698)
Phe-Val-Pro-Ile-Phe-Thr-Tyr-Gly-Glu-Leu-Gln-Arg-Met-Gln-Glu-Lys-Glu-Arg-Asn-Lys-Gly-Gln

Pancreatic polypeptides (36 amino acids, mol wt 4,226)
Ala-Pro-Leu-Glu-Pro-Gln-Tyr-Pro-Gly-Asp-Asp-Ala-Thr-Pro-Glu-Gln-Met-Ala-Gln-Tyr-Ala-Ala-Glu-Leu-Arg-Arg-Tyr-Ile-Asn-Met-Leu-Thr-Arg-Pro-Arg-Tyr-NH_2

Somatostatin (14 amino acids, mol wt 1,639)
H-Ala-Gly-Cys-Lys-Asn-Phe-Phe-Trp-Lys-Thr-Phe-Thr-Ser-Cys-OH

Bombesin (14 amino acids, mol wt 1,620)
Glp-Gln-Arg-Leu-Gly-Asn-Gln-Trp-Ala-Val-Gly-His-Leu-Met-NH_2

Source: Go VLW, Owyang C. Radioimmunoassay of gastrointestinal hormones. In: Glass GB, ed. *Progress in Gastroenterology*, vol 3. New York: Grune and Stratton, 1977:156. Reprinted by permission.

PRESUMED MECHANISM OF HORMONAL ACTION

Peptide hormones bind to specific receptors on target cell membranes. This first step in mediation of the effect of the hormone on specific cells has been demonstrated in a number of instances, examples of which are the binding of ^{125}I-gastrin to canine antral smooth muscle, and of ^{125}I-secretin to hepatocytic plasma membranes. Binding alone is only a first step, since non-specific or inhibitory binding may also occur. Some further alteration of target cells, proportional to the amount of hormonal binding, must occur—the hormonal response. One such measurable response is the intracellular activation of the enzyme adenylate cyclase at cellular membranes, with the resultant production of adenosine 3′5′-monophosphate (cyclic AMP) from cytoplasmic adenosine triphosphate (ATP). But Gardner (1979) has pointed out that this response may not correlate with the observed functional changes in the cell, and that target cells may respond to stimulation with specific hormones by means other than the generation of cAMP. However, where hormone binding, cAMP release, and effector cell responses all occur proportionately and at the same time in the same system, a clear cause and effect relationship can be assumed. Since these conditions have been met infrequently in the case of gastrointestinal hormones, our understanding of their mechanisms of action is only presumptive at present. The variety of actions attributable to gastrointestinal hormones is summarized in Table 2–3.

ESTABLISHED GASTROINTESTINAL HORMONES

Secretin, CCK, and gastrin have been identified, characterized, and proved to have important physiologic significance. They are thus agreed to be established gastrointestinal hormones. Since pancreozymin has been found to be identical to CCK, it is no longer considered as a separate hormone.

Secretin

Secretin [molecular weight (mol wt) 3,073, 27 amino acids] is the first of all hormones to have been discovered, its effects on the pancreas having been noted by Bayliss and Starling in 1902. It is secreted throughout the small intestinal mucosa by granular intervillous cells (S-cells) that are concentrated mainly in the duodenum and jejunum. Secretin is released primarily by hydrogen ions in a concentration below pH 4.5, a response that is probably enhanced by cholinergic innervation.

The major effect of secretin is in stimulating the secretion of bicarbonate and water by the pancreatic ductal system, thereby washing preformed pancreatic digestive enzymes already in the ductal system into the upper small intestine. The hormone also stimulates the secretion of pepsinogen, increases the tone of the pyloric sphincter, and enhances the action of CCK on the gall bladder. In physiologic amounts it also has the following inhibitory effects: reduction of the release of glucagon and gastrin, reduction of the amount of hydrochloric acid secreted by the stomach in response to a dose of gastrin, inhibition of the tonic contraction of the lower esophageal sphincter and of peristalsis of the stomach and intestine, and reduction of the absorption of water from the small intestine.

Table 2–3. Effects of Gastrointestinal Hormones on Digestive Tract

Effect	*Lower Esophageal*	*Stomach*					*Pancreas*		
Hormone	*Sphincter*	*Acid*	*Pepsin*	*Motility*	*Pylorus*	*Trophism*	*Ducts*	*Acini*	*Trophism*
Secretin	I	I	S	I	S		S	see Other Effects	
Cholecystokinin	I	S	?I	S-empty I-full	S	?S	S	S	S
Gastrin	S	S	S	S		S	S	S	S
Motilin	S		S	S					
Vasoactive Inhibitory Polypeptide	I	I	I	I			S		
Gastric Inhibitory Polypeptide		I	I	I					
Enteroglucagon	I	I		I				I	
Pancreatic Polypeptide		S			I		see Other Effects	I	
Chymodenin								see Other Effects	
Bulbogastrone		I	I	I					
Entero-oxyntin		S							
Somatostatin		inhibits release of gastrin, motilin, secretin, VIP, glucagon							
Enkephalin		S					I	I	

Main effects are indicated. For physiologic importance of each, see text. S = stimulatory; I = inhibitory.

Table 2-3. Effects of Gastrointestinal Hormones on Digestive Tract (Continued)

Effect	Gall Bladder		Small Intestine					
Hormone	Motility	Secretion	Motility	Water Absorption	Secretion	Blood Flow	Trophism	Other Effects
Secretin	S		I	I				Enhances CCK effect on pancreas; inhibits its release of gastrin
Cholecystokinin	S	S	S	I		S	S	Weakly stimulates, competitively inhibits gastrin; potentiates secretin; stimulates Brunner glands
Gastrin	S	S	S		?S	S	S	Circulates in several forms; G 17 more potent than G 34
Motilin			S					
Vasoactive Inhibitory Polypeptide	I	S			S			Causes marked vasodilatation; delays release of gastrin
Gastric Inhibitory Polypeptide					S			Inhibits gastrin release; enhances release of insulin and gastrin; physiologic effect on stomach questionable

Table 2–3. Effects of Gastrointestinal Hormones on Digestive Tract (Continued)

Effect	*Gall Bladder*		*Small Intestine*					
Hormone	*Motility*	*Secretion*	*Motility*	*Water Absorption*	*Secretion*	*Blood Flow*	*Trophism*	*Other Effects*
Enteroglucagon			I		S		?S	
Pancreatic Polypeptide	I							Potentiates low doses of secretin; inhibits high doses
Chymodenin								Stimulates release of chymotrypsinogen only
Bulbogastrone								
Entero-oxyntin								
Somastostatin								
Enkephalin	I		I		I			

Cholecystokinin

Cholecystokinin (mol wt 3,918, 33 amino acids) is synthesized maximally in the jejunum and to a lesser degree in the duodenum and ileum in large, round, dense mucosal I cells. CCK has also been found in the cerebral cortex of rats (Pinget et al 1978). CCK is released maximally by fat; L-amino acids and peptides are also effective. Hydrochoric acid causes a lesser release of CCK.

The major physiologic effects of CCK are the stimulation of contraction of the gall bladder, and the release of enzyme-containing zymogen granules from pancreatic acinar (A) cells. CCK also potentiates the effect of secretin on the pancreas, stimulates motility, acid secretion, and pyloric contraction in the stomach, motility, bile, and Brunner gland secretion in the intestine, growth of the pancreas (trophic effect), blood flow in the inferior mesenteric artery, and the release of insulin. It inhibits peristalsis in the full stomach, contraction of the lower esophageal sphincter and the sphincter of Oddi, and the absorption of fluid and electrolytes from the small intestine.

Gastrin

Gastrin (mol wt 2,190, 17 amino acids) is primarily synthesized in G cells in the antrum of the stomach, and also in the duodenum and jejunum. These mucosal cells are granular and variable in size. Gastrin has been identified in a number of molecules of different size: minigastrin (G 14), gastrin (G 17), and big gastrin (G 34). A larger molecule, big, big gastrin, is probably not found in nature. Various fragments of gastrin have also been identified in the blood of patients with gastrin-secreting tumors, but these fragments are often inactive because they do not contain the entire C-terminal four-peptide chain. G 14 and G 17 are more potent physiologically than G 34. Trace amounts of gastrin have also been identified in the brain and in the delta cells of pancreatic islets.

The release of gastrin is stimulated by peptides and amino acids in the stomach and by cholinergic stimulation. Distention of the canine antrum also causes the release of gastrin, but this does not appear to be the case in normal humans. Elevation of serum calcium and epinephrine levels stimulate the release of gastrin, but they may not play a role in healthy subjects. The release of gastrin is progressively inhibited by lowering pH in the gastric antrum below 3.0, and is abolished at pH 1.5. The release of gastrin is also inhibited by large doses of hormones of the secretin family, and by calcitonin and somatostatin. It has already been stated that CCK reduces the effect of gastrin on oxyntic cells by competitive receptor binding.

Gastrin is the major hormone responsible for the stimulation of hydrochloric acid secretion in the stomach. It also has trophic effects on gastric and intestinal mucosa, increases tonus in the lower esophageal sphincter and peristalsis in the stomach, increases blood flow to the pancreas, stomach and intestines, and stimulates pancreatic, intestinal, and biliary secretions. Although these effects have been shown to occur with physiologic doses of gastrin, their importance in normal homeostasis has not been fully ascertained.

CANDIDATE GASTROINTESTINAL HORMONES

A number of other peptide hormones have been identified, each of which possesses measurable effects on the alimentary tract. Since their true place in normal human physiology has not been fully adduced, they are considered to be candidate hormones. A number of these hormones (VIP, GIP, somatostatin, glucagon, and pancreatic polypeptide) have been identified as the mediators of effects on the gastrointestinal tract produced by adenomata of neural crest origin, and are thus important in those pathologic states.

Somatostatin

Somatostatin (mol wt 1,658, 14 amino acids) is, of course, not strictly a gastrointestinal hormone since its largest source is in hypothalamic (D) cells. However, similar cells are also located in the upper gut and stomach, and somatostatin has been shown to inhibit the release of gastrin, glucagon, motilin, secretin, and VIP. While the physiologic significance of these effects is not established, somatostatin may well be the gastric inhibitory chalone released by acidification of the gastric antrum.

Motilin

Motilin (mol wt 2,700, 22 amino acids) is secreted by chromaffin cells (EC2) in the duodenum and jejunum, and appears to be released in humans by acidification of or introduction of fat into the duodenum. Motilin stimulates gastric and intestinal contractions, accelerates gastric emptying, increases tone in the lower esophageal sphincter, and increases the secretion of pepsinogen.

Vasoactive Intestinal Polypeptide

Vasoactive intestinal polypeptide (mol wt 3,326, 28 amino acids) is secreted by specific endocrine (D_1) cells widely distributed throughout the intestinal tract and pancreas, mainly in the lower small intestine and colon. VIP secreting cells have also been found in the cerebral cortex and hypothalamus. The mechanism of its release is not clear, but it has been implicated convincingly as the causative agent in most, if not all, cases of the

Verner-Morrison syndrome (watery diarrhea, hypokalemia, hypochlorhydria) in which functioning adenomata or carcinomas have been found to contain large amounts of VIP. This hormone has also been found to be present in certain squamous-cell carcinomas of the lung and in ganglioneuroblastomas.

VIP has marked vasodilator and hypotensive effects. It also stimulates glycogenolysis and the release of insulin. It causes a heavy secretion of water and electrolytes from the small intestine, pancreas, and gall bladder by releasing adenylate cyclase and raising mucosal levels of cyclic AMP. VIP inhibits the secretion of acid and pepsinogen by the stomach, delays the release of gastrin, and relaxes smooth muscle in the esophagus, the lower sphincter, stomach, and gall bladder.

Enteroglucagon

Enteroglucagon (mol wt 3,489, 29 amino acids) is probably identical to pancreatic glucagon, although it is produced by (A) cells in the gastric fundus. Another hormone much like enteroglucagon (enteroglucagonoid, mol wt 2,900) is produced by alphalike (G) cells in the small intestine and colon. It is released by feeding.

Actions of enteroglucagon on the alimentary tract include marked inhibition of intestinal motility, esophageal sphincter tone, and secretion of enzymes by the pancreas. This hormone also appears to stimulate the secretion of water in the small bowel and colon, and may have trophic effects on the small intestine.

Pancreatic Polypeptide

Pancreatic polypeptide (mol wt 4,200, 36 amino acids) is produced primarily in D_2 cells of pancreatic islets in chickens, hogs, cattle, and sheep as well as humans. It is released by the action of dietary fat and protein, by insulin hypoglycemia, and by GIP, VIP, and CCK.

Pancreatic polypeptide stimulates the secretion of hydrochloric acid in the basal state, but inhibits the response to gastrin. It also has paradoxical effects on the pancreas, stimulating the effects of low doses and inhibiting the effects of high does of secretin. It also inhibits pyloric tone, gall bladder contractions, and the secretion of pancreatic enzymes.

Gastric Inhibitory Polypeptide

Gastric inhibitory polypeptide (mol wt 5,105, 43 amino acids) is formed in specific (K) cells in duodenal and jejunal mucosa. It is released in two peaks: 45 minutes after the ingestion of glucose, and 2 to 3 hours after the ingestion of fat. Its release is not affected by acidification of the duodenum.

GIP appears to enhance the release of insulin and glucagon, and may be responsible for some cases of hypoglycemia. It stimulates small intestinal secretion, and inhibits the basal and stimulated secretion of acid by the stomach, the secretion of pepsin, the release of gastrin, and the motility of the stomach.

Chymodenin

Chymodenin (mol wt approx. 5,000) is found in duodenal extracts rich in secretin and CCK. It has the unique attribute of having only a single identified function, and of stimulating the release of only one enzyme, chymotrypsinogen, from the pancreas. Prior to the discovery of this effect, it had been assumed that no monospecific stimulant like chymodenin existed. Now there is a realistic possibility that other such hormones will be discovered.

Enkephalins and Endorphins

Using immunoassay, Polak et al (1977) demonstrated the presence of opiate compounds and their receptors in digestive endocrine cells and myenteric plexi, especially in the gastric antrum and duodenum, but also in the gall bladder, pancreas, ileum and colon. These compounds resemble fragments of beta-lipotropin, a pituitary polypeptide containing 91 amino acids. The two enkephalins presently identified are pentapeptides which occur towards the C-terminus of the larger complex, containing tyrosine-glycine-glycine-phenyl alanine and, at the C-terminal, either leucine (Leu-enkephalin) or methionine (Met-enkephalin). Removal of either the leucine or methionine moiety reduces the biological activity of these compounds markedly but does not affect their binding affinity, while removal of the N-terminal tyrosine molecule leads to total inactivity. Endorphins are larger peptide fragments of lipotropin which contain the Met-enkaphalin pentapeptide at their N-termini.

While the physiological actions of opiate peptides on the digestive system are still being appraised, it has been shown that Met-enkephalin does increase gastric acid secretion in dogs, independent of gastrin (Konturek 1980). Other studies indicate that enkephalins decrease the meal-stimulated secretion of bicarbonate and enzymic protein by the pancreas, reduce small intestinal secretions, relax the gall bladder, contract the sphincter of Oddi, and reduce myoelectrical activity in the intestine. There is a growing body of evidence suggesting that the antidiarrheal effect of exogenous opiates may be largely due to reduction of small intestinal secretion rather than, as formerly thought, to reduced intestinal motility alone.

PUTATIVE GASTROINTESTINAL HORMONES

A number of gastrointestinal responses have been described that appear to be mediated hormonally. In at least two instances, the responsible hormone has been named but not identified, much as was the case previously with gastrin and secretin, whose effects were noted long before they themselves were purified and defined.

Bulbogastrone

It has been noted that acidification of the bulb (first portion) of the duodenum inhibits the production of acid in the denervated stomach stimulated by food and gastrin. Motility of the stomach is diminished and the release of pepsin is also inhibited. This effect does not occur if the duodenum below the bulb is acidified, and it does not seem to depend on the release of secretin, VIP, or GIP. The effect appears to be mediated by a hormone, and bulbogastrone may be either a member of the family of gastric secretory inhibitors called enterogastrones, or identical with some other already defined hormone, such as somatostatin (Schusdziarra et al 1979).

Entero-Oxyntin

The third, or intestinal, phase of gastric secretion appears to be hormonally mediated, since introduction of protein digests into the small intestine evokes a brisk secretion of acid from the denervated stomach. This effect appears to be greater than the gastric response to the release of CCK and is not associated with elevation of serum gastrin levels. Other evidence for the existence of entero-oxyntin will be presented in Chapter 4.

HISTORICAL DIGRESSION

Personages mentioned without further reference in this chapter include: Sir William Maddock BAYLISS (1860–1924), British physiologist, London; Johann Conrad BRUNNER (1653–1727), German anatomist, Mannheim, Heidelberg; Ruggero ODDI (1864–1913), Italian surgeon, Bologna; and Ernest Henry STARLING (1866–1927), British physiologist, London. The Verner-Morrison syndrome is named after John Victor VERNER, Jr. (1927–) American internist, Durham, North Carolina, and Lakeland, Florida; and after Ashton MORRISON (1922–). Ulster-American pathologist, Belfast, Durham, Philadelphia, and Bound Brook, New Jersey. Their original description of a pancreatic tumor secreting a gastrointestinal hormone was published under the title, "Islet cell tumor and a syndrome of refractory watery diarrhea and hypokalemia," Am J Med 25:374-80, 1958.

SELECTED REFERENCES

Chey, WY, Gutierrez JG. The endocrine control of gastrointestinal function. Adv Intern Med 23:61–84, 1978.

Gardner JD. Receptors for gastrointestinal hormones. Gastroenterology 76: 202–214, 1979.

Glass GBJ, ed. *Gastrointestinal Hormones.* New York: Raven Press, 1980.

Konturek SJ. Somastostatin and opiate peptides: their action on gastrointestinal secretions. In: Glass GBJ, ed. *Gastrointestinal Hormones.* New York: Raven Press, 1980, pp 693–716.

Pinget M, Straus E, Yalow RS. Localization of cholecystokinin-like immunoreactivity in isolated nerve terminals. Proc Nat Acad Sci USA 75:6324-26,1978.

Polak JM, Sullivan SN, Bloom SR, et al: Enkephalin-like immunoreactivity in the human gastrointestinal tract. Lancet 1:972–74, 1977.

Rayford PL, Miller TA, Thompson JC. Secretin, cholecystokinin, and new gastrointestinal hormones. N Engl J Med 294:1093–1101, 1157–64, 1976.

Schusdziarra V, Romiller D, Harris V, et al. Release of gastric somatostatin-like immunoactivity during acidification of the duodenal bulb. Gastroenterology 76:950-53, 1979.

Walsh JH, Grossman MI. Gastrin. N Engl J Med 292:1324–34, 1377–84, 1975.

DISCUSSION QUESTION

Gastrointestinal responses to polypeptide hormones may be elicited by pharmacologic or physiologic doses. Discuss the implications of these types of response to possible pathophysiology or to therapy.

CHAPTER 3

The Esophagus

The squamous epithelium of the esophagus differs strikingly from the columnar epithelium of the remainder of the alimentary canal. There are also far fewer mucosal glands in the esophagus than in the stomach and intestine. Its normal function is to transmit swallowed material from the pharynx to the stomach, while preventing gastric contents from regurgitating into the esophagus and, with associated structures, preventing swallowed material from entering the respiratory tree. The secretion of mucus probably serves both to protect the mucosa and to lubricate swallowed boluses of food.

HISTOLOGY

There is an abrupt histologic change from squamous to columnar epithelium at the anatomic esophagogastric junction. The thick squamous epithelium contains a narrow basal layer in which mitotic activity occurs. This basal layer is thrown at intervals into folds, called rete pegs, which project no more than halfway into the covering layer of epithelium (Figure 3–1). The lamina propria contains scattered round cells, lymphocytes, plasma cells, and histiocytes, and is subtended by a thin muscularis mucosae which is gently contracted at rest and casts the mucosa into blunt linear folds. These mucosal folds rest on loose submucosal connective tissue which allow for mucosal expansion during swallowing, thereby facilitating the passage of large boluses of food.

Below the submucosa of the esophagus, just as in the stomach and small intestine, there are two layers of muscle, an inner layer of circular muscle, and an outer layer of longitudinal muscle. In the upper third of the esophagus, these layers are composed entirely of striated muscle, while the lower third is composed solely of smooth muscle fibers. The middle third of the esophagus is a transitional zone of mixed striated and smooth muscle, the former type being predominant in the proximal portion and smooth muscle predominating in the distal portion. Myenteric ganglion cells (Auerbach plexi) are scattered throughout the esophageal muscularis between the circular and longitudinal muscles. The concentration of these cells increases progressively from the upper to the lower esophagus.

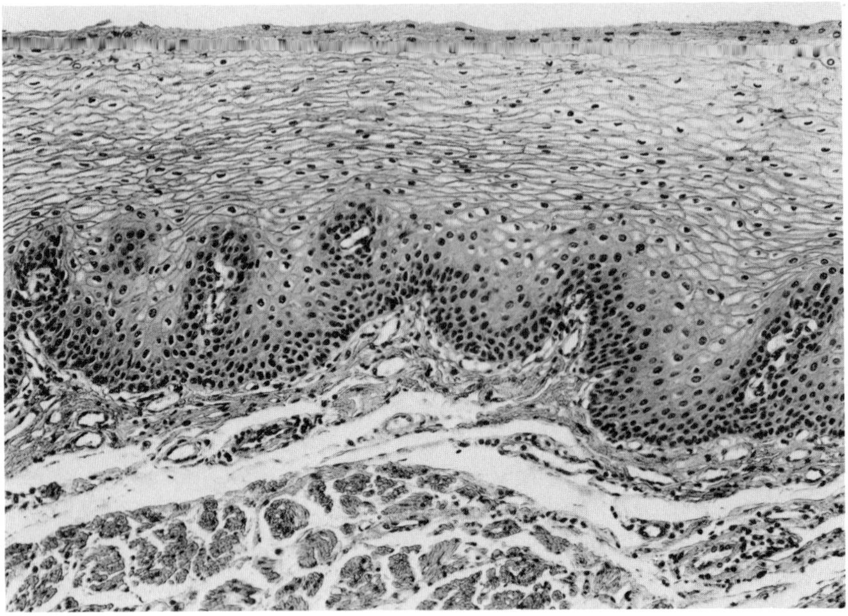

Figure 3-1. Biopsy specimen from a normal esophagus. Note that the basal layer of the squamous epithelium is thin, and that rete pegs extend less than halfway to the surface. Compare with Figure 3-6. (Original magnification x80).

Sphincter muscles can be readily identified in the pharynx and upper esophagus. In fact, individual upper, middle, and lower constrictors have been delineated in the pharynx. Distal to these is the upper esophageal sphincter (UES), which consists of the cricopharyngeal muscle posteriorly and the cricoid cartilage anteriorly. No such specialized sphincteric muscle can be demonstrated at the lower end of the esophagus, although physiologically sphincteric function clearly occurs in that location. Thus, the UES is both an anatomical and a physiologic sphincter, while the lower esophageal sphincter (LES) is physiologic alone.

External to the muscularis of the esophagus, there is a sheath of loose areolar tissue. Unlike most of the remainder of the luminal alimentary tract, the esophagus has no clearly defined serosal layer, and this loose tissue sheath allows for considerable distensive and axial movement.

Extrinsic Neural Control

A paired swallowing center has been identified in the reticular substance of the brainstem, close to the midline, between the facial nucleus and the inferior olive. This center appears to be essential for initiation of the pharyngeal component of swallowing. Effective relaxation of the UES following contraction of the distal pharynx and the initiation of peristalsis in the upper esophagus are also dependent on an intact swallowing center, but not exclusively so. There appears to be some intrinsic control of these activities as well. Although the vagus nerve influences peristaltic activity in areas of the lower esophagus where smooth muscle predominates, this portion of the esophagus can function well without extrinsic innervation. Thus, distention of the upper portion of a denervated (vagotomized) esophagus will result in normal peristalitic flow distally and appropriate relaxation of the LES. Vagal stimulation in the intact animal causes relaxation of the tonically contracted LES. One may conclude that extrinsic innervation is essential for normal function of the UES and for peristalsis in the striated muscular portions of the esophagus, while intrinsic innervation controls peristaltic activity in the lower or smooth muscle portions of the esophagus and in the LES, despite the fact that the vagus nerve also exerts some supervisory effects.

The effects of pharmacologic agents on esophageal motility differ at different levels, and attest to the presence of cholinergic, adrenergic, and noncholinergic, nonadrenergic innervation. In those portions of the esophagus dominated by striated musculature, the upper esophageal sphincter and the upper esophageal body, the motor nerves are similar to those of skeletal muscle elsewhere in the body and appear to be cholinergic and responsive to nicotine. In the smooth muscle of the body of the esophagus, there appear to be both cholinergic (muscarine-responsive), and noncholinergic, nonadrenergic (peptidergic) receptors. It has been suggested that the transmitter agent for the latter receptors may be the hormone, vasoactive intestinal polypeptide (VIP). In the LES, there appears to be a variety of receptors. Cholinergic agonists appear to increase LES pressure in humans as do adrenergic α-receptors; β-receptors are inhibitory; and relaxation of the sphincter after a swallow appears to be solely peptidergic. There has also been the suggestion that esophageal peristalsis may be subserved at least partially through myogenic control systems, in which electrical activity is propagated directly from cell to cell without chemical or neural intermediaries.

Physiology

Simply put, the esophagus can be considered to be a peristaltic tube with a tonically contracted sphincteric zone at each end. The UES is an area of high pressure at rest interposed between the pharynx, wherein pressure is atmospheric, and the body of the esophagus whose intraluminal pressure is equal to the intrathoracic pressure. This sphincter prevents the passage of air into the esophagus with inspiration.

Swallowing is initiated centrally when a chewed bolus of food is passed by the tongue from the mouth into the relaxed oropharynx. The soft palate elevates against the nasopharynx, thereby preventing the bolus from entering the nose. The three hypopharngeal sphincters then contract sequentially from above downward, first closing the epiglottis, then passing the bolus into the area of the UES, which relaxes as the bolus approaches and closes with the termination of the swallow.

Peristalsis

Following the swallow, a primary peristaltic wave commences in the upper esophagus and sweeps the contents along, arrival of the bolus at any area of the esophagus being followed by the primary contraction wave. This wave of peristalsis appears to be of multiple origins. Initially, distention of the esophagus produces a brief contraction of the circular muscle, which does not appear to be dependent on intrinsic innervation. Following this comes a sustained contraction of the longitudinal coat, consequent to myenteric nerve stimulation. This, in turn, is followed by a further contraction of circular muscle that is initiated by relaxation of the longitudinal muscle (off response), following a latent period which is longer in the upper esophagus than it is in the lower segments (Goyal et al 1976).

The Lower Esophageal Sphincter

The LES, which usually lies anatomically at the level of the diaphragmatic hiatus, is about 3 to 4 cm in length, and, when open, consists of an upper ring (the inferior esophageal sphincter) and a lower ring (the constrictor cardiae) separated by a 2–3-cm area called the esophageal vestibule. The LES is tonically contracted at rest, producing pressures that range from 10 to 35 mm Hg higher than those obtaining in the chest or stomach. As a peristaltic wave approaches, pressure in the LES falls to intragastric levels, allowing the bolus to pass into the stomach (Figure 3–2). Failure of this fall to occur results in retention of all or a portion of the bolus in the lower esophagus. Should any material reflux upward from the stomach to the esophagus during LES relaxation, a secondary wave of peristalsis (induced by the distention resulting from the refluxed contents) sweeps the material back into the stomach.

The cause for the tonic closure of the LES at rest is not known, since it does not appear to depend on either extrinsic or intrinsic innervation. That some hormonal influence plays a part is apparent from the fact that the administration of gastrin, or the ingestion of substances such as protein or alkalis which release gastrin from the antrum of the stomach, leads to a prompt increase in LES pressures. This response does not appear, however, to be dose related, and the increased tone induced by the ingestion of alkali may not be accompanied by a corresponding rise in serum gastrin levels. But

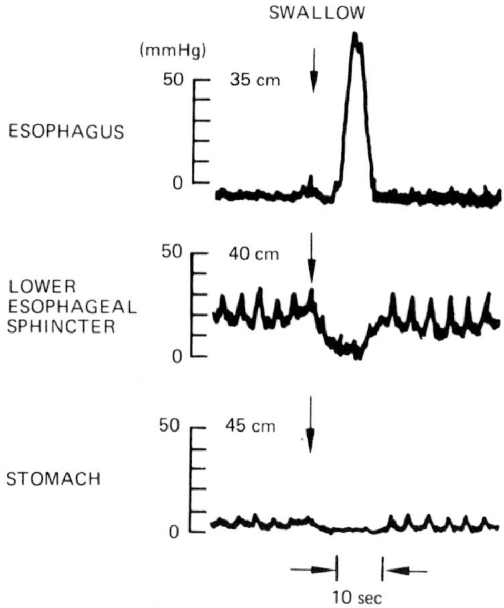

Figure 3–2. Manometric study of a normal lower esophageal sphincter. The high-pressure zone in the LES (middle lead) separates the gastric pressure (lower lead) and the intraesophageal pressure (upper lead). Swallowing (arrow) causes a prompt fall in pressure (relaxation). The figures in centimeters indicate distances from the incisors. From Goyal RK. Viewpoints Dig Dis 8:1–4 (Dec), 1976. Reprinted by permission.

to carry the relationship between gastrin and sphincter tone further, it has also been found that the introduction of acid into the stomach, which reduces gastrin secretion, is accompanied by reduction of LES pressure. A fatty meal also reduces basal pressures in the LES and diminishes the response to a dose of gastrin. This action of fat is doubtless due to its release of cholecystokinin (CCK) from the duodenum, since the effects of CCK, or its terminal octapeptide, are the same as the effect from fat. CCK alone is a mild stimulant of LES contraction, but reduces the response to gastrin when both hormones are given simultaneously. This observation has led to the supposition that CCK is avidly taken up by gastrin receptors in the LES, and indeed displaces gastrin from these receptors.

Basal LES tone is not reduced by exogenously administered or endogenously released secretin, although both of these methods of raising blood secretin levels will inhibit the increase of LES pressure produced by gastrin. The responses to glucagon administration on basal and stimulated LES pressures are essentially the same as those of secretin. The failure of secretin or glucagon alone to reduce LES pressures, while at the same time being able to inhibit the action of gastrin, indicates that these hormones must interact with gastrin in mitigating its effects.

LES pressure is also increased by compression of the upper abdomen, a response which is greatly diminished in cases where the sphincteric area has slipped upward into the chest. This response is abolished by vagotomy. Cigarette smoking and the ingestion of alcohol, caffeine, and chocolate will considerably reduce resting pressures in the LES. Manometric characteristics of the normal LES are as follows:

1. Resting pressure 10–35 mm Hg greater than intragastric.
2. Pressure falls promptly to zero after a swallow; returns to resting levels in 10–15 seconds.
3. Pressure increases 40–50 percent more than intragastric with abdominal compression.
4. Pressure increases with administration of gastrin; falls with secretin or cholecystokinin.

The Aging Esophagus

Most of the observations of normal esophageal function have been made on young to middle-aged healthy people. Observations which have been made in elderly individuals without esophageal symptoms indicate that aging alone may be associated with pharyngeal weakness, decreased peristaltic strength in the body of the esophagus in response to a swallow (primary contractions) and decrease also in response to distention (secondary contractions). Furthermore, several studies indicate that there is an increased tendency for spastic, nonpropulsive (tertiary) contractions to appear in healthy people over the age of 65. Studies on the LES in a geriatric population suggest that resting pressures in the sphincter may be reduced and that the relaxation of the LES in response to a swallow tends to be prolonged over normal. Each of these observations suggests that esophageal striated and smooth muscle activity lessens with aging.

SYMPTOMS OF ESOPHAGEAL DISEASE

Beyond noting a tendency to swallow involuntarily and frequently throughout the day, the normal observant individual rarely has occasion to think about esophageal function. The limits of esophageal compliance will occasionally come to the fore when a large bolus, poorly masticated and inadequately moistened with saliva, is swallowed, and its slow progression through a stretched esophagus is manifested by a painful sensation commencing in the upper chest and progressing gradually downward. The discomfort terminates when the esophagus rids itself of the bolus by passing it into the more commodious stomach. Esophageal protest in the form of a pronounced substernal burning sensation often follows the ingestion of very hot or highly seasoned foods. Similarly, the normal esophagus may occasionally complain of acid reflux from the stomach after a fatty meal, smoking, or the ingestion of alcohol, by causing heartburn, a low substernal transitory burning sensation. When any of these symptoms is rare, is clearly related to an identifiable cause, disappears spontaneously after a short time, and is nonrecurring, one need not be concerned about the possibility of underlying disease. However, the recurrence of even mild symptoms should alert both patients and physicians to the need for further study.

The most prominent symptoms of esophageal disease are difficulty on swallowing or after swallowing (dysphagia), pain on or after a swallow (odynophagia), heartburn (pyrosis) either spontaneous or postprandial, belching, and bleeding. Loss of blood may be manifest dramatically by vomiting (hematemesis), altered blood in the stools causing a black discoloration (melena), or occult bleeding with resultant anemia. Each of these symptoms may occur singly or in concert with others. Loss of weight and strength may also be ancillary symptoms of esophageal disease.

Dysphagia

Dysphagia, the most important symptom of significant esophageal disease, may occur only with certain kinds of food. Thick, dry, or pasty boluses, such as meat or bread, are most apt to cause trouble, while more liquid substances may be swallowed normally. If the disorder producing dysphagia is located in the pharynx or upper esophagus, patients may be able to locate the level of dysfunction with fair precision. For lesions in the mid or lower esophagus, however, localization is often imprecise and is generally referred to the mid or upper substernal area, even for disorders that primarily affect the lower esophagus.

Dysphagia occurs in five categories of pharyngoesophageal disease:

1. Neuromuscular disorders involving the pharynx and hypopharynx, which make it difficult to initiate swallowing. Any disorder which interferes with the innervation of striated muscle, such as myasthenia gravis, will interfere with the initiation of swallowing. Disorders of the brainstem which ablate the vagal nuclei, including disseminated sclerosis, medullary strokes, or bulbar poliomyelitis, and neuronal disorders like diphtheritic neuronitis, are also commonly associated with this sort of dysphagia. Similar functional loss occurs with striated muscular disorders, including polymyositis, dermatomyositis, and myotonic muscular dystrophy. The common denominator in all these disorders is the reduced or total inability to carry through with a voluntary or involuntary swallow. As a consequence, patients will

commonly have trouble swallowing their own saliva and may either aspirate it or expectorate frequently. Where the soft palate is also unable to contract and close off the nasopharynx from the oropharynx during a swallow, patients may also experience uncomfortable nasal reflux of food at times.

2. Disorders in which the upper esophageal sphincter fails to relax properly or closes prematurely in response to a swallow. Although not a common complaint, occasionally, patients will note difficult passage of food in the area of the lower neck, despite an unimpaired ability to initiate a swallow.
3. Disorders in which propulsive motility in the body of the esophagus is impaired. These include neural disorders, such as achalasia of the esophagus and diabetic enteropathy, or diseases like scleroderma or polymyositis, in which the cause is primarily muscular. Patients complain of slow passage of food after a swallow, marked difficulty in swallowing against gravity, and often regurgitation of food eaten some time earlier. In other patients, spasms of the esophageal musculature will interfere with smooth propulsion of a bolus.
4. Disorders in which the lumen of the esophagus is compromised by an intrinsic or extrinsic lesion. This category includes such intrinsic lesions as cancer, strictures or inflammation of the esophagus, and extrinsic lesions, such as bronchogenic carcinoma, mediastinal tumors, or aneurysms of the aorta. The degree of dysphagia varies directly with the amount of obstruction and is usually worse for solid foods than it is for liquids. Loss of weight is a commonly associated symptom. Dysphagia often does not appear until the degree of constriction is well advanced.
5. Disorders in which the lower esophageal sphincter does not relax in response to a swallow. This is usually associated with reduced propulsive motility as well and is the characteristic finding in achalasia of the esophagus and in Chagas disease. One suspects the existence of such a disorder in patients who complain of frequent reflux of ancient food residues, unmixed with acid gastric contents, as well as dysphagia. Characteristically, both liquids and solids are handled with difficulty.

Patients with true dysphagia do not as a rule complain of any sensation suggesting a lump in the throat, or globus. Where this sensation does exist, swallowing and its aftermath are usually normal and loss of weight rarely occurs. There is some evidence that patients with a globus sensation may have increased pressure in the cricopharyngeus muscle, but this is not always so, and the sensation itself is most commonly related to psychogenic disorders.

Odynophagia

Odynophagia occurs most commonly with dysphagia, but may at times appear alone. Its presence usually implies the existence of an ulcerative lesion in the esophagus, such as an ulcerated neoplasm, candidiasis, or peptic ulceration. Odynophagia is a common early complaint following the ingestion of caustic agents, and may also appear as a result of strong esophageal spasms.

Heartburn

Heartburn, a sensation of burning substernal discomfort commencing at the level of the lower sternum and radiating upward, is probably the most common symptom of esophageal disease. It may be associated with the simultaneous or subsequent complaint of acid or sour regurgitation into the oropharynx, and almost invariably results from relaxation of the lower esophageal sphincter with resultant regurgitation of acidic gastric contents into the esophagus. However, minor degrees of reflux noted during contrast X rays of the esophagus or during esophageal manometry, are not invariably associated with heartburn. The symptom does not appear to develop unless the esophagus has also lost its ability to respond to reflux with a strong wave of secondary peristalsis, which normally sweeps regurgitated material back into the stomach. In the absence of an effective peristaltic response to reflux, the acidic and bile-containing material remains in the esophagus for long periods and leads to esophagitis. It is felt currently that heartburn results when acid-bile reflux occurs into an area of preexisting esophageal inflammation. Thus, true heartburn is a fairly reliable symptom of decreased pressure of the lower esophageal sphincter with associated esophagitis. It is frequently relieved promptly by standing upright, which facilitates esophageal emptying, or by the ingestion of antacids.

Belching

Belching may merely result from the involuntary or conscious introduction of air into the hypopharynx, followed by forcible expulsion. In some parts of the world, this voluntary act after a particularly pleasant meal is a sign of high regard for the host or hostess. In others, it is a sign of bad manners. Belching after ingestion of carbonated beverages is most commonly the result of overdistention of the gastric fundus, with resultant forcible relaxation of the inferior sphincter and upward movement of the gas. None of these types of belching is a symptom of disease. However, belching may at times be subconsciously induced by patients suffering from angina pectoris, diffuse esophageal spasm or heartburn, in an effort to gain relief from their discomfiture, and physicians should learn to recognize its possible importance in these cases. The presence of a foul odor to the refluxed gas should also raise the possibility of esophageal or gastric retention as a cause of the belching.

Bleeding

Bleeding from the esophagus may appear in a variety of ways, depending on the rapidity of blood loss and the direction in which the blood is conveyed once it enters the esophagus. If the hemorrhage is brisk and associated with vomiting, as might be the case when dilated submucosal veins (varices) are ruptured in the lower esophagus, the vomitus will contain freshly shed blood (hematemesis). This symptom is not diagnostic of esophageal hemorrhage, however, since it may also occur in patients with actively bleeding gastric or duodenal lesions, such as peptic ulcers. Furthermore, not all brisk esophageal hemorrhage is associated with hematemesis. In many cases, the blood passes directly into the stomach and small intestine, and the first symptoms experienced by the patient are those of depleted blood volume (faintness, sweating, thirst, tachycardia, air hunger) followed eventually by the appearance of grossly bloody or tarry (melenic) stools.

If bleeding from an esophageal disorder is slow and chronic, as it might be with extensive inflammatory or destructive lesions of the esopahgeal mucosa, such as esophagitis or carcinoma, the patient may have no early symptoms at all. Only when a specimen of stool is checked for occult blood and found to be positive, or when a blood count shows evidence of iron deficiency anemia, or when symptoms of anemia force the patient to apply for treatment will the true severity of the underlying disease become apparent. This is the first of many situations in gastroenterology where the importance of routinely testing all individuals for occult intestinal bleeding becomes apparent. It is crucial to keep clearly in mind the fact that numerous life-threatening diseases of the alimentary canal, especially cancer, manifest themselves in their early and most treatable stages only with occult bleeding, and that the appearance of more intrusive symptoms such as pain, indigestion, and loss of weight often means that the underlying disease has progressed well beyond the limits of curable treatment.

CLINICAL STUDY OF THE ESOPHAGUS

History and Physical Examination

The use of confirmatory diagnostic studies is indicated in any patient whose symptoms suggest the presence of esophageal disease. The physical examination by itself is not usually diagnostic, although it may be helpful in confirming a history of loss of weight and malnutrition which frequently accompanies serious esophageal lesions. Thus, atrophy of the papillae of the tongue suggests a nutritional deficiency of B vitamins, thiamin, niacin, or riboflavin. A heavily coated tongue frequently accompanies significant disease of the upper gastrointestinal tract, including the esophagus. Absence of salivation and consequent dysphagia are common consequences of Sjögren syndrome, a chronic inflammatory disease of salivary and lacrimal glands, accompanied often by arthritis. Observation of a patient while swallowing water will often document neurologic or muscular disorders affecting the swallowing process.

Scleroderma, a collagen disorder that usually reduces esophageal peristalsis to a great degree and will be discussed below, is frequently manifested by tightness and inelasticity of the skin of the hands, wrists, forearms, and face. Patients with scleroderma commonly complain also of Raynaud phenomenon, which is due to vasospasm of arteries in the hand on exposure to cold, causing whiteness, pain, and occasionally ulcerations of the fingertips. Other collagen disorders, such as rheumatoid arthritis and dermatomyositis, occasionally reduce motility in the esophagus and may be documented by examination.

Esophagitis due to infections with *Candida* or herpes viruses, occurs commonly in patients receiving immunosuppressive therapy for other disorders, such as lymphomas. Candidiasis can be confirmed occasionally by the observation of white patches of exudate in the mouth, tongue, or throat. Bleeding esophageal varices are often suggested by the finding of an enlarged liver and spleen, abdominal ascites, or cutaneous signs of chronic liver disease, such as spider nevi on the face or shoulders, ecchymoses, glossitis, or enlarged subcutaneous veins in the upper abdominal or lower chest areas, representing collateral venous flow around obstructed portal pathways.

Where neurologic disorders are suspected as a cause of reduced ability to initiate voluntary deglutition, a great variety of clinical signs may be present. The patient with amyotrophic lateral sclerosis will show evidence of muscular fasciculations, particularly in the arms and shoulders. Patients with cerebrovascular accidents involving the brainstem and patients with parkinsonism are often found to have difficulty swallowing their own saliva; patients in the former group will usually have oculomotor palsies, palatal weakness, and difficulty with movements of the tongue as well. Diabetic patients with disturbances of esophageal motility almost invariably show signs of associated peripheral neuropathy.

Examination of the mouth in patients with obstructive disorders of the esophagus, such as a Zenker diverticulum of the cervical esophagus, achalasia, or carcinoma, often reveals the malodorous smell of decaying food. While this is not a pleasant finding for the examiner, its diagnostic importance is great. Examination of the base of the neck, especially on the left side, for hard, fixed, enlarged lymph nodes containing metastatic tumor (Virchow nodes) is extremely important in patients suspected of having cancer of the lower esophagus or upper stomach.

X Ray

With the use of a swallowed radiopaque substance, such as barium, for a contrast medium, the lumen of the hypopharynx and esophagus can be studied by fluoroscopy and by films which stop the action and provide a permanent record (Figure 3–3). Intrinsic lesions, such as neoplasms, are identified by the indentations that they make on the barium column. The tumor itself is radiolucent, but its mass subtracts a corresponding amount of opacity from the barium column, and is called a "negative" filling defect. Abnormal taperings or narrowings of the esophagus can also be demonstrated with contrast studies. Diverticula, which are outpouchings of the wall of the esophagus, or ulcers, which are breaks in the mucosa of the esophagus, allow barium to proceed into areas not normally entered. These are called "positive" filling defects.

Fluoroscopy with barium may demonstrate peristaltic abnormalities or spasms in the esophagus. Occasionally these abnormalities, while clinically significant, may not be demonstrable with ordinary thin barium but can be demonstrated by the swallowing and progress of a bolus of thick barium paste, or a cracker or large marshmallow coated with barium. Permanent records of esophageal motility (cineroentgenograms) can also be made, but the amount of exposure to ionizing radiation does not often justify the use of this procedure.

Roentgenologic procedures are readily available, rapid, relatively cheap, highly diagnostic, and afford essentially no discomfort to the patient. They are risky only in patients who might be expected by their history to have tracheobronchial aspiration after swallowing. In such patients, it is best to perform roentgenography with a water-soluble contrast medium. This is more expensive than barium, and affords less fine mucosal detail, but its added safety in these patients warrants its use. Radiologic procedures are the most common and simplest approaches to the study of patients with esophageal disease.

Endoscopy

The application of fiberglass optics to the field of endoscopy has revolutionized the direct diagnosis of diseases of the esophagus, stomach, duodenum, and colon. The rigid and semirigid instruments of the past have been replaced by fully flexible endoscopes that transmit intense cold light for viewing purposes into the gastrointestinal tract from an external source,

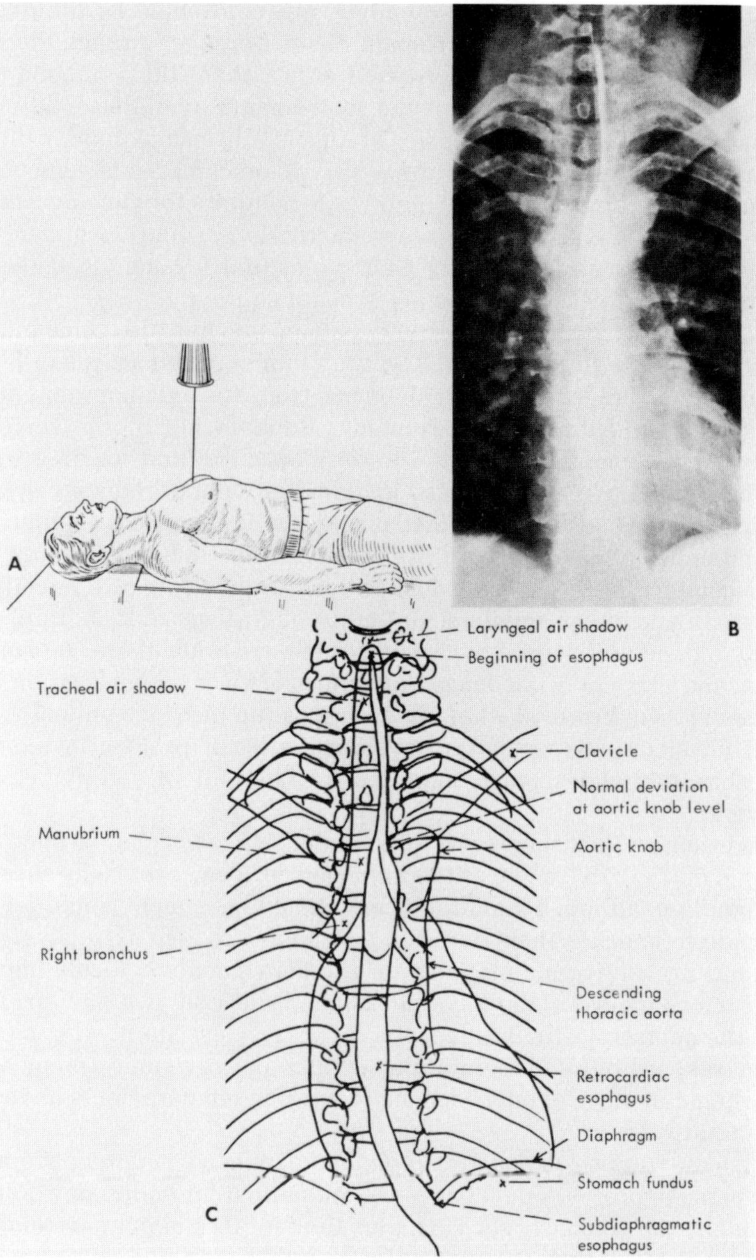

Figure 3–3. Anteroposterior radiograph of esophagus. *A*, positioning of patient; *B*, radiograph of barium-filled esophagus; *C*, labeled tracing of *B*. From Meschan I. *Synopsis of Roentgen Signs II*. Philadelphia: WB Saunders, 1966. Reprinted by permission.

and return excellent images to the examiner through a second fiber bundle bound into the instrument. These images are unaffected by the degree of bending or twisting that the instrument has undergone to reach the area of disease, and they can be photographed with either still or motion picture cameras (Figure 3–4). Almost all the instruments available today can be used for obtaining adequate biopsies of almost any lesion, and for the surgical removal of polyps in their entirety. Television cameras have been developed for transmitting endoscopic pictures to monitors for viewing by several observers simultaneously. Studies are currently in progress to devise safe methods for fulgerating bleeding gastrointestinal lesions via endoscopes, either by high-voltage electric or laser beam cautery.

With improvement of endoscopic instruments has also come increased comfort and safety to the patent. The use of an external source of light has eliminated the danger of mucosal burns from the incandescent internal sources used in outmoded instruments. Refinements of the instrument-maker's art have made it possible to develop third- and fourth-generation endoscopes that have been reduced in diameter without reducing the clarity of the image or the utility of the instrument itself. The present upper gastrointestinal endoscope for general use is only 11 mm in diameter, and causes little discomfort to the patient. Most patients require no local anesthesia in the pharynx and only a small amount of preoperative sedation. Dangers are very few indeed and consist of rare cases of aspiration of oral secretions or vomitus, and extremely uncommon instances of visceral perforation. Experience has shown, however, that endoscopy is the province only of the well-trained physician. Expertise is developed after a prolonged, supervised traineeship, and endoscopists must learn to be patient and painstaking in their work.

Endoscopes themselves are quite expensive, averaging around $7,000 in today's market, exclusive of the light source. They are easily susceptible to mishandling, although manufacturers should be complimented for the efforts made to improve their durability. Repairs are also expensive, and hygienic and preventive maintenance of the instruments is highly important. These factors almost alone have occasioned the rise of a new profession, that of the gastrointestinal diagnostic laboratory assistant, who is charged with the responsibility of maintaining a full, operative unit—no mean challenge when a number of endoscopists of varying temperaments have access to the facilities!

High start-up costs, long training, and expensive maintenance have all tended to make professional charges to the patient for endoscopy quite high, occasionally outrageously so. This, plus the fact that upper gastrointestinal endoscopy is more time-consuming for the physician and more uncomfortable for the patient, has led most gastroenterologists to prefer radiography as the first-line diagnostic tool in patients with suspected esophageal or gastroduodenal disease, except in cases of major upper gastrointestinal hemorrhage, or intestinal bleeding from an unknown site where endoscopy

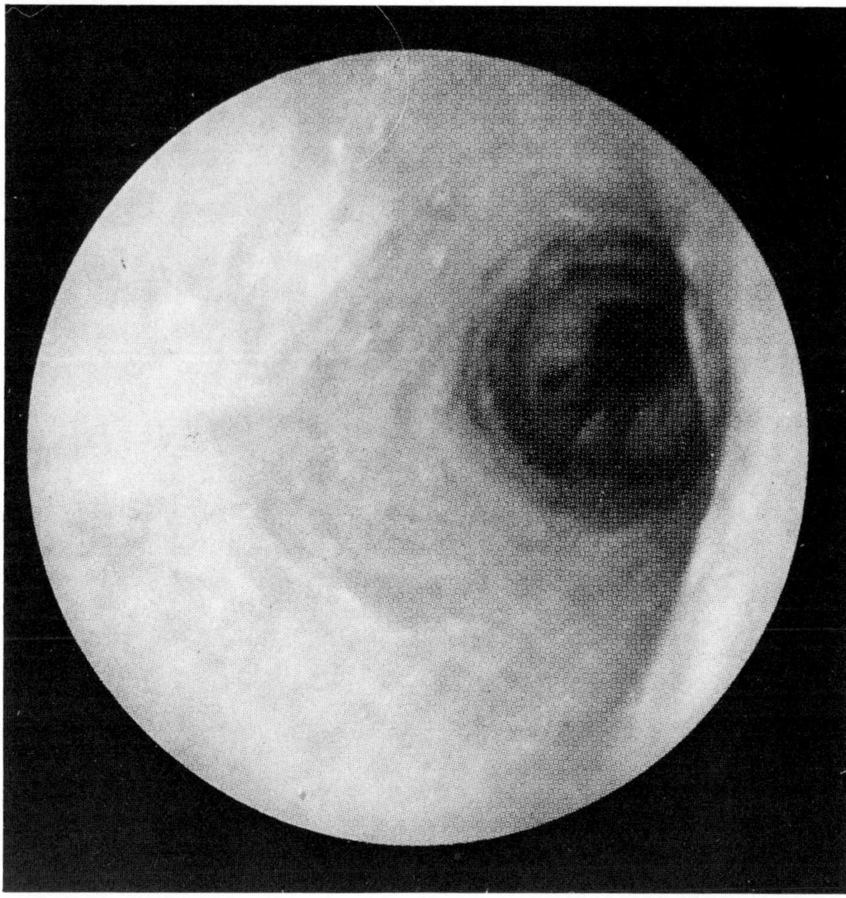

Figure 3–4. Endoscopic view of normal lower esophagus. The cardia appears in the distance. From Demling L et al. *Endoscopy and Biopsy of the Esophagus and Stomach: A Color Atlas*. Philadelphia: WB Saunders, 1972. Reprinted by permission.

holds a decided edge over radiography in its ability to arrive at a precise diagnosis.

The primary indication for upper gastrointestinal endoscopy is for further clarification of lesions documented by X ray. It is often indicated also in symptomatic patients whose X rays are negative. In some esophageal and duodenal disorders, a positive radiographic study alone is adequate for diagnosis without endoscopy. However, in most cases of esophageal and gastric disease demonstrated by radiography, subsequent endoscopy is advisable to confirm the presence of benign disorders, to rule out possibly malignant disease, and to diagnose the extent and severity of disorders detected by radiography. In making the decision to perform an endoscopy, physicians must be continuously alert to the patient's discomfort and to cost effectiveness, and must keep goals of the procedure clearly in mind.

Manometry

Since many disorders of the esophagus produce abnormalities in muscular tone or peristalsis, and since radiography and endoscopy are often unable to document these abnormalities precisely, esophageal manometry has long been used as a research tool and has recently been used clinically to provide more precise physiologic information in patients with propulsive esophageal disorders. Unfortunately, the techniques used in esophageal manometry often differ from one laboratory to another, and pressure measurements tend to be higher when larger tubing is used. Thus, clinicians must be thoroughly familiar with specific laboratory standards and with their recording techniques before attempting to interpret the results.

As practiced today, a three- to seven-lumen polyvinal tube is employed in esophageal manometry. The outer diameter of the completed assembly is approximately 6 mm. In the seven-lumen assembly six recording tubes, each containing a pressure sensor and each with a recording port at a different level, are arranged radially around the seventh central tube. This central lumen is employed only for the aspiration of secretions, not for the recording of pressure. The lowermost three ports, each cut into one of the tubes, are arranged at different points on the circumference of the assembly, in order to record anteroposterior and lateral pressures, and are separated from one another by 1 cm distances longitudinally. Ports into tubes three to six are spaced at 5-cm intervals. Fidelity of pressure recordings is obtained by a slow mechanical infusion of water into each tube, the pressure wave being conveyed through the column of water.

The tube assembly is passed through the subject's nose until the central tube opening rests in the stomach. Separate studies are then succesively made of the resting pressure and swallowing relaxation response in the LES, the peristaltic response of the body of the esophagus to a wet or dry swallow, and the resting and swallowing dynamics of the UES. Sphincteric pressures are measured through the lowermost three ports, while motility in the body of the esophagus is recorded at a different time from the upper four ports. The resting pressure in the LES ranges normally between 10 and 35 mm Hg greater than intragastric pressure. It falls to zero about 2 seconds after a swallow, and then returns to the resting level in another 6 to 12 seconds. Since the lower esophagus moves upward with a swallow, this relaxation response must be recorded at each of the lower three ports to avoid being misled by the artificial fall that occurs when the lowermost port of the recording tube is displaced into the stomach by esophageal contraction. The zone of high pressure in the LES is approximately 3 to 4 cm long, and is located at a depth of 42 to 44 cm from the nares. External pressure on the epigastrium increases resting pressure in the normal LES. Since the esophagus is flattened anatomically so that the anteroposterior diameter is shorter than the side-to-side diameter, pressures recorded at ports directed anteroposteriorly are normally considerably higher than the pressures recorded at lateral ports. Representative ranges of LES pressure in health and disease are as follows:

Condition	*mm Hg*
achalasia	50.5 ± 4.6
Zollinger-Ellison syndrome	27.2 ± 2.1
normal	15.0 ± 1.7
pernicious anemia	9.9 ± 1.4
gastroesophageal reflux	7.3 ± 0.5
scleroderma	5.8 ± 0.6

The body of the esophagus extends manometrically for a distance of 21 cm between the lowermost portion of the UES and the upper border of the LES. Resting pressures in the body of the esophagus are at zero, and they may actually fall below zero during inspiration if the zero reference point is intragastric rather than intrathoracic pressure. Peristaltic contractions in the body of the esophagus are successively recorded at each of the four upper recording ports in response to a swallow. The wave of contraction moves more rapidly in the proximal body and in the midesophagus, slowing at the level of the aortic arch and in the lower esophagus, the speed ranging from 1 to 5 cm per second. The pressure of the contraction waves also varies between 60 and 100 mm Hg, and tends to decrease with age.

Pressures in the UES are also recorded from the closely spaced lower ports. As in the LES, lateral pressures are lower than anteroposterior pressures. The normal antero-posterior pressure at rest may be 80 mm Hg or higher, and relaxation occurs within 0.2 to 0.5 seconds after a wet swallow. The UES is located 18 to 19 cm below the nares.

Figure 3–5 defines the normal esophageal manometric pattern in response to a swallow. It can be referred to again as motility disorders of the esophagus are discussed below.

Intraesophageal Monitoring of pH

In patients suspected of having esophagitis resulting from the reflux of acidic gastric contents into the esophagus, producing recurrent bouts of pyrosis, fluoroscopy alone may not always demonstrate this reflux, despite such maneuvers as observing a swallow in the Trendelenberg position (elevation of abdomen and lower extremities above the chest). The observation of pH changes during prolonged periods by way of an electrode in the lower esophagus will demonstrate times where highly acidic levels (below pH 3.0)

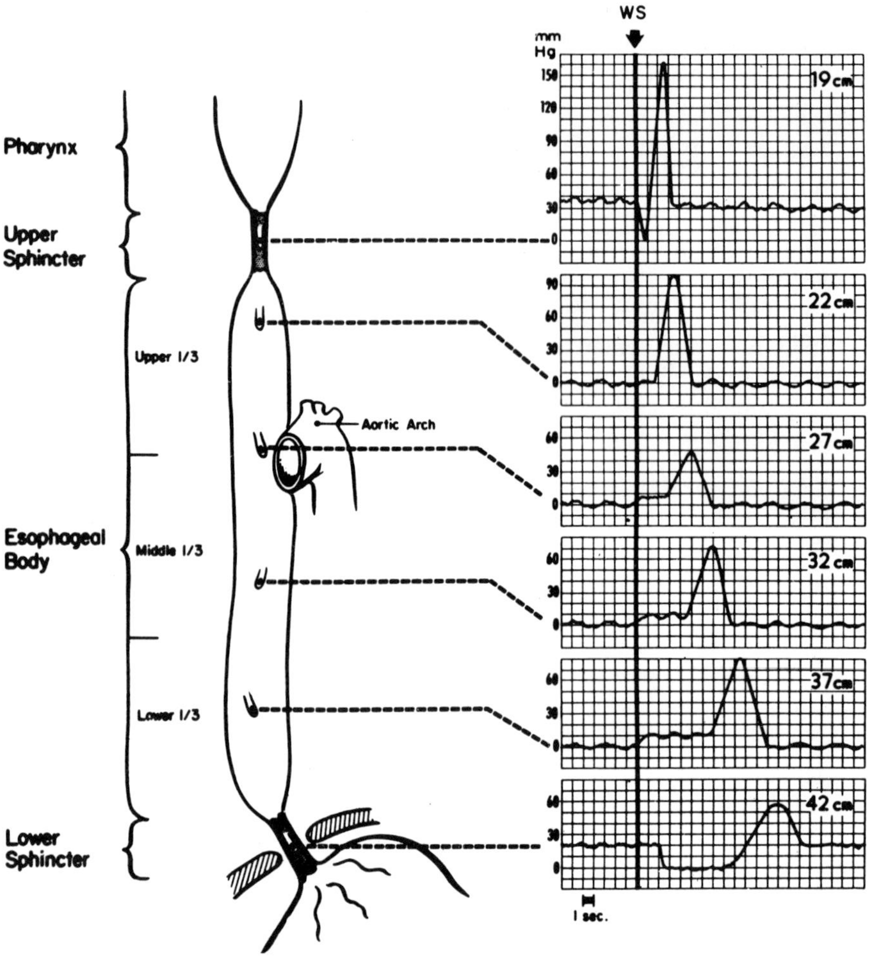

Figure 3-5. Schematic representation of esophageal pressures at rest and after a wet swallow. From Dodds WJ. Arch Intern Med 136:515–23, 1976. Copyright 1976, American Medical Association.

are attained. If such periods are frequent, prolonged, and accompanied by heartburn, the diagnosis of acid-reflux esophagitis is confirmed.

Where the test remains negative despite the Trendelenberg maneuver, a provocative test using the intragastric instillation of 300 ml of 0.1 N hydrochloric acid may be employed. Under these circumstances, 80 percent of normal individuals will not show evidence of reflux after 10 to 15 minutes, and 20 percent will show asymptomatic reflux. On the other hand, 20 percent of patients with true reflux esophagitis might not demonstrate a fall in intraesophageal pH after the intragastric infusion of acid (Pope 1972).

Acid Perfusion of the Esophagus (Bernstein Test)

In cases where patients complain of symptoms suggesting heartburn and radiographic studies are normal, or in patients with documented gastroesophageal reflux whose symptoms are not typical of pyrosis but might be anginal or skeletal, 300 ml of 0.1 N hydrocholoric acid may be dripped slowly into the midesophagus. During the course of this slow intraesophageal drip, patients with esophagitis will almost invariably note that their symptoms are strongly reproduced, and that they disappear shortly after the infusion is changed to distilled water. To avoid subjective errors in this test, it is best performed under circumstances wherein neither the subject nor the observer are aware of the nature of the fluid being instilled.

I have had occasional experiences where, in treating physicians or other medically sophisticated patients who were known previously to experience gastroesophageal reflux, I have suspected that new symptoms of substernal, often radiating pain, were actually due to angina pectoris. The patient is often reluctant to accept this new diagnosis, and would far rather be treated for esophagitis. In such cases, the acid perfusion test has proved to be helpful in confirming that esophagitis is not the problem, and in directing therapy more appropriately.

Esophageal Scintigraphy

Using a gamma camera to record counts over the chest and upper abdomen following the ingestion of ^{99m}Tc sulfur colloid, it has recently become possible to quantitate esophageal motility with considerable accuracy (Tolin et al 1979). After successive swallows, the normal individual clears the esophagus of the radioisotope within 10 to 15 seconds, while patients with motor dysfunctions of the esophagus require much longer periods. This procedure has the advantage of requiring much less radiation exposure than does cineradiography, and may simulate normal conditions better than barium, which has a higher viscosity than does saliva and gastric juice and may alter motility characteristics somewhat.

MOTOR DISORDERS OF THE ESOPHAGUS

Many prominent esophageal diseases are primarily neuromuscular in origin. To varying degrees they can result from overactivity or underactivity of the upper and lower sphincters and of the body of the esophagus, either singly or in combination (Cohen 1979). The variety of disorders associated with LES disfunction, peristaltic abnormalities, or both, is suggested in Table 3-1.

Table 3-1. Disorders Related to Alterations in Esophageal Peristalsis and Lower Sphincter Tones

Peristalsis	*Lower Esophageal Sphincter*		
	Hypoactive	*Normal*	*Hyperactive*
Hypoactive	esophagitis scleroderma	neuropathy aging	true achalasia
Normal	asymptomatic reflux	normal state	early achalasia
Hyperactive	variant diffuse spasm	true diffuse spasm	vigorous achalasia

Reduced Resting Pressure in the Lower Esophageal Sphincter

A large number of patients are seen in whom resting pressures in the LES are at or below 10 mm Hg. Furthermore, the pressure in this sphincter does not show the normal increase that would be expected in response to exertion of pressure on the epigastrium, to the administration of exogenous gastrin, following alkalinization of the gastric antrum or after a high protein meal. The LES appears to have lost its intrinsic myogenic tone and, as a consequence, contents easily reflux into the esophagus from the stomach.

Gastroesophageal reflux does not cause symptoms in all patients, and may only be discovered incidental to upper gastrointestinal X ray studies. Those patients who are symptomatic appear also to have diminished secondary esophageal peristalsis, so that the distention caused by reflux does not promptly provoke a wave that forces the contents back into the stomach. Heartburn is the major symptom of reflux, and its presence usually correlates well with the finding of esophagitis on biopsy.

The proximate cause of esophagitis, whether acid or bile salts, or both, is not certain, and the degree of esophagitis does not correlate well with the severity of the patients' complaints, nor with the X ray findings. Thus, several of the studies mentioned above, such as endoscopy and acid perfusion testing, are frequently necessary to confirm the clinical impression.

Pope (1972) has described the histologic changes that take place in reflux esophagitis. Normal esophageal mucosa has a thin basal layer of young squamous cells overlying the submucosa, and dermal pegs (epithelial growth centers) that reach less than halfway to the surface of the epithelium from the basal layer. This basal layer is thickened in patients with symptomatic reflux, and the rete pegs are broader and longer (Figure 3-6), reaching to the surface of the mucosa—changes indicating mucosal proliferation. In the most severe cases, signs of inflammation, including infiltration with inflammatory cells and breaks in the epithelial layer (ulcerations), are seen. Endoscopically, the early changes of esophagitis are not usually detectable; in more advanced cases one sees hyperemia of the mucosa, exudation, and occasionally, ulcers and hemorrhage.

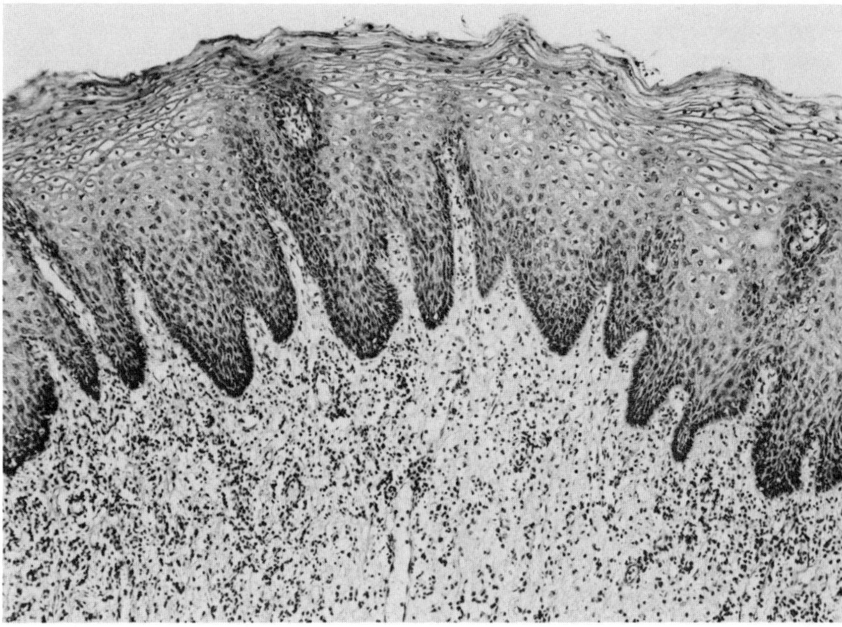

Figure 3-6. Biopsy specimen from patient with reflux esophagitis. Hyperplasia of the squamous mucosa is manifested by broad and long rete pegs and thickening of the basal layer. Hyperemia and lymphocytic infiltration are present in the submucosa. (Original magnification x80).

There appears to be general agreement at present that prolonged exposure to gastric reflux may eventually lead to metaplasia of the esophageal mucosa (Barrett epithelium). This appears microscopically (Figure 3-7) as an epithelium composed of tall columnar cells and goblet cells that may rarely contain gastric chief and parietal cells in the distal esophagus. More proximally, however, Barrett epithelium is often like intestinal mucosa, and is cast in something like a villous pattern, with glandular aggregations interspersed. This epithelium may also be stratified and has been considered to be a premalignant lesion leading to adenocarcinoma of the esophagus. Barrett mucosa may also show ulcerations and underlying inflammatory infiltrate (Paull et al 1976).

Scarring and stricture formation in the esophagus is a late consequence of chronic esophagitis, with or without metaplasia. Patients in whom strictures have occurred generally note a decrease in the frequency and severity of their pyrosis, along with progressive dysphagia, resulting in a gradually decreasing ability to ingest solid foods and an increased dependency on liquids.

Therapeutic Mechanisms in Esophagitis. The avoidance of recumbency, especially after meals, can help reduce the frequency of refluxive symptoms. So

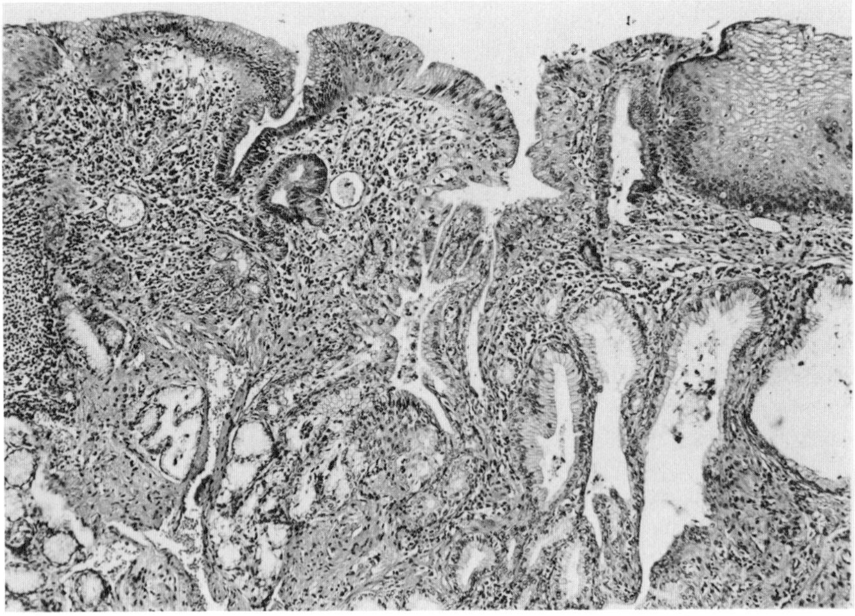

Figure 3-7. Biopsy specimen from a patient with chronic esophagitis and resultant metaplasia of the mucosa (Barrett epithelium). Note the normal squamous epithelium at right and the metaplastic columnar epithelium, resembling that of the gastric mucosa, on the remainder of the specimen. Mucous glands resembling gastric antral tissue are present in the submucosa, and a heavy lymphocytic infiltrate is present throughout. (Original magnification x80.)

too, can the avoidance of foods, such as chocolate, fat, and alcohol, which reduce LES pressures. Direct irritants, such as citrus juices and vesicant spices, should be omitted. Cigarette smoking and drugs that reduce sphincter tone, such as anticholinergics and isoproterenol, should also be avoided. Antacids are helpful in assuring that whatever contents are refluxed from the stomach will be at a pH level, generally above 4.0, at which further mucosal irritation is least likely to occur. Antacids are generally prescribed to be taken when acid levels are expected to be highest, approximately one hour after meals, and at bedtime. The use of antacids containing aluminum salts is enjoying increased popularity because of the avidity with which bile acids combine with that element.

Certain success has attended the use of drugs that have been shown to increase resting pressures of the LES in patients with incompetent sphincters. Among these are the cholinergic agonist, bethanechol (Urecholine), which is well tolerated in oral doses of 25 mg qid, and the recently synthesized direct stimulant of smooth muscle, metoclopramide. Fortunately, this drug is presently available for therapeutic use in an oral form. Cimetidine, which blocks acid-stimulatory histamine (H_2) receptors on gastric parietal cells, has also been found to be very beneficial in the symptomatic

Opération L.E.S

management of patients with reflux esophagitis. The benefit of cimetidine parallels its ability to reduce the secretion of acid by the stomach.

The therapy outlined above will provide symptomatic relief in the bulk of patients with reflux esophagitis and esophageal ulcer, even in those who may have had considerable bleeding. Ancillary treatment with progressively larger esophageal dilators may also be necessary in patients with esophageal strictures, but this too is commonly effective. Surgery is reserved for those patients whose symptoms recur promptly as the intensity of therapy is reduced, or in the small percentage who do not respond to treatment. Where surgery is contemplated, particularly in patients who have not responded to medication, it is essential that tests previously described have shown conclusively that symptoms are indeed due to the esophagitis. No more than 10 percent of patients with reflux esophagitis should require surgery.

Surgical management has fortunately emerged from an era of uncertainty about the correct operative technique. When hiatal hernias were felt to be the major cause of reflux esophagitis, many surgeons were content with a simple hernial repair. Unfortunately, this operation was attended by a very high incidence of nonhealing or recurrent esophagitis and has been abandoned. Present-day surgery is contrived at increasing pressure in the LES, and this is accomplished by invaginating the distal esophagus into the fundus of the stomach, wrapping the fundus partially or completely around the esophagus, suturing it in place, and securing the esophagus to the diaphragm so that the esophagogastric junction remains in an intra-abdominal position (procedures of R.H.R. Belsey, L.D. Hill and R. Nissen). Postoperative studies have shown that this procedure leads to healing of esophagitis and strictures, and that it is attended by LES pressures significantly higher than preoperative levels. The response of the LES to increased intra-abdominal pressure is improved, as is the response to the exogenous administration of gastrin. It has been suggested also that Barrett epithelium may regress toward normal after successful antireflux surgery, although this has not been completely substantiated. A recent study by Brand and colleagues (1979) indicates that some deterioration of benefits, including increasing symptoms and increasing reflux, may occur starting five years after successful surgery.

Hiatal Hernias. Protrusions of the stomach above the diaphragm may be associated with, but are certainly not the cause, of incompetence of the LES (see review in Cohen 1979). They are considered here because of their common association with reflux esophagitis, and because hernias of the direct type may actually aggravate reflux in patients with LES incompetence by the consequent displacement of the esophagogastric junction into the low-pressure inthrathoracic environment.

Eighty-five percent of hiatal hernias are of the purely sliding variety, in which the esophagogastric junction slips above the diaphragm, pulling the stomach in its train (Figure 3–8). Because the pressure that exists within t

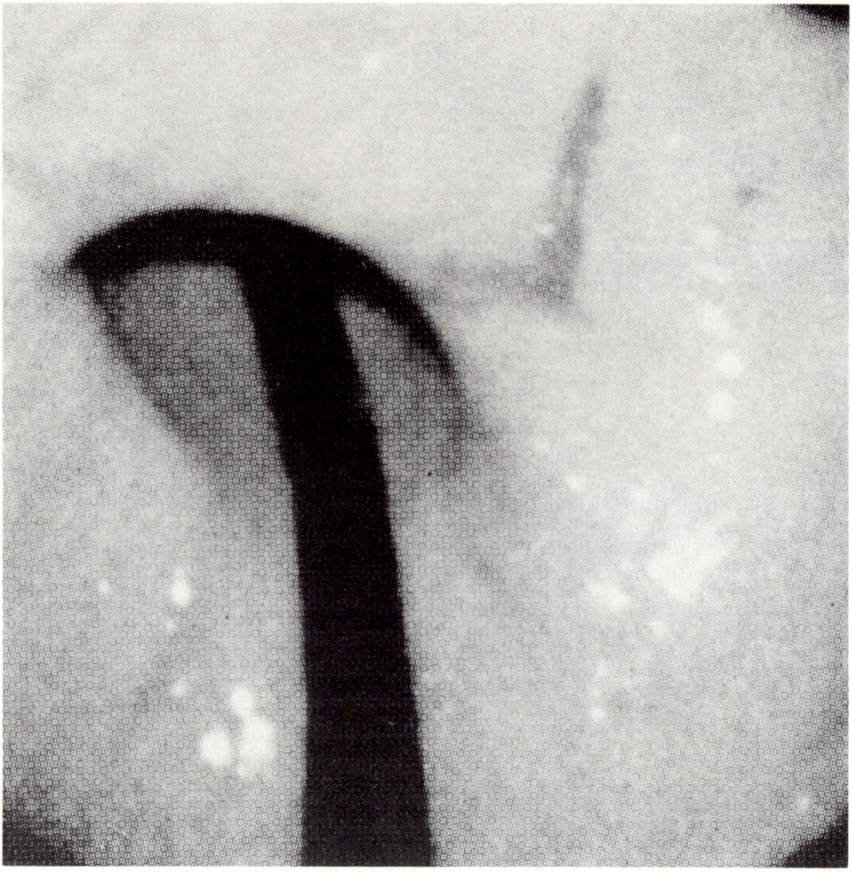

Figure 3–8. Endoscopic view of sliding hiatal hernia seen from below. Note the proximal portion of the gastroscope entering the stomach and the upward protrusion of the stomach through the diaphragm. From Demling L et al. *Endoscopy and Biopsy of the Esophagus and Stomach: A Color Atlas*. Philadelphia: WB Saunders, 1972. Reprinted with permission.

peritoneal cavity is greater than intrathoracic pressure, there is an upward force continuously exerted by the abdominal viscera against the diaphragmatic hiatus. This force is normally resisted by ligaments which bind the esophagus snugly to the diaphragm. The effects of these structures, however, can be overcome by the weakening effects of aging, as well as by conditions that increase intra-abdominal pressure such as obesity, pregnancy, and ascites. Sliding hernias may be very large, allowing as much as half of the stomach to protrude into the thorax; in the main, however, they are usually much smaller and involve only a fraction of the stomach. Symptoms are almost nil unless there is coexisting incompetence of the LES, or unless food or gastric contents are retained in the upper stomach in patients with very large hernias. Such patients may suffer from occasional regurgitation, vomiting, or lower chest distress due to gastric distention. Rarely, ulcers may occur in the herniated portion of the stomach as a probable result of the retention.

In the less common (5 percent of all hiatal hernias) paraesophageal hernias, the stomach protrudes into the chest alongside the esophagus, allowing the gastroesophageal junction to remain in its normal position astride the diaphragm. These hernias often result from upper abdominal trauma, and may be large enough to include the entire stomach. As the stomach enters the sac of a paraesophageal hernia, the greater curve of that organ, being less fixed anatomically than the lesser curve, migrates upward and becomes the leading edge. Thus, in a total paraesophageal herniation of the stomach into the chest, the stomach is truly upside down. Furthermore, the stomach rotates 180 degrees on its vertical axis in a total herniation and may actually obstruct the passage of food into the stomach from the esophagus, and of secretions into the duodenum. Such obstructions require immediate surgical repair, as do the strangulations of the stomach that may occur when arterial blood supply is comprised sufficiently in large paraesophageal hernias. For these reasons, large paraesophageal hernias should probably be operated on when diagnosed, while large sliding hernias may be treated conservatively. Any type of hernia is considered to be either reducible, if it disappears when the patient stands erect, or incarcerated, if it remains in place. Incarcerated paraesophageal hernias are most likely to be symptomatic.

The remainder of hiatal hernias (15 percent) are mixed sliding and paraesophageal, their symptoms depending on which type predominates. In most instances, little treatment of the hernias themselves is required, although weight control particularly may help prevent complications.

Progressive Systemic Sclerosis (Scleroderma). Well over half of all patients with this disorder, and most specifically those who have associated Raynaud phenomenon, are visited by esophageal disease as well. The disease involves both the LES, which becomes progressively incompetent, and the smooth muscle of the lower two-thirds of the esophagus, which becomes progressively aperistaltic. Histologically, the smooth muscle layer in both areas shows varying degrees of atrophy, although the muscular lesion may not be visible microscopically in patients with early physiologic abnormalities. Patients with other collagen vascular disorders, such as systemic lupus erythematosus, dermatomyositis, rheumatoid arthritis, and idiopathic Raynaud phenomenon may manifest similar abnormalities. In scleroderma, the esophageal symptoms may precede cutaneous induration and thickening by months or years. Histologic evidence of esophagitis is found in patients who suffer from advanced degrees of incompetence of the LES. The fact that Raynaud phenomenon is seen in almost all patients with esophageal dysfunction suggests that chronic vasospasm may be etiologically involved.

Symptoms of esophageal scleroderma depend on the extent of the lesion. Where the body of the esophagus alone is affected, the patients will note a form of dysphagia typified by a sensation of slow passage of the bolus after a swallow. The discomfort is worst with solid foods and may be relieved by washing food downward with a liquid, or by successive dry swallows. The most severe symptoms are experienced by patients who have hypotonia of the lower sphincter, for this lesion plus aperistalsis of the esophagus are the prime requisites for the development of esophagitis. They thus note frequent heartburn, and may have odynophagia as well, resulting from ulcers of the distal esophagus, and progressive dysphagia, resulting from strictures.

Management of scleroderma of the esophagus is similar to that outlined above for reflux esophagitis, and is often quite successful. Repeated dilatation of strictures may be necessary, and in cases where this approach is not successful or needs frequent repetition, antireflux surgery has been beneficial.

Other Causes of Reflux Esophagitis. Decreased LES tone with symptomatic reflux appears to be frequent in other settings. In infancy, the disorder called esophageal chalasia generally resolves spontaneously during postnatal development but is occasionally severe enough to require medication or even surgery. The cause of the LES incompetence is unknown. In pregnancy, sphincter weakness seems to be related to levels of estrogen and progesterone which appear to reduce smooth muscle tone. Symptoms almost invariably disappear in the postpartum period.

It has been clearly shown that prolonged nasogastric intubation can lead to reflux of gastric contents into the stomach, presumably because of induced incompetence of the LES. Subsequent complications, such as esophageal ulcer and bleeding and aspiration pneumonia, can be life threatening. While treatment is often effective, preventive measures, such as the conservative use of indwelling tubes, elevation of the patient's head and chest while on nasogastric suction, and even the prophylactic administration of cimetidine can avoid this difficulty. Similarly, esophagitis, esophageal ulcers and softening and rupture of the esophagus have been seen in patients with extensive burns. Here again, intubation and supination are probably important causes, but nutritional and circulatory factors probably also have an etiologic role.

Increased Resting Pressures in the LES, With Failure to Relax (Achalasia) After a Swallow

Pathophysiology. These are the criteria of a common idiopathic disorder of the esophagus, called achalasia or cardiospasm. This disorder is associated with moderate to marked decreases in the number of ganglion cells in esophageal myenteric (Auerbach) plexi. Ganglionic destruction has also been found in the dorsal nuclei of the vagus nerves, and the nerve trunks themselves have been found to be abnormal, suggesting that the disease results from a neurotropic, possibly viral, agent. The disease is worldwide in distribution, is unassociated with other disorders, and appears to be unassociated with age or sex.

Denervation of the esophageal musculature results in (1) the disappearance of effective peristalsis in the body of the esophagus; (2) failure of the LES to relax in response to a swallow; (3) increased resting pressure in the LES; (4) increased contractile response of the denervated muscle to parasympathomimetic drugs, such as acetylbeta methylcholine (Mecholyl); and (5) increased contractile sensitivity to the administration of the gastric antral hormone gastrin, or its analogues. The latter two responses are probably a direct reaction to denervation, as described by Cannon. With progressive obstruction due to achalasia, the proximal esophagus dilates and elongates, and the wall often hypertrophies, resulting in a condition called *megaesophagus.*

Symptoms. Patients with achalasia often complain initially of difficulty in swallowing liquids as well as solids, while in patients with disorders that narrow the lumen of the esophagus, such as strictures or carcinoma, difficulty occurs first with solids alone. This is probably due to the fact that liquids are just as likely to be unable to negotiate the unrelaxed LES as are more solid foods. Awaiting the spontaneous emptying of the esophagus might provoke so much discomfort that the patient may stop eating or vomit spontaneously for relief. Such vomitus is distinctive, since it contains no gastric acid and does not taste sour. Loss of weight is a common consequence of the dysphagia. Sharp chest pain is not usually experienced in typical achalasia.

When the esophagus dilates and is able to accommodate larger quantities of food, dysphagia may abate for a time, but the danger exists that esophageal contents will regurgitate upon lying down and be aspirated into the tracheobronchial tree. Resultant acute or chronic aspiration pneumonitis is a well recognized complication of advanced achalasia.

Diagnosis. The diagnosis of achalasia can usually be made on fluoroscopic examination of the esophagus. There is a narrowed distal segment, representing the area of the LES, between the esophagus and the stomach, and the esophagus itself is mildly to markedly dilated and aperistaltic (Figure 3–9). Often the esophagus is immense in size, and an air-fluid interface, representing the level of retained fluid in the esophagus, can be seen on a conventional lateral X ray of the chest without use of a contrast agent. When proximal dilatation of the esophagus is only slight, however, there may be some difficulty in distinguishing between achalasia, carcinoma, and stricture of the esophagus. Here again, the absence of proximal peristalsis in the esophagus favors a diagnosis of achalasia.

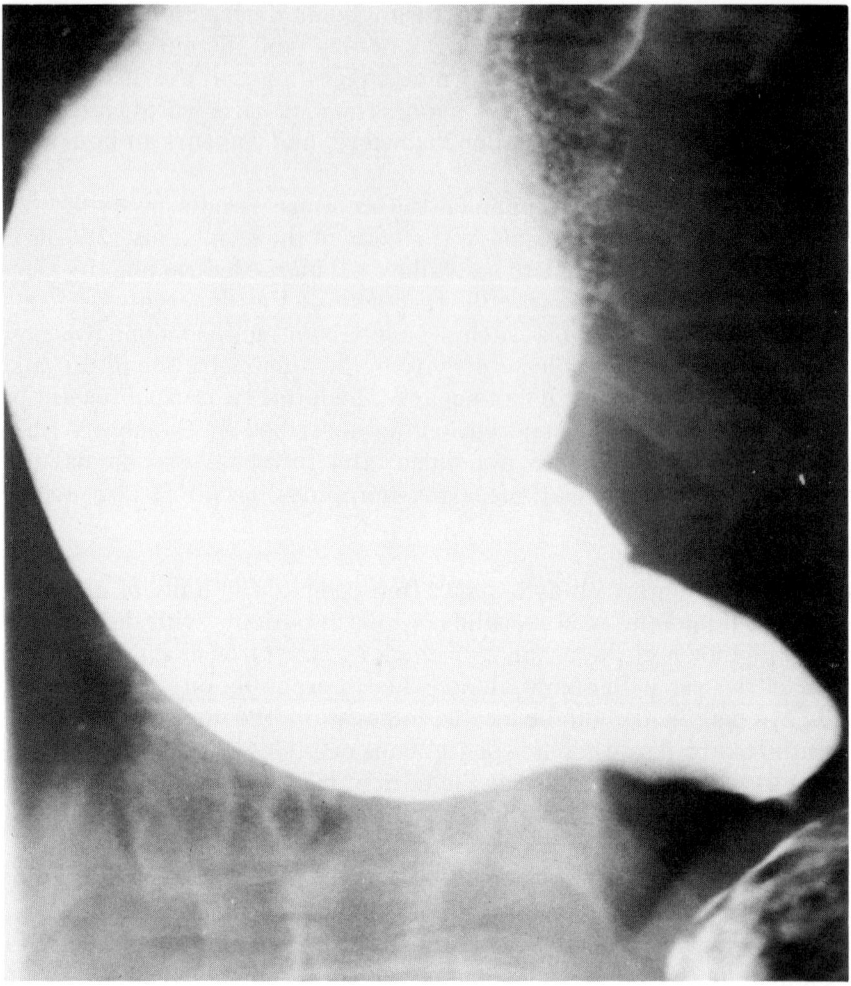

Figure 3–9. Barium contrast radiograph of the lower esophagus in a patient with achalasia and megaesophagus. The lower esophagus is markedly dilated and tapers smoothly to a blunt termination at the level of the contracted lower esophageal sphincter. Courtesy of Dr. Renate Duchesneau.

Typical achalsia can be clearly documented by esophageal manometry. Recordings from the LES show resting pressures about two times or more greater than normal (40 to 60 mm Hg instead of 15 to 20 mm) (Figure 3–10). These resting pressures increase markedly in response to the administration of gastrin or methacholine. Furthermore, after a wet swallow, LES pressures in achalsia fall somewhat, but not nearly to intragastric levels, thus illustrating the mechanism responsible for the functional obstruction. In evaluating the body of the esophagus manometrically in patients with acha-

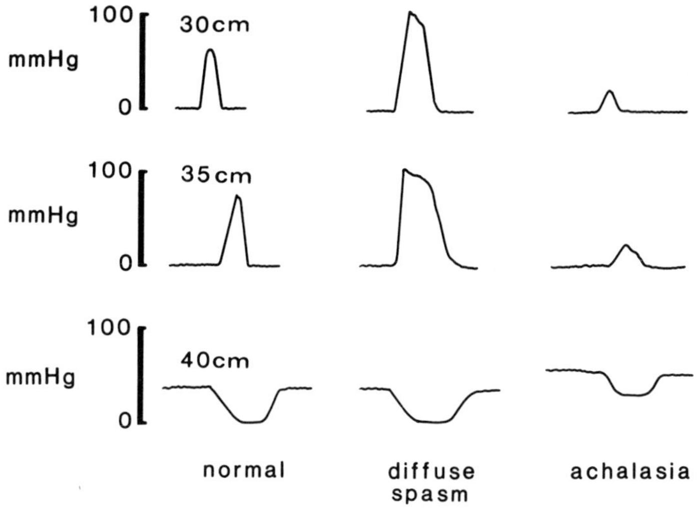

Figure 3–10. Simplified typical normal esophageal motility and pressure patterns (stylized) compared with those found in diffuse spasm and achalasia. Note in the normal state that contraction occurs first after a swallow at the more proximal site (30 cm) and shortly after at 35 cm, while in diffuse spasm contractions occur at the two sites simultaneously, and are longer in duration and much higher in pressure. Pressure at the LES (40 cm) falls to intragastric levels (0 mm Hg) as the contraction wave reaches the lower esophagus in both the normal state and in diffuse spasm. In achalasia, the resting LES pressure is high and, when relaxation occurs, sphincteric pressures remain higher than intragastric, thus prohibiting the passage of esophageal contents into the stomach.

lasia, either aperistalsis or markedly reduced peristalsis is seen after a swallow.

Endoscopic examination after removal of esophageal contents by aspiration is indicated in all patients who have been newly discovered to have achalasia, because cancers of the fundus of the stomach can occasionally infiltrate the lower esophagus in such a way that the physiologic changes of achalasia are induced. Typically, secondary peristalsis is absent endoscopically in patients with achalasia, and the LES appears to be tightly closed. However, the tip of the instrument can invariably be passed into the stomach with slightly increased pressure, and the gastric cardia and fundus can then be examined carefully from below. Patients with long-standing achalasia have been shown to have an increased incidence of esophageal carcinoma, perhaps resulting from chronic stasis. Thus, any change or aggravation of symptoms in patients known to have this disease is probably a justification for endoscopy.

Therapy of achalasia with medication is not very successful, although occasional benefit is achieved from large doses of anticholinergic drugs, which may reduce resting LES pressures. The calcium-transport inhibitor, nifedipine, which reduces smooth muscle spasm, has been shown to reduce LES pressure and improve symptoms in some patients (Bortolotti and Labo 1981) Present treatment is designed to weaken the sphincter in one of two ways. Muscle fibers in the LES may be ruptured by forcible dilatation with a water- or air-filled balloon placed fluoroscopically, or they may be partially transected during an open operation (Heller myotomy). Both procedures have been successful. Hydrostatic or pneumatic dilatation risk rupturing of the esophageal wall, and patients who have had this procedure done should be observed closely for 24 hours after the procedure, looking for evidence of subcutaneous emphysema in the chest or neck. It is also advisable to X ray these patients again in a day to evaluate the results of the dilatation and to look for leaks of barium from the esophageal wall. After myotomy, approximately 20 percent of patients will develop gastroesophageal reflux, unless an antireflux procedure was performed at the same time. Presently, it is my practice to treat patients first with hydrostatic dilatation, unless they are under 15 years of age. If successful, this may be repeated at three- to four-year intervals if necessary. Myotomies are advised for young patients and for patients in whom dilatation has not been effective.

As yet unexplained, is the now substantiated observation of Vantrappen et al (1979), that a number of patients with achalasia experience a return of esophageal motility following pneumatic dilatation and Heller procedures. This rather surprising finding suggests that, at least in some individuals, the myenteric network above the LES is merely dormant and not absent when achalasia is present.

Chagas Disease. This disorder, common in northern Brazil and in parts of Central America, results from infection with the organism *Trypanasoma cruzi.* The infection produces in the esophagus disturbances which are physiologically identical to those of achalasia, except that the resting pressure in the LES may be normal. The organism appears to elaborate a neurotoxin which selectively destroys myenteric plexi in many parts of the body, including the heart, colon, bronchi, and ureters, as well as the esophagus. It is involvement of these other organs which distinguishes Chagas disease from primary achalasia.

Idiopathic Intestinal Pseudo-obstruction. In the past decade, a syndrome has been described in which all portions of the intestinal tract, including the esophagus, suffer from motility disturbances which result in motor weakness, distention, and retention of contents (Sullivan et al 1977). The disorder is often familial, and some of the patients have shown evidences of degeneration of myenteric plexi, while others have demonstrated no histologic abnormalities and are presumed to have uncharacterized physiologic disorders. Because of inadequate small intestinal mixing, these patients commonly have bacterial overgrowth in their small intestinal tracts and resulting malabsorption.

The esophageal disorder in this disease is characterized by normal or low resting pressures in the LES, with failure to relax after a swallow. The body of the esophagus may display aperistalsis, as in achalasia, or simultaneous non-propulsive spasms. In most cases, esophageal retention is not the major symptom, although it may at times be highly significant.

Zollinger-Ellison Syndrome. Patients with gastrin-secreting tumors of the pancreas or surrounding organs commonly have multiple peptic ulcers and diarrhea, as will be discussed in Chapter 5. They have also been found to have increased resting pressures in the LES, which usually respond normally to a swallow. Occasionally, they may also have dysphagia. The LES hypertonia has not been directly related to the hypergastrinemia, although it does return to normal in conjunction with successful removal or obliteration of the tumor mass. Not all patients with hypergastrinemia have increased LES pressure, however, and gastrin levels do not correlate with LES pressure (McCallum, Walsh 1979). The hypergastrinemia of patients with pernicious anemia and other types of atrophic gastritis is often associated with lower than normal pressures. The explanation for this seeming paradox is not clear, although it is felt that the gastrin circulating in these patients may not be in a functionally active form.

Repetitive Non-propulsive Spasms in the Body of the Esophagus (Diffuse Esophageal Spasm)

Sustained contractions of the esophagus, occurring simultaneously at different levels, and often of high amplitude, may be seen occasionally during manometric examination in asymptomatic patients (Figure 3–10). Such contractions appear to be more common in elderly subjects and may be responsible for the tertiary spasms seen on fluoroscopy (Figure 3–11). When such contractions occur after at least one-third of all swallows and are associated with substernal pain and dysphagia, a diagnosis of diffuse esophageal spasm (DES) is justified. The main pathologic correlate of this disorder is the presence of inflammatory infiltrates around myenteric plexi and variable degrees of degeneration in esophageal branches of the vagus nerves. The body of the esophagus normally shows no response to the administration of intravenous gastrin, while high-amplitude contractions are induced in patients with DES by this hormone, another probable example of Cannon's observations on the supersensitivity of denervated muscle. Patients do not experience pain and dysphagia with every swallow, and most often have normal peristaltic responses. They are most comfortable when their food is well chewed and swallowed slowly. Their symptoms are frequenty ameliorated by the use of sublingual nitroglycerine (0.3 to 0.6 mg), and may be prevented by the regular administration of longer acting nitrites. In cases where symptoms are severe and unremitting, surgical myotomies of the distal esophagus have been found to be effective.

Typically, patients with DES have normal function of the lower esophageal sphincter (LES), and there is no delay in passage of food into the

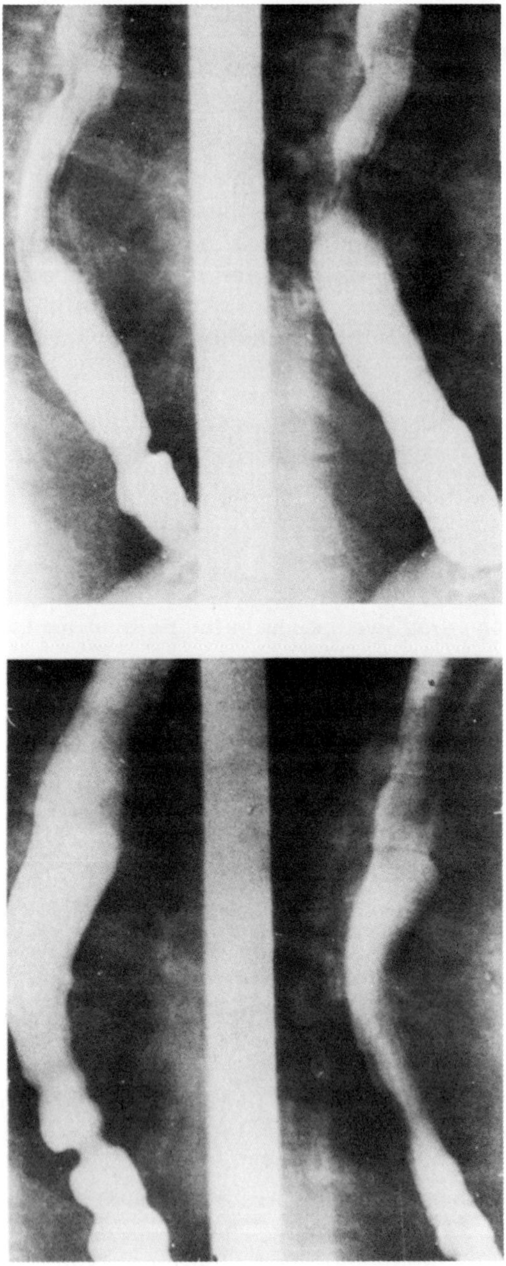

Figure 3–11. Tertiary contractions of the esophagus of the type commonly seen in diffuse esophageal spasm. From Pope CE. Motor Disorders. In: Sleisinger MH, Fordtran JS. *Gastrointestinal Disease.* Philadelphia: WB Saunders Company, 1973. Reprinted by permission.

stomach once the spasm in the body of the esophagus has disappeared. Patients do not lose weight and are usually relieved to learn that their substernal discomfort does not indicate the existence of coronary arterial disease. However, at times patients with DES may display the typical responses of achalasia in the LES, high resting pressures and failure of adequate relaxation upon swallowing. In these cases, food lingers in the esophagus and weight loss and regurgitation may occur, just as in true achalasia. Because of the esophageal spasms, these patients complain more often of severe substernal pain than do most patients with achalasia, and some investigators have accordingly labeled their disorder as vigorous achalasia.

A few patients with previously diagnosed DES have been found to progress to true achalasia, an observation which supports the thought that these two disorders may be somewhat different manifestations of the same underlying abnormality, progressive disease of myenteric plexi, vagus nerves, and vagal nuclei. This conclusion makes sense since it provides a single explanation for the complete spectrum of esophageal motor dysfunction, even though the proximate cause remains obscure.

Failure of Relaxation of the Upper Esophageal Sphincter (Cricopharyngeal achalasia)

The UES has not been studied as thoroughly as the lower sphincter, and one is much less able to speak authoritatively about its dysfunction. Resting pressures tend to be much higher than in the LES, ranging from 40 to 80 mm Hg, and the relaxation response to a swallow comes considerably earlier. Some patients with pharyngeal dysphagia, and often with tracheobronchial aspiration as well, have been found to have achalasia of the UES on manometric study. Tracings may show adequate relaxation after a swallow, followed by an earlier than normal contraction that does not allow the entire bolus to pass. Many of these patients also have posterior outpouchings of the pharyngeal mucosa, or pulsion diverticula (Zenker), through the latticelike striated muscular coat of the hypopharynx, above the site of the cricopharyngeus muscle. These diverticula may become quite large and push the pharynx forward, thereby obstructing it, as they fill with food. It is not clear presently whether all patients with Zenker diverticula have cricopharyngeal achalasia as well. Their symptoms are usually relieved totally by surgical removal of the diverticulum alone, although cricopharyngeal myotomy may also be indicated at times.

An analog to Zenker diverticula, epiphrenic diverticula, may occur just above the diaphragm in occasional patients, some of whom also have achalasia of the esophagus. These too are believed to be caused by increased intraluminal pressure, but they are rarely symptomatic because they do not significantly compress the esophagus.

Disturbances of Motility in the Hypopharynx and Body of the Esophagus

While almost all of the motility disorders described heretofore have been confined primarily to the esophagus, there is a large variety of systemic disease as well which may adversely affect pharyngeal and esophageal motility, generally by decreasing muscular contraction. Pharyngeal dysphagia is common in patients with disorders of the brainstem or striated musculature, such as vascular disease, dermatomyositis, disseminated sclerosis, muscular dystrophy, myasthenia gravis, amyloidosis, and amyotrophic lateral sclerosis. Pharyngeal weakness and weakened peristalsis in the body of the esophagus are seen also in patients with diabetic neuropathy and hypothyroidism. The strength of pharyngeal contraction appears to decrease with age as well.

Any of these patients is subject to the combined dangers of tracheal aspiration and malnutrition. Where the underlying disease is not responsive to treatment, it may become necessary to perform tracheostomies to prevent aspiration, and to feed the patient through indwelling nasogastric tubes.

MISCELLANEOUS ESOPHAGEAL DISORDERS

Traction diverticula of the esophagus occur in the body of the esophagus when mediastinal inflammatory lesions, such as tuberculous lymph nodes, adhere to its outer wall, contract by fibrosis, and pull a localized segment of the wall out of line. These diverticula have a wide mouth, do not become obstructed, and cause symptoms rarely. In contrast with Zenker and epiphrenic diverticula which protrude through the muscularis and consequently contain no muscular tissue in their wall, traction diverticula are classified as true diverticula since they contain all layers of the esophagus.

Esophageal webs are inflammatory changes with thin strands of fibrosis found in the hypopharynx and cervical esophagus of some patients, usually women, with iron deficiency anemia, stomatitis, atrophy of the tongue, and thin, soft, spoon-shaped fingernails. This syndrome, described by Plummer and Vinson, is often associated with cervical dysphagia which may respond only to dilatation. The disorder seems to be a response to iron deficiency, and is usually treated effectively by replacement of iron stores. Patients with Plummer-Vinson syndrome appear to be at increased risk for the development of cancer of the hypopharynx or cervical esophagus.

Corrosive strictures of the esophagus result from the accidental or intentional ingestion of strong acids or alkalis, such as lye. Initially, the mucosa of the esophagus becomes necrotic and ulcerates, and perforations of the esophagus into the mediastinum may occur. Within several days, fibrosis commences, with consequent extreme narrowing of the esophageal lumen. The resultant strictures are commonly very long and may involve all of the body of the esophagus.

If the patient is seen early, diagnosis is made by the history and often the observation of ulcerations in the hypopharynx or palate. At this stage, saline lavage should be attempted and the patient should be asked to swallow a long strand of umbilical tape to be used later for the passage of dilators, should that become necessary. There is also some evidence that administration of glucocorticoids at this stage may prevent or reduce later stricture formation. Any sign of esophageal perforation, such as fever or the appearance of subcutaneous emphysema, should indicate the immediate addition of antibiotics to the regimen. It is my custom to omit endoscopy at this time in an effort to prevent instrumental perforation.

If strictures are demonstrated after the first week, periodic dilatation of the esophagus should be commenced. While this will often not prevent later motility disturbances, dilatation can obviate the development of severe obstruction. In cases where strictures are highly symptomatic and unresponsive to dilatation, bypass surgery, employing a segment of transverse colon placed subcutaneously in the anterior chest, is the only acceptable alternative.

Ringlike strictures of the lower esophagus may be responsible for partial lower esophageal obstruction, and are of two types (Figure 3-12). The uppermost type corresponds with the inferior esophageal sphincter, and probably results from hypertrophy of those fibers. The lower type is a mucosal ring, containing no fibers from the muscular layers of the esophagus, and occurring at the level of the constrictor cardiae muscle, which is also the junction of esophageal squamous and upper gastric columnar mucosa (Goyal et al 1971). Neither type of ring shows associated inflammation. One or both of these rings occur in around 10 percent of asymptomatic patients; only a small number of subjects with lower esophageal rings are symptomatic. Esophageal dilatation is usually effective in controlling their symptoms.

Esophagitis due to candidiasis and herpes simplex are truly diseases of "medical progress" since they occur almost solely in patients receiving immunosuppressive therapy for a variety of serious illnesses. Immunoincompetence secondary to malnutrition may also precede the appearance of *Candida* and herpes esophagitis. These disorders may not be associated with lesions in the mouth, so it is essential to perform esophageal X rays whenever an immunosuppressed or poorly nourished patient newly complains of dysphagia or odynophagia.

The radiological picture is often pathognomonic, showing a long segment of mid esophagus containing numerous small, but deep, ulcerations. These changes give a furry appearance to the margins of the esophagus. Marked mucosal friability, hyperemia, and ulceration is seen on endoscopy, and biopsy or scrapings of the mucosa generally reveal the responsible organism.

Therapy of esophageal candidiasis or herpes demands reduction of immunosuppressive therapy and institution of hyperalimentation, either orally or intravenously. Nystatin orally may be beneficial in early stages of

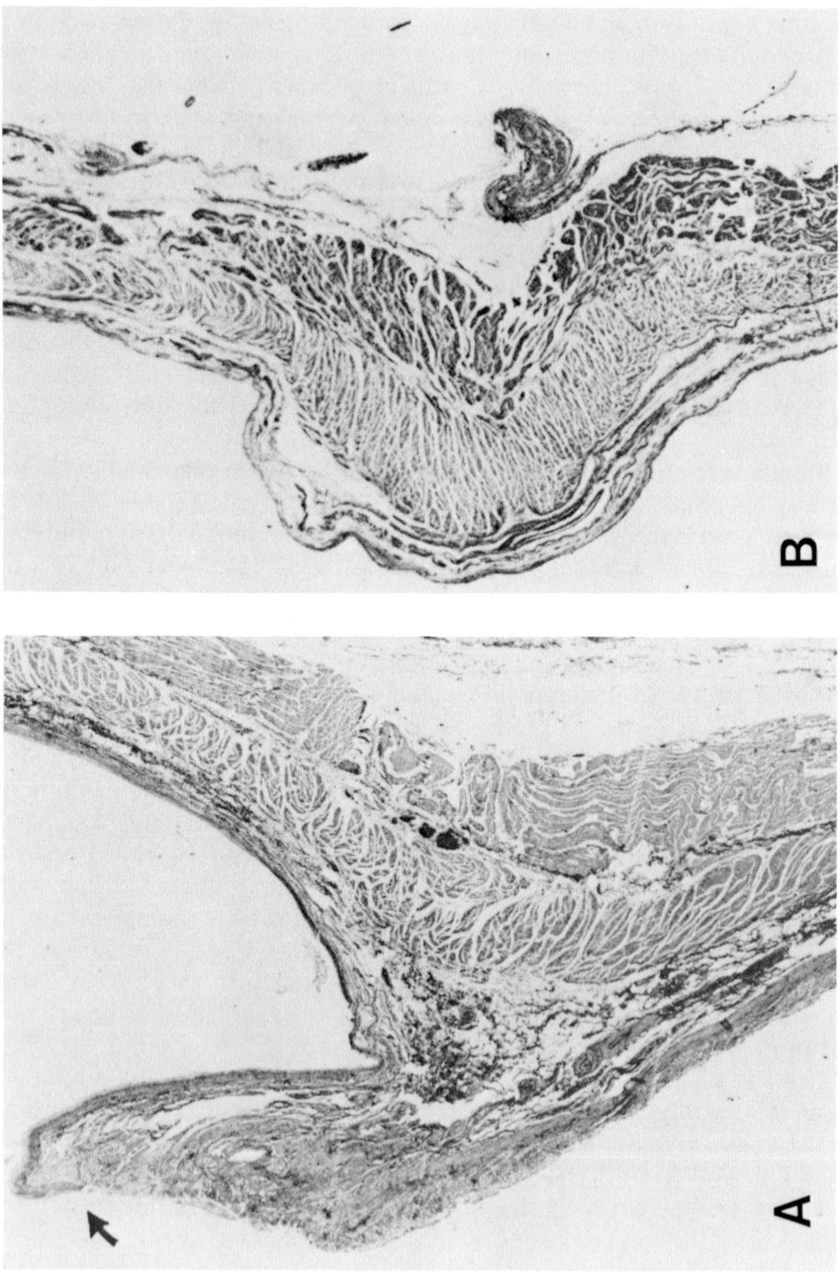

Figure 3-12. Sections of two types of lower esophageal ring. *A*, a mucosal ring, with arrow placed at squamocolumnar junction. Note that the muscularis does not participate in this ring. *B*, a muscular ring. From Goyal RK, Bauer JL, Spiro HM. N Engl J Med 284: 1175–80, 1971. Reprinted by permission.

candidiasis, but most patients with severe disease will require treatment with amphoterecin B.

NEOPLASMS

Carcinoma

Squamous cell (epidermoid) carcinoma (Figure 3-13) is the most common form of esophageal neoplasm. It tends to occur more commonly in men than in women, and has been reported to have an increased incidence among certain peoples such as Eskimos and blacks. The incidence is also increased among alcoholics, patients with achalasia, mucosal metaplasia in the esophagus (Barrett epithelium), lye strictures, and the Plummer-Vinson syndrome. According to American Cancer Society estimates, 8,800 new cases of esophageal carcinoma and 7,600 deaths occurred among Americans in 1980.

Although squamous cell carcinomas are the most common malignancy in the uppermost 90 percent of the esophagus, adenocarcinomas occur in the area just above the gastroesophageal junction. Most of these are probably cancers in metaplastic tissue, but they may also have extended upward from sites in the cardia of the stomach. It has been previously stated that such cancers may present with symptomatic and radiologic features of achalasia.

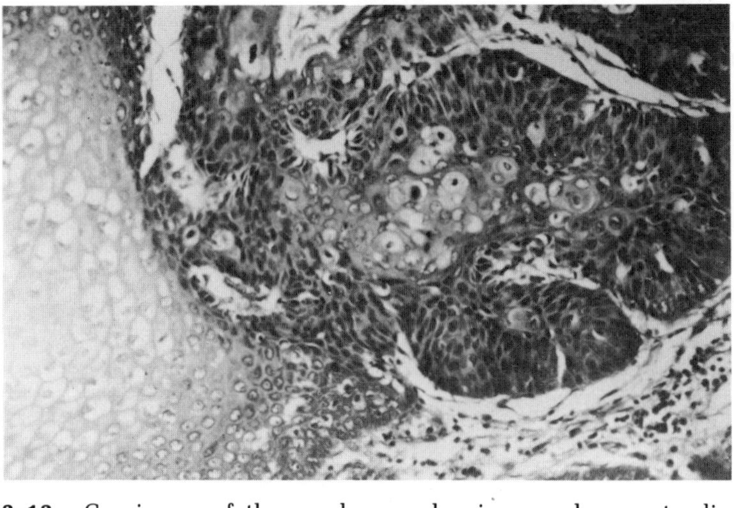

Figure 3-13. Carcinoma of the esophagus, showing neoplasm extending from basal cells of the normal mucosa on the left. Original magnification x63.

Since the esophagus is an elastic and distensible organ, carcinoma does not usually interfere with swallowing until it has involved a large portion of the circumference of the lumen. Since the esophagus has no outer serosal layer, cancer tends to spread more readily to adjacent areas and organs. Thus, the disease is usually far advanced and inoperable by the time it becomes symptomatic. Since esophageal lymphatics are located in the submucosa and cancer spreads longitudinally through these channels, the true area of involvement of the esophagus with tumor is often considerably more extensive than appears to be the case on fluoroscopy. Cancers in the lower portions of the esophagus tend to cause symptoms earlier in their course, because the lumen is narrower at this point than it is in the mid esophagus.

Dysphagia usually appears first with solid foods, while liquids may pass without difficulty until the later stages. Pain is not common. The mildness of these symptoms often encourages patients to postpone seeking medical guidance. Dysphagia soon progresses to restriction of intake, and often to prodigious losses of weight. Patients may also regurgitate and aspirate swallowed food, and may develop hoarseness if the recurrent laryngeal nerves are trapped in the tumor mass.

Even though the diagnosis is usually confirmed by history and by X ray, esophagoscopy and biopsy should be done to confirm it and to document its extent accurately. Surgical resection is the treatment of choice, but the results are discouraging primarily because of the extent of the tumor at the time of diagnosis. The five-year survival rate for patients who are able to undergo surgical resection is about 15 percent for lesions below the aortic arch and only 3 percent for those above it. Supervoltage X ray therapy is probably indicated in all cases, since epidermoid tumors are highly radiosensitive. Occasionally, this treatment alone may induce very long remissions of the disease but the risk of radiation pneumontis is great. At this writing, chemotherapy has little to offer, but possibly helpful agents such as 5-fluorouracil and adriamycin may be tried.

Leiomyoma

Although rare, this tumor is the most common benign tumor of the esophagus. Most often, it is noted incidentally on X ray as a smooth-surfaced, dome-shaped, 2–3-cm defect on the margin of the lower esophagus. The overlying mucosa is usually intact in asymptomatic patients, and no treatment is required. The diagnosis should be confirmed by endoscopy. Esophageal hemorrhage due to ulceration of the mucosal surface by enlarging tumor is the most common symptom, and surgical incision is indicated if this occurs. The development of leiomyosarcoma is rare and is heralded by symptoms of dysphagia and enlargement of the tumor mass.

HISTORICAL DIGRESSION

Personages mentioned without further reference in this chapter include: Leopold AUERBACH (1828–1897), German physiologist, Breslau; Norman Rupert BARRETT (1903–), British surgeon, London, described mucosal metaplasia in esophagitis, 1950; Lionel BERNSTEIN (1923–), American gastroenterologist, Chicago, Washington; Walter Bradford CANNON (1871–1945), American physiologist, Boston; Carlos CHAGAS (1879–1934), Brazilian bacteriologist, Rio de Janeiro; Gonçalves CRUZ (1872–1917), Brazilian bacteriologist, Rio de Janeiro; Edwin Homer ELLISON (1918–1970), American surgeon, Columbus, Ohio and Milwaukee, codiscoverer of gastrinoma syndrome, 1955; Ernst HELLER (1877–1964), German surgeon, Breslau, described esophageal myotomy procedure with Georg Gottstein in 1913; James PARKINSON (1755–1824), British physician and surgeon, wrote, "An essay on the shaking palsy," 1817; Henry Stanley PLUMMER (1874–1936), American internist, Rochester, Minnesota, described esophageal webs and iron deficiency anemia, 1915; Maurice RAYNAUD (1834–1881), French internist, Paris, described syndrome of digital vasospasm on exposure to cold environment, 1862; Friedrich TRENDELENBERG (1844–1924), German surgeon, Rostock, Bonn, Leipzig; Porter Paisley VINSON (1890–1959), American internist, Rochester, Minnesota, Richmond, Virginia; Rudolf VIRCHOW (1821–1902), German pathologist, Würzberg, Berlin; Freidrich Albert Ritter von ZENKER (1825–1898), German pathologist, Dresden, Erlangen; Robert Milton ZOLLINGER (1903–), American surgeon, Columbus, Ohio, codiscoverer of gastrinoma syndrome.

SELECTED REFERENCES

Bortolotti M. Labo G. Clinical and manometric effects of nifedipine in patients with esophageal achalasia. Gastroenterology 80:39–44, 1981.

Brand DL, Eastwood IR, Martin D, et al. Esophageal symptoms, manometry and histology before and after antireflux surgery. Gastroenterology 76:1393- 1401, 1979.

Cohen S. Medical progress. Motor disorders of the esophagus. N Engl J Med 301:184–192, 1979.

Fisher RS, Malmud LS, Roberts GS, et al. The lower esophageal sphincter as a barrier to gastroesophageal reflux. Gastroenterology 72:19 22, 1977.

Goyal RK ed. Symposium on esophageal motility. Arch Intern Med 136:511–601,1976.

Goyal RK, Bauer JL, Spiro HM. The nature and location of the lower esophageal ring. N Engl J Med 284:1175–80, 1971.

Livstone EM, Sheahan DG, Behar J. Studies of esophageal epithelial cell proliferation in patients with reflux esophagitis. Gastroenterology 73: 1315–19, 1977.
McCallum RW, Walsh JH. Relationship between lower esophageal sphincter pressure and serum gastrin concentration in Zollinger-Ellison syndrome and other clinical settings. Gastroenterology 76:76–81, 1979.
Paull A, Trier JS, Dalton MD, et al. The histologic spectrum of Barrett's esophagus. N Engl J Med 295:476–80, 1976.
Pope II CE. Recognition and management of gastroesophageal reflux. Viewpoints. Dig Dis 4:1–4 (Jan), 1972.
Sullivan MA, Snape WJ Jr, Matarazzo SA, et al. Gastrointestinal myoelectrical activity in idiopathic intestinal pseudo-obstruction. N Engl J Med 297:233–38, 1977.
Tolin RD, Malud LS, Reilley J, et al. Esophageal scintigraphy to quantitate esophageal transit. Gastroenterology 76:1402–8, 1979.
Vantrappen G, Janssens J, Hellemans J, et al. Achalasia, diffuse esophageal spasm and related motility disorders. Gastroenterology 76:450–57, 1979.

CLINICAL CONFERENCE 1

A 53-year-old white woman was admitted to the hospital complaining of progressively severe pain in her chest and regurgitation shortly after eating throughout the previous year. Food appeared to stick in the subxiphoid area after almost every meal and at times while she was eating. She experienced trouble with both liquids and solids. Regurgitation often occurred within 10 to 15 minutes after eating, and was productive of food chunks that tasted much as they did upon swallowing. There was no nausea, abdominal distress, or heartburn. She ate six to seven times a day in order to maintain her weight, but had lost 20 pounds in spite of this.

Chest pain was related to meals, but also occurred at other times without any relation to exertion or position. The pain was moderately severe in intensity, was localized to the substernal area, and did not radiate. Episodes usually lasted about five minutes and occurred several times daily.

Eight years prior to admission, she had consulted a physician after having experienced a single episode of pain in her chest. An electrocardiogram was normal, and an upper gastrointestinal series showed a small herniation of her stomach into her chest.

She had been treated for nervousness occasionally during the past 10 years, and had been given sedatives for this difficulty and experienced some relief. For the past 3 years she had noted that her hands and fingers became white and painful when exposed to the cold. The patient was born in Brazil and had moved to the United States with her family at age 10. Divorce had followed a brief marriage, and she had never been pregnant.

On examination, she was a well-developed middle-aged woman showing evidence of moderate loss of weight, but no apparent distress. Her skin was not remarkable. Positive physical findings were limited to the abdomen where there was a slight tenderness to pressure in the epigastrium. The edge of the liver descended one finger breadth below the right costal margin on deep inspiration and was firm, sharp, and nontender. The area of percussion dullness over the liver was 11 cm wide. The spleen was not palpable.

Her hematocrit was 36 percent, hemoglobin 12.4 g per dl, and her white blood count 8,700. Urinalysis and liver function tests were normal. Esophagrams and chest X rays were taken. Two representative films are shown in Figure 3–14. Esophagoscopy showed a considerable amount of detritus in the esophagus but was otherwise normal. The cardioesophageal junction was identified 40 cm from the incisors. No signs of esophagitis or stricture were demonstrated.

1. What are the possible causes of this patient's dysphagia? How are these supported or contradicted by her history, laboratory findings, and esophagoscopy?
2. Indicate the most likely cause of her dysphagia and suggest any other procedures which could be usefully employed to confirm this. How would these aid in making the diagnosis?
3. Propose a therapeutic regimen and indicate the reason for each component of the program.

CLINICAL CONFERENCE 2

Part 1

A married white man was seen for the first time at the age of 54 years. Epigastric pain which had troubled him for several years was his major difficulty, although he also complained of dysphagia and belching. The dysphagia was a feeling of fullness below the lower part of his sternum, usually following the ingestion of solid foods. It was often accompanied by the regurgitation of food without vomiting. Food seemed to stick in his lower chest at times. The patient also said that he had once vomited red blood many months before. There was no history of weight loss, and the dysphagia was neither persistent nor progressive. Physical examination and routine laboratory work, including blood counts, were normal. Films from an upper gastrointestinal series are shown in Figure 3–15.

The patient was placed on a bland diet plus antacids. In spite of this treatment, he continued to complain of epigastric distress associated with a burning pain which radiated upward. Sour acrid fluid would occasionally appear in the back of his throat. Dysphagia continued to be mild and intermittent, and no weight loss or bleeding appeared. Four months after the first

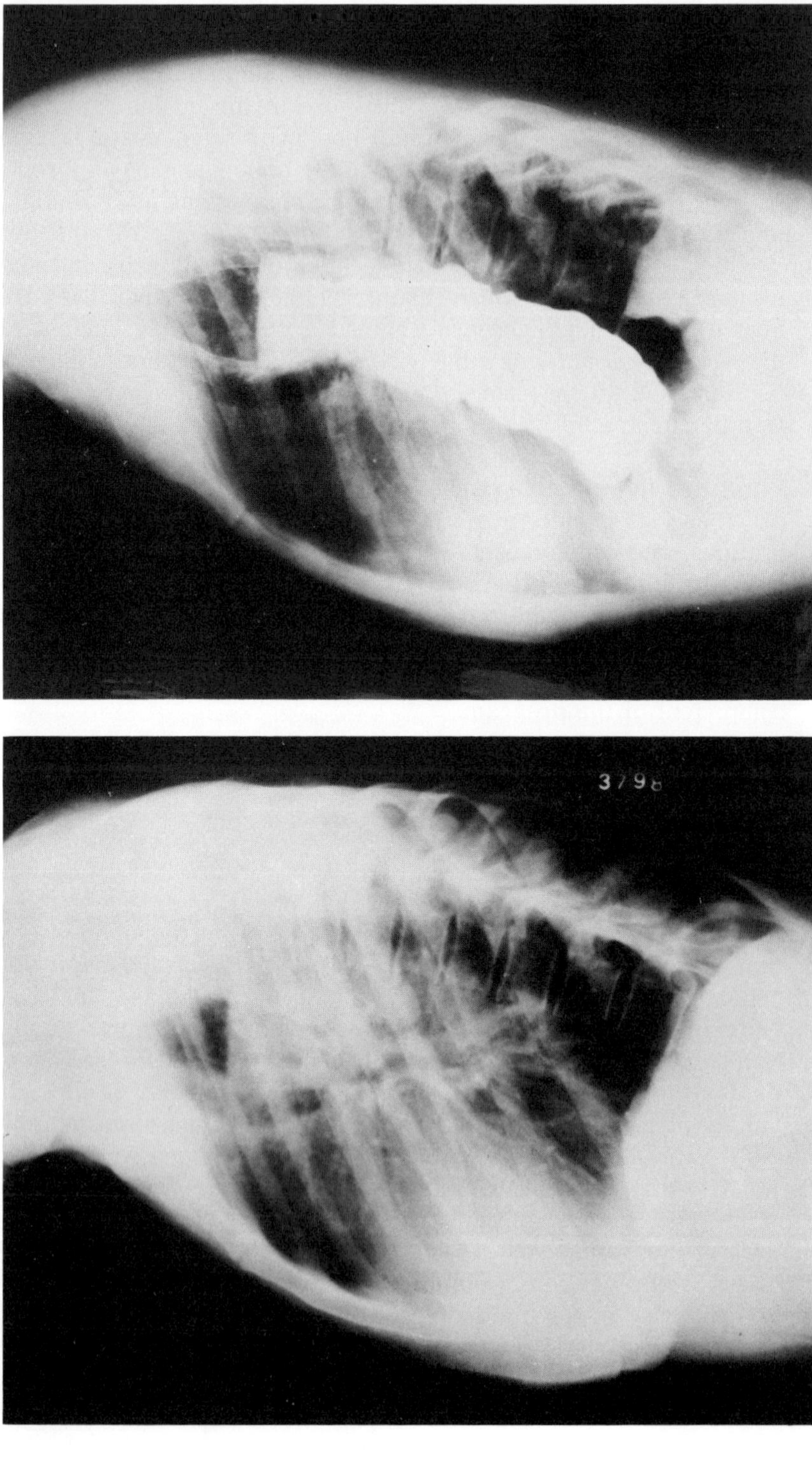

Figure 3-14. Plain lateral chest film (*left*) and film of the barium-filled esophagus (*right*), Clinical Conference 1.

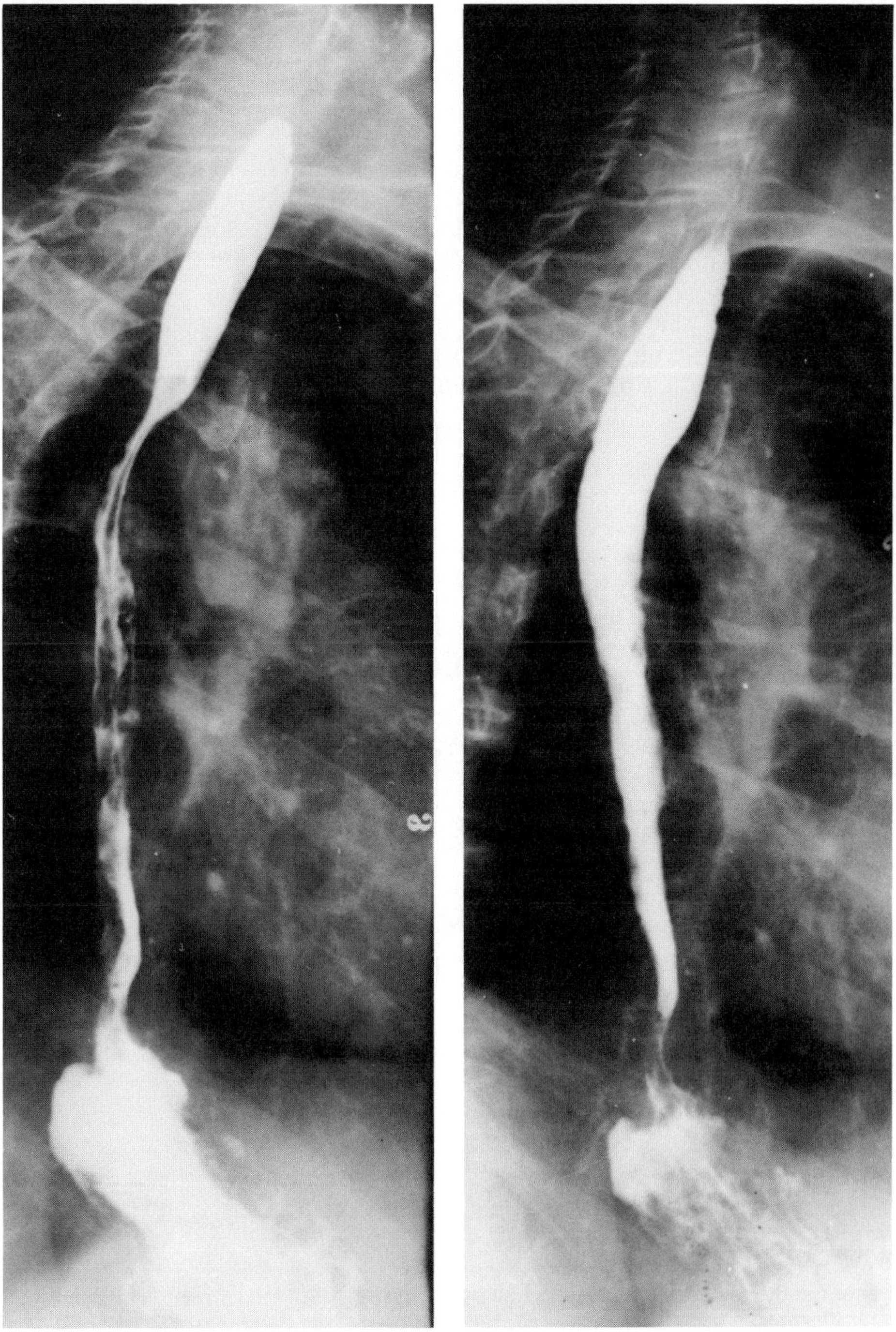

Figure 3–15. Oblique esophagrams, Clinical Conference 2, Part 1. Courtesy of Dr. Bertram Fleshler.

visit, an esophageal acid perfusion (Bernstein) study was performed and was considered to be unequivocally positive. Esophagoscopy showed gastric rugae at a distance of 36 cm from the incisors. The gastric tissue was slightly friable, and the mucosa of the distal esophagus was extremely friable and bled from the slightest pressure or from mere scraping by the esophagoscope. No stricture or tumor was seen, but gastroesophageal reflux was present. A biopsy was performed (Figure 3–16).

The patient was not seen again for 10 months, after which he again complained of substernal sticking and burning. He stated that a "stomach operation" had been performed elsewhere eight months before. He felt better for some time after surgery but was now experiencing his former symptoms again. Examination was normal, except for the presence of a recent left paramedian upper abdominal scar. Another esophagoscopy was

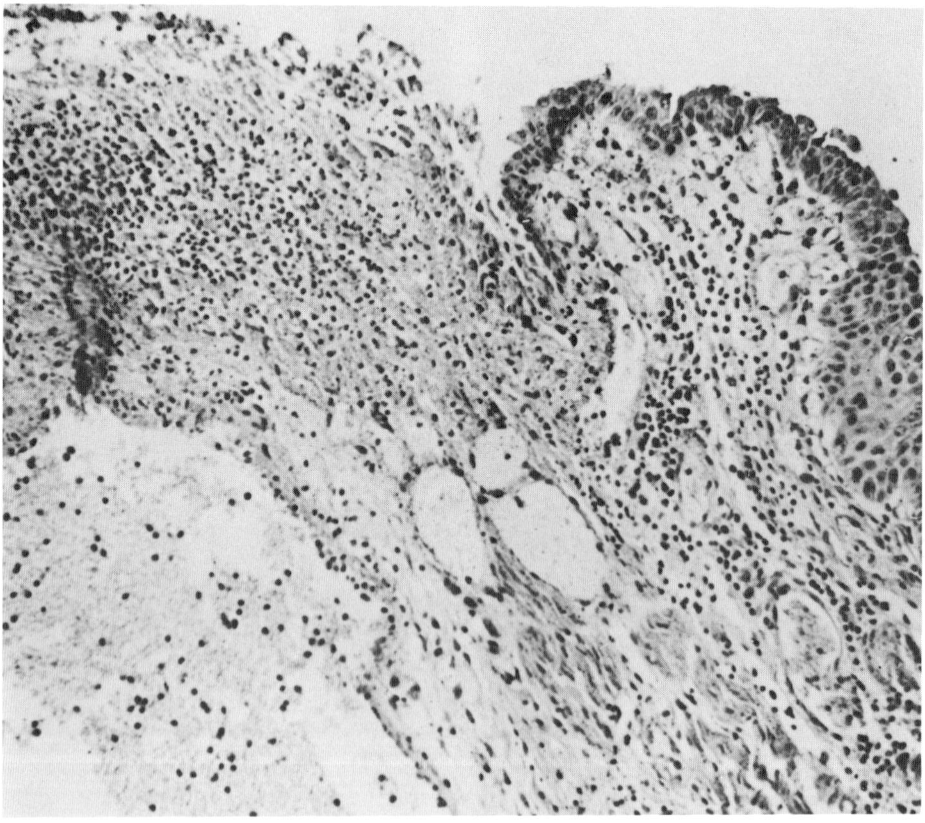

Figure 3–16. Esophageal biopsy, Clinical Conference 2, Part 1. Courtesy of Dr. Bertram Fleshler.

performed, and the mucosa at the cardioesphageal junction was red, edematous, and friable. Two superficial erosions were seen in the area of friability. The lesion was confined to the distal few centimeters. Normal mucosa was seen at 35 cm and above.

1. What are the diagnostic possibilities in this patient? State which diagnoses are most likely. Give both positive and negative evidence for these possibilities.
2. Discuss the medical management indicated.
3. What indications were there for surgery in this patient, and what kinds of surgery might have been considered?

Part 2

The patient reappeared nearly four years after his last examination, complaining of recurrent dysphagia for the previous 10 months. Symptoms of burning epigastric pain and dysphagia had occurred intermittently in the intervening period, but about 10 months later they became more persistent. Initially he had difficulty with solid foods, which caused a sticking sensation in the lower retrosternal area. Eventually he was able to eat soft foods only with some difficulty, although liquids passed fairly well. His appetite had remained reasonably good through this period, but a weight loss of 18 pounds was recorded.

Physical examination was within normal limits. The hematocrit was 33 percent and the hemoglobin 8 g per dl. The white count and other laboratory studies were within normal limits. Two esophagrams are shown in Figure 3–17. At esophagoscopy, a constricting lesion was encountered at about 30 cm from the incisors. Submucosal nodularity was seen at the site of the narrowing and immediately proximal to it. The mucosa appeared normal. The major site of narrowing seemed to be in the right lateral wall. Two biopsies were obtained. Figure 3–18 was taken at 32 cm and Figure 3–19 at 24 cm from the incisors. Esophageal washings for cytology on three occasions showed no tumor cells.

1. What are the differential diagnostic possibilities? Give supporting data for the diagnostic possibilities listed and indicate which diagnosis you favor.
2. In light of your diagnosis, what management would you recommend?

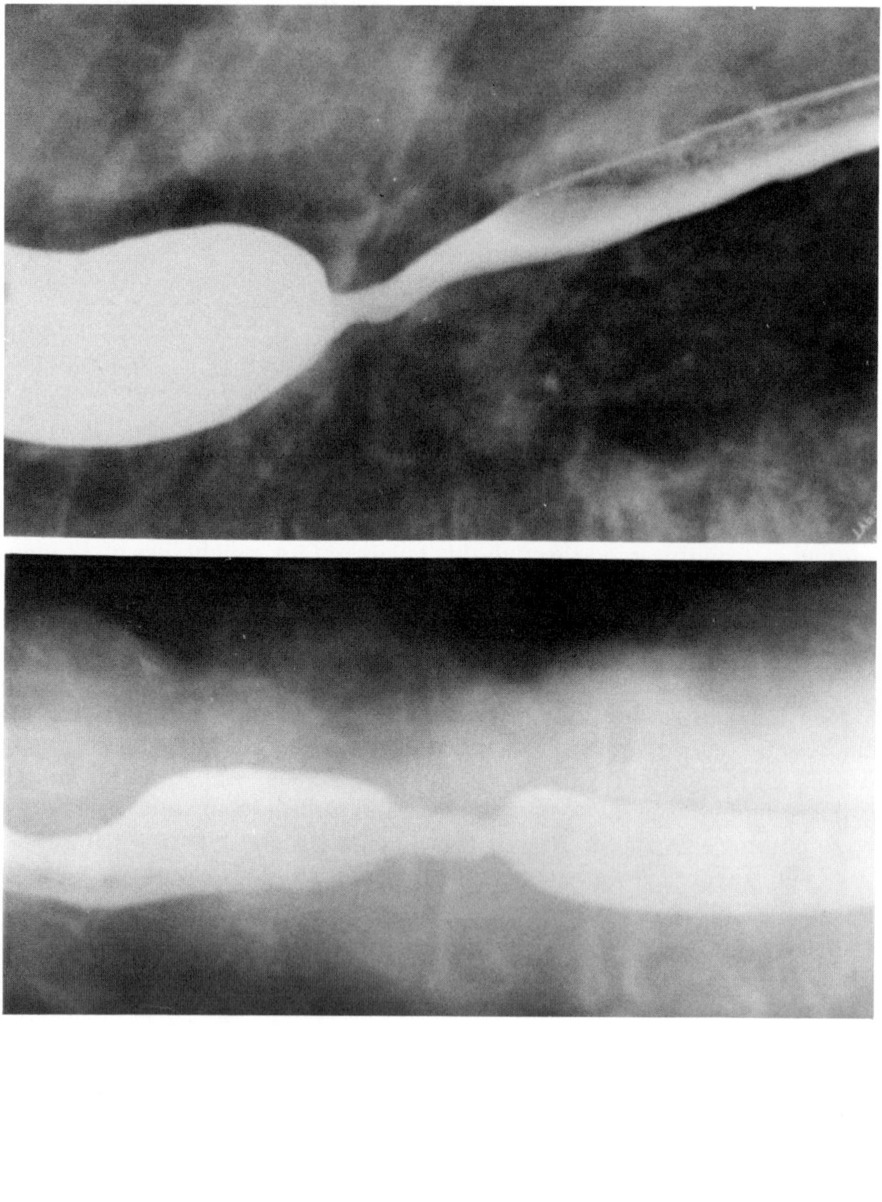

Figure 3-17. Mid esophageal X rays, Clinical Conference 2, Part 2. Courtesy of Dr. Bertram Fleshler.

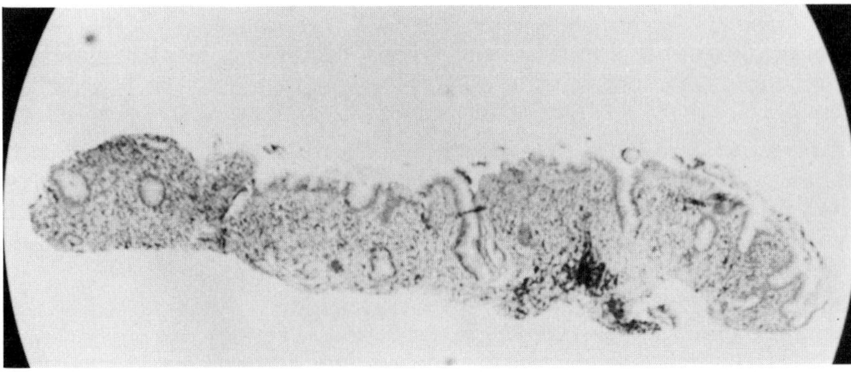

Figure 3–18. Biopsy of esophagus at 32 cm from incisors, Clinical Conference 2, Part 2. Original magnification x25.

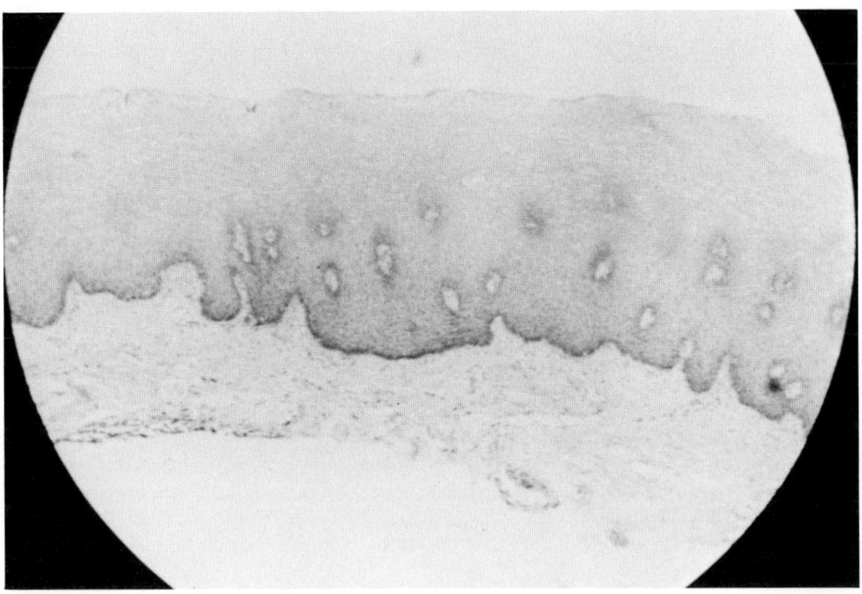

Figure 3–19. Biopsy of esophagus at 24 cm from incisors, Clinical Conference 2, Part 2. Original magnification x25.

CHAPTER 4

Functional Characteristics of the Stomach

Voltaire has written, "Thought depends absolutely on the stomach, but in spite of that, those who have the best stomachs are not the best thinkers." In actuality, a number of our best thinkers have expended much effort on furthering our understanding of gastric function. The ignorance existing a century and a half ago is summarized by a statement attributed to William Hunter, "Some physiologists will have it, that the stomach is a mill, others, that it is a fermenting vat, others, again, that it is a stew-pan; but, in my view of the matter, it is neither a mill, a fermenting vat, nor a stew-pan; but a stomach, gentlemen, a stomach."* Commencing with the observations of Beaumont who proved that the stomach secreted hydrochloric acid, that it had its own motility characteristics and was able to digest proteins, and that both motility and secretion varied with the emotional state of his subject, and of Pavlov, who showed the effect of vagal influences on gastric function, much has been learned. And, while gaps still exist in our knowledge of the stomach, a remarkably complete picture of its function and diseases is available to us today.

It is a much more complex organ than the esophagus, and elaborates a number of exocrine and endocrine substances that figure in digestion, immunosurveillance, and intestinal absorption. In recent years, histology has been fairly closely related to function and has provided a rather clear basis for the understanding of pathophysiology in numerous diseases involving the stomach. Among the important substances elaborated in different parts of the stomach, some are produced exclusively, or nearly exclusively, there, while the remainder are formed in other organs as well. Those formed exclusively or preponderantly in the stomach are hydrochloric acid, intrinsic factor, pepsinogens and gastrin; those formed elsewhere as well include mucus, immunoglobulin A (IgA), histamine, 5-hydroxytryptamine (serotonin, 5-HT) and prostaglandins. Each has a part to play in health maintenance, disease pathophysiology, or both.

---

*Quoted by William Osler. In William Beaumont. A pioneer American physiologist. New York: Dover Publications. Reprinted, 1959.

FUNCTIONAL HISTOLOGY AND PHYSIOLOGY

The human stomach may be divided into five geographic areas (Figure 4–1): the *cardia,* a small segment several centimeters in width that surrounds the esophagogastric junction; the *fundus,* the uppermost portion of the stomach, distal to the cardia but superior to it anatomically; the *body,* which extends distally from the fundus to the level at which the gastric lumen assumes a transverse direction; the *antrum,* which is the peristaltic portion of the stomach distal to the body; and the *pylorus,* the sphincteric portion just proximal to the duodenum. These areas are not sharply demarcated anatomically, and are different from the histologically distinct areas, but they are useful in the localization of gastric lesions by radiography or endoscopy, and at surgery.

Microscopy reveals only three histologically distinctive portions of the stomach, the cardia, the oxyntic or acid-pepsin-secreting area (Figure 4–2), and the antral or pyloric gland area (Figure 4–3), from which gastrin is secreted. Mucosa of the cardia consists of a columnar epithelium, folded into convoluted glands which secrete mucus. This area includes no more than 5 percent of the entire mucosal surface of the stomach.

The Oxyntic Gland Area

This region occupies up to 80 percent of the gastric mucosa, more on the anterior and posterior wall and greater curve than on the lesser curve. Also covered by columnar epithelium, the thick oxyntic mucosa dips downward into multiple, deep, rather tightly packed pits, called *foveolae* (Figure

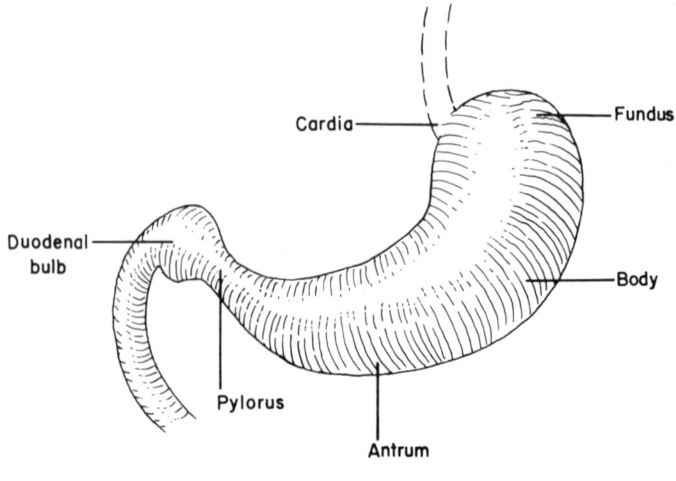

Figure 4–1. Schematic outline of geographic regions of the stomach.

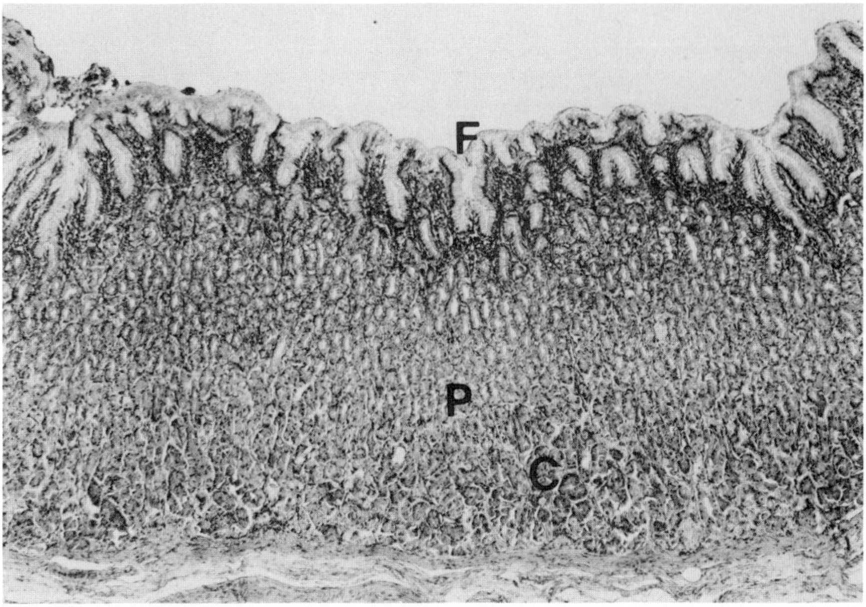

Figure 4-2. Fundic mucosa of the stomach (also called oxyntic or acid-pepsin-secreting mucosa) consists of foveolar cells (F), parietal cells (P) with granular eosinophilic cytoplasm, and chief cells (C) with basophilic zymogen granules. Original magnification x50.

4-4). Each foveola traverses about one-quarter of the width of the oxyntic mucosa, and serves as the outlet for the secretions of approximately four straight, elongated, tubular glands. The junctional area between the deeper gastric glands and the more superficial foveola is called the *mucous neck area*, and is the site where epithelial mitosis and cell differentiation occurs. Cells which migrate upward from the neck area into the foveola become slightly basophilic, mucous-secreting and probably prostaglandin-secreting cells. This migration is rapid, and complete cellular turnover in the foveola occurs every 5 to 7 days. Those cells which migrate downward into the tubular glands become oxyntic or parietal cells, chief cells, and argentaffin (Kultschitsky) cells. Oxyntic cells secrete both hydrochloric acid and intrinsic factor, are slightly eosinophilic, and predominate in the upper portions of the glands. Chief cells secrete at least two varieties of pepsinogen, contain a granular, basophilic cytoplasm, and predominate in the lower portion of the glands. Argentaffin cells produce serotonin and probably histamine, contain silver-staining cytoplasmic granules, and are much less numerous than either chief or oxyntic cells. The half-life of oxyntic cells is around 23 days, and the half-life of chief cells is somewhat longer. None of these cells undergoes mitosis, since replication occurs only in the mucous neck area. Oxyntic cells account for around 32 percent of the volume of the mucosa of the body

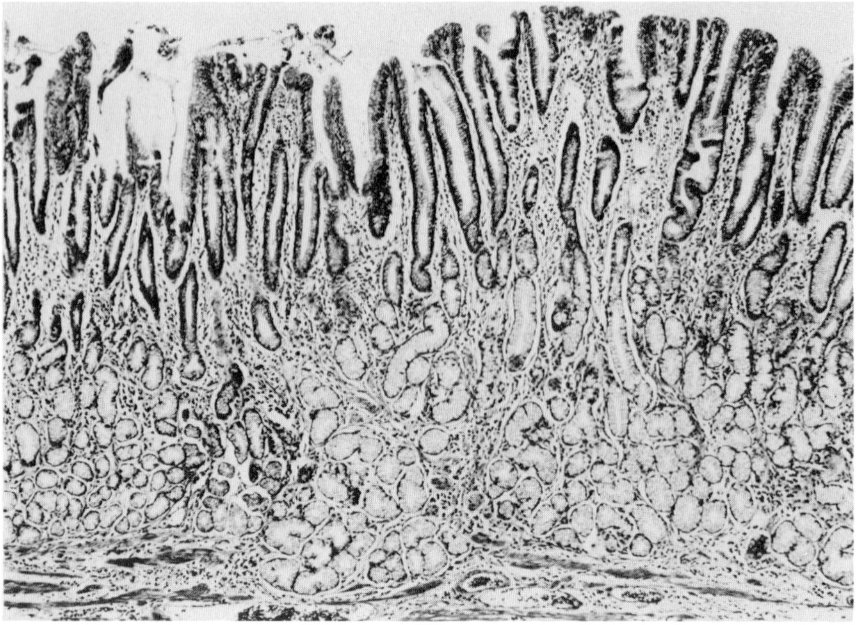

Figure 4–3. Antral mucosa consists of foveolar cells and mucous glands with clear cytoplasm. Gastrin (G) cells are also present in this area of the mucosa but are not identifiable by H and E staining. Original magnification x55.

of the stomach, chief cells, 26 percent; surface mucous cells, 17 percent; and mucous neck cells, 6 percent.

Electron microscopy shows that mucous cells characteristically contain numerous stippled cytoplasmic (? pepsinogen) granules, while the resting chief cell is typified by large cytoplasmic zymogen granules, presumably pepsinogen, each surrounded by a thin membrane. Following stimulation with histamine or gastrin, pepsinogen secretion occurs and the number of cytoplasmic granules diminishes. Parietal cells in the resting state are packed with mitochondria, each containing numerous cristae; they also contain a network of cytoplasmic tubules and canaliculi containing microvillae (figure 4–5). After stimulation with histamine, mitochondrial cristae decrease, and the villous lined canaliculi expand, with a decrease in the number of tubulovesicles. This indicates that the tubules are an essential portion of the secretory network in the parietal cell and can expand remarkably in response to a stimulus. The large number of mitochondria indicates the availability of an abundance of adenosine triphosphate (ATP) for the energy-dependent processes of hydrogen ion removal from tissue fluids, and secretion of hydrochloric acid in 180 mM concentrations.

The Production of Hydrochloric Acid. The normal oxyntic mucosa at rest secretes from 0 to 5 mEq HCl per hour; when maximally stimulated, this

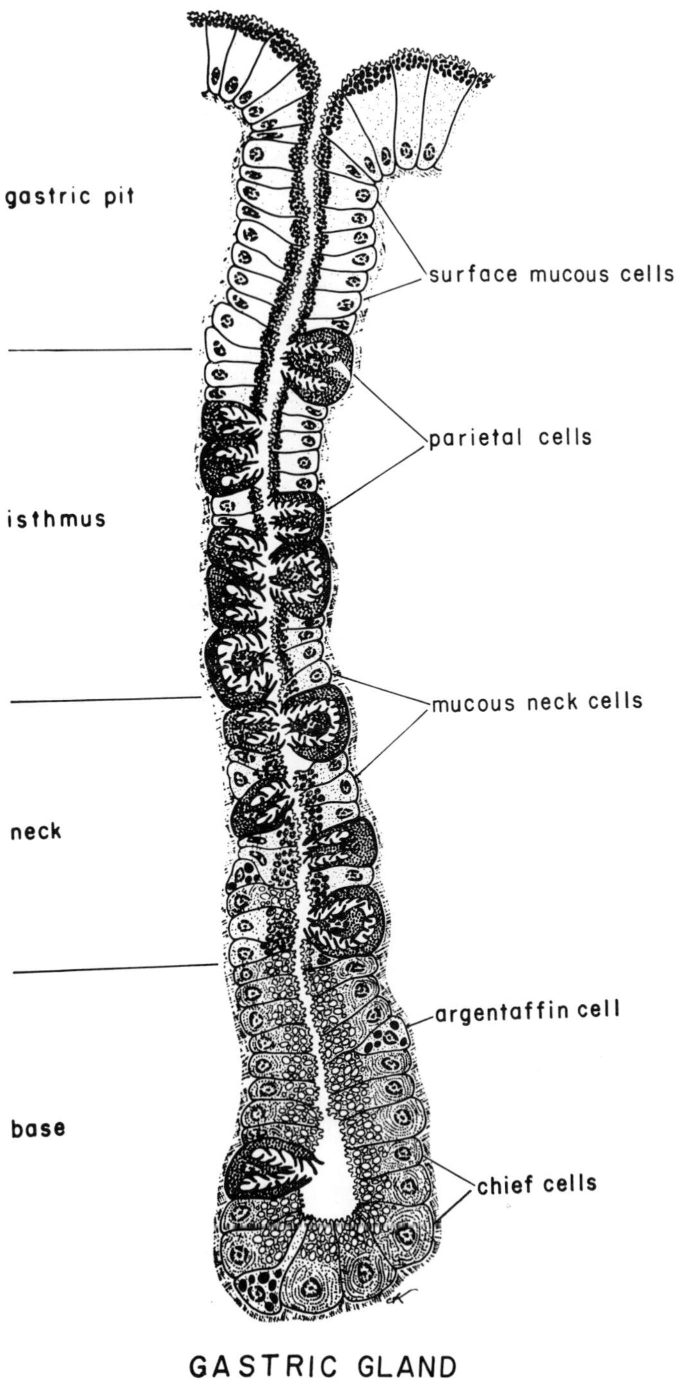

Figure 4-4. Diagram of gastric foveola, showing location of different cell types. From Ito S, Winchester RJ. J Cell Biol 16:541, 1963. Reprinted by permission.

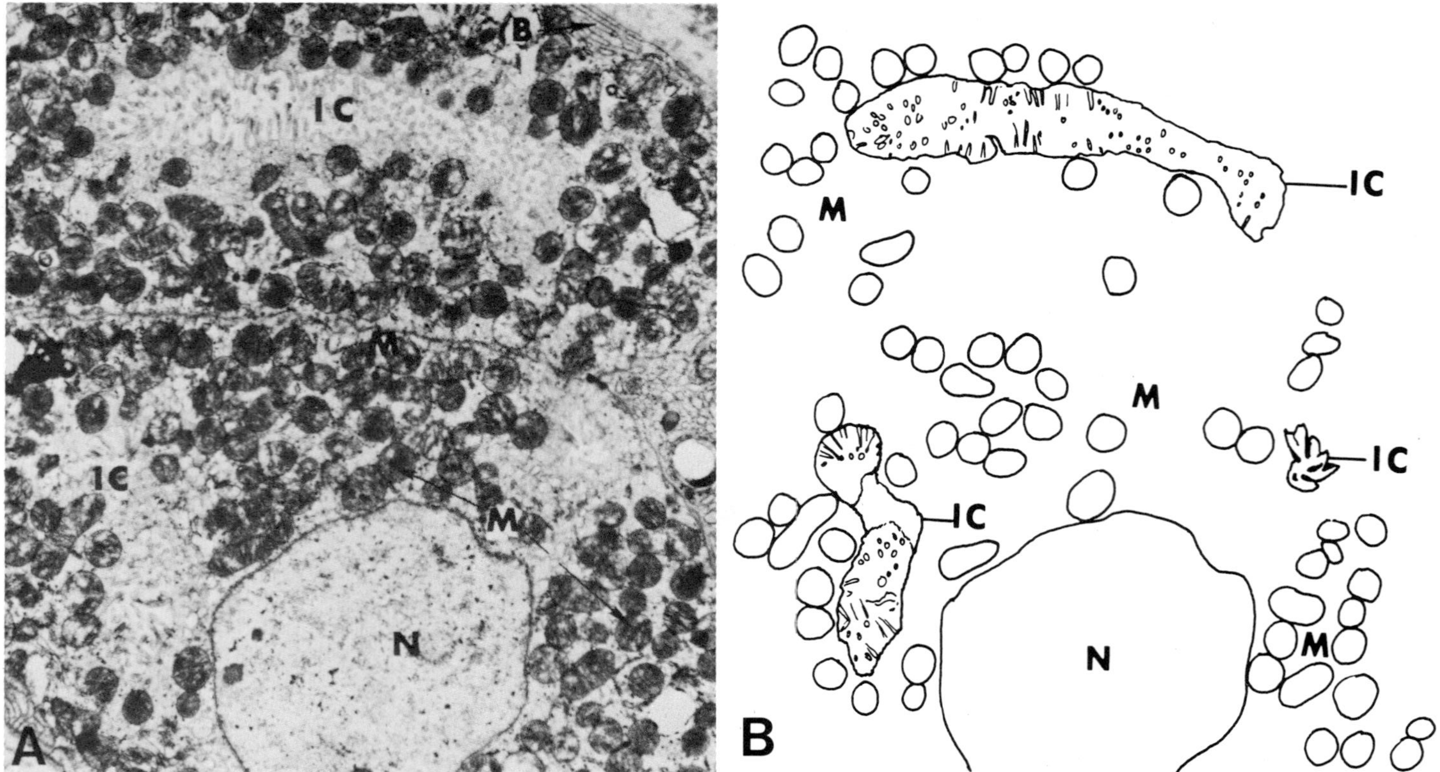

Figure 4–5. *A*, electron photomicrograph of an oxyntic cell. Between numerous oval mitochondria (M), parts of the intracellular canaliculus (IC), lined by numerous microvilli, may be seen. Basal infoldings (B) of the plasma membranes are located at the edge of the cell. The nucleus (N) appears in the lower portion of the picture. Original magnification x9000. From McGuigan JE. Anatomy. In: Sleisinger MH, Fordtran JS. *Gastrointestinal Disease.* Philadelphia: WB Saunders, 1973. Reprinted by permission. *B*, Diagram of *A*, highlighting the abundant mitochondria of the resting oxyntic cell and the extensive network of intracellular canaliculi which dilate markedly while acid is being secreted.

secretion normally peaks at 25 to 30 mEq per hour. At rest, gastric secretions contain about 100 mEq of Cl^-, 90 mEq of Na^+, 6-7 mEq of K^+ and 3–4 mEq of H^+ per liter. When maximally stimulated, hydrogen ion secretion increases greatly, chloride increases moderately, potassium increases slightly, and sodium falls precipitously, concentrations being about as follows: Cl^-, 160 mEq; Na^+, 3-4 mEq;; K^+, 16–17 mEq; and H^+, 140 mEq, per liter.

Stimulation of the oxyntic cell produces a ready supply of energy by the breakdown of high energy phosphate bonds, as evidenced by the conversion of ATP to AMP by ATPase. This energy is used by the cell to form carbonic acid intracellularly from H_2O and CO_2 in tissue fluids, in company with the enzyme, carbonic anhydrase. Hydrogen and chloride are pumped into the gastric gland lumen, while HCO_3^- leaves the cell by way of venous channels, causing a rise in pH (alkaline tide) in this system. Three different ATPases have been identified in the oxyntic cell, and are thought to be involved in both the secretion of bicarbonate into the intracellular fluid and the secretion of potassium into the glandular lumen.

Back-diffusion and the Mucosal Barrier. Gastric mucosa transports water very poorly in either direction, regardless of the tonicity of gastric contents. It does, however, normally allow small amounts of acid to diffuse back into the mucosa from the lumen (Ivey 1971). The barrier to more extensive back-diffusion and resultant damage or destruction of gastric mucosa by the concentrated acid with which it is in contact, might possibly be maintained by tissue prostaglandins (E, A, $F_{2\alpha}$), 20-carbon oxygenated fatty acids formed in mucosal cells from arachidonic acid. As will be mentioned later, prostaglandins E and A inhibit the formation of acid by oxyntic cells, while $F_{2\alpha}$ does not. However, all three forms appear to have a cytoprotective function as well, which is exhibited at dosage levels much lower than those which inhibit acid secretion. Prostaglandins protect against gastric ulcers ordinarily produced by absolute ethanol and boiling water, and there is evidence that they are produced endogenously in response to dilute irritants. The mechanism of this cytoprotection is not clear, but it is obviously very important in the intact animal, since previous exposure to prostaglandin inhibitors increases the possibility of mucosal damage very greatly.

The defense against the massive backflow of acid and consequent mucosal destruction has been called the mucosal barrier, owing to former thinking that gastric mucus may itself be somewhat protective against acidic damage. That this may be at least partially true is illustrated by the fact that continuous removal of mucus by a cotton pledget from exposed gastric mucosa in humans and animals does result in visible damage within 15 to 30 minutes. Mucus itself is secreted throughout the stomach and is a complex mixture of tenacious glycoproteins, blood group substances, and even small amounts of serum albumin.

The Concept of Parietal or Oxyntic Cell Mass (OCM). There is considerable variation from person to person in the amount of gastric mucosal area occupied by oxyntic glandular tissue. In some subjects, oxyntic tissue occupies nearly the entire mucosa, whereas in others antral tissue might encompass as much as half of the greater curve area, and nearly all of the lesser curve. These observations form the basis for the concept of OCM and help to explain why there is such variability in the range of hydrochloric acid produced in normal subjects by a maximal stimulus with histamine or gastrin (maximal acid output, MAO). In healthy human subjects, MAO ranges from 5 to 45 mEq per hour (mean 20–25 mEq). So-called maximal doses of histamine are 40 μg/kg per hour intravenously or a single dose subcutaneously; of betazole (a histamine analog causing fewer side effects), 1.5 mg/kg subcutaneously; of pentagastrin (the synthetic C-terminal pentapeptide of gastrin) 6 μg/kg subcutaneously or intramuscularly. A clear positive correlation has been made between OCM and MAO by doing careful oxyntic cell counts on resected specimens of stomach and comparing these to MAOs previously obtained.

OCM is affected by internal changes in the body. Thus, not only has it been found that patients with gastrin-producing tumors (Zollinger-Ellison syndrome) have a markedly increased oxyntic cell mass and that patients who have undergone antral resection, which greatly reduces gastrin-producing tissue, develop a reduction in OCM, but trophic effects of gastrin have been demonstrated in a variety of in vitro and in vivo research projects. Pentagastrin increases cell numbers in tissue cultures of gastric mucosal cells, increases the labeling of messenger RNA, and hastens the incorporation of labeled thymidine into DNA. This trophic effect of gastrin is not confined to oxyntic cells but appears to affect chief cells and small intestinal mucosa as well. The effect does not see to be merely the result of acid stimulation alone, since an equally potent acid secretory agent, like histamine, does not show the same trophism. However, some patients with tumors of histamine-secreting cells (mastocytomas) have been shown to have increased populations of oxyntic cells, and a similar observation has been made in dogs given regular doses of histamine in beeswax for extended periods. All of these observations support the conclusion that OCM is a dynamic feature of the oxyntic mucosa and is capable of gradual alteration from time to time as stimuli change.

Production of Intrinsic Factor. When vitamin B_{12} is ingested, it binds to salivary proteins which form a complex resistant to gastric acidity. These salivary proteins are called r binders, because they show rapid electrophoretic migration. The complex is unbound in the duodenum, largely due to the action of pancreatic trypsin, and the released free B_{12} is quickly rebound to a mucoprotein, intrinsic factor, formed in oxyntic cells. The B_{12}–intrinsic factor complex remains intact until the lower portion of the ileum is reached. At that level, the complex binds to mucosal receptors, and the vitamin B_{12} is released from the intrinsic factor and absorbed. In some cases of pancreatic insufficiency, where the r factor–B_{12} complex remains intact, B_{12} is unable to complex with intrinsic factor and is not absorbed in the ileum, leading to a deficiency state. The secretion of intrinsic factor parallels the secretion of hydrochloric acid, and patients without oxyntic cells develop pernicious anemia, which is the result of advanced B_{12} deficiency. The name, intrinsic factor, was given to this substance long before its composition was known. In the second decade of this century, Minot and coworkers recognized that pernicious anemia could be treated by injections, but not by the oral ingestion, of crude liver extracts. They assumed that some factor, intrinsic to the process of absorption, was lacking, and discovered eventually that pernicious anemia patients would improve in response to oral crude liver extracts, if these were mixed with gastric juice from healthy subjects.

Production and Actions of Pepsinogens. The zymogen granules of chief cells contain a homogenous protein whose molecular weight is about 42,000. From these, at least two families and numerous subvarieties of polypeptide proteases, pepsinogen I and II, are elaborated. Both of these pepsinogens become active enzymes in the presence of acid through the hydrolytic loss of several peptide radicals; they are denatured at pH levels above 7. The conversion of pepsinogen to pepsin below pH 5.5 becomes autocatalytic after it is first initiated. Group I pepsinogens are distinguished from those of group II by their more rapid electrophoretic mobility, and by the fact that they are secreted in oxyntic tissue only. They also appear to have different pH optima. Pepsinogen II is produced in mucous cells of the oxyntic gland area and in antral glands, as well as in chief cells. At pH levels above 3.5, pepsin has weak enzymatic activity, but at levels below this it splits primary peptide linkages, and thus becomes a strong, though not essential, proteolytic enzyme.

Argentaffin and Mast Cells. Serotonin and histamine are produced by the argentaffin cells which reside in the oxyntic epithelium, while histamine and heparin are produced by mast cells in the lamina propria of the oxyntic and antral areas. Tissue histamine and its methyl derivatives are very strong stimulants of the oxyntic cells and appear also to be important mediators of the stimulatory effects of gastrin and acetylcholine on this tissue. Whether histamine itself is the final common mediator of all stimuli to acid secretion, or whether it merely facilitates their effects, is not clear. At any account, if the so-called histamine (H_2) receptors on oxyntic cells are blocked competitively by a nonstimulatory analog of histamine (metiamide, cimetidine), the effects of gastrin, acetylcholine, and histamine itself are diminished tremendously. The importance of heparin and serotinin in normal mucosal metabolism is not clear.

The Antral or Pyloric Gland Area

This portion of the gastric mucosa is thinner than oxyntic mucosa, foveolae are deeper, and the tubular glands are coiled rather than straight. The glands themselves are composed of only a single type of cell, which looks like a mucous cell and appears to secrete group II pepsinogens and mucus. Gastrin-producing G cells are located in the lamina propria of the antrum, adjacent to the tubular glands. They have been found in many species, including humans, have large cytoplasmic granules, predominate in the lower two-thirds of the antrum and react positively when exposed to fluorescent antigastrin antibodies. They are similar morphologically and in staining characteristics to nonbeta (delta) cells in the islets of the pancreas, and to the tumor cells of patients with the Zollinger-Ellison syndrome. The predominant form of gastrin produced in the antrum of the stomach is the 17-peptide variety, although some big gastrin (G 34) is also produced (Walsh and Grossman 1975).

THE REGULATION OF GASTRIC SECRETION

Gastric secretion of acid and pepsin is regulated by complex interactions, not all well understood, between vagus nerves, gastrin, and other peptide hormones. Traditionally, the entire process of gastric secretion has been divided in an arbitrary fashion into three phases: cephalic, gastric, and intestinal. This classification was based on early observations of a preprandial rise in gastric acidity associated with contemplation of a meal, a secondary rise after food actually entered the stomach, and a tertiary rise sometime after a meal began to enter the small intestine. That these phases are interrelated and, to a certain extent, mediated by similar stimuli became apparent as further investigations were undertaken.

The Cephalic Phase

Stimulation of either vagus nerve, the left more than the right, provokes a brisk outpouring of acid, pepsin, and mucus from the stomach. This fact was first demonstrated by Pavlov in dogs with pouches of the body of the stomach which had been surgically isolated from the remainder of the stomach without disturbing their nerve supply, and has been documented repeatedly since. Heidenhain devised a pouch similar to that of Pavlov, except that the vagus nerve supply was interrupted. Stimulation of the vagus after this procedure evoked no secretory response in the stomach. The vagal response in Pavlov preparations is reduced, but not abolished, by previous removal of the antrum of the stomach. This suggests that the vagus operates partially by direct stimulation of the oxyntic cells, and partially by the release of a hormone, presumably gastrin.

In most animals and in humans, the vagal mechanism is stimulated by hunger, anger, pleasant food odors, hypoglycemia, and conditioning. It is inhibited by a full stomach, fear, anticholinergic agents, elevations of blood glucose levels, and of course by vagotomy. Interruption of the vagi also reduces the secretory response of the stomach to histamine and to gastrin.

Thus, the cephalic phase of gastric secretion is mediated entirely by the vagus nerves and disappears when they are transected. By acidifying the antrum of the stomach, the cephalic phase reduces the release of gastrin in the next phase and probably accounts for the fact that the rise of gastric acidity after a meal is gradual rather than sudden.

The Gastric Phase

The secretion of acid during the cephalic phase also facilitates the conversion of the simultaneously released pepsinogens to active proteolytic enzymes. Ingestion of protein, and its splitting into polypeptides by pepsin, causes the elaboration of more acid and pepsin in the stomach through the release of antral gastrin. Fat and carbohydrate meals do not lead to a release of antral gastrin. While distention of the antrum also causes gastrin release in dogs, it does not seem to do so in humans. However, vagal afferent fibers in the antrum are stimulated by distention and account for a vagal contribution to the secretion of acid and pepsin during the gastric phase (vagovagal reflex). Even after vagotomy, there is a small rise of gastric acidity with antral distention, apparently due to local cholinergic reflexes in the stomach wall. Greater amounts of acid and pepsin are produced during the gastric phase of secretion than during the cephalic and intestinal phases. Blood levels of gastrin also rise during this phase.

The Intestinal Phase

Some investigators believe that a distinct hormone, entero-oxyntin, is responsible for the rise in gastric acid secretion after food has entered the intestine. That this substance is not intestinal gastrin seems to be confirmed by the fact that perfusion of the upper intestine with liver extracts in dogs and humans, causes gastric secretion to rise without a corresponding rise in serum gastrin levels (Kauffman and Grossman 1979). Thus, the existence of entero-oxyntin is inferential; it has not been isolated or characterized as yet. It appears to be a weak stimulant of acid secretion when given alone, but it potentiates the stimulatory effects of gastrin, histamine, and bethanechol in animals. It appears to be much more effective in animals whose gastric antra are intact. The effect of this agent is interrupted by cholinergic blockade, but not by vagotomy, indicating its probable mediation through cholingic reflex arcs. The intestinal phase of gastric secretion is markedly enhanced in animals whose portal blood is shunted around the liver, indicating that entero-oxyntin is probably inactivated by the liver in the normal state.

Konturek (1980) has been unable to demonstrate intestinal phase secretion in animals unaccompanied by a rise in serum gastrin as well, the gastrin being released presumably from the duodenum. Since these observations give to gastrin a primary role in intestinal phase secretion, the physiologic role of entero-oxyntin is still in doubt.

There are a number of factors which appear to keep the intestinal phase of gastric secretion in check. Among these are the intestinal hormones, cholecystokinin (CCK) and secretin, and the putative hormone, bulbogastrone. Furthermore, a normal bile-acid pool, normal digestion, and absorption of ingested fats in the intestine, and an intact upper small intestine seem to keep gastric secretion under some degree of control (Konturek 1977).

When administered alone in fairly large doses, CCK is a mild stimulant of acid secretion. However, both CCK and secretin in physiologic doses are capable of reducing the acid-stimulatory effects of gastrin, but not of histamine. It is believed that CCK displaces gastrin from receptors on the oxyntic cell. Acidification of the duodenal bulb in dogs also reduces gastrin-stimulated responses, due to the action of bulbogastrone, but there is some question about the applicability of these observations to normal human subjects. Another form of enterogastrone appears to be released by the presence of fat in the gut. That this reduces histamine-stimulated acid secretion in Heidenhain animals strongly implies that CCK and secretin are not the responsible agents, since they have been shown to reduce only gastrin-stimulated acidity. There is some evidence that this agent may be either vasoactive intestinal polypeptide or gastric inhibitory polypeptide, because they are elaborated in the small intestine, released by fat, and inhibit both gastrin- and histamine- induced secretion.

Any agency that reduces the bile acid pool, such as interruption of the enterohepatic circulation of bile salts or diverting bile salts from their ileal site of absorption, leads to an increase in acid secretion by the stomach. The mechanism of this effect is not clear, but it does not appear to be related to gastrin excess. Thus, a normal bile acid pool keeps the secretion of acid in check, while a reduced pool leads to increased output. On the other hand, the increase in gastric secretion after massive resection of the small intestine has been shown to be associated with increases in serum gastrin. This may be due either to the removal of factors inhibiting the release of gastrin, or to decreased gastrin removal from the blood.

The Effects of Other Hormones and Prostaglandins

Potential relationships between the secretions of extra-alimentary endocrine glands and gastric secretion have been the subject of innumerable reports. Conclusive data have been difficult to obtain, because responses to similar stimuli seem to be subject to considerable variation in different species, and because different studies have employed different techniques of evaluation and often nugatory controls. The more valid studies referring to this subject have focused on disorders of the adrenal cortex and the parathyroids.

The Adrenal Cortex. The incidence of peptic ulcer in adrenal or pituitary insufficiency, or following adrenalectomy in humans, approaches zero, and the secretion of acid and pepsin in patients with these disorders is very low indeed. The converse of this observation, that hypersecretion and peptic ulcer are prominent features in patients with excesses of adrenocortical hormone, does not appear to be true. In fact, Conn and Blitzer (1976) have reviewed extensively many reports dealing with the relationships of glucocorticoids to peptic ulcer and have concluded that there is no relationship between the two, at least in patients receiving adrenocorticosteroid therapy.

The output of acid is decreased in cats, rats, and dogs following adrenalectomy, or after the administration of metyrapone, an agent which blocks the 11 beta-hydroxylation of corticoids in the adrenal cortex. The secretion of pepsin is reduced in cats, but not in dogs. Normal gastric secretion, but not hypersecretion, is restored in these animals by the administration of glucocorticoids, but not by mineralocorticoids (desoxycorticosterone, aldosterone) or epinephrine. Adrenalectomy reduces the concentration, but not the volume, of acid. The secretory change is not associated with obvious atrophy of the gastric mucosa, nor is it due to destruction of the mucosal barrier, since back-diffusion of hydrochloric acid is not increased.

It may be concluded that glucocorticoids are necessary to facilitate the effects of trophic agents on the oxyntic and possibly the chief cells, but acting alone they are apparently not trophic. They do reduce gastric mucosal mitoses and enhance back-diffusion of acid caused by aspirin and bile salts (Chung et al 1978).

Parathormone. Interest in the relationship between parathormone and gastric secretion was stimulated by the common observation that the incidence of peptic ulcer in patients with hyperparathyroidism is much higher than the expected incidence in the general population, 20 to 25 against 5 to 7 percent. A number of observers have found that increased concentrations of hydrochloric acid and pepsin and increased volumes of gastric secretion appear rapidly when the levels of serum calcium are elevated by administration of calcium salts in healthy subjects to levels seen in patients with hyperparathyroidism. Barreras (1973) recounts that the basal output of acid can be increased more than fourfold by this method, to a level which is nearly 30 percent as high as the peak output. Without calcium, or with saline alone, the basal output is about 6 percent of the peak response. The effect of calcium is blocked by the administration of magnesium, atropine, or the histamine$_2$ blocking agent, cimetidine, and is nil in Heidenhain pouches. The stimulatory effect of calcium is associated with a rise in serum gastrin levels, is mediated by the release of antral gastrin, and is blocked by antrectomy. Thus, hypercalcemia, whether due to hyperparathyroidism or induced artificially, releases gastrin and stimulates the secretion of acid. This response appears to require the mediation of intact cholinergic pathways.

Antidiuretic hormone has been reported to reduce the volume of gastric secretion, but not the concentration of hydrochloric acid. Reductions of up to 70 percent of basal secretory volume have been obtained by its use.

Thyroid Relationships. Miller, Gorman, and Go (1978) have summarized reports on the relationship of thyroidal diseases to gastric secretion. Although most clinical reports suggest that both hyperthyroidism and hypothyroidism are associated with a reversible hypoacidity, the results are far from unanimous. Gastritis is, however, common in both disorders, and may explain an autoimmune fall in OCM.

Prostaglandins. Reference has already been made to the fact that the gastrointestinal tract, including the stomach, produces prostaglandins in large amounts. They are released from the mucosa by vagal stimulation, and animal and human studies alike have shown that numerous natural prostaglandins of the E and A type, when given intravenously, inhibit the secretion of hydrochloric acid after a variety of stimulants. Synthetic methylated prostaglandins can be given orally or applied topically and reduce histamine-, gastrin- and peptone-stimulated acid secretion in man and animals (Robert 1977). They do not affect the secretion of pepsinogen, their action is not reduced by vagotomy, and it does not appear to be related to reductions in blood flow. Thus, the effects of prostaglandins in reducing acid secretion appear to be the result of direct action on the oxyntic cells, possibly through interference with the production of cAMP.

THE ESTIMATION OF GASTRIC ACIDITY IN HUMANS

In patients with certain diseases, such as peptic ulcer, pernicious anemia, and malignant disorders of the stomach, it is often desirable to evaluate the ability of the stomach to secrete acid. One wishes to know not only whether the stomach is capable of secreting any acid at all, but also the amount of acid it is able to produce in response to a maximal stimulus. Maximal stimulatory doses of histamine, betazole, or pentagastrin are those beyond which further increments will not evoke greater production of acid. The maximal doses of these agents have been given earlier in this chapter, and the relationship of MAO to parietal cell mass has been described.

Accurate clinical estimation of acid production requires that a nasogastric tube be passed and fluoroscopically positioned so that the tip of the tube rests in the most dependent portion of the body of the stomach in order to facilitate complete aspirations. The measurement of basal acid output (BAO) is the first goal of a conventional gastric analysis. The amount of gastric secretion obtained in one hour of continuous aspiration, with the patient in a basal (fasted and rested) state, is an adequate estimation of basal capacity. The pH of the gastric contents is obtained and results are expressed as milliequivalents of HCl produced per hour. In our laboratory, the normal BAO ranges from 0 to 6 (mean 2.0) mEq. Levels tend to be higher than normal in patients with duodenal ulcer and other hypersecretory states. They are extremely high, up to 100 mEq per hour, in patients with gastrin-secreting tumors. BAO tends to decrease with aging, conditions associated with atrophy of the gastric mucosa, and after vagotomy.

Measurement of the capacity of the stomach to secrete acid after a maximal stimulant is called MAO if expressed as the total acid produced in a full hour after receiving the stimulus, and the peak acid output (PAO) if expressed as twice the maximal 30-minute output obtained after the stimulus is administered. For all practical purposes, there is little advantage of PAO over MAO determinations, as long as the laboratory is consistent in reporting its results. Similarly, the type of stimulus used makes no difference in the final result, as long as the dosage is maximal. Most laboratories presently are employing the synthetic *N*-terminal pentapeptide of gastrin, pentagastrin, because it is so well tolerated and produces minimal, if any, side effects. If the maximal or peak output is measured carefully, results are surprisingly consistent from time to time in the same patient.

Values for MAO in our laboratory in normal subjects average about 20 mEq per hour, with a large range of from 5 to 45 mEq. With aging alone, MAO falls, often to below 10 mEq. Patients with duodenal ulcer tend to have MAO levels about 30 percent above normal, while patients with ulcers of the body of the stomach have levels 20 to 25 percent below normal. In patients with pernicious anemia, no HCl at all is produced in response to a maximal stimulus, while in patients with the Zollinger-Ellison syndrome the MAO is often only 10 to 15 percent higher than the BAO, because the stomach is being stimulated almost maximally, even in the basal state, by endogenously produced gastrin. Most patients with cancer of the stomach have a lower than normal MAO, due largely to the oxyntic cellular atrophy which is so commonly associated with this disease. But the results of maximal stimulation in patients with cancer of the stomach cannot be used diagnostically because they overlap so greatly with results in normal individuals, especially older subjects, and in patients with benign ulcers of the stomach. Although the determination of BAO and MAO provide a fine measure of the functional capacity of the resting and stimulated stomach, their most important clinical applications are confined to the confirmation of a diagnosis of the Zollinger-Ellison syndrome or of pernicious anemia.

Clinical use is made occasionally of the fact that hypoglycemia causes marked vagal stimulation with resultant increase of gastric acidity. In patients who have had therapeutic vagotomies for the treatment of peptic ulcer, it is occasionally useful to know whether the vagotomy has been performed adequately. In these cases, moderate hypoglycemia is induced by the intravenous injection of 10 units of regular insulin while maintaining gastric suction (Hollander test). Gastric secretion increases in normal subjects within 15–20 minutes after the blood glucose level falls below 50 mg per dl, but does not increase in patients who have had an adequate vagotomy. Any increase in acid output greater than 20 mEq above the basal rate is considered a normal response.

MEASUREMENT OF SERUM GASTRIN LEVELS

Serum gastrin levels should be measured by radioimmunoassay (RIA) in patients suspected of having a hypersecretory hypergastrinemic disorder. This possibility arises whenever the BAO is greater than 10 mEq per hour, and especially when the BAO is 40 percent or more of the MAO. Serum gastrin should also be measured in patients with recurrent peptic ulcer after surgical treatment, in patients whose peptic ulcers do not respond well to conventional medial management, and in those whose ulcers are in unusual locations, beyond the first part of the duodenum.

There are a number of RIA techniques for measuring serum gastrin (Strauss 1978). To prepare the antigen, either synthetic or purified human gastrin is conjugated to bovine serum albumin. Antibodies are produced by injecting this antigen into rabbits or guinea pigs. The resulting antibody is incubated with tracer amounts of ^{125}I-gastrin distributed in diluted serum containing unknown amounts of gastrin. Both labeled and unlabeled gastrin bind competitively to the antibody, forming labeled and unlabeled antigen-antibody complexes. The percentage of label bound to the antibody declines as the amount of gastrin in the unknown solution increases. Final determination of bound to unbound gastrin is made by measuring radioactivity levels and comparing the amount of reduction of binding of the label to standard curves. The bound and unbound fractions are separated by one of several techniques, such as absorption on charcoal, filtration on a Sephadex column, or precipitation of rabbit gamma globulin with antirabbit goat serum. RIA techniques reflect total levels of minigastrin (G 13), gastrin (G 17), big gastrin (G 34), and to variable extents, big, big gastrin, and gastrin peptide fragments, but do not distinguish among them. The different fractions can, however, be distinguished electrophoretically. The clinical significance of this separation is not apparent, although it is known that minigastrin and gastrin are more active secretory stimulants than are big and big, big gastrin.

As might be expected from the fact that there are so many different techniques for measuring serum gastrin levels, there is considerable lack of reproducibility between laboratories. However, it is only the numbers that differ, and if each laboratory is used as its own standard, results are quite consistent and diagnostic. The average normal level of fasting serum gastrin is about 50 pg per ml, and ranges from 20 to 100 pg. The upper limit of normal is 200 pg, and in the presence of gastrinoma (Zollinger-Ellison syndrome), fasting levels may rise to over 7,000 pg (70–80 percent, G 34). Levels are not elevated in fasting patients with duodenal ulcers, but after a protein meal gastrin concentrations normally increase by over 50 percent and remain elevated longer in ulcer patients than in normals. The slow intravenous infusion of calcium ions at the rate of 5 mg per kg per hr increases levels of gastrin at least twofold in patients with gastrinomas, but does not elevate them above 300 pg per ml in patients with duodenal ulcers. The administration of intravenous secretin to patients with gastrinomas causes a doubling of gastrin levels within 15 minutes, a reaction of unexplained cause which is almost specific for this disorder. Other conditions in which hypergastrinemia accompanies hypersecretion of hydrochloric acid include: hyperplasia of antral G cells; antral distention due to pyloric scarring or inflammation; and retention of antral tissue in communication with alkaline duodenal contents after inadequate surgery for peptic ulcer (McGuigan 1974). In these disorders, gastrin levels do not increase in response to secretin (Korman et al 1972).

Gastrin (G 17) levels are elevated strikingly in many patients with gastritis, and especially in patients with pernicious anemia who have circulating antibodies to oxyntic cells and little inflammation in the antrum. Levels of G 34 are elevated in patients with intestinal obstruction, unassociated with hypersecretion of acid. Hypergastrinemia without hyperacidity also often accompanies chronic renal insufficiency.

GASTRIC MOTILITY

As is also true in the case of the esophagus, the control of gastric motility is under neural, myogenic, and hormonal influences. Kelly (1976) has pointed out that muscular activity differs between the upper and lower stomach. Thus, the fundus and upper body (proximal part) of the stomach function as a unit capable of marked receptive relaxation in response to the volume of a meal, and of slow tonic contractions after the meal. The lower body and antrum (distal stomach) are the site of regular peristaltic waves (three per minute) which mix and grind gastric contents, moving chyme distally while retaining large particles and moving them proximally. The pacesetter for this peristaltic activity has been localized to a group of myenteric cells on the upper portion of the greater curve of the stomach.

The ability of the proximal stomach to relax receptively with distention is evidenced by the fact that intragastric pressure at rest is 0 cm water, rises to 10 cm after the introduction of 500 ml of air or water, and remains unchanged if that volume is doubled. Tonic contractions of the proximal stomach appear to be under vagal control, while sympathetic stimulation reduces these contractions. Gastrin and cholecystokinin also inhibit contractions in the proximal stomach and decrease intragastric pressure.

Peristalsis in the distal stomach is preceded by a wave of depolarization, the rate and the intensity of the motility varying somewhat with the volume and qualities of the gastric contents. Waves are stimulated by vagal impulses, inhibited by sympathetic impulses. While gastrin inhibits motility of the proximal stomach, it stimulates peristalsis in the distal organ, as does cholecystokinin. Secretin, bulbogastrone, and glucagon inhibit peristalsis.

Density, pH, and osmolar receptors in the upper portion of the duodenum also regulate peristalsis in the distal stomach and gastric emptying. The greater the acidity and caloric density of gastric contents, and the more that their osmolarity varies from that of body fluids, the more slowly does the stomach empty. Thus, a saline or an isotonic sugar solution empties almost immediately. Water empties more slowly than saline, and increasing the concentration of sugar solutions slows motility proportionately. Fats move the most slowly of all basic dietary constituents, while solid foods must be ground down to an optimal size before the pylorus will relax enough to transmit them. The effects of duodenal receptors on gastric emptying are probably mediated both hormonally and through reflex arcs. The rate of gastric emptying, all other things such as density and character of contents being equal, is also influenced by pressures induced in the proximal stomach. Any gastric contents leave the stomach more rapidly when the stomach is full than they do as it empties.

Measurement of Gastric Emptying

There are a number of occasions where it becomes useful to document the rate of gastric emptying and the character of gastric peristalsis in humans. Among these are instances of gastric retention due to inflammatory or malignant diseases of the distal stomach and motor disorders of the stomach, such as scleroderma and amyloidosis where the muscular layer is infiltrated by disease, or diabetic enteropathy where the myenteric neuronal network is impaired.

The rate at which barium solutions leave the stomach can be measured qualitatively by fluoroscopy or radiography at fixed intervals. Normally, a barium solution commences to leave the stomach within 15 to 20 minutes, and has completely emptied in four hours. Efforts have been made to reproduce clinical situations by mixing barium with standardized meals, but these approaches have not been generally employed. With a meal of average fat content, gastric emptying may not commence until one hour after ingestion and not be completed until six hours have elapsed.

A saline load test has also been devised, employing 750 ml of isotonic salt solution administered by nasogastric tube. Normally, no more than 300 ml remain in the stomach 30 minutes after its introduction. In patients with gastric retention, the volume aspirated at 30 minutes is commonly larger than the amount introduced.

Scintigraphic scanning can be employed to measure the gastric emptying rates. Employing different radiolabels for liquids and solids. Heading et al (1976) were able to show that liquids emptied more rapidly than solids, and that the former cleared at an exponential rate while the latter exited in a more linear fashion.

HISTORICAL DIGRESSION

Personages referred to in this chapter without further reference include: William BEAUMONT (1785–1853), American military surgeon, Fort Mackinac, Plattsburgh, St. Louis, published "Experiments and observations on the gastric juice and the physiology of digestion" in 1833; Rudolf Peter Heinrich HEIDENHAIN (1834–1897), German physiologist, Breslau, described denervated gastric pouch, 1878; Franklin HOLLANDER (1899-1966), American physiologist, New York, described insulin test for vagal continuity, 1943; Nicholas KULTSCHITZKY (1856–1925), Polish histologist, Cracow; George Richards MINOT (1885–1950), American internist, Cambridge, Massachusetts, Nobel laureate in medicine, 1934; Ivan Petrovich PAVLOV (1849–1936), Russian physiologist, St. Petersburg (Leningrad), Nobel laureate in physiology, 1904.

SELECTED REFERENCES

Barreras RF. Calcium and gastric secretion. Gastroenterology 64:1168–84, 1973.

Chung RSK, Field M, Silen W. Effects of methylprednisolone on hydrogen ion absorption in the canine stomach. J Clin Invest 62:262–70, 1978.

Conn HO, Blitzer BL. Non-association of adrenocorticosteroid therapy and peptic ulcer. N Engl J Med 294:473–79, 1976.

Heading RC, Tothill P, McLoughlin GP, et al. Gastric emptying rate measurement in man. A double isotope scanning technique for simultaneous study of liquid and solid components of a meal. Gastroenterology 71:45–50, 1976.

Ivey KJ. Gastric mucosal barrier. Gastroenterology 61:247–57, 1971.

Kauffman GL, Grossman MI. Serum gastrin during intestinal phase of acid secretion. Gastroenterology 77:26–30, 1979.

Kelly KA. Gastric motility in health and after gastric surgery. Viewpoints Dig Dis 8:1–4, 1976.

Konturek SJ. Intestinal mechanisms regulating gastric secretion. In: Glass GBJ, ed. Progress in Gastroenterology, Vol 3. New York: Grune and Stratton, 1977: 395–438.

Konturek SJ. Gastrin and intestinal phase of gastric secretion. (Letter). Gastroenterology 78:193–94, 1980.
Korman MG, Scott DF, Hansky J, et al. Hypergastrinemia due to an excluded gastric antrum: A proposed method for differentiation from the Zollinger-Ellison syndrome. Aust N Z J Med 2:266–71, 1972.
McGuigan JE. Disorders of gastrin secretion. Adv Int Med 19:175–93, 1974.
Miller LJ, Gorman CA, Go VLW. Gut-thyroid interrelationships. Gastroenterology 75:901–11, 1978.
Robert A. The inhibitory effects of prostaglandins on gastric secretion: Their possible role in the treatment of gastric hypersecretion and peptic ulcer. In: Glass GBJ, ed. Progress in Gastroenterology, Vol 3. New York: Grune and Stratton, 1977:777-802.
Strauss E. Radioimmunoassay of gastrointestinal hormones. Gastroenterology 74:141–52, 1978.
Walsh JH, Grossman MI. Gastrin. N Engl J Med 292:1324–34, 1377–84, 1975.

DISCUSSION QUESTIONS

1. A Heidenhain pouch dog is conditioned to expect a feeding when a bell is sounded. What should happen to the pH of pouch secretions when the bell rings? Why? How might the fine structure of the parietal cells change after the bell is sounded? Would responses be any different in a Pavlov pouch dog? Why?
2. What effects would you expect pentagastrin to have on Heidenhain pouch secretion if it were injected intravenously when the antrum contained a small amount of consomme madrilenne? When the antrum was empty? Would the amount of pentagastrin injected per unit time make any difference? Why?
3. A 40-year-old man consults you because of recurrent ulcer pain two years after having had a vagotomy for similar complaints. X rays confirm the presence of a duodenal ulcer. What other tests would now be helpful to you in outlining a plan of treatment? How would the results affect your advice to the patient?
4. You are called by a radiologist who informs you that an elderly patient you had referred for X rays because of epigastric pain and weakness is found to have an ulcer in his stomach. His hematocrit was 27 percent, red blood count 1.8×10^6, white blood count 4,200. What findings would you anticipate on gastric analysis? What are the most likely diagnoses? Why?

CHAPTER 5

Gastritis and Gastric Mucosal Hypertrophy

The mucosa of the stomach may be injured by a variety of agents, ethyl alcohol, aspirin, other inhibitors of prostaglandin (PG) synthesis, bile salts, and certain bacterial toxins being prominent offenders. Where the period of exposure to the injurious agent is short and not repeated, mucosal damage invariably disappears within a brief period, although its acute effects may have been very severe. To a degree, the damage is also dose related and obligatory. Thus, a large fraction of patients taking even small doses of aspirin by mouth have been found to develop a bit of asymptomatic gastrointestinal bleeding, demonstrated by the appearance of occult blood in their stools. The amount of blood loss increases directly with the time of exposure but reaches major proportions in only a small percentage of patients. Indeed, it has been truthfully stated that were aspirin submitted to the Federal Drug Agency today for approval as a new drug it would doubtless be turned down.

Tissue damage in acute gastritis is usually superficial, involving only the mucosa and upper submucosa. It may also be associated with erosions, consisting of interruptions of the epithelium which do not penetrate the entire mucosa. Where the exposure to noxious agents is protracted, chronic persistent inflammatory changes may occur, particularly in the antrum or at the antral-oxyntic junction. Chronic gastritis of the fundus and body, on the other hand, appears to be predominantly the result of autoimmune phenomena.

SUPERFICIAL AND EROSIVE GASTRITIS

Pathophysiology

Certain agents, such as heat, bile salts, ethyl alcohol, and aspirin have been shown to be capable of damaging the gastric mucosa of experimental animals and, in some instances, of humans as well (Smith et al 1971).

Possible Role of Prostaglandin in Preventing Injury. The effect of tissue PG in preventing or reducing this sort of injury in the laboratory has already been described. Since nonsteroidal anti-inflammatory compounds, such as aspirin and indomethacin, are known to inhibit PG synthesis by blocking the enzyme which transforms arachidonic acid into endoperoxides, it is reasonable to presume that this inhibition results both in decreased cytoprotection and increased acid secretion in exposed individuals. Since germ-free animals do not develop gastric mucosal damage on exposure to aspirin, it has been suggested that bacteria or their toxins are mediators of the pathologic effects of aspirins. Glucocorticoids, which inhibit PG production by delaying the release of arachidonic acid from phospholipid stores by phospholipase A, have also been implicated as a cause of erosive gastritis. Despite these relevant observations, the precise role of PG in preventing mucosal injury is not established.

Effects of Disruption of Mucosal Barrier. Davenport (1978) has summarized the mechanisms and consequences of the disruption of the gastric mucous barrier by aspirin. At gastric pH levels below 3.5, aspirin in un-ionized and penetrates into the fatty component of epithelial cell membranes. Upon exposure to higher intracellular pH, aspirin ionizes and damages the cell enough to permit increased back-diffusion of hydrocholoric acid. Intramucosal HCl stimulates myenteric plexi to induce gastric contractions, fosters the secretion of pepsinogen, and releases histamine from tissue mast cells. The histamine induces further secretion of acid and also causes vasodilatation and increased permeability of mucosal capillaries. This last step leads to tissue edema, loss of plasma into the gastric lumen, disruption of capillary walls, and bleeding. Thus, acute damage to gastric epithelium can lead to dire, severe, and self-propagating immediate consequences. Since ethanol, bile acids, and lysolecithin (produced in the duodenum by the action of pancreatic phospholipase A on lecithin in bile) are also capable of breaching the mucosal barrier, results of mucosal exposure to these agents is similar to those produced by aspirin. Pretreatment of animals with PG before exposure to glucocorticoids, aspirin, or bile greatly inhibits the development of erosive gastritis. This effect appears to be distinct from the acid-inhibitory action of PG, although pretreatment with antacids also protects gastric mucosa from chemical injuries.

Reduction of Injury from Mucosal Damage. Kivilaakso and Silen (1979) have shown that even though luminal acidity is essential to the production of mucosal ulcers following exposure to agents that breach the mucosal barrier, much less damage appears if the injury occurs while acid secretion is being actively stimulated. They have demonstrated that such stimulation leads to alkalinization of the lamina propria because of the alkaline tide (rise of luminal H^+ offset by rise in tissue HCO_3^-) resulting from oxyntic activity. This tissue alkalinity protects mucosa from acidic damage. Conversely, systemic and tissue acidosis worsens damage in the injured mucosa. Adequate mucosal blood flow also restricts mucosal damage, and tissue pH falls when blood flow is inhibited.

Stress Ulcers. A form of erosive gastritis of the body of the stomach frequently appears in patients who have undergone periods of transient ischemia of the gastric mucosa in association with hypotension, severe injury, extensive burns, and complicated surgery. Multiple superficial erosions appear in the body of the stomach, and bleeding is often extreme. The presence of acid in the stomach is essential to the development of these lesions. Presumably, the ischemia develops from slowing of capillary flow or from the opening of arteriovenous shunts in response to hypotension, so that blood flow bypasses the gastric mucosa, thereby disrupting the mucosal barrier. Acid then back-diffuses as in aspirin-induced disruption, and damage ensues. The incidence of this complication is diminished greatly by pretreatment of patients at risk with intragastric antacids, or with the H_2-blocking agent, cimetidine. Stress ulcers induced in rats by restraint or forced exertion can also be prevented by pretreatment with PGE_2. The type of stress ulcer associated with extensive burns was described by Thomas Blizard Curling in 1842, and has since borne his name even though the lesions he described were confined to the duodenum. An obituary in 1888 describes Curling as "never what is called brilliant" and "by nature somewhat cold," but "always painstaking and accurate," with a "character of singular honesty and straight-forwardness, and—a kind heart."*

Mallory-Weiss syndrome, while not strictly speaking a form of gastritis, was described in 1929 as consisting of several mucosal tears in the cardia of the stomach often extending into the lower esophagus, consequent to a short period of heavy retching or vomiting. All of the original 15 patients were alcoholics, as are most of the patients seen today. Occasionally, however, Mallory-Weiss tears occur in patients who have been vomiting for other reasons, especially with salicylate-induced gastritis. It is a reasonable assumption that retching places great stress on the upper gastric mucosa, and that tears are likely to result if cytoprotective mechanisms have been subverted by drugs or toxins, such as alcohol. It is not, in fact, uncommon to see patients who show simultaneous findings of both erosive gastritis and mucosal tears, thus suggesting a common etiology for these disorders. Since the lacerations are commonly quite deep, the tendency to bleed severely is very great indeed.

Pathology

Superificial gastritis (Figure 5–1) may be diffusely distributed throughout the stomach, and consists of hyperemia and edema, especially of the lamina propria, with some extension into the submucosa. There is moderate

*British Medical Journal, 1:563-64, 1888.

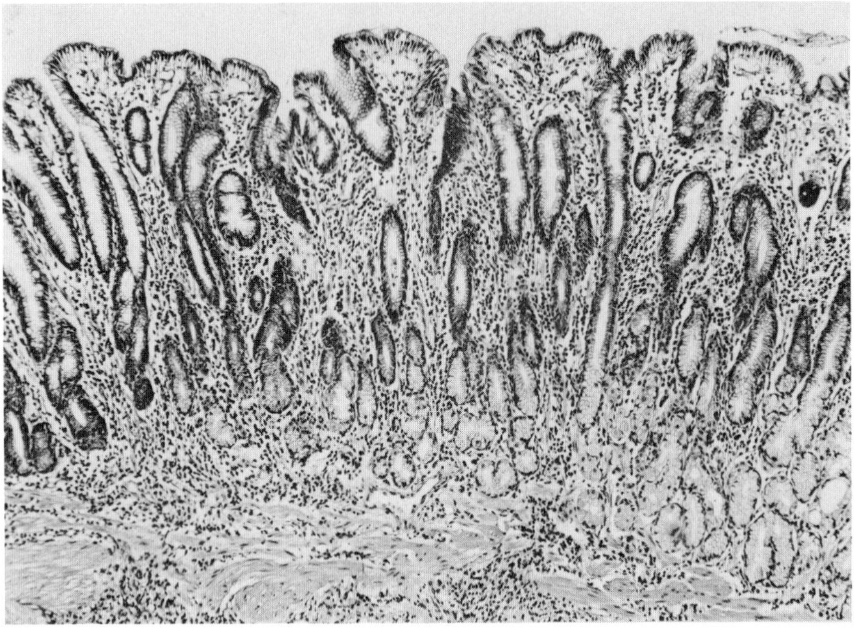

Figure 5–1. Superifcial gastritis. The lamina propria is edematous. Inflammatory cells have infiltrated the lamina propria, muscularis mucosae, and submucosa. The epithelium is intact. Original magnification x80.

infiltration of segmented granulocytes and a slight focal degranulation, but not disruption, of the surface epithelium.

Erosive gastritis (Figure 5–2) is similar to superficial gastritis except that the delicate neck region of the gastric gland tends to undergo necrosis so that in addition to the changes described above, there is also focal sloughing of the mucosa. Autodigestion then takes place at the denuded surface, and the acid of the stomach discolors the hemoglobin in the exposed vessels so that multiple, superficial black erosions result. These tend to be small, round, and widely scattered. They remain above the intact muscularis mucosae and are thus defined as erosions rather than ulcers. Erosive gastritis tends to heal readily and leave no scar.

Mallory-Weiss tears of the cardia of the stomach often extend somewhat into the lower esophagus and present grossly as multiple (usually three to five) fissures, 10 to 25 mm in length and 2 to 3 mm wide, extending deeply into the submucosa of the stomach and occasionally into the muscularis. Rarely, they may penetrate through the wall of the esophagus (Boerhaave syndrome). Blood clots or open vessels are commonly seen in the fissure itself. Microscopically, the fissure is noted to extend deep to the mucosa, and contains fibrin and an exudate of polymorphonuclear leukocytes at its base, as in any acute ulceration. The mucosa adjacent to the fissure may be slightly edematous but appears otherwise to be normal.

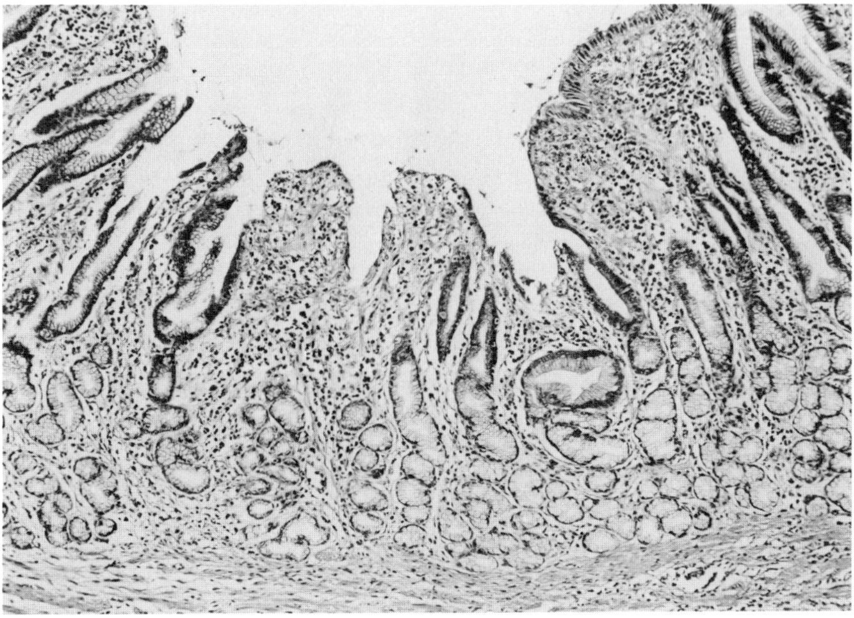

Figure 5–2. Gastric erosion in pyloric gland area of stomach. Note that the surface epithelium and mucosal pit cells have sloughed in one area. The lamina propria is infiltrated with inflammatory cells. Original magnification x80.

Symptoms and Course

While occasional patients complain of epigastric burning discomfort from acute gastritis, and some patients with Mallory-Weiss lacerations may apply for care because of vomiting, the primary reason for seeking medical help is upper gastrointestinal bleeding (Figure 5–3). The blood loss may manifest itself as hematemesis or as the passage of red-to-melenic, usually foul-smelling, stools. With extensive blood loss, symptoms of hypovolemia, such as tachycardia, shortness of breath, weakness, faintness, and sweating are noted. Faintness and dizziness are accentuated by assumption of an erect or sitting position. With large amounts of blood in the intestine, patients commonly experience frequent peristaltic rushes in the abdomen, often preceding an urge to defecate. In some patients with erosive gastritis, the bleeding ceases spontaneously in a short time; patients with lacerations of the cardia usually require further treatment.

Treatment

Management of acute gastritis consists of controlling blood loss (see below), identifying and discontinuing any noxious agents, and providing a

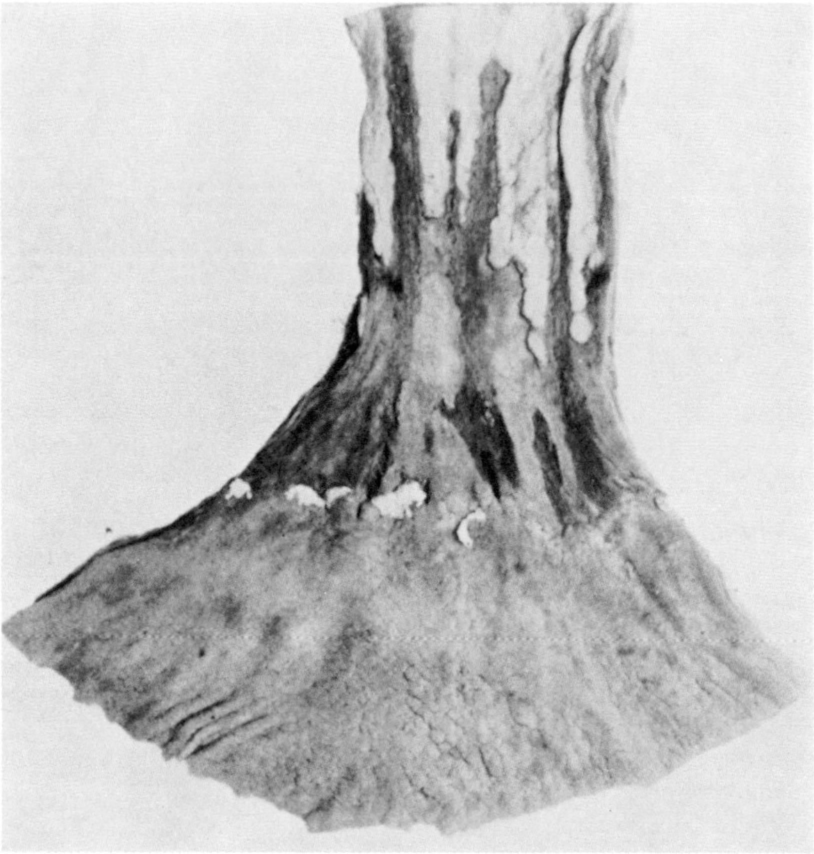

Figure 5–3. Mallory-Weiss tears. Several fissurelike longitudinal ulcerations can be seen in the lower portion of the esophagus. Two were deep, the others rather superficial. From Mallory GK, Weiss S. Am J Med Sci 178:506–15, 1929. Reprinted by permission.

milieu for the gastritis or lacerations to heal. This latter aspect of treatment is usually managed adequately by reducing the secretion of acid with cimetidine (300 mg every six hours, orally or intravenously), or by raising intragastric pH with doses of oral antacids capable of neutralizing 100 mEq HCl every two to four hours. While they are potentially attractive therapeutic agents, methylated prostaglandins are not yet available for clinical use. As stated earlier, erosive gastritis and lacerations of the cardia have a great natural tendency to heal rapidly once bleeding has stopped, so prolonged therapy is not necessary, as long as the causative agent is identified and removed.

The best management of either of these disorders is to prevent their occurrence by identifying patients at risk (e.g., those who have had massive injuries or burns, patients with acute alcoholic intoxication, patients receiving nonsteroidal anti-inflammatory agents), and treating them with regular doses of antacids or cimetidine. For patients at long-term risk, doses of these agents may be reduced gradually as tolerated.

MANAGEMENT OF MAJOR UPPER GASTROINTESTINAL HEMORRHAGE

Massive upper gastrointestinal hemorrhage may arise from a variety of diseases, some of which have not as yet been discussed. However, since it is a major problem occurring among patients with erosive gastritis, stress ulcers, and Mallory-Weiss syndrome, its management will be discussed here. The causes of massive upper gastrointestinal bleeding vary considerably from one institution to another. A hospital which treats a large number of accident victims will see many patients with bleeding stress ulcerations. One in which alcoholism is a prominent habit among its patients will have a major percentage of bleeding from esophageal varices associated with cirrhosis of the liver, and in hospitals with a large proportion of patients over age 65, gastric ulcer and superficial gastritis will be frequent causes. Colcher (1975) has tabulated the causes of upper gastrointestinal hemorrhage from a number of studies where the diagnosis was made at endoscopy. Duodenal ulcers were responsible for 15 to 40 percent of massive hemorrhages; esophageal varices, 10 to 30 percent; gastric ulcer, 10 to 20 percent; erosive gastritis (including stress ulcers), 10 to 35 percent; Mallory-Weiss syndrome, 5 to 15 percent; esophagitis 5 to 10 percent; gastric tumors, 3 to 5 percent. In approximately 5–10 percent of patients, the site of hemorrhage remains undiagnosed or is diagnosed erroneously. Generally, this figure becomes smaller where the diagnostic workup is most vigorous. However, the prudent physician may not, as discussed below, wish to pursue diagnostic studies energetically in those patients whose bleeding stops and whose X rays show no indication of serious disease.

While there is some difference of opinion among gastroenterologists about the fine points of management in patients with major upper gastrointestinal bleeding, most agree on the broad, general principles and their order of precedence. First and foremost is the restoration of circulating blood volume, followed immediately by or simultaneous with efforts to control bleeding. Attempts to diagnose the cause and site of bleeding should be undertaken only after volume is actually being restored and the patient's condition has commenced to stabilize. Let us discuss the steps in order.

Restoration of Circulating Blood Volume. The patient with major gastrointestinal bleeding should immediately have a large catheter placed into as large a peripheral vein as can be found, and blood should be drawn for typing, cross-match, and coagulation studies. Intravenous fluids are started immediately, using artificial plasma expanders if the patient is in shock, or 5 percent dextrose in saline, if hypovolemia is not accompanied by shock.

Whole blood or packed cells are started as soon as they become available. Circulating volume depletion is best measured by frequent monitoring of the pulse rate and its character, and the blood pressure. If shock does not respond promptly to these measures, pressor agents such as vasopressin may be necessary, although these run the risk of reducing blood flow to coronary, mesenteric, and renal arteries. The major consideration initially should be to maintain cerebral blood flow and to prevent acidosis and cardiac arrest.

As hypovolemia begins to correct, pulse rate slows and pulse pressure decreases toward normal. It may be difficult at such times to determine whether the supine patient is still hypovolemic. Under these circumstances, a check of pulse and pressure with the patient sitting upright will provide the answer; patients with mild hypovolemia show an increase in pulse rate and pulse pressure in this position. Measurement of blood counts and hematocrit at this early stage of blood loss is not helpful in determining the extent of hemorrhage, since significant hemodilution and fall in hematocrit do not occur until at least 24 hours after massive bleeding commences.

Efforts to Control Bleeding. When the patient presents with a history of hematemesis, or when a nasogastric aspirate shows red blood or acid-hematin (coffee-grounds coloration) content, an upper gastrointestinal site of hemorrhage (source above the duodenal-jejunal junction) can be assumed. In these cases, lavage with iced water or iced saline can often reduce mucosal bleeding by causing constriction of mucosal arterioles. Absence of bloody or coffee-grounds contents does not rule out a lower gastric or duodenal site of bleeding, and lavage may still be a good plan at this point. If coagulation studies demonstrate a shortage of platelets or coagulation factors, transfusions with platelets or with fresh frozen plasma may be indicated. Many centers presently administer cimetidine to all patients with upper gastrointestinal hemorrhage, and studies indicate its probable value.

If bleeding appears to stop in response to these measures, therapy can be reduced in intensity, antacids can be added to the program under the assumption that the disorder is related to acid-peptic factors, and simple diagnostic studies can be undertaken when convenient. If bleeding continues, further measures become necessary. These include nonspecific measures such as constricting mesenteric and gastric blood flow by the use of a vasopressin drip and urgent measures to diagnose a specific bleeding point.

Diagnosing the Cause and Site of Bleeding. The patient's history is often very helpful in diagnosing the cause of bleeding. Thus, a patient who has been consuming frequent and large doses of aspirin probably has erosive gastritis, a patient who has been in the hospital for a few days subsequent to receiving injuries in an automobile accident probably has stress ulcers, and a patient who has been vomiting or retching after an alcoholic debauch probably has Mallory-Weiss lacerations. Similarly, a history of epigastric pain relieved by meals for days or weeks before the hemorrhage suggests the presence of a peptic ulcer, and signs of hepatomegaly, jaundice, and an abdominal collateral venous pattern support an impression of bleeding esophageal varices.

But things are often not what they appear to be—the cirrhotic patient may be bleeding from a duodenal ulcer, and the salicylate-ingester may have high gastric lacerations. Thus, continued or recurrent bleeding is a clear indication for upper gastrointestinal endoscopy. This procedure can provide an answer regarding the site of upper gastrointestinal hemorrhage in around 90 percent of patients, and it is well tolerated by even the most ill. Endoscopic findings may be equivocal in patients who are bleeding so heavily that the field of vision is obliterated, and in some patients whose bleeding has actually stopped and no clear points of disease remain. Previous nasogastric suction may produce erosions that can usually be distinguished from those occurring spontaneously. By and large, endoscopy is most effective and provides valid information quickly.

With continued bleeding and negative endoscopic findings, selective angiography of the celiac axis vessels will demonstrate a bleeding point if bleeding is active at the time of the study. If a bleeding point is identified, the catheter can be left in place and used for the introduction of vasopressin, which may reduce bleeding by causing arterial vasospasm.

Surgery. Surgery is indicated for the control of upper gastrointestinal hemorrhage if the measures outlined above—volume replacement, ice-water lavage, H_2 blocking agents, antacids, vasospastic agents—are non-availing, or if hemorrhage is so massive that losses cannot be compensated for by intravenous replacement. The type of surgery performed depends on the nature of the lesion. Surgery for gastritis often requires resection of the involved portion of the stomach, surgery for peptic ulcer will be discussed in the next chapter, and surgery for Mallory-Weiss lacerations usually consists of oversewing of the tears themselves.

For the patient who stops bleeding spontaneously or in response to therapy, diagnostic measures can be undertaken at leisure. The procedure performed is usually a matter of personal preference. I lean, in such patients, to the undertaking of a careful series of contrast barium X rays, an upper gastrointestinal series, for this is a highly accurate diagnostic procedure, well tolerated by almost every patient and not extremely expensive to perform. If a specific lesion is found, therapy is instituted or continued as indicated. If the study is completely normal, patient and physician can feel assured that no ominous lesion has been overlooked and that bleeding resulted from either gastric erosions or, in apposite cases, Mallory-Weiss lacerations. Performance of an endoscopy in such patients should, in my estimation, be undertaken only if radiologic studies detect an abnormality of uncertain cause. Others prefer to endoscope all patients who have bled since 20-percent of ulcers may be missed on X rays. A recent controlled study, however, has shown that routine endoscopy in patients whose upper GI bleeding ceases in hospital provides no benefit over no endoscopy (Peterson et al 1981). Endoscopy can also be useful in distinguishing between benign and malignant gastric ulcers, leiomyomata, and gastric anomalies which may become sites of bleeding.

In summary, the patient with major upper gastrointestinal bleeding constitutes a true medical emergency. First steps should be directed at reducing the major potential cause of death, hypovolemia, and diagnostic and therapeutic efforts not directly restorative of hypovolemia should be postponed. Efforts to stop bleeding by the use of lavage, pressor agents, and coagulation factors can proceed along with efforts to restore blood volume, but should never precede them. Diagnostic measures are of tertiary importance after volume and bleeding control measures have been instituted. Discontinuation of bleeding allows for the undertaking of diagnostic procedures at leisure, while continued bleeding requires that they be performed on an urgent basis.

CHRONIC ATROPHIC GASTRITIS

Two general categories of chronic gastritis have been distinguished by Strickland and Mackay (1973). The first is an inflammatory process causing thinning of the mucosa and epithelial metaplasia primarily in the fundus and body of the stomach, called type A. The second, type B, is a form of chronic gastritis which involves the antrum primarily, and in which the mucosa of the body and fundus may show only focal inflammation. While some cases of chronic gastritis cannot be clearly classified as either type A or type B, their numbers are quite small.

Pathophysiology

Type A Gastritis. The antral mucosa may be slightly involved in the chronic inflammatory reaction of type A gastritis, but usually it is not. By definition, all patients with this disorder have circulating antibodies to oxyntic cell membranes, and often demonstrate antibodies to intrinsic factor and thyroid epithelial cells as well, along with antinuclear antibodies occasionally. Furthermore, they may also show at the time of diagnosis or later evidence of other probable autoimmune disorders such as Hashimoto thyroiditis, hyperthyroidism and hypothyroidism, hypoparathyroidism, insulin-dependent diabetes mellitus, Addison disease, and vitiligo. The strength of this association is demonstrated by the fact that it operates in both directions; thus, patients with thyroiditis, Addison disease, and hypoparathyroidism commonly also have antibodies to oxyntic cells. First-degree relatives of patients with atrophic gastritis, type A, show a considerably higher than normal incidence of parietal antibodies as well (Table 5-1).

Patients with type A gastritis have very low secretions of gastric acid, or none at all, since the disease progressively destroys oxyntic cells. There is a reciprocal rise in levels of serum gastrin, probably in response to sustained elevations of antral pH coupled with the fact that antral gastrin cells are not destroyed by inflammation in this type. Some patients with type A gastritis, and not only those who secrete antibodies to intrinsic factor, develop malabsorption of vitamin B_{12} and eventually, pernicious anemia. All patients with pernicious anemia have type A gastritis, show a striking

Table 5-1. Chronic Atrophic Gastritis*

	Type A Immunogenic	*Type B Nonimmunogenic*
Frequency	approx. 5% (adults)	approx. 20% (adults)
Gastritis, fundus, and body	diffuse	none to focal
Gastritis, antrum	none to slight	diffuse
Circulating antibodies		
To parietal cells	all (by definition)	none (by definition)
To intrinsic factor	15%	< 10%
To antral G cells	none	7%
To thryroid	frequent	< 10%
Fasting serum gastrin	elevated	low to normal
Achlorhydria or hypochlorhydria	marked	slight to moderate
Vitamin B_{12} malabsorption	frequent	rare
Associated autoimmune diseases	increased	not increased
Gastric antibodies in relatives	increased	not increased
Pernicious anemia	common	none
Abdominal discomfort	none	frequent
Gastric ulcer	none	occasional
Gastric cancer	5–10% (20 years)	10% (20 years)
Ethanol, salicylate ingestion	not increased	increased
Protein-losing gastropathy	yes	probably
Cellular immunity	reduced in pernicious anemia	unknown
Mucosal IgA cells	reduced 90% in pernicious anemia	unknown
Mucosal IgG cells	increased 15% in pernicious anemia	unknown

*Does not include a small percentage of cases with antral gastritis and parietal cell antibodies.

reduction in gastric mucosal IgA-secreting cells, and have reduced cellular immunity.

The evidence seems clear then, that type A gastritis is familial, that it is probably the result of chronic autoimmune cellular destruction, and that it is frequently associated with other autoimmune disorders. It is interesting to note that the two major diseases first described by Thomas Addison, pernicious anemia and idiopathic atrophy of the adrenal cortex, are now believed to be the result of autoimmune processes. Addison himself thought that pernicious anemia was caused by adrenocortical disease.

Type B Gastritis. This form of gastritis, involving primarily the antrum, occurs with four times the frequency of type A and is commonly associated with some possible exogenous etiology, such as chronic intake of alcohol, heavy smoking, or ingestion of salicylates. That this is not nearly as likely as type A gastritis to have an autoimmune etiology is demonstrated by the fact that patients and their families demonstrate no evidence of increased incidence of other autoimmune antibodies or diseases. Vandelli et al (1979) have shown that some patients, 8 out of 106, with type B gastritis do indeed carry autoantibodies to gastrin-producing cells and tend to have lower than normal levels of circulating serum gastrin. There might thus be a small percentage of type B patients in whom an autoimmune reaction is operative, but this does not appear to be the case in the great bulk of patients.

Patients with chronic antral gastritis have a higher than expected incidence of gastric ulcer, probably occurring as a result of chronic inflammation, and seem to have a higher than normal incidence of gastric carcinoma as well. They rarely develop vitamin B_{12} malabsorption, and never contract pernicious anemia.

Pathology

Gross examination of the stomach of a patient with atrophic gastritis reveals a fragile wall and a markedly thin mucosa underneath which rugae are often difficult to identify. Mucosal involvement in type A appears primarily in the upper stomach; in type B, mainly in the antrum. The surface of the involved areas is flat, and the mucosa, while intact, is thin and has a translucent quality so that a tracery of submucosal veins can be seen if the stomach is transilluminated. Clusters of lymphocytes are scattered throughout the submucosa. Chief and parietal cells are either greatly decreased in number, or absent entirely, depending on the severity of the process. Goblet or mucous cells are abundant in the surface epithelium, and basophilic microcysts appear in the deepest portions of the glands. The mucosa often resembles that of the ileum, and the change is described as "intestinalization" of the gastric mucosa (Figure 5–4). Epithelial cells often develop a brush border typical of intestinal epithelium. Other changes include an increased cellularity and density of the connective tissue of the lamina propria, and often a thickening of the muscularis mucosae.

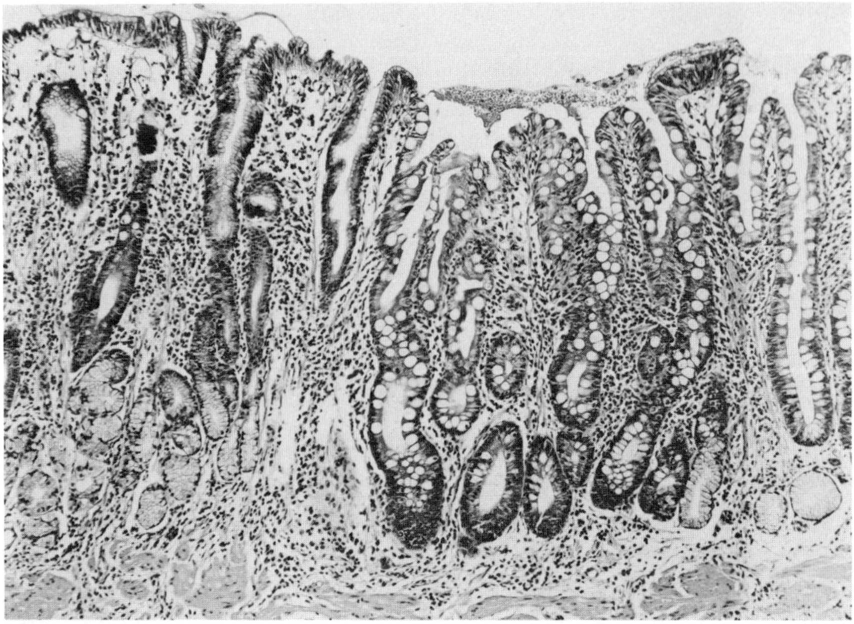

Figure 5-4. Chronic atrophic gastritis with intestinalization. The antral mucosa (*left*) is replaced by absorptive intestinal cells and goblet cells. A heavy inflammatory infiltrate is present. Original magnification x80.

Symptoms

There are no typical symptoms associated with type A gastritis. Most patients with untreated pernicious anemia have no gastrointestinal complaints other than for occasional anorexia, which is probably due to vitamin B_{12} deficiency rather than gastritis. Patients with chronic antral (type B) gastritis, do frequently have complaints of upper abdominal fullness and discomfort after meals, with occasional pain responsive to antacids. The picture is quite variable from patient to patient, and many patients with antral gastritis have no abdominal complaints. Acute or chronic gastrointestinal bleeding may be the first indications of chronic gastritis.

Diagnosis

Radiologic studies show no consistent abnormalities in type A gastritis, although some radiologists feel that decreased prominence of gastric rugal folds can be detected in patients with advanced mucosal atrophy. In antritis (type B), however, there is often narrowing of the antrum, distortion of its mucosal folds, and decreased peristalsis. At times, the findings are also suggestive of an infiltrating cancer of the antrum, so endoscopic evaluation is indicated.

Endoscopy can clearly distinguish the presence of mucosal atrophy, primarily by the absence of rugal folds and by the translucence of the gastric mucosa in areas that are involved by the process. A tracery of submucosal veins, not normally visible, is a clear indication of atrophy. In the antrum, the mucosa often appears to be thickened somewhat and slightly reddened. The smooth passage of peristaltic waves through the antrum is a helpful sign of benignity in a patient suspected of having an antral carcinoma. Occasionally small antral erosions are visible endoscopically in a patient with symptomatic antral gastritis (Figure 5–5).

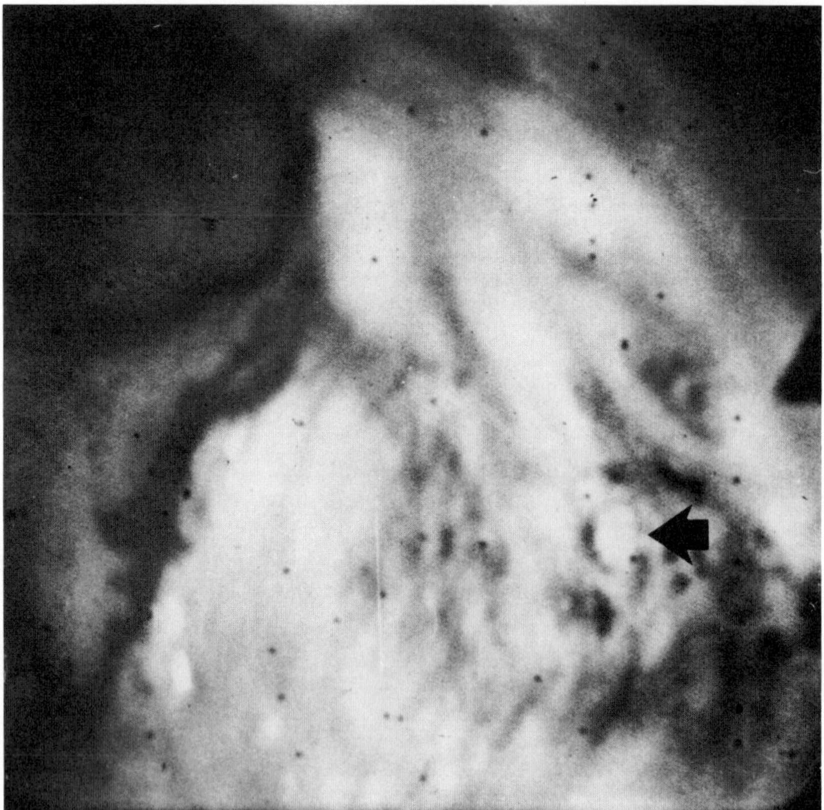

Figure 5–5. Hemorrhagic and erosive gastritis. This view of the posterior wall of the stomach shows hemorrhagic areas, irregular black smudges, and a central acute erosion (arrow). The small black spots are caused by broken fibers in the endoscopic bundle. (Courtesy of Dr. Kevin Geraci).

Treatment

Evidence of superficial active or erosive gastritis in patients with type B gastritis indicates that antacid therapy may be worthwhile. If acidity is high in the symptomatic patient, cimetidine should be given for a period of four to six weeks. Patients should be instructed to stop alcohol intake, avoid salicylates, and discontinue smoking. Atrophic gastritis of the body of the stomach (type A) requires no treatment, except of vitamin B_{12} injections if malabsorption exists. It has been shown that patients with autoimmune gastritis will develop improved acid secretion and increased absorption of vitamin B_{12} after receiving glucocorticoids for a time. But the side effects of the therapy heavily outweigh its benefits in this situation, and the observation is of no therapeutic value, although it does help confirm the autoimmune nature of type A gastritis.

Consequences of Chronic Atrophic Gastritis

Cancer of the Stomach. It has been recognized for many years that patients with pernicious anemia (type A gastritis) run an increased risk of developing cancer of the stomach, amounting to 5 to 10 percent over 10 or more years. It has been felt that the intestinal metaplasia seen in this condition may well be premalignant, and that patients with pernicious anemia should regularly be studied with upper gastrointestinal radiography. Since this recommendation is risky in itself because of the radiation hazard, it is presently advised that patients with this disease simply have their stools checked for occult bleeding, an early sign of cancer, twice yearly. Another observation bearing on this matter (Shearman et al 1966) is the fact that many patients presenting with cancer of the stomach have reduced blood levels of vitamin B_{12}, a number of them even having circulating antibodies to oxyntic cells. Thus, among patients with cancer of the stomach are those who have preclinical pernicious anemia.

Although the reason for the association of type A atrophic gastritis and cancer of the stomach is not known, MacLaurin (1979) has reviewed evidence showing that patients with pernicious anemia may suffer from impaired T-lymphocyte function, leading to failure of control of the B-lymphocyte response to self-antigens. He has also demonstrated impaired cellular immunity in patients with pernicious anemia. It is possible that decreased immunosurveillance predisposes patients to the development of cancer.

I am not aware of similar studies in patients with antral (type B) atrophic gastritis, although the incidence of gastric cancer appears to be increased in them as well. Thus, 10 percent of Strickland's patients with type B gastritis developed cancer of the stomach during 10 years of follow up. Another observation that attests to the etiologic importance of chronic gastritis in the genesis of cancer of the stomach is the increased incidence of cancer of the gastric remnant in patients who have had partial gastric resections for peptic ulcer in the remote past. Gastritis, due to the post-operative chronic reflux of bile and lysolecithin into the gastric remnant, is almost invariably seen in these patients.

Almost all patients with cancer of the stomach show a degree of accompanying chronic atrophic gastritis. The present presumption is that the gastritis preceded the cancer. While the incidence of cancer of the stomach has shown a decrease of about two-thirds among American men and women in the last quarter-century, it is still far from being eliminated (Figure 5-6). The American Cancer Society estimates that 23,000 new cases appeared and 14,000 deaths occurred in the United States in 1980. Furthermore, cancer of the stomach is the most common malignancy seen among men and women in Japan and Chile, occurring at rates seven to eight times more frequent in those countries than it does in the United States. It is presumed that exogenous factors, such as nitrosamines in food, are the cause of these dif-

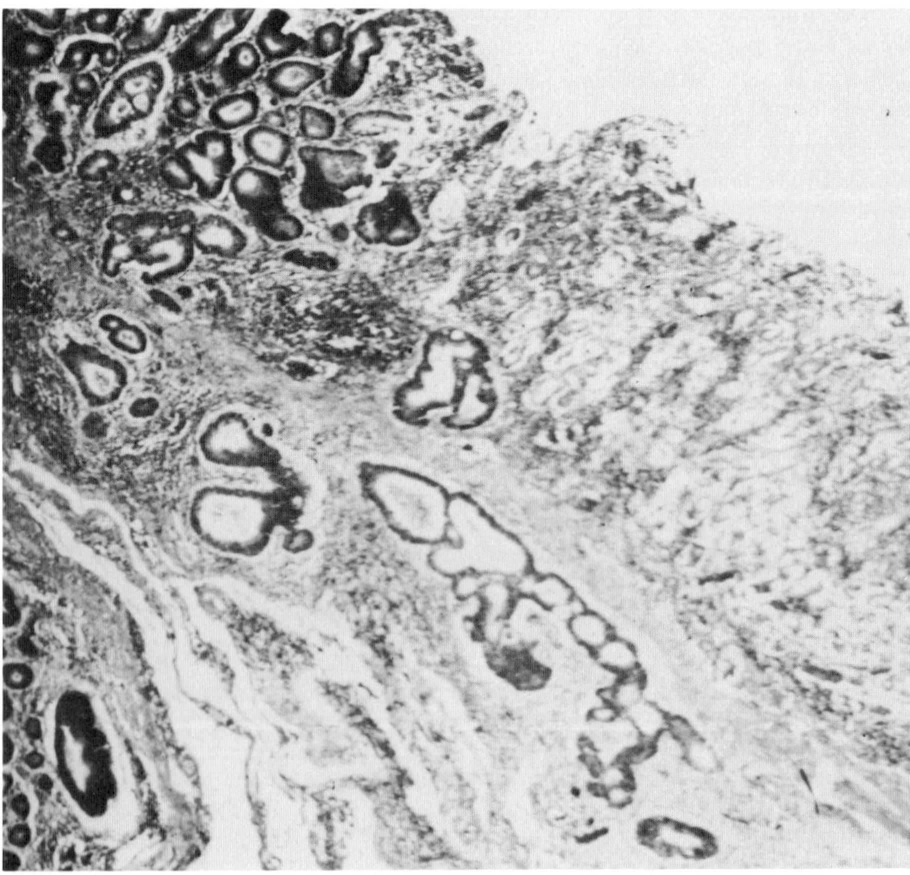

Figure 5-6. Adenocarcinoma of the stomach. Irregular mucosal glands at left have infiltrated deeply into the submucosa. Original magnification x40.

ferences, since the incidence of type B gastritis appears to be more common in Japan at least than in the United States.

Chronic Protein Loss. Chronic atrophic gastritis is often associated with the increased exudation of plasma proteins, especially albumin, into the gastric lumen. This may result at times in hypoalbuminemia and edema in patients with atrophy, although not as frequenty as it does in patients with gastric mucosal hypertrophy. It is believed that the inflammatory process leads to partial disruption of the mucosal barrier, secondary capillary damage, and resultant exudation. This is one of a large number of protein-losing enteropathies.

GASTRIC MUCOSAL HYPERTROPHY

There are two distinct nonmalignant disorders leading to hypertrophy of the gastric mucosa, one of which is associated with hypersecretion of hydrochloric acid and the other with either hypochlorhydria or achlorhydria (Table 5–2). In the former type, which is most commonly seen in the Zollinger-Ellison syndrome, hypertrophy of all glandular elements occurs, but the major influence is on the chief and oxyntic cell population. The latter type, first described by Menetrier (1888) and more clearly delineated by Hurst and Stokes (1926), is quite rare and consists primarily of hypertrophy of epithelial mucous cells above the foveolar neck, the remainder of the mucosa being either normal or partially replaced by mucous cells. Inflammation appears to be a minor factor in both disorders; when present, it is usually not extensive and tends to be patchy. Because of this, the term *mucosal hypertrophy* or *gastropathy* seems preferable to hypertrophic gastritis (Figure 5–7).

Table 5–2. Gastric Mucosal Hypertrophy

	Zollinger-Ellison Type	*Menetrier-Hurst Type*
Primary site of hypertrophy	oxyntic and chief cells	epithelial mucous cells
Serum gastrin	elevated	probably normal
Gastric acidity	extremely high	low to absent
Albumin loss	no	yes
Peptic ulcer	often multiple	no
Diarrhea	common	common
Bleeding	often acute, massive	slow, chronic
Hypoalbuminemia	rare	frequent
X ray findings	ulcer(s); giant rugae	giant rugae
Treatment	cimetidine, anticholinergics, surgery	surgery observation

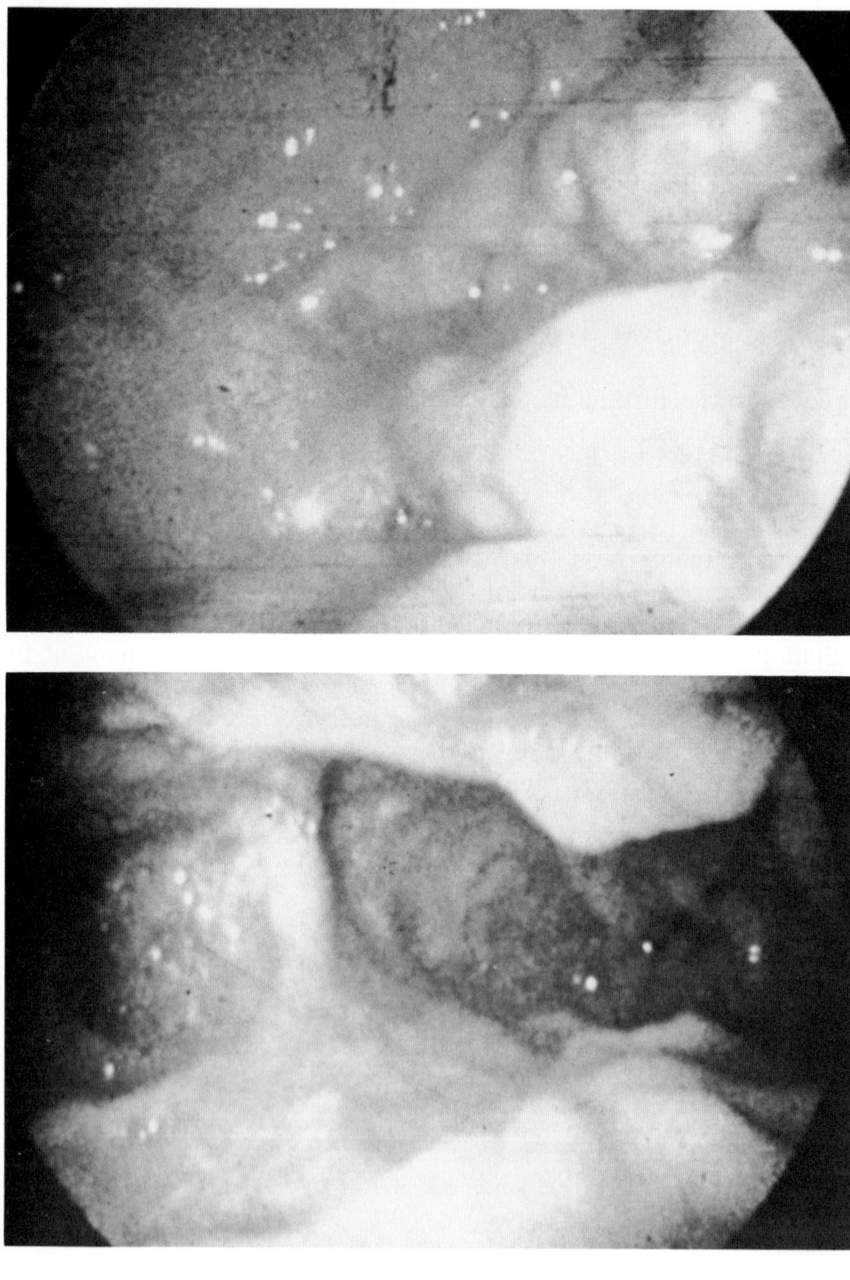

Figure 5–7. Giant gastric rugae. Large boggy rugal folds are present on the anterior and posterior walls (A) and the greater curve (B) of the stomach. From Umeda N. *Diagnosis by Gastrophotography.* Philadelphia: WB Saunders, 1971. Reprinted by permission.

Pathology and Pathophysiology

Zollinger-Ellison (ZE) Syndrome. The gastric mucosa and submucosa are often several times the normal thickness. Mucosal folds are enlarged, tightly packed, and tortuous and resemble, as Hurst remarked, the convolutions of the brain. The stomach wall is grossly soft and edematous. The process is diffuse, especially in the body and cardia of the stomach, and the large rugal folds are easily noted on radiography and endoscopy. Histologically, one is again impressed by the thickening of the mucosa, and the gastric foveolae are seen to be very deep, while gastric glands contain an increased number of chief and oxyntic cells (Figure 5-8). There may also be lymphocytic infiltrates in the lamina propria, but inflammation is scanty.

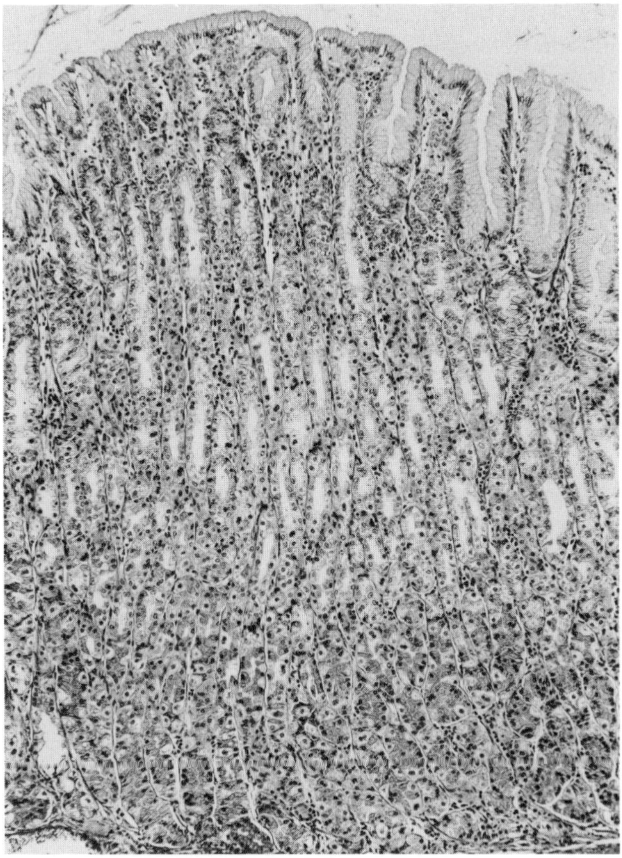

Figure 5-8. Gastric fundal biopsy in patients with the Zollinger-Ellison syndrome. Note the markedly increased depth of gastric foveolae and the increased numbers of parietal cells. Compare with normal mucosa in Figure 4-2. Original magnification x80.

The glandular hypertrophy is now believed to result from the trophic effect on the gastric mucosa of the large amounts of gastrin being secreted in these patients. The hypergastrinemia arises from either benign or malignant gastrinomas, usually arising in the pancreas, or hyperplasia of antral G cells. In addition to high serum gastrin levels, patients characteristically have markedly increased basal acid outputs, relentless and often multiple ulcers in the duodenum, and diarrhea resulting primarily from acidification of the duodenum and consequent inactivation of pancreatic digestive enzymes.

Menetrier-Hurst (MH) Disease. Grossly, the gastric mucosa is indistinguishable from that seen in Zollinger-Ellison patients. The wall of the stomach is thick and soft. Microscopically, the hypertrophy in MH disease is confined to the mucus-secreting cells above the foveolar neck, the foveolae themselves elongating remarkably into frondlike structures (Figure 5–9). Chief and oxyntic cells do not proliferate, and the latter may actually disappear. In Hurst's patient, there was also great thickening of the muscularis mucosae and the deep muscular layers of the stomach, but this is not an invariable finding.

The chief functional consequences of MH disease are the remarkable loss of albumin secreted from the hypertrophic mucosal glands, and the iron deficiency and anemia resulting from the slow chronic loss of blood through the edematous mucosa. The amount of albumin secreted daily into the stomach of patients with MH disease can be very high (Citrin et al 1957). Levels of acid secretion are usually normal or low, though occasionally patients will have pentagastrin-fast achlorhydria. Diarrhea is also a common complaint. Peptic ulcers are not seen in these patients and gastrin levels are normal. The cause of the mucosal hypertrophy is not known.

Symptoms

Patients with the ZE syndrome present most commonly with typical symptoms of peptic ulcer, differing from the more common type in that they are less responsive to therapy with antacids, recur promptly after healing, and are commonly either multiple or else located in portions of the duodenum distal to the bulb, areas in which simple peptic ulcers are most unusual. Diarrhea is a frequent complaint, often associated with malabsorption of fats and loss of weight. These symptoms are also unusual in patients with simple peptic ulcers. Gastrointestinal hemorrhage from bleeding ulcers is a frequent problem in patients with the ZE syndrome.

Alimentary symptoms in patients with MH disease are often vague, consisting primarily of poor appetite and upper abdominal discomfort after meals. Diarrhea is often troublesome, but there is usually no malabsorption of fat. Weakness due to anemia and edema due to hypoalbuminemia may be

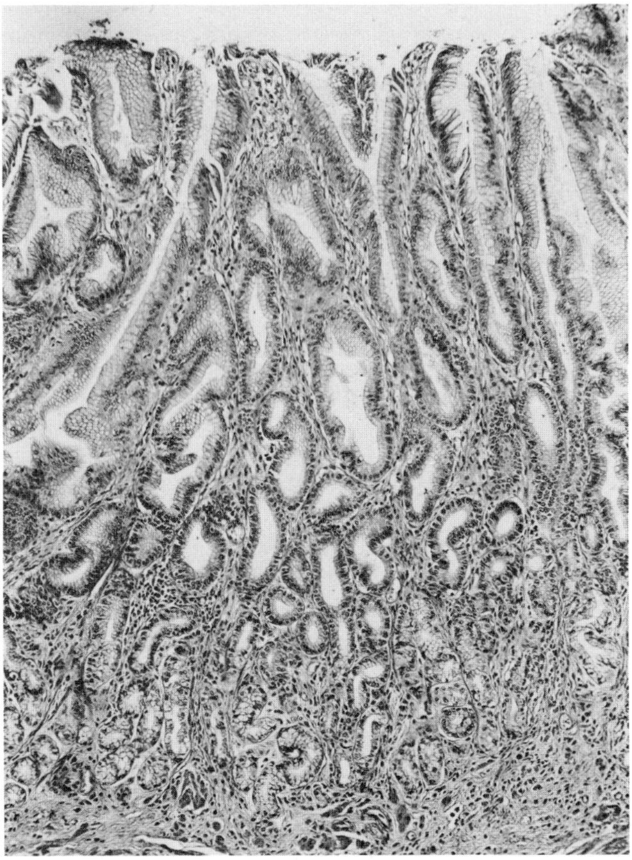

Figure 5-9. Menetrier-Hurst disease. In contrast to the Zollinger-Ellison syndrome, the thickened gastric mucosa is due primarily to an increase of mucous-secreting cells with papillary projections. Oxyntic cells are not increased. Original magnification x80.

severe and are often the primary complaints of patients seeking medical assistance. The anemia is often associated with occult blood in the stools. Massive hemorrhage is not seen.

Diagnosis

The diagnosis of these disorders rests on radiologic findings, endoscopic confirmation, and laboratory results. ZE syndrome is associated with large rugal folds, multiple peptic ulcers, and frequently edema of the mucosa of the upper small intestine. The radiologist may wish to have confirmation that the enlarged rugae are not due to an infiltrative lymphosarcoma, so endoscopy and biopsy may be useful confirmatory studies. Patients may have already undergone partial gastric resections for previous intractable peptic ulcers, and be found on X ray to have recurrent ulcers at or near to the gastroenterostomy site (marginal ulcers). Hypersecretion of acid and hypergastrinemia are almost invariably found. If serum gastrin levels are not diagnositc, their marked increase after administration of calcium, secretin, or both, is often confirmatory.

MH disease may appear similar to ZE syndrome on X ray and endoscopy. However, the absence of peptic ulcers and hypersecretion of acid, the normal levels of serum gastrin, and the commonly associated hypoalbuminemia are of great diagnostic help.

Treatment

ZE Syndrome. Until recently, the accepted treatment for patients with ZE syndrome was total gastrectomy. This was based on the argument that the causative gastrinoma was most commonly a slowly growing malignant neoplasm which could not be extirpated completely, or could not be fully delineated at surgery. Therefore, it was deemed necessary to remove the entire target, the stomach, in order to avoid further peptic ulcerations. Fortunately, a recent report (McCarthy 1978) of 61 patients with ZE syndrome indicates clearly that cimetidine, the H_2-blocking agent that binds to histamine receptors on oxyntic cells, can be highly effective. Fifty-two out of 61 patients were treated successfully with the long-term use of cimetidine, although often in doses twice as large (600 mg qid) as amounts needed in conventional duodenal ulcers. Five additional patients responded well when anticholinergic drugs (propantheline, 15 mg qid, or glycopyrrolate 1 mg qid) were added to the cimetidine. Only 5 of these patients developed gynecomastia from the cimetidine, a complication that seems to result from testosterone-inhibiting effects of the drug, and that often subsides with reduction of the dose. There have also been suggestions that cimetidine may induce mild reductions in sperm counts, but this has not as yet proved to be a major reason for its discontinuation, especially in patients as seriously ill as those with the ZE syndrome. Four of McCarthy's patients died from metastatic gastrinoma, but there is some evidence that this condition may respond to the simultaneous administration of streptozocin. This drug, a glucosomine nitrosourea, is administered once weekly intravascularly at a dose of 1.0 g/m^2, for four weeks. Although streptozocin is mildly diabetogenic and causes bone marrow suppression in 20 percent of patients, its usefulness is limited more by the fact that it commonly leads to severe damage to proximal renal tubules.

Thus, the best approach to treatment in the ZE syndrome would commence with the use of cimetidine and, if needed, anticholinergics. When ulcers have healed, patients should be carefully studied for metastases, and a good case can be made for surgical exploration with removal of as much of the tumor mass as possible at that time. Use of streptozocin would depend on the findings at surgery.

MH Syndrome. This can be treated definitively only by surgery, with total or subtotal gastrectomy, depending on the amount of stomach involved. The indications for this treatment are either severe chronic albumin loss, or severe anemia, usually the former. Anemia alone, responsive to the administration of iron, is probably not a surgical indication because the operation itself in such cases is worse than the disease. Since the rugal hypertrophy in this disease is not believed to be a premalignant lesion, there is no need for surgery in patients whose symptoms are mild or controlled with iron alone. Because this condition may also undergo spontaneous regression, surgery should not be performed until a period of observation has confirmed its chronicity (Berry et al 1980).

HISTORICAL DIGRESSION

Persons referred to in this chapter include: Thomas ADDISON (1793–1860), British physician, London, described adrenal necrosis, 1849; Herman BOERHAAVE (1668–1738), Dutch physician, Leyden, professor of theory of medicine, botany, chemistry; Thomas Blizard CURLING (1811–1888), British surgeon, London, described ulcerations of the stomach in burn patient, 1842; Hakaru HASHIMOTO (1881–1934), Japanese pathologist, Tokyo, described thyroiditis, 1912; Sir Arthur Frederic HURST (1879–1944) British gastroenterologist, London; Frank Burr MALLORY (1862–1941), American pathologist, Boston; Pierre Eugene MENÉTRIER (1859–1935), French physician, Paris; Soma WEISS (1899–1942), German-American physician, Boston, Hersey Professor of Medicine, Harvard University.

SELECTED REFERENCES

Berry EM, Ben-Dov Y, Freund U. Spontaneous remission of protein-losing gastropathy associated with Menetrier's disease. A plea for conservative management. Arch Intern Med 140:99–100, 1980.

Citrin Y, Sterling K, Halsted JA. Mechanism of hypoproteinemia associated with giant hypertrophy of gastric mucosa. N Engl J Med 257:906–12, 1957.

Colcher H. Guidelines for fiberoptic examination in upper gastrointestinal bleeding. Adv Int Med 20:399–423, 1975.

Davenport HW. A digest of digestion, 2nd ed. Year Book Medical Publishers Chicago, 1978.

Hurst AF, Stokes A. Case of hypertrophic gastritis (gastritis polyposa): recovery after gastrectomy. Guys Hosp Rep 76:351–61, 1926.

Kivilaakso E, Silen W. Pathogenesis of experimental gastric-mucosal injury. N Engl J Med 301:364–69, 1979.

McCarthy DM. Report on the United States' experience with cimetidine in Zollinger-Ellison syndrome and other hypersecretory states. Gastroenterology 74:453–58, 1978.

MacLaurin BP. The stomach-pernicious anaemia and gastritis. In: Asquith P. Immunology of the gastrointestinal tract. Edinburgh: Churchill Livingstone, 1979:55–65.

Mallory GK, Weiss S. Hemorrhages from lacerations of the cardiac orifice of the stomach due to vomiting. Am J Med Sci 178:506–15, 1929.

Menetrier P. Des polyadenomes gastriques et de leurs rapports avec le cancer de l'estomac. Arch de Physiol Norm et Path (4th ser), 1:236–62, 1888.

Peterson WL, Barnett CC, Smith HJ et al. Routine early endoscopy in upper-gastrointestinal-tract bleeding. A randomized, controlled trial. N Engl J Med 304:925–29, 1981.

Shearman DJC, Finlayson NDC, Wilson R, et al. Carcinoma of the stomach and early pernicious anemia. Lancet 2:403–5, 1966.

Silen W, Skillman JJ. Stress ulcer, acute erosive gastritis and the gastric mucosal barrier. Adv Int Med 19:195–212, 1974.

Sleisinger MH. Illuminating the antrum. N Engl J Med 300:1436–37, 1979.

Smith, BM, Skillman JJ, Edwards BG, et al. Permeability of the human gastric mucosa. Alteration by acetylsalicylic acid and ethanol. N Engl J Med 285:716–21, 1971.

Strickland RG, Mackay IR. A reappraisal of the nature and significance of chronic atrophic gastritis. Am J Dig Dis 18:426–40, 1973.

Vandelli C. Bottazzo GF, Doniach D, et al. Autoantibodies to gastrin-producing cells in antral (Type B) chronic gastritis. N Engl J Med 300:1406–10, 1979.

Zollinger RM, Ellison EH. Primary peptic ulcerations of the jejunum associated with islet cell tumors of the pancreas. Ann Surg 142:709–28, 1955.

DISCUSSION QUESTION

A 40-year-old woman with mild epigastric discomfort after meals and tiredness for six months has a normal physical examination. Urinanalysis is normal, hematocrit 30 percent, stools negative for occult blood. An upper gastrointestinal series is negative. Because of persistent symptoms a gastroscopy is performed and diffuse mucosal atrophy is found in the fundus and body of the stomach. What further studies should be performed? How should this patient be followed?

CHAPTER 6

The Pathophysiology of Peptic Ulcer

We have seen that the major exocrine secretions of the gastric mucosa are hydrochloric acid, two families of pepsinogens, and several varieties of mucus. Acidity facilitates the conversion of pepsinogens to their active proteolytic forms, and provides the optimal pH levels for these enzymes to perform their work. Mechanisms for controlling the rate and quantity of acid and pepsin secretion are complex and often interdependent. They involve the stimulatory effects of the vagi, gastrin, and entero-oxyntin, and the inhibitory effects of the various enterogastrones (such as vasoactive intestinal peptide (VIP), gastric inhibitory peptide (GIP), and somatostatin), secretin, cholecystokinin, and possibly a chalone produced in the gastric antrum itself. The elements that drive these stimulatory and inhibitory effects are not clearly understood and involve genetic, environmental, and experiential factors. The net result is that the secretion of acid varies from person to person, depending among other things on the oxyntic cell mass, and patterns of secretion vary from time to time in any one individual, depending on the state of hunger or emotional stress, diet to a certain extent, and the coexistence of certain diseases. Those effects which increase the production of acid and pepsin can be considered to be *ulcerogenic*, while those which reduce their secretion are felt to be *mucoprotective*.

Prime among the elements that serve to protect the mucosa of the stomach and duodenum from damage are the rapidity with which gastric epithelium above the foveolar neck replaces itself and the cytoprotective effects of mucosal prostaglandins. Other protective factors include the alkalinity of the lamina propria, the adequacy of mucosal blood flow, the rate and quality of the mucus secreted in the upper digestive tract, and the alkalinity of Brunner glandular secretion in the duodenal mucosa. When cytoprotection is reduced by the administration of prostaglandin-inhibiting agents, or when epithelial mitosis is arrested by the administration of RNA destructive agents, such as the alkylating drugs used in the chemotherapy of cancer, mucosal damage is likely to ensue. Erosion or ulceration of gastric or duodenal mucosa can then be considered to be the result of an increase of ulcerogenic factors, a decrease in mucoprotective factors, or both. The lesions are termed *peptic* ulcers or erosions if they appear in mucosa exposed to acid-peptic secretions.

EXPERIMENTAL PEPTIC ULCERS AND EROSIONS

In order to determine the mechanisms by which the upper gastrointestinal tract may become susceptible to peptic injury and to measure the preventive or therapeutic effects of various chemical agents, peptic lesions have been produced experimentally in a variety of animals. Unfortunately, most of the lesions so induced have been acute ones, either erosions or ulcers, most are located in the stomach, and most heal without scarring. Thus, they differ considerably from the most common peptic lesion of humans, which is a chronic cicatricial ulceration of the first portion (bulb) of the duodenum. However, these experimental lesions have suggested mechanisms by which mucosal injury occurs acutely and leave one with the impression that they might well presage more chronic lesions.

Spontaneous Peptic Ulcers in Animals

Spontaneously occurring acid peptic disease in animals is extremely rare. However, Brodie (1968) observes that 80 to 100 percent of a strain of inbred mice develop peptic ulcers within 26 months of life. The incidence of spontaneous esophagogastric ulcers in swine is also considerable, but this may be due to restraint or nutritional factors rather than to hereditary predisposition.

Induced Hypersecretion of Acid and Pepsinogen

Gastroduodenal ulcers can be produced regularly in dogs and other animals given prolonged treatments with histamine. The effect is increased by the simultaneous administration of carbachol, which is a strong muscarinic stimulant of acid secretion in dogs. Among rats pretreated with histamine and a liquid diet, immersion stress produces a high incidence of ulcers and a decrease in mucosal DNA (Takuchi and Johnson 1979). However, the use of pentagastrin instead of histamine in doses producing equivalent amounts of acid results in a significantly lower ulcer index and a much smaller fall in mucosal DNA after stress. This difference is believed to be the result of trophic and cytoprotective effects of gastrin, not shared by histamine.

Pyloric ligation in rats commonly leads to the hypersecretion of acid, perforating ulcers in the proximal gastric rumen, and hemorrhagic erosions in the distal glandular stomach. These lesions are prevented by vagotomy, anticholinergics, and drugs which block peptic activity. Methylated prostaglandins also greatly reduce their incidence (Robert et al 1976).

Deviations of duodenal secretions to the lower small intestine and gastroenterostomy produce gastric hypersecretion followed within a few weeks by deep, perforating ulcers at the stoma in dogs (Mann and Williamson, 1923). The mechanism of the hypersecretion is not clear, but it may be related to the decrease in the size of the bile acid pool resulting from the operation.

Induced Stress

Central nervous system effects have been shown to be capable of producing duodenal erosions in some Rhesus monkeys forced into a pattern of avoidance behavior. Twelve hours daily for four weeks, each of nine animals was restrained and subjected to a regular electrical shock which could be avoided only by pressing an easily accessible lever. The two animals whose acid-secretory levels were the highest in the group developed duodenal erosions (Polish et al 1962). Similarly, acute hemorrhagic stress erosions are seen in a large proportion of rats subject to tight restraint for 4 to 24 hours, the frequency of erosions being proportional to the degree of restraint and being greater if restraint is carried out during the night, a time when rats are most active physically. The severity of these lesions is reduced greatly by prestress vagotomies, anticholinergic drugs, methylated prostaglandins, and tranquilizers.

Engel (1974) has summarized work by Ader which indicates that restraint ulcers occur more frequently in rats with high levels of circulating pepsinogen, who have been raised in groups rather than singly, and who have not been handled in the preweaning period. It has also been shown that restrained rats subjected to recurring electrical shocks are less likely to develop ulcers when they have a lever handy by which they can prevent the shocks. Stress ulcers are then multifactorial in etiology, depending on the genetic makeup of the animal, early care, upbringing, and reaction to the stressful situation. Engel concludes that one of the important psychological factors contributing to lowered disease resistance is "loss of the ability of the organism to predict and maintain control over its environment." But even such major losses in independence as this are more stressful in some animals than in others.

The application of these observations to the human condition is clear. They indicate a number of the complexities involved in our attempts to understand the pathogenesis of the peptic ulcer diathesis.

Induced Damage to the Gastric Mucosal Barrier

The fact that aspirin can breach the mucosal barrier of the stomach, permit an increase in the back-diffusion of acid, and lead to gastric erosions has already been discussed. The administration of aspirin can cause gastric erosions in both large and small laboratory animals, whether the drug is given orally or intravenously. These erosions can be prevented by a previously performed vagotomy, by administering the aspirin in liquid form with antacids, and by previous ligation of the common bile duct. The latter procedure leads to a reduction of gastric acid secretion (Guth et al 1976), probably by preventing the reflux of biliary taurocholate, a stimulant of gastrin release, into the gastric antrum (Sekine et al 1980). Aspirin also inhibits prostaglandin synthetase, but it is not clear whether this effect relates to its ulcerogenic properties. Other nonsteroidal anti-inflammatory agents such as indomethacin, naproxen, and ibuprophen can also cause gastric erosions in humans and animals, but their ability to breach the gastric mucosal barrier has not been fully demonstrated. Ethanol, and bile acids as well, also disrupt the mucosal barrier of the stomach and produce gastric erosions, but have not been widely used in the study of experimental ulceration.

PATHOGENESIS OF PEPTIC ULCER

It has been estimated that at some time in the lives of 5 to 10 percent of the population of the Unites States and Great Britain resistance to peptic ulceration is overcome. Ulcers appear most commonly in the duodenal bulb, less often in the stomach. Approximately 70 percent of peptic ulcers are duodenal, 20 percent gastric (three-fourths in the antrum, and one-fourth in the remainder of the stomach), 7 to 8 percent in the esophagus among patients with gastroesophageal reflux, 1 to 2 percent beyond the duodenal bulb, and the remainder occur as anastomotic or marginal ulcers in the jejunum following a surgically established gastrojejunostomy. Mendeloff (1974) has described an "endemic" of duodenal ulcer which commenced in the 1930s and started to decline in the 1960s, to the point where it now seems to be half as great as it was a few decades ago.

Classification of Peptic Ulcer Patients

Patients with peptic ulcer can usually be distinguished as falling into one of two categories (Table 6–1) on the basis of functional, demographic, sexual, and genetic characteristics. Most patients with duodenal ulcer and most with ulcers in the gastric antrum could be placed in what might be called category A. These are usually associated with increased oxyntic cell

Table 6–1. Classification of Peptic Ulcer Patients

	Category A	*Category B*
Location of ulcer	duodenal bulb, antrum	body of stomach, some in bulb some in antrum
Oxyntic mass, acid output	increased	normal to decreased
Serum pepsinogen I	increased	normal
Serum gastrin		
Fasting	normal	elevated
Postprandial	elevated	—
Family history	positive	usually negative
Age of onset	1st-4th decades	beyond 5th decade
Sexual predominance	men > women	men = women
Associated gastritis	normal frequency	increased
Ulcerogenic drugs	normal frequency	increased
Stress factors	increased	normal frequency

mass, increased peak acid output, higher levels of serum pepsinogen I, more disposition to occur also among first-degree relatives and among men, and less chronic gastritis. Category B would include the remainder of patients with gastric ulcers, primarily those in the body of the stomach, and less than 35 percent of patients with duodenal ulcer. In these patients there is either a normal or reduced oxyntic cell mass and peak acid output, normal pepsinogen I levels, little familial clustering, approximately equal incidence among men and women, and a high incidence of ulcerogenic drug ingestion and associated chronic gastritis. Emotional stresses seems to be greater in category A patients. In this category, the increased secretion of acid and pepsin appears to be of more pathogenetic consequence than is a decrease in mucosal resistance; in category B the opposite is true. It is important to keep clearly in mind, however, that all patients with peptic ulcers must be secreting at least small amounts of acid, and that all must have passed the limits of mucosal resistance. A small number of patients with benign gastric ulcer and apparent anacidity have been described, but their very rarity suggests that the ulcers are probably not truly peptic lesions. This classification of peptic ulcers attempts to distinguish them more on a pathogenetic than an anatomical basis.

Genetic Factors. These include levels of serum gastrin and pepsinogen I, ABO blood types, and HLA types. Fasting serum gastrin levels tend to be normal in category A (duodenal) ulcer patients and elevated in category B patients, reflecting in the latter group probable chronic gastritis leading to higher antral pH levels and increased antral G cell secretion. After meals, however, serum gastrin levels rise to well above normal in category A patients, indicating increased sensitivity of the gastrin secretory mechanism to protein stimulation. It has been suggested also that patients with duodenal ulcers tend to respond less well to mechanisms which normally inhibit gastrin secretion. Thus, Walsh et al (1975) showed that such patients respond to acidification of the antrum with less than half of the acid secretory inhibition seen in normal subjects. This finding, however, has been disputed (Thompson and Swierczek 1977).

Group I pepsinogens are secreted only in the oxyntic mucosa, and Samloff et al (1975) have presented evidence that serum pepsinogen I levels parallel peak acid output levels in about two-thirds of patients with duodenal ulcers. There is also some evidence that first-degree relatives of some duodenal ulcer patients have higher than normal levels of pepsinogen I and that this tendency seems to fit the criteria for a hereditary autosomal dominant characteristic (Rotter et al 1979). This measurement may turn out to be a useful screening test for ulcer susceptibility among relatives of category A patients. The fact that many patients with duodenal ulcer do not have hyperpepsinogenemia supports the notion that numerous factors are involved in its etiology.

Blood type A, B, and H glycoproteins are secreted into the gastric mucus and in saliva by nearly 80 percent of all persons studied. Nonsecretors who also have blood type O have been shown to have a 50 percent greater risk of developing duodenal ulcers than do persons with other blood types. Type O secretors show a lesser, but still distinctly increased risk. Rotter et al (1977) have also shown that individuals with HLA type B5 show a thrice-normal incidence of duodenal ulcer when compared to age-matched controls of other HLA types. How these two observations interrelate among themselves, and with other factors such as oxyntic cell mass, is not known. But they do indicate that certain members of the population carry hereditary tendencies which increase their hazard of developing category A ulcers.

Demography. There is clearly something curious about the apparent decrease now being noted in the incidence of duodenal ulcer in America and Great Britain. During 1970-78 hospitalizations for duodenal ulcer decreased 43 percent in the United States, deaths from peptic ulcer decreased 31 percent and the male:female ratio has fallen to 1.2 for hospitalizations (Elashoff and Grossman 1980). It is also noteworthy that gastric ulcer was so much more common and duodenal ulcer almost an oddity at autopsy at the turn of the century. The incidence of duodenal ulcer is considerably higher in urban than in rural inhabitants; there is a male predominance for the disease although the incidence among employed women, particularly those with family responsibilities, appears to be rising; and there is no particular occupational clustering. There are some areas of the world in which the prevalence of gastric ulcer is much greater than duodenal ulcer, such as in Japan and Chile. It is interesting that these countries also show higher incidences of gastric cancer as well, indicating that the chronic gastritis that is so prevalent in both patients with gastric ulcer and gastric carcinomas may be of etiologic importance in both disorders. The prevalence of cigarette smoking and alcoholism probably also have a positive effect on the incidence of peptic ulcer. Approximate prevalence rates for all peptic ulcers are about 7 percent among men and 2 percent among women, at least in Western Europe and the United States (Mendeloff and Dunn 1971). The mortality rates from duodenal ulcer in the United States during 1958–1964 were 4.7 per 100,000 population among men, 1.4 among women, and from gastric ulcer 4.5 among men and 1.8 among women.

Associated Diseases. Much has been made of the increased incidence of peptic ulcers in patients with chronic obstructive lung disease, cirrhosis of the liver, and rheumatoid arthritis. It is not clear what etiologic significance these associations have, although it is possible that alcohol and a number of medications taken for treatment of other disorders may have induced the ulcer problem. Alcohol and certain of the anti-inflammatory agents are capable of breaching the gastric mucosal barrier, while glucocorticoids and aminophylline are known to cause digestive symptoms but have not been shown to be ulcerogenic. The presence of vascular shunts that bypass hepatocytes in patients with cirrhosis of the liver may lead to higher serum gastrin levels and increased acid secretion.

Psychosomatic factors are clearly related to the activation of ulcer symptoms in some patients, particularly those with category A lesions, and perhaps contribute also to their chronicity. But no one has truly demonstrated the extent of this influence. Patients frequently describe a deep emotional conflict, or feelings of depression or frustration immediately preceding the onset of an ulcer attack, and resolution of these stresses may hasten recovery. Clearly, there is no single personality type which increases the liability to peptic ulcer. It is most likely that emotional trials are merely one of a number of variables already described which participate in the pathogenesis of the disease, for just as there are many ulcer patients under stress preceding an attack, there are a considerable number as well in whom no such pressures can be documented.

Pathology of Peptic Ulcer

A mucosal interruption in the stomach or duodenum is called a peptic ulcer only if it is deep enough to penetrate through the entire mucosa. Any lesser penetration is called an erosion. This distinction is of considerable clinical importance because erosions cannot usually be detected by radiography and are much less likely to be associated with recurrences.

Grossly, an ulcer is a discontinuity of mucosal surface with an inflammatory base. Erosions tend to be soft as well as superificial with an infiltration of neutrophilic leukocytes, whereas chronic ulcers tend to be deep and firm with lymphocytic infiltration and conspicuous fibrosis. As previously related, acute erosions in the stomach are common, multiple, superficial, and transient, healing without scarring. The chronic gastric or duodenal ulcer is entirely different. It tends to be single, deep, firm, and persistent and is associated with massive scarring. Whereas almost all acute ulcers are self-healing, chronic ulcers are more likely to be persistent, seriously distressing to the patient, difficult at times to treat, and attended by more chronic complications.

The chronic ulcer (Figure 6–1) in the stomach occurs principally along the lesser curvature, usually in antral mucosa and often at the junction of the antrum with the foveolar mucosa. The shape is round or oval. The size is usually small, with most measuring around 1 cm in diameter. Although an occasional ulcer is large and referred to as a giant ulcer, analysis reveals that 50 percent measure less than 2 cm in diameter and 75 percent are accommodated within a diameter of 3 cm. The rim is firm and only slightly raised, with the edges at times overhanging the tissue beneath. The rim is also uniform throughout its entire circumference, thus distinguishing a benign from a malignant lesion. The base is deep and the walls are steep in benign lesions; carcinomatous ulcers tend to be shallower and more spreading with less steep walls. The proteolytic activity of gastric juice tends to digest debris, so that the surface of the ulcer base is either clean or contains a smooth whitish yellow exudate. When the ulcer has penetrated deeply, it

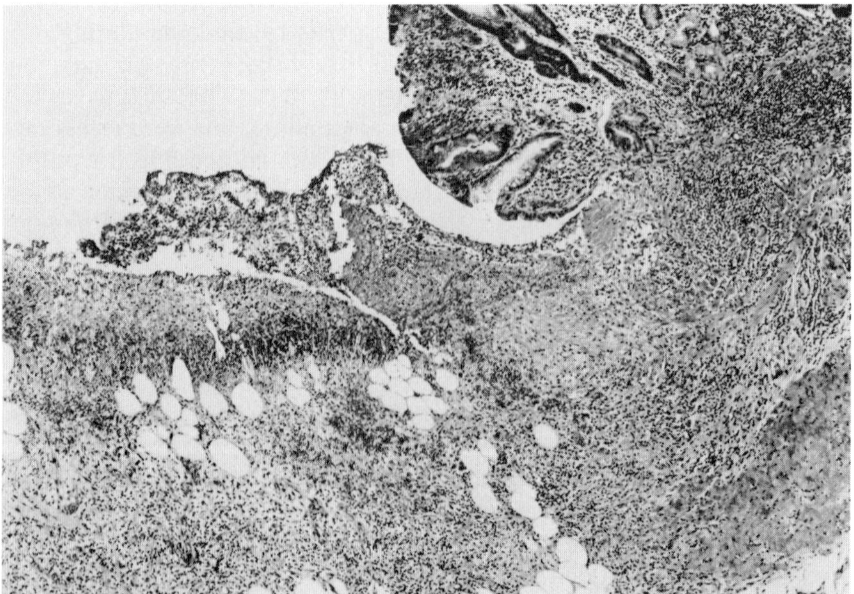

Figure 6–1. Chronic gastric ulcer of antrum. Original magnification x50.

is often possible to identify muscle fibers or pancreatic lobules in the base by gross examination. When the proteolytic activity encounters an artery, its wall may also be eroded, and the ruptured vessel is often clearly apparent at the ulcer base.

Microscopically, a chronic ulcer regularly reveals four distinct layers which can be seen on scanning power view of the transected surface (Figure 6–2):

1. The most superficial, proceeding from the mucosal side, is a layer of exudate consisting of masses of polymorphonuclear leukocytes interlaced with strands of fibrin.
2. Beneath this a layer of necrotic debris that is amorphous and deeply eosinophilic. This layer is finely particulate, and specific cells are not identifiable.

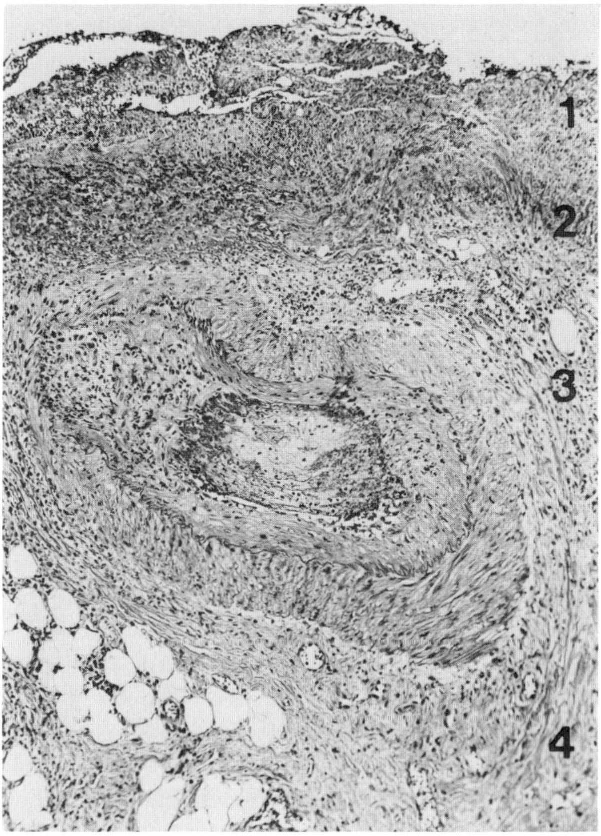

Figure 6–2. Bed of chronic gastric ulcer. There are four distinct layers: (1) neutrophilic exudate, (2) necrotic debris, (3) granulation tissue, and (4) scar. A thrombosed artery with arteritis is shown in the center. Original magnification x80.

3. Under this is a granulation layer composed of loose areolar tissue infiltrated with delicate capillaries. Granulation tissue signifies the presence of an active reparative process.
4. The deepest layer of the chronic ulcer is the scar. This constitutes the base and sides of the defect and gives the lesion its firm consistency. The dense fibrous tissue of the scar interrupts the external muscle layers, overlies the base, and extends for a short distance laterally through the gastric or duodenal wall and to the serosa, which becomes scarred if the surface is free, or adherent to some adjacent structure if it is not.

In summary, the four regular layers which form when the ulcer is chronic are exudate, necrosis, granulation, and scar.

Two other changes are commonly present in the base or margins of the ulcer wall. One is an arteritis, the other neuritis. Both of these terms refer to a fibrous proliferation that arises in the subintimal layer of arterial walls and encompasses nerves, probably in response to long-standing inflammation. Clinically, the neuritis may be a cause of ulcer pain, and the arteritis may limit the extent of hemorrhage in the event of arterial erosion. These changes are usually seen in the marginal tissue of the ulcer.

It is characteristic of peptic ulcers that they heal with scarring. The scar is a focus of dense fibrous tissue that radiates outward from a central nidus, which was previously the site of the ulcer base. The mucosa has extended over the surface, but usually has fewer glands than normal mucosa, and the base has filled in with connective tissue. Not infrequently, a band of connective tissue extends outward from the ulcer site and on contraction of this scar, a permanent indentation of the gastric or duodenal contour is formed. When this process becomes pronounced in the stomach, especially after the healing of giant gastric ulcers, a circular constriction may develop around the entire circumference of the stomach, dividing it into two chambers connected by a much narrower passageway. When seen on X ray, this dual chamber contour is referred to as an hourglass stomach. A similar process in the first portion of the duodenum leads to a deformity of the duodenal bulb, which gives it the contours of a three-leafed clover, easily demonstrable also on radiography (Figure 6–3). Such scarring is a hallmark of previous ulceration in that area.

The Zollinger-Ellison syndrome is usually associated with extensive mucosal hypertrophy of the glandular portions below the foveolar neck in the proximal stomach. Multiple duodenal and jejunal ulcers are commonly found. In patients with G cell hyperplasia, cells which stain positively with gastrin antiserum are seen in increased numbers in the antral mucosa. In patients with gastrinomas in the pancreas or elsewhere, the tumors contain sheets of cells resembling normal antral G cells, cells containing atypical granules, or mixture of typical and atypical cells. Some agranular cells are also seen. These cells produce G 13, G 17, and G 34 (Dawson 1976).

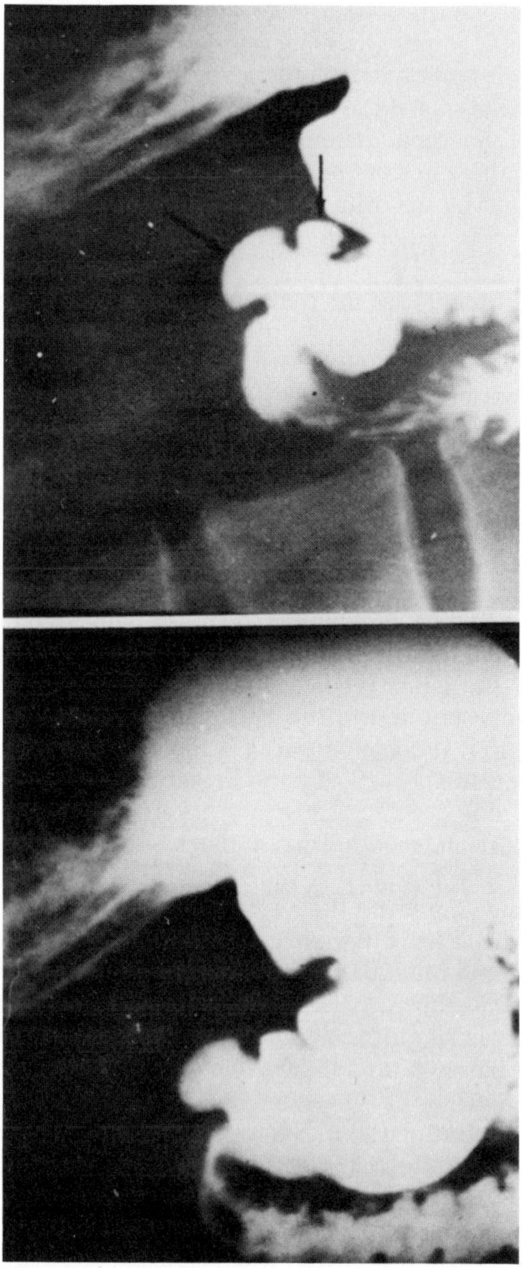

Figure 6-3. Cloverleaf deformity of the duodenal bulb due to scarring from previous ulceration. Two projections (arrows) change in configuration in various exposures and represent pseudodiverticula. From Stein GN, Finkelstein AK, Markowitz RI. In: Bockus HL, ed. Gastroenterology, vol 1, 3rd ed. Philadelphia: WB Saunders, 1974:671. Reprinted by permission.

Symptoms

In evaluating symptoms in patients with peptic ulcer, it is essential to recall that as many as one-third or more of patients have no particular symptoms until an actual complication, such as hemorrhage or perforation, occurs. That so many patients are asymptomatic is not difficult to understand considering that the gastric and duodenal mucosa are not supplied with pain-sensory fibers. Visceral distention may cause a variety of discomfort, but true pain probably does not occur until sensory nerves deep in the visceral wall are irritated by the inflammatory process, or until the ulceration has penetrated to adjacent viscera, such as the pancreas or the underside of the liver.

Students are often taught that the pain of ulcer disease is intermittent, relieved promptly by meals or antacids, recurs two to three hours after meals, and commonly awakens patients during the night. The pain is said to be localized to the uppermost portion of the epigastrium, just below the xiphoid process of the sternum, and it may radiate directly through to the back, especially in patients whose ulcers have penetrated into the pancreas. To a certain extent, this description is valid, but there is great variability of symptoms between patients.

Abdominal Pain. The important feature about pain in patients with peptic ulcer—and this appears to be true whether the ulcer is located in the stomach or the duodenum, since the two cannot be distinguished on symptomatic grounds alone—is that the primary discomfort appears in the *upper* abdomen rather than being confined to the epigastrium, that it does indeed tend to be intermittent, that it commonly wakes the patient from sleep, and that it is usually relieved temporarily by the ingestion of antacids, but not necessarily by meals (Table 6–2).

One of the studies performed on this subject is reported by Earlham (1976) who interviewed 100 patients in the London Hospital with symptomatic duodenal ulcer and compared their complaints to those of a group of control patients hospitalized for minor surgical conditions unrelated to peptic ulcer, esophagitis, or gall bladder disease. The control group was similar to the ulcer group in every other way (sex, occupation, age, habits, etc.), except for weight, which was significantly lower in the study group. So much for an older notion that patients tend to be overweight because they "feed" their ulcers to relieve pain!

Earlham discovered that of 120 primary pain sites in the 100 patients, 81 were located in the upper epigastrium, 7 were in the lower epigastrium, 17 in the right and 3 in the left hypochondrium, and 12 in the umbilical area. Heartburn was a common secondary pain, and back pain, usually between the scapulae or in the upper lumbar area, was reported as a secondary site 48 times.

Periodicity of pain was reported in 85 patients, although it did not always disappear completely during periods of remission. Worry tended to

Table 6-2. Characteristics of Pain in Peptic Ulcer

1.	located in abdomen above umbilical level
2.	may be predominantly right or left sided, or central
3.	frequently penetrates to back
4.	commonly occurs during sleep
5.	tends to wax and wane or disappear
6.	temporarily relieved by antacids
7.	aggravated by worry
8.	not necessarily seasonal or relieved by meals

aggravate symptoms in three-fourth of the patients, but vacations did not seem to provide relief. Neither was there any great seasonal variation of symptoms.

Patients felt that a wide variety of foods caused aggravation of pain. Pastry and fried foods were commonly indicted, but gravies, beer, chocolate, coffee, and tea were not considered to be common offenders. A bland diet was helpful to only about 20 percent of patients. Antacids, however, relieved symptoms rapidly in 76 of 88 patients.

Nocturnal pain is indeed a common complaint among patients with ulcer. Eighty-eight percent of Earlham's patients and none of his controls noted this discomfort.

Family history of duodenal ulcer among first- and second-degree relatives was 46 percent among patients and only 8 percent in controls.

Thus, what one gains from this careful study of ulcer pain is that the location is usually upper abdominal, though the point of most intense pain is quite variable, that the intensity varies considerably during the day, that it is commonly relieved by antacids but not by food, and that it often wakes the patient from sleep. Rather surprisingly, pain is seldom aggravated by the ingestion of acid secretagogues, such as ethyl alcohol and caffeine. I have, in fact, interviewed many patients whose ulcer pain is relieved by alcohol and coffee.

The cause of ulcer pain is not at all clear, adherents being found to support any of several notions: that it is due to hypermotility of the gastroduodenum, to acid bathing the ulcer crater, or to both. Intragastric drips of 0.1 N HCl have been shown to induce pain in patients with peptic ulcer, but so too have agents which increase motility. Oral antacids, which cause prompt symptomatic relief, unfortunately for this discussion both elevate intraluminal pH and slow motility, so the debate remains unsettled and perhaps even moot since, as will be seen, its resolution does not appear to be essential to providing an excellent treatment program.

Other Symptoms. Symptoms other than pain do not play a large part in the perception of peptic ulcer. As has been seen, heartburn is a common secondary complaint, while nausea is not. Patients will commonly note water brash that is either a reflux of acidic gastric contents without vomiting or increased salivation. However, this symptom also occurs without peptic ulcer. Vomiting, usually with relatively small volumes of gastric contents, may occur when pain is intense, and occasionally relieves the pain. It is not a common symptom and is to be distinguished from the massive vomiting associated with gastric retention or the bloody vomiting of arterial perforation, which are major complications of peptic ulcer. As already mentioned, loss of small amounts of weight is a frequent though not invariable symptom. Changes in bowel habits are similarly nonspecific, except for the major diarrhea often seen in patients with Zollinger-Ellison syndrome, usually malabsorptive in type and associated with loss of weight. At times, diarrhea may also be complained of by patients taking large doses of antacids containing magnesium. Constipation, on the other hand, may be reported by patients taking calcium or aluminium-containing antacids.

COMPLICATIONS OF BENIGN PEPTIC ULCER

Bleeding, perforation, and gastric retention are the major complications of peptic ulcer. Significant complications occur in about 30 to 40 percent of all patients.

Bleeding

Gastrointestinal bleeding is the most common complication of peptic ulcer, occurring in upward of 75 percent of patients at some time during the course of their illnesses. Most often, the degree of bleeding is mild, associated with no particular symptoms, and diagnosed only by finding occult blood in the stools or an iron deficiency type of microcytic hypochromic anemia. Peptic ulcer rarely causes continuous blood loss, but the effects of repeated small losses are cumulative and may reflect themselves in such symptoms as weakness, easy fatigability, and tachycardia on exertion. Major acute hemorrhages occur in about 25 to 30 percent of ulcer patients and are, of course, dramatic episodes. Chronic repetitive blood loss is usually the result of capillary bleeding adjacent to the ulcer, while massive hemorrhages result from erosions into submucosal arteries.

The rapidity of blood loss determines the patient's presenting symptoms. When the hemorrhage is heavy and rapid, the patient appears with signs of hypovolemia, varying from dizziness, sweating, and orthostatic hypotension to complete vascular collapse and shock. The bleeding may present clinically as hematemesis, during which the patient vomits either fresh blood or blood containing hemoglobin that has been changed into acid hematin by contact with gastric acid and thus appears to have a brown, or coffee-grounds color. On the other hand, blood may appear solely in the stools. Large volumes of blood entering the alimentary tract causes intestinal hypermotility, and the resulting stools may be dark red, usually having a strong foul odor. If the blood has remained in the intestinal tract for longer periods, which may be the case if bleeding is submassive, the resulting stools appear to be shiny black in color, resembling tar in sheen and consistency, a finding called melena. Although there are numerous other causes of upper gastrointestinal bleeding (see Chapter 5) when hemorrhage occurs in a patient known to have had a previous peptic ulcer or who has had prior symptoms compatible with ulcer, it is most likely due to an ulcer.

Tachycardia, oral dryness, air hunger, and hypotension vary directly with the extent of blood loss. Systolic pressure commonly increases during early stages of hypovolemia, associated with tachycardia. This widening of pulse pressure usually occurs before hypotension supervenes, except in older patients who are less likely to respond to blood loss with appropriate tachycardia. Since gastrointestinal bleeding is often severe enough to compromise coronary and renal blood flow, it is important to monitor urinary output and the electrocardiogram during severe hemorrhage. This is particularly true among patients over age 50 in whom cardiac, renal, and cerebral complications of hemorrhage are more frequent than in younger patients.

Perforation

Ulcer perforation is of two kinds: (1) that which occurs through the serosa and directly into the peritoneal cavity, a free perforation; and (2) that which occurs through the wall of the stomach or duodenum and into an adjacent viscus, such as the pancreas or liver, a confined perforation or penetration. Free perforations occur in 3 to 5 percent of all peptic ulcers; penetrations are considerably more common.

Free anterior perforation of a peptic ulcer causes immediate soiling of the peritoneal cavity by gastric and duodenal contents, leading to an acute chemical peritonitis from the action of acid, pepsin, bile acids, and pancreatic enzymes. This process spreads rapidly to involve the upper peritoneal cavity, although its extent is often limited to a degree by action of the greater omentum. Both visceral and parietal layers of the peritoneum become acutely inflamed, and since the latter is very well supplied with sensory receptors, the resulting pain is immediate and intense. There is associated marked reflex spasm of the striated musculature of the abdominal wall, which immediately develops the boardlike rigidity characteristic of this disorder. Because the contents of the stomach and duodenum are usually sterile, especially in patients with hyperacidity, the peritoneal exudate resulting from perforation is rarely infected during the first few hours after the perforation occurs. Bacterial contamination usually does appear within 12 hours, after which surgical closure of the perforation is more hazardous to the patient.

Because of the dramatic nature of symptoms associated with a free perforation, diagnosis is usually an easy matter, although it may be somewhat more obscure in a patient who has not had symptoms of peptic ulcer previously. The pain is most likely to be confused with the severe symptoms of acute pancreatitis or intestinal infarction, both of which may also cause acute peritonitis. Occasionally, acute cholecystitis may cause similar pain. Identification of rigidity of abdominal musculature, and of the absence of bowel sounds supports the impression of parietal peritonitis.

Since perforation of the alimentary tract, especially of the stomach or duodenum, is usually associated with the passage of air from the viscus into the peritoneal cavity, one can often substantiate the impression of perforation by noting tympanites on percussion over the liver, which is normally quite dull to percussion. An upright film of the abdomen (Figure 6–4), or a film taken with the patient lying on the right side (lateral decubitus), will commonly show free air in the abdominal cavity. These are much more sensitive studies than physical examination alone.

Posterior penetration of a peptic ulcer is a much more common complication than free perforation, probably because peptic ulcers are more

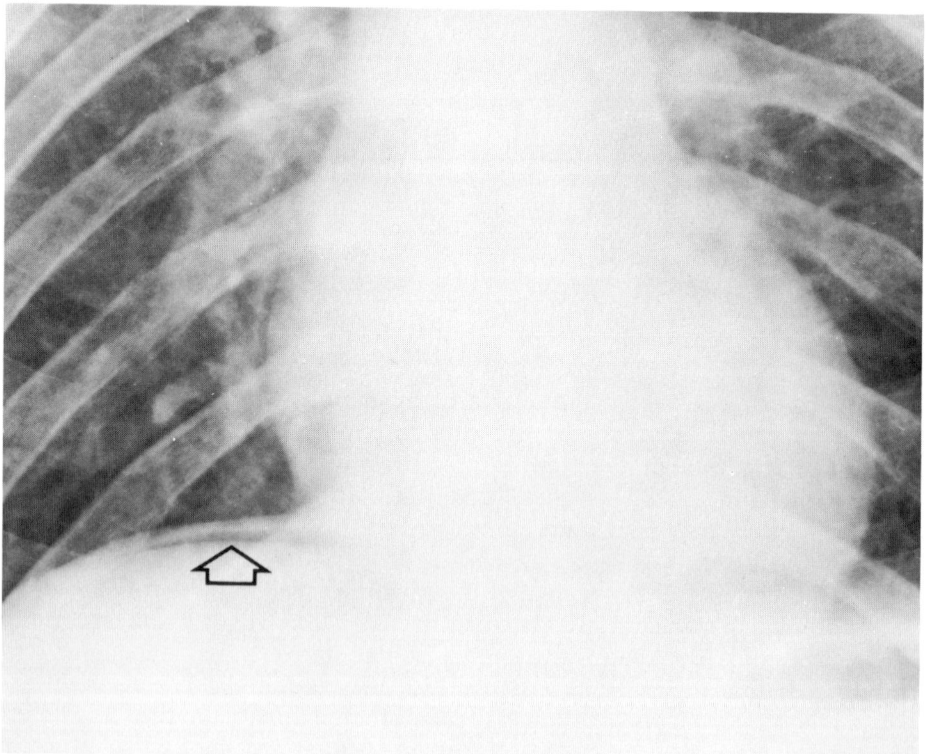

Figure 6–4. Perforation of duodenal ulcer. This upright film of the chest shows an accumulation of free air under the right leaf of the diaphragm, from anterior perforation of the ulcer.

commonly located on the posterior wall of the duodenum and stomach. This complication should be suspected when a patient's previous pain is replaced by a more intense, continuous pain most commonly located in the back. The increased focusing of pain is believed to be due to a shift from visceral to somatic receptors, the latter being more precise and more sensitive than the former. Pain is often so severe that the patient cannot stand or sit fully erect and tends to flex the spinal column. The pain of a posterior penetration is usually less responsive to antacids than is the pain of an uncomplicated ulcer.

Treatment of free perforations should be by surgical plication (closure) of the perforation as soon as possible. Whether a more definitive operation for ulcer, such as vagotomy and antrectomy, should be done at the same time is still debatable, but the availability of better medical therapy today probably makes surgery beyond simple plication unnecessary. Considerable therapeutic success has been attached to nonoperative therapy in patients whose perforations have occurred more than 12 hours prior to examination, and in older patients who may be less well able to tolerate an operation. This involves placing the patient on intravenous alimentation, constant nasogastric suction, and if needed, aerobic and anaerobic antibiotics. The rationale of this treatment is based on the knowledge that the greater omentum covers a perforation spontaneously after it occurs and may form a very effective seal, provided that simultaneous efforts are made to reduce intestinal secretions and contents and nutrition is adequate. Penetrations are often well managed by conventional, nonsurgical ulcer therapy. Surgery is considered only if this treatment is shown to be ineffective.

Gastric Retention

Between 10 and 20 percent of patients with peptic ulcer disease in the gastric antrum or duodenal bulb experience gastric retention of varying degrees. This is most commonly the result of mucosal edema and smooth muscle spasm in the pyloroduodenal area, and occasionally fibrotic strictures in this segment. The retention associated with edema and spasm is frequently responsive to medical therapy; that associated with scarring probably requires surgery, particularly when the antral or pyloric channel is narrowed to less than 0.5 cm in diameter.

Vomiting is one of the primary symptoms of gastric retention. The pattern of vomiting might differ considerably from patient to patient, depending somewhat on the functional activity of the stomach. If retention is associated with edema and inflammation and gastric muscular tone is good, vomiting is generally frequent and occurs soon after eating. Vomitus contains only food which has been recently ingested. If the obstruction is of longer duration, especially in patients with pyloric stenosis, gastric dilatation occurs after a time, and peristalsis weakens and may disappear. In such instances the patient may vomit infrequently, though copiously, the vomitus containing residues of food often eaten one or more days prior to the emesis. The patient may no longer experience ulcer pain, noting instead a discomfort after meals that increases with the amount of food eaten. This discomfort may be compensated for by reduction of the intake of food, resulting in loss of weight. Emesis or gastric suction causes great relief of the distress.

Patients with gastric retention often become quite dehydrated and suffer from electrolytic depletion. Loss of H^+ ions in the vomitus leads to alkalosis. A modest degree of hyponatremia also may occur, but this is limited by the exchange of Na^+ for H^+ in the gastric mucosa, and by increased release of aldosterone to conserve Na^+. Hypochloremia is severe in most cases, as is hypokalemia. K^+ is lost both in gastric contents and in the urine due to increased aldosterone release. Thus the characteristic metabolic picture in patients with advanced gastric retention is one of a metabolic hypochloremic, hypokalemic alkalosis. Azotemia may also be associated if circulating blood volume has been decreased enough to reduce renal blood flow, or if tubular damage has occurred as a result of hypokalemia.

Physical findings vary from almost none at all to marked dehydration, tetany, confusion, and even coma. There may also be evidence of recent loss of weight, and occasionally an ill-defined mass may be palpable in the epigastrium or left upper quadrant of the abdomen. It may also be possible in thin patients to see the outline of the mass against the abdominal wall and at times to see peristaltic waves moving from left to right in this area. A splashing sound may be elicited by grasping each iliac crest and suddenly shaking the supine patient. This succussion splash is produced by the presence of both air and water in the obstructed stomach. When present, tetany is due to alkalosis rather than to hypocalcemia.

Treatment involves gastric suction, replacement of fluid and electrolytes, and therapy of the underlying peptic disease. Decompression of the stomach often allows it to regain normal tone and peristaltic activity within 48 to 72 hours, especially when the gastric retention is due primarily to inflammation and edema. Gastric emptying can then be measured by use of the saline-loading test described earlier; if emptying appears to be adequate, conventional ulcer therapy can then be applied, though without the use of anticholinergic agents, since they may exacerbate the retention. It is my practice to perform an endoscopic examination after the suction period, for this is the most practical way to evaluate the diameter of the pyloroduodenal segment quickly and with minimal discomfort to the patient. Much hospital time can be saved by this procedure, since the likelihood that medical treatment will be successful is very small in those patients whose pyloric segments cannot be negotiated by the endoscope. These patients are better advised to have an early operation than to waste time in a trial of medical therapy.

THE SPECIAL PROBLEM OF GASTRIC ULCER

Distinctions between gastric and duodenal ulcers have already been considered in the discussion of categories A and B patients. The present discussion is confined primarily to patients with category B ulcers in whom gastric hyposecretion and chronic gastritis are commonly associated. The problem is to distinguish definitively between a benign peptic ulcer and a malignant ulcer.

Differential Diagnosis

Fortunately, this is much more precise at present than it has been in the past, largely because of advances in diagnostic techniques. The history is rarely useful in distinguishing benign from malignant gastric ulcers, since upper abdominal pain, relieved by antacids and aggravated at night, is common to both types of lesion. Gastric analysis is helpful only if there is total anacidity after maximal stimulation, this being strong evidence of malignancy. Hypochlorhydria, even if it is marked, does not rule out a benign ulcer, and hyperchlorhydria may occur with malignant lesions. Radiologic examination of the upper gastrointestinal tract may be quite definitive (Nelson 1969). The benign ulcer tends to be sharply demarcated from surrounding tissue, symmetrical, and deep, its apex often protruding beyond the margins of the gastric wall. The base of the ulcer is usually smooth, and there is often a ring of mucosa overhanging the mouth (Figure 6–5). Peristaltic waves often pass smoothly through the ulcerated area. The malignant lesion (Figure 6–6) is more likely to be irregular in outline, asymmetrical, shallow, and surrounded with a wall that is indurated and nonperistaltic. It is less likely to have the collar-button outline of the typical benign lesion. The rugal folds tend to run around a malignant ulcer, being spread apart by the underlying tumor, while they seem to radiate outward from a benign lesion, having been pulled together by the underlying scar (Table 6–3). Save for the fact that benign ulcers rarely occur on the greater curve of the stomach above the antrum, location of the lesions is not distinctive.

Endoscopy provides further basis for differential diagnosis by allowing a direct look at the lesion where, once again, the benign lesion is sharply punched out and symmetric with a smooth yellowish white exudate (Figure 6–7). Malignant ulcers are irregular in outline, often show nodularity in the surrounding mucosa, and produce a grayish green exudate, often containing small amounts of blood (Figure 6–8). The pattern of rugal folds is the same as that seen on X ray. Most endoscopists recommend that biopsies be taken from each quadrant of the rim of a gastric ulcer, since cancer may be detectable in only a small area. For this reason, some also like to take brushings of the ulcer base for cytologic study. Malignant cells are more deeply staining, show frequent mitotic figures, and have a high nuclear to cytoplasmic ratio.

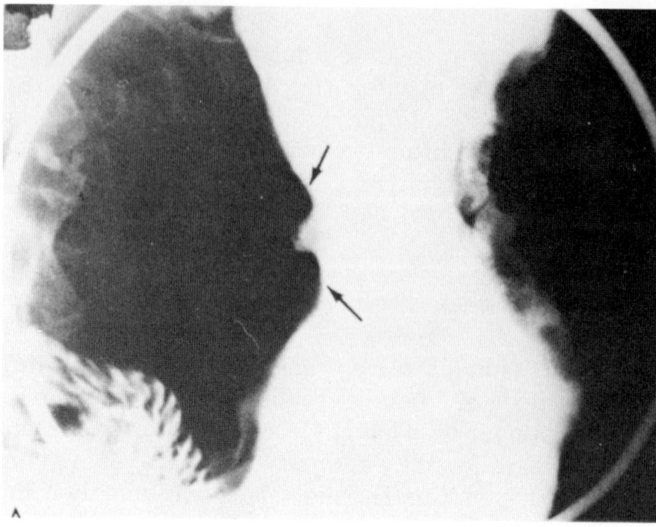

Figure 6–5. An ulcerating lesion is noted along the lesser curve of the body of the stomach. A narrow radiolucent band (Hampton line) parallels the base of the crater. Note the smooth, symmetrical concavities (ulcer mounds) above and below the crater. These signs indicate a benign ulcer. From Stein GN, Finkelstein AK, Markowitz RI. In: Bockus HL, ed. Gastroenterology, vol. 1, 3rd ed. Philadelphia: WB Saunders, Reprinted by permission.

With present diagnostic capabilities, it is possible to identify all but 1 or 2 percent of malignant ulcers at the time of initial studies. However, because some cancers will be missed by the most complete evaluation, it is advisable to follow the course of ulcer healing during treatment. A properly responding benign ulcer should show a 50 percent decrease in size after three weeks of therapy, and complete healing within eight weeks. If response is significantly slower than these rates, surgical resection is advisable. While most ulcers so removed turn out to have been benign, the operation has not been in vain, because such benign ulcers generally have a high rate of prompt recurrence, greater than 50 percent in the first year.

The response to therapy is measured by disappearance of symptoms, which should occur during the first week, and follow-up radiologic examinations. While malignant ulcers may rarely "heal" or disappear by X ray criteria, there is usually enough residual abnormality remaining, such as induration or tumor of the gastric wall, to make the examiner suspicious that all is not well, and that further studies are needed.

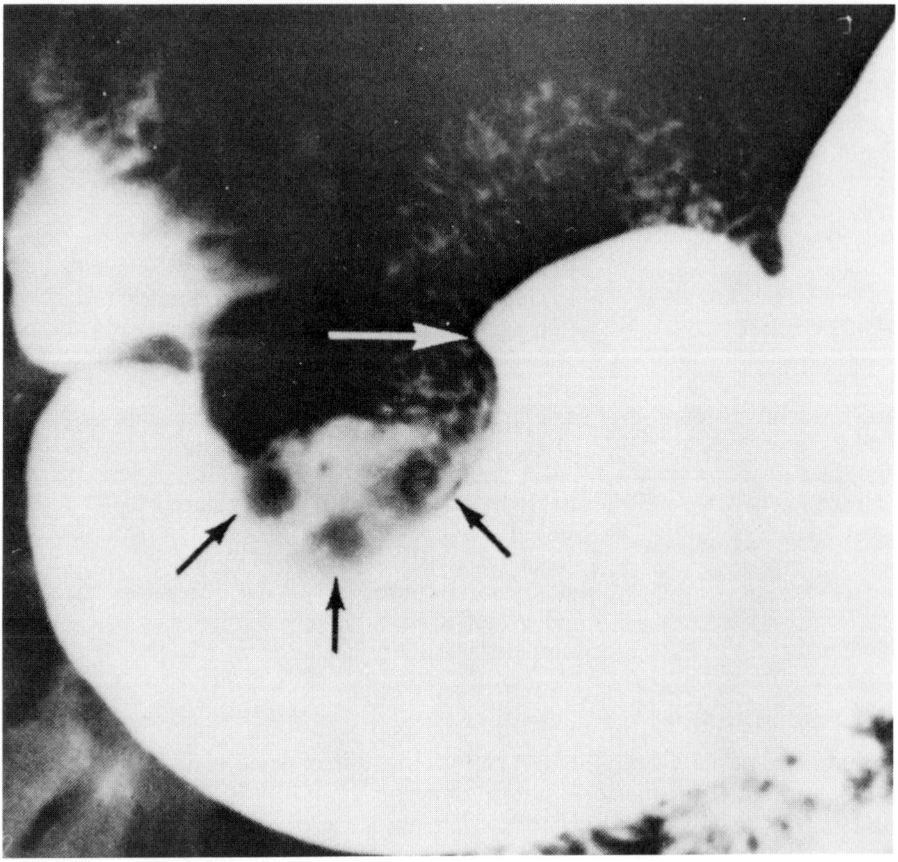

Figure 6-6. A prone radiograph of the gastric antrum showing an ulcerating carcinoma. The barium collection is irregular and does not extend outside the projected lumen of the stomach. It is surrounded by coarsely nodular and asymmetric radiolucent filling defects (arrows) that are sharply demarcated from the rest of the stomach. The mass makes a sharp angle with the adjacent gastric wall (vertical arrow). From Stein GN, Finkelstein AK, Markowitz RI. In: Bockus, HL, ed. Gastroenterology vol. 1, 3rd ed. Philadelphia: WB Saunders, 1974. Reprinted by permission.

Risk of Future Cancer

The problem of gastric ulcer is complicated by the fact that a number of patients develop carcinomas of the stomach many years following the appearance of the original lesion. It is unrealistic to suppose that the original ulcer was malignant and has just lain fallow for 15 to 20 years. It is more likely that metaplasia has occurred in the chronically inflamed gastric mucosa, followed by anaplasia, the ulcer being an early stage in this con-

Table 6–3. Radiologic Characteristics of Gastric Ulcers

	Benign	*Malignant*
Margins of crater	sharp, smooth, symmetric	irregular, nodular, asymmetrical
Rim of ulcer	overhanging, thin (Hampton line), or thick (collar-button deformity)	no overhanging rim
Walls and base of ulcer	smooth, usually symmetric	nodular, commonly asymmetric
Depth of crater	often penetrates beyond to normal gastric wall	rarely penetrates beyond gastric wall (ulcerated mass)
Tissue mound surrounding crater	smooth, rises gradually from surrounding gastric wall	often irregular, arises abruptly from gastric wall
Character of gastric wall	pliable	indurated
Rugal folds	radiate outward from tissue mound	separated by tissue mound
Peristalsis	usually normal through ulcerated area	not transmitted through area
Healing	often leaves a scar	rarely heals

tinuum, the cancer being a late manifestation. Severe antral gastritis and much evidence of intestinal metaplasia was found by Johansen (1976) in all but 2 of 64 cases of macroscopic carcinomas of the stomach, exophytic (fungating) and ulcerative.

THERAPEUTIC APPROACHES IN PEPTIC ULCER

As is true in other areas of endeavor, it is also useful in medical therapeutics to pause occasionally and reflect on where we are today, where we were yesterday, how we have arrived at the one point from the other, and where we are going. The treatment of peptic ulcer is a case in point. Older notions of care have been found to be wanting, and are being replaced by newer ideas and methods that seem to revolutionize therapy but may have drawbacks of their own. There is thus a need to look toward the future as well.

Previous Attitudes

At the close of World War II, a generation ago, diet, rest and antacids were the cornerstones of ulcer therapy. Acid-pepsin and an area of de-

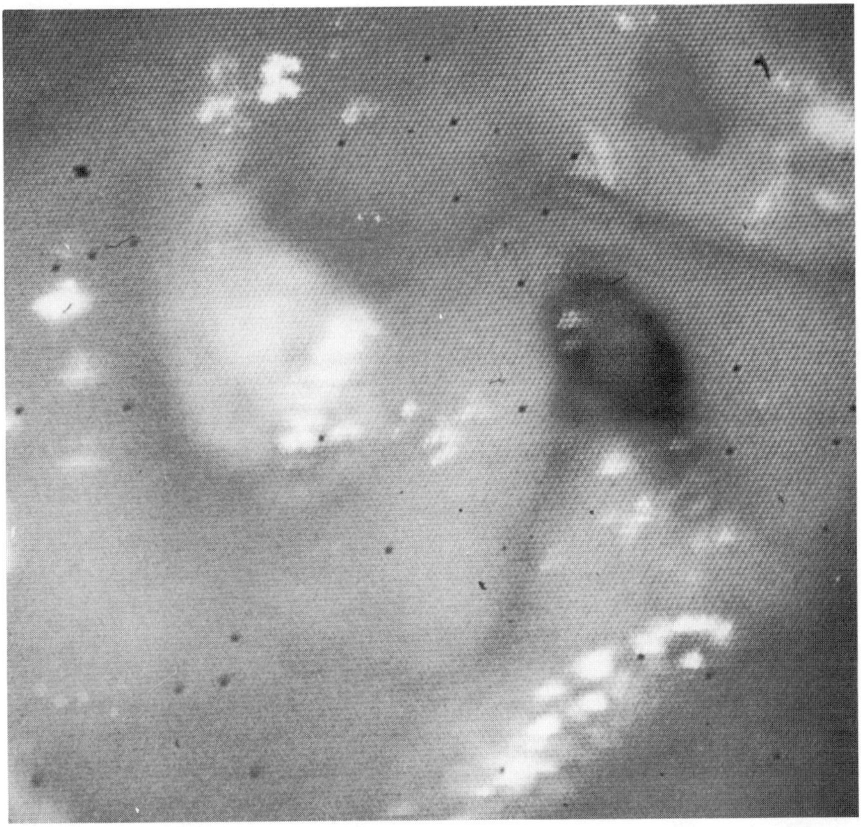

Figure 6-7. A benign antral ulcer seen by endoscopy just proximal to the pylorus. Ulcer edges are smooth and well defined, and homogeneous yellowish white exudate fills the crater.

creased resistance were felt to be the root causes of peptic ulceration, as they are today, and therapy was primarily directed at blocking the former, because very little was known about mucosal resistance and cytoprotection and the reasons that the normal stomach does not digest itself. Accordingly, numerous poorly absorbable antacids were made available and used heavily, preference being given to those containing calcium because of their higher neutralizing capacity and their relatively poor absorption, which served to prevent the onset of systemic alkalosis. Diet was also considered highly important: its blandness was believed to contribute to reduction of appetite-stimulated gastric secretion, and major secretagogues, such as caffeine, chocolate, meat proteins, alcohol, and spices, were forbidden. Feedings were kept small and frequent to avoid overdistention of the stomach and hunger.

The antisecretory effects of belladonna on both acid and pepsin secretion were well known, but therapeutic use of this drug and of atropine was

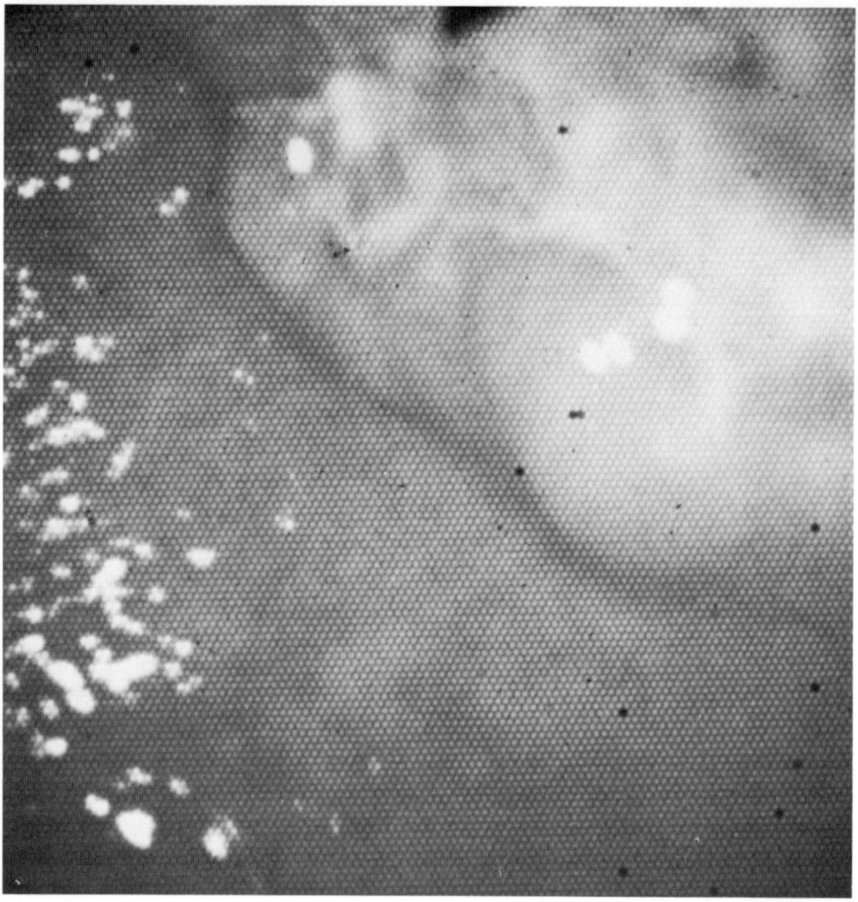

Figure 6–8. An ulcerating carcinoma in the fundus of the stomach. Note the tumor mass and the irregular borders of the ulceration. The floor of the crater appears to be uneven.

limited by its side effects. Physicians hoped that new anticholinergics that did not cause oral dryness or visual blurring would soon be synthesized. Propantheline, isopropamide, quarzan, glycopyrrolate, poldine, and many other synthetics did indeed emerge from pharmaceutical laboratories in the next 15 years, but they could not achieve more than a 35 percent reduction in postprandial gastric secretion without causing serious adverse effects. Accordingly, anticholinergics were never adopted uniformly into the therapeutic regimen for peptic ulcer, although many physicians did employ them especially to reduce nocturnal gastric secretion. It was a major disappointment when the analogs of histamine, discovered to have antihistaminic effects in the 1940s, were found incapable of reducing the effects of histamine on gastric secretion. It was concluded that histamine must produce its target effects through more than a single mechanism.

Psychosomatic factors assumed great importance in the post-war years, and stress was assumed to play a major part in the etiology of peptic ulcer. Accordingly, therapeutic regimens featured rest, reassurance, changes in lifestyles and often of jobs, and sedatives as prominent components.

The use of diet, rest, and antacids a generation ago was far from unsuccessful in treating peptic ulcer and allowed prominent gastroenterologists to speak glowingly of their results. Walter Lincoln Palmer, while pointing to the importance of a patient's cooperation in therapy and of "the physician's knowledge, personality, tact, enthusiasm, persistence, resourcefulness, and painstaking care," could conclude that, "in few chronic diseases are the results more definite or more gratifying."* Obviously, the treatment of peptic ulcer in those days required great stamina and dedication from both patient and physician, but the results could be favorable, although statistics were rarely given and most reports were anecdotal. Henry L. Bockus echoed Palmer's thoughts when he wrote, "I have stated repeatedly that the patient with uncomplicated duodenal or gastric ulcer will become symptom-free promptly on an adequate regimen and will remain so if intelligently followed-up for a period of six months to one year."** But despite these optimistic pronouncements, all clinicians were concerned about the rigorousness and extent of the recommended diets and about the high rate of recurrence of peptic ulcer, which ranged from 45 to 95 percent in five years. There was clearly room for improvement.

Present Attitudes

In evaluating the results of ulcer therapy today, it is of the utmost importance to recognize the indispensability of having parallel data on a simultaneously studied control population, matched as nearly as possible in age, sex, race, social status, and stage of disease with the patients being evaluated. One of the major problems confronting clinicians in the evaluation of newer therapies is the great natural tendencies which ulcers have to heal spontaneously. Thus, Scheurer et al (1977) have determined that among patients seen early in an ulcer attack and given only placebo therapy including antacids when wanted, the size of gastric ulcers will be reduced by one-half in 1.7 weeks, and of duodenal ulcers in 1.9 weeks. Twenty-seven percent of gastric ulcers and 53 percent of duodenal ulcers healed completely in less than three weeks, while in less than 6 weeks 83 percent of gas-

*Palmer WL. In: Portis SA. Disease of the digestive system, 2nd ed. Philadelphia: Lea and Febiger, 1944:234.

**Bockus HL. Gastroenterology, vol. 1, 1st ed. Philadelphia: WB Saunders, 1944:471.

tric ulcers and 73 percent of duodenal ulcers had healed. Lest too much be made of these results, it is important to remember that this study was done in only one center, on a limited group of patients, and that no data on recurrence rates are given. The data do, however, provide important information relating to the natural history of peptic ulcer in at least one community.

Diet. The discussion of diet by Bockus required 9 out of the 41 pages devoted to therapy of uncomplicated ulcer, and Palmer required 5 out of 13 pages. By contrast, one of the current textbooks of gastroenterology uses a half page to discuss dietotherapy and begins by stating, "No form of dietary treatment has been shown to be helpful in healing ulcers or preventing recurrences."* Smoking cigarettes and using aspirin are deplored, but even the use of coffee and alcohol, strictly forbidden in years past, has not been found to be critically harmful to the peptic ulcer sufferer.

The present state of dietary nihilism is based on results from a number of controlled studies (Buchman et al 1969) comparing healing of duodenal ulcers in patients on unrestricted diets with others on bland diets. Each shows no significant benefit from either dietary restrictions or small feedings, and rather thoroughly destroys those formerly supreme tenets of peptic ulcer therapy.

Rest. Easing tension, repose, placidity, and even hospitalization for the purpose of removing patients from daily aggravations are mentioned by earlier authors as prominent elements of therapy in uncomplicated peptic ulcer. But here again, a generation of experience has disclosed no particular benefit of rest in ulcer therapy, to the point where it is barely mentioned in modern texts. This is not to deny that anxiety and tension may exacerbate ulcer symptoms, for many patients do indeed note this association. It simply implies that other elements are of greater importance.

Antacids. Oral antacids continue to be relied on today in the treatment of ulcer, their use having been shown to be clearly beneficial in wide clinical experience. A carefully structured study (Peterson et al 1977) has documented their efficacy in healing duodenal ulcers in 78 percent of patients in four weeks, as compared with a 45 percent rate of healing among controls. There is a great deal of difference in neutralizing capacity among the many antacid preparations available commercially, and liquids appear to be much more effective than tablets. Calcium-containing antacids should be avoided because of the rebound hypersecretion which they often induce, due to the stimulation of gastrin release by the small amount of calcium absorbed from the intestine (Levant et al 1973).

Antacids must be ingested frequently enough throughout the day to maintain gastric pH levels about 4.0 to 4.5 most of the time. Their effects

*Sturdevant RAL, Walsh JH. In: Sleisinger MH, Fordtran JS. Gastrointestinal disease, 2nd ed. Philadelphia: WB Saunders, 1978:852.

vary directly with the time of gastric emptying. Each dose should be capable of neutralizing 100 mEq of HCl. Considerations of taste, bowel effects, and sodium content enter into the choice of specific antacids, and the volume of each dose will vary depending on the neutralizing capacity of the preparation selected.

Current Recommendations. For active gastroduodenal ulcers, a dose of antacid capable of neutralizing 100 mEq HCl should be ingested seven times daily, one and three hours after each meal and at bedtime, for eight weeks or until healing of ulcer is demonstrated radiographically. To minimize recurrence, it is advisable to give the same dose twice daily, indefinitely, thereafter. Whether this will fully avoid recurrences is not clear, but it will certainly reduce their frequency.

Toxicity of antacids is rarely of serious consequence today, although the diarrhea produced by large amounts of magnesium and the constipation caused by aluminum salts may occasionally become problems. These can usually be managed by adjusting the intake of these two elements as required. It is also important to recognize that aluminum hydroxide can interfere with the intestinal absorption of drugs administered simultaneously, especially of oral antibiotics. It is thus not advisable to give these drugs together.

Since aluminum-containing antacids also interfere with the absorption of phosphorus, it is important to monitor serum phosphorus levels in patients taking these medications for extended periods. Chronic hypophosphatemia may lead to osteomalacia and myopathy, the onset of which can be forestalled by adding phosphorus to the diet or by using phosphorus-substituted antacids. Since small amounts of aluminum are also absorbed from antacids and normally excreted into the urine, it is advisable to minimize the intake of aluminum-based antacids in patients with chronic renal failure, unless they are essential to reduce hyperphosphatemia. In uremics, aluminum can cross the brain barrier and has been implicated in the etiology of uremic encephalopathy.

Formerly, when absorbable antacids, such as bicarbonate of soda, and large amounts of milk were used in the therapy of peptic ulcer, the milkalkali syndrome was a common complication. Hypercalcemia followed by precipitation of calcium in renal tubules and renal insufficiency were the hallmarks of this iatrogenic illness. Today, alkalosis is rarely seen as a complication of using poorly absorbed antacids, and the incidence of hypercalcemia has been greatly reduced by the shift away from high calcium diets and calcium-containing antacids.

Antisecretory Drugs

Anticholinergic Agents. After more than a generation of trial, these drugs do not as yet have a clearly defined place in the therapy of peptic ulcer, al though they are still used frequently (Ivy 1975). Since they do reduce the basal secretion of acid by half, anticholinergics are often helpful in patients with persistent nocturnal pain. They also potentiate the benefits of antacids and cimetidine, and their value has already been discussed in management of the Zollinger-Ellison syndrome. The widespead use of anticholinergics has been limited by the side effects of oral dryness, urinary retention, and visual blurring, by their therapeutic limitations, and most of all by the advent of more effective antisecretory agents.

Blockers of Histamine-Induced (H_2) Acid Secretion. There are two active sites on the histamine molecule (Figure 6–9), the imidazole ring and the ethylamine side chain (Feldman and Richardson 1978). When the charged ammonium ion on the side chain adheres to an appropriate receptor, it produces the prominent (H_1) effects of allergy, such as vasodilatation and edema. The imidazole ring is responsible for acid secretory and cardiac (H_2) effects when it binds to appropriate receptor sites. Conventional antihista-

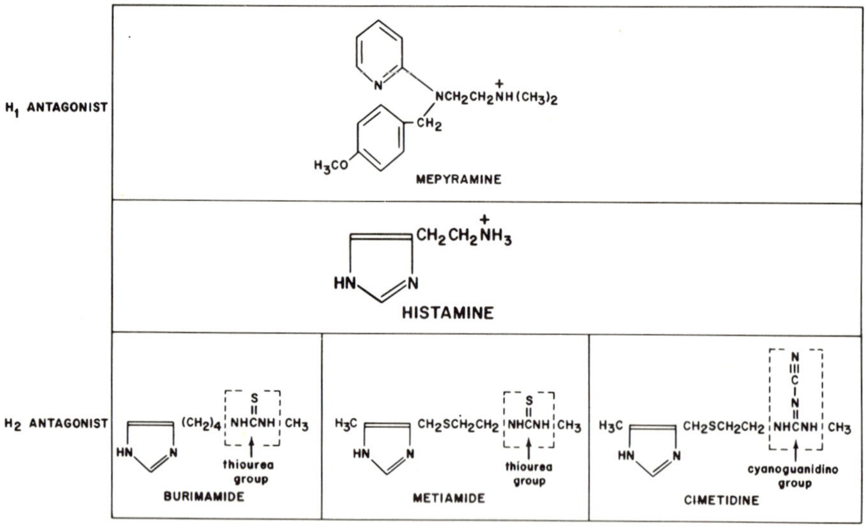

Figure 6–9. Chemical structure of histamine, an H_1-receptor antagonist (mepyramine), and H_2-receptor antagonists (burimamide, metiamide, and cimetidine). H_1 antagonists contain a charged ammonium group (like histamine) and aryl side groups; H_2 antagonists possess (like histamine) an imidazole ring and side chain. Differences in chemical structure between H_1 and H_2 antagonists may explain the individual selectivity for the respective receptors. Reproduced with permission from Feldman M, Richardson CT. Histamine H_2 receptor antagonists. In: Stollerman GH, et al, eds. Advances in Internal Medicine, vol 23. Copyright © 1978 by Year Book Medical Publishers, Inc., Chicago.

minics contain charged ammonium groups on their side chains and bind competitively with histamine to H_1 receptors. Several of the H_2 receptor antagonists synthesized to date contain an imidazole ring and compete with that portion of the histamine molecule for imidazole receptor sites on oxyntic and other cells. However, newer H_2 blocking agents have thiazole or furan rings and are most effective. The mechanism by which these drugs inhibit the action of histamine on oxyntic cells is not certain, but may involve receptor blockade, inhibition of adenylate cyclase action, or increased destruction of histamine by induction of imidazole N-methyltransferase activity.

There is clear and ample evidence that H_2 receptor antagonists cause marked inhibition of oxyntic cell responses to histamine, insulin hypoglycemia, gastrin, parasympathomimetic agents, caffeine, and food. Maximal doses reduce food-stimulated secretion of acid by 75 to 85 percent in three hours. The newest H_2 blocking agents, ranitidine and tiotidine, are at least twice as effective as cimetidine against basal- and gastrin-stimulated acid secretion, on a weight-for-weight basis (Lohrmann et al 1980; Richardson et al 1981). While they are much more effective than anticholinergic drugs acting alone, the effect of H_2 blockers is potentiated by anticholinergics. While these drugs cause increased postprandial hypergastrinemia, they have not been shown to lead to increases of oxyntic cell mass after extended use. H_2 blocking agents also reduce the stimulated levels of intrinsic factor secretion but do not appear to reduce its basal secretion. They do not appear to affect the rate of pepsin secretion or of gastric motility. There is evidence that one of these agents, cimetidine, appears to be cytoprotective in that its use in doses less than those required to reduce acid secretion improves gastric resistance to ulceration (Guth et al 1979). Pretreatment of animals with cimetidine also reduces the incidence of stress and aspirin-induced ulcerations.

Duodenal Ulcer Therapy. Cimetidine has proved to be strikingly effective in the treatment of duodenal ulcer. In a multicenter study of 300 patients who were allowed to take antacids as needed, 56 percent of hospitalized patients treated with cimetidine showed endoscopic evidence of ulcer healing after two weeks, as compared with 37 percent of controls (Binder et al 1978). Among outpatients, the respective two-week healing rates were 46 and 26 percent. In another study, healing rates of pyloric and duodenal (category A) ulcers were 84 percent after six weeks of treatment with cimetidine and 38 percent with a dummy (Hetzel et al 1978). Relapse rates within a year after ending therapy were similar in the two groups, 43 percent with cimetidine and 37 percent with the dummy. Among 36 patients with healed ulcers in whom the dose of cimetidine was reduced by half, there was no relapse in 80 days. In this same interval, relapses were found among 45 percent of patients whose ulcers had healed under dummy treatment. These results have been extended in later studies and indicate a minimal relapse of healed ulcers among patients carried on doses of cimetidine reduced to 25 percent of the therapeutic amount during a period of two years. Discontinuation of cimetidine at that time, however, led to a high rate of recurrence of peptic ulcer.

A comparison between healing rates for duodenal ulcers treated with antacids or cimetidine showed no significant difference at four weeks, albeit with a slight advantage to cimetidine (Ippoliti et al 1978). Symptoms were relieved promptly by both treatments, and side effects were confined to the antacid group, where one-fourth of patients experienced occasional diarrhea.

Gastric Ulcer Therapy. Cimetidine also appears to be helpful in the treatment of gastric (category B) ulcers (Freston 1978). Owing to a concern that it may be unjustified to allow some patients to receive no treatment for even a limited period, no pure controls were included in two multicenter studies in the United States. Instead, cimetidine alone was compared with antacids alone and healing rates were not significantly different at six weeks, though there was a trend favoring cimetidine. Healing rates ranged from 41 to 70 percent in various groups. In a few European studies, cimetidine was significantly better than antacids in healing gastric ulcers, but the amounts of antacids prescribed were quite small by American standards. A study by Gwyn Morfam et al (1978) showed complete healing of gastric ulcer in all of 26 patients treated with cimetidine for three months, but this was similar to the healing rates with carbenoxylone (see below).

A cautionary note on the use of cimetidine in the treatment of gastric ulcer is sounded by a report of two patients whose gastric ulcers healed completely during therapy and were later found to have carcinoma in situ after a prompt relapse. Similar findings were obtained in two other patients whose ulcers had grown much smaller on cimetidine therapy, though they had not healed completely (Taylor et al 1978). Thus, it is probably prudent to perform endoscopic examinations on all patients whose gastric ulcers have appeared to heal on treatment.

Use of cimetidine in the Zollinger-Ellison syndrome is discussed in Chapter 5.

Toxicity of Cimetidine. In a small number of cases, cimetidine has been found to cause granulocytopenia (Freston 1979), gynecomastia (Kruss and Littman 1978), transient male sterility (van Thiel et al 1979), mental confusion (Schentag et al 1979), and adverse drug-drug interactions with warfarin (Silver and Bell 1979). Granulocytopenia has been reported in 26 of 1.3 million patients in the United States, and has almost invariably occurred in patients with severe complicating disorders, such as renal failure or sepsis. The mechanism is not clear, and may involve reduced DNA synthesis in stem cells. Gynecomastia and transient sterility are attributed to the fact that cimetidine is antiandrogenic and competitively inhibits testosterone binding to receptor sites in the prostate, seminal vesicals, and testes (Winters et al 1979). While both of these adverse effects appear to be dose related and reversible with discontinuation of cimetidine, one would hesitate to use the drug for long-term maintenance treatment of young and middle-aged men without careful monitoring of testicular size and sperm counts. Hypersensitivity hepatitis has been reported in one patient exposed to cimetidine on several occasions (Villeneuve and Warner 1979).

Mental confusion appears to occur only in patients with renal and hepatic dysfunction who develop high blood levels of cimetidine. This effect may be the result of binding to H_2 receptor sites in the central nervous system, for cimetidine has been shown to be capable of passing the blood brain barrier. Particular care must also be taken in patients receiving coumarinlike anticoagulants while taking cimetidine, for the anticoagulant effects may be sharply increased.

Cimetidine in Older Patients. Gugler and Somogyi (1979) report that plasma clearance of cimetidine is reduced by more than half in patients over age 50; they suggest that this may make smaller dosages advisable. This may also increase the incidence of side effects in older patients. Bradycardia due to blockage of H_2 sinus node receptors does not, fortunately, appear to be a significant problem.

In summary, cimetidine is an effective, well-tolerated drug in patients with duodenal and gastric ulcers, and in the Zollinger-Ellison syndrome. Its long-term use at reduced dosage shows promise of preventing recurrences. Its ability to reduce complications and the need for surgery is potentially very great, although not proved at present. The cost to the patient of daily therapeutic amounts of cimetidine is somewhat less than the cost of proprietary antacids in recommended doses. The acid reducing effects of a single dose lasts more than twice as long as a single dose of antacids. Choice between antacids and cimetidine rests with the physician and the patient; their effects on ulcer healing appear to be similar.

Current Recommendations. In duodenal and gastric ulcer, 300 mg is given four times daily, with meals and at bedtime, for at least six weeks in patients with duodenal ulcer and until endoscopic healing has been demonstrated with gastric ulcers. Maintenance therapy with 400 mg at bedtime is probably advisable for at least one to two years after healing. A bedtime dose of an anticholinergic agent may be employed for patients with nocturnal pain, and antacids should be added if any patient is not free of pain within a few days after commencing cimetidine. Since there is evidence that at least one antacid reduces the absorption of oral cimetidine given simultaneously, these two agents should probably not be administered together (Steinberg and Lewis 1980). Dosage should be reduced by half in patients with hepatic or renal insufficiency and possibly in the elderly, blood counts should be checked every two weeks during the first two months of treatment, and male patients should be observed for antiandrogenic effects.

Other Therapeutic Modalities

Carbenoxolone. A derivative of the glycyrrhizic acid fraction of licorice, carbenoxolone, has been shown to be quite effective in healing gastric ulcers during the past 20 years, and to reduce recurrences (Baron and Sullivan 1970). It has very little effect on acid secretion and may be either directly cytoprotective or function primarily by increasing the secretion of gastric mucus. Carbenoxolone is similar in its electolytic effects to aldosterone and often leads to sodium retention, hypertension, and potassium loss; such effects can be relieved by simultaneously administering thiazide diuretics. The drug is not available in the United States and has not been shown to be more effective than cimetidine in the management of gastric ulcer.

Radiation of the Stomach. In the past, irradiation of the gastric fundus with up to 2,000 rads in a total of five doses has been employed to reduce acid secretion in patients with resistant or recurrent ulcers. The treatment has been effective in many instances, but it has never attained wide popularity because of objections to the use of radiation for benign illnesses, plus the fact that acid secretion usually returns to pretreatment levels within 6 to 12 months, and that gastric ulceration has occurred occasionally after irradiation.

Prostaglandins. In the future, it is possible that the cytoprotective and acid inhibitory effects of type E prostaglandins may be useful in ulcer therapy and prophylaxis. Methylated forms are active orally, but their tolerance may be limited because of the diarrhea that is often associated with their use (Robert 1979). The results of clinical trials are awaited with interest.

SURGERY FOR PEPTIC ULCER

The need for surgery in peptic ulcer therapy varies inversely with the efficacy of nonsurgical modalities. It is still too early to say how greatly the widening use of cimetidine will forestall the need for surgery, but it is probably safe to say that about 15 percent of patients with chronic peptic ulcer will eventually require an operation. Except for the fact that the approach is more direct, the physiologic avenues of therapy open to the surgeon are similar to those available to the physician. These are the removal of vagal influences by disrupting the vagus nerve, the removal of gastrin effects by antrectomy, and, rarely now, the reduction of acid secretory capacity by removal of portions of the proximal stomach. The advantages and disadvantages of the various forms of surgical manipulation can be understood by a consideration of the history of surgical procedures for peptic ulcer.

Gastrojejunostomy

Simple gastrojejunostomy without tissue resection is no longer employed. Since gastric secretion continues unabated after this operation, and may even be increased, and since the jejunum, which is less resistant to ulceration than the duodenum or stomach, is directly exposed to acid and peptic activity, the incidence of ulcers occurring around the gastrojejunal stoma is prohibitively high.

Gastric Resection

Gastric resection with gastroenterostomy is one of two types, the Billroth I type, in which the remaining stomach is anastomosed end to end with the transected duodenum, and the Billroth II type, in which the duodenal stump is closed, and the transected end of the stomach partially closed and then attached end to side to the upper jejunum distal to the ligament of Treitz. The loop of jejunum is brought up to the stomach either in front of the transverse colon (antecolic) or through the mesocolon (retrocolic). Originally, these operations were designed to remove all of the antrum and a large amount of the proximal stomach as well (subtotal gastrectomy), but the complications were too great. While the recurrence of peptic ulcer was small, the incidence of weight loss, rapid gastric emptying and fatigue was so great that high gastric resections have been abandoned. Efforts to remove the antrum alone (hemigastrectomy) reduced the incidence of nonulcer complications, but were associated with a high rate of recurrent ulcer (up to 50 percent).

Vagotomy with Drainage Procedure

In an effort to preserve gastric function while reducing acid secretion, efforts were directed at transecting the two vagal trunks at the level of the lower esophagus (truncal vagotomy) and compensating for the resultant gastric atony by enlarging the pyloric valve (pyloroplasty) or by establishing a gastrojejunostomy. While this procedure is well tolerated, the incidence of recurrent ulcer is about 20 percent, and many patients continue to have gastric retention despite the drainage procedure. Furthermore, the gall bladder often becomes hypotonic after a truncal vagotomy, and duodenal and small intestinal motility is disturbed frequently enough to cause troublesome diarrhea.

Truncal vagotomy with hemigastrectomy is an effective operation in keeping recurrences to about 1 percent and is still being widely used. It is, however, associated with some rapid-emptying problems (dumping syndrome) and diarrhea.

Selective vagotomy with drainge procedure essays to sever only those vagus fibers going to the stomach, and thus is intended to avoid problems with abnormal postoperative small intestinal and gall bladder motility. Gastric retention continues to be a problem with this procedure, but the incidence of recurrent ulcer is acceptably low, as is the overall incidence of unsatisfactory results (5 percent).

Superselective (proximal gastric) vagotomy is a tedious procedure which was developed in an attempt to remove only those vagal fibers supplying oxyntic tissue, without affecting antral contractility, and obviating a drainage procedure and associated dumping syndrome. The last objectives have indeed been met, but the reduction of acidity is only about half of the decrease achieved by selective vagotomy, so a higher recurrence rate of ulcer is anticipated (Welch and Malt 1979).

Indications for Surgery in Peptic Ulcer

Pyloric stenosis due to stricture, uncontrollable or recurrent bleeding, and perforation of the stomach or duodenum are clear indications for gastric surgery. Similarly, the failure of ulcer healing after a reasonable trial with adequate therapy, or the continuation of symptoms during therapy also mandate this approach. Most disputes between physicians and surgeons come in trying to decide upon therapeutic recommendations for the patient with a recurrence of ulcer. Here it is highly important to consider the patient's own desires, and to provide a clear understanding of the alternatives, their advantages and disadvantages. Once this is done, consensus can generally be obtained.

It is important to bear in mind that prompt recurrence or slow healing of peptic ulcers is commonly seen in patients with hypercalcemia and in the Zollinger-Ellison syndrome. Proper tests should be performed to learn if either of these disorders is present.

Complications of Gastric Surgery

Acute complications are becoming increasingly uncommon as surgical competence increases. But one must be alerted to the possibility that malnourished or immunosuppressed patients may heal their wounds poorly and are subject to leaks and abscesses around anastomoses and sutured duodenal stumps. Intravenous hyperalimentation has reduced this danger considerably, although the patient's temperature and white blood count must be watched carefully in the postoperative period. Similarly, attention should be given to pulmonary toilet, since aspiration of mucus and atelectasis are major problems in patients after subdiaphragmatic surgery.

Chronic complications are still of considerable importance. Generally, the greater the amount of stomach removed at surgery, the more likely the patient is to experience loss of weight and strength afterward. But fortunately, this problem is reduced by the fact that large resections of the stomach are now rarely performed. So too is the problem of retained gastric antrum, in which gastric transection is performed too proximally and antral tissue is left attached to the duodenal stump. Where this occurs, patients develop hypergastrinemia and prompt appearance of anastomotic ulcerations.

Dumping Syndrome. The dumping syndrome stills occurs in 5 to 10 percent of antrectomies or pyloroplasties. This problem develops whenever the stomach suddenly empties hypertonic contents directly into the small intestine, leading to the sudden movement of fluids from the vascular compartment into the intestinal lumen, and causing distention of the bowel, signs of acute hypovolemia, and diarrhea. Patients learn that symptoms are often precipitated by the ingestion of hypertonic fluids and can be minimized by avoiding sugar and liquids with meals. The use of serotonin antagonists, such as methysergide or cyproheptidine, may also be helpful.

Gastric Retention. Gastric retention continues to be a problem in patients with selective and truncal vagotomies. The use of proximal gastric vagotomy seems to lessen its incidence. Where symptoms continue to be a major complaint, and when recurrent ulceration and pyloric strictures are not complicating features, the smooth muscle stimulant, metoclopramide, tends to relieve the gastric retention.

Stomal Gastritis. Stomal gastritis commonly occurs in the gastric mucosa adjacent to a gastrointestinal stoma. This chronic inflammation may be the site of recurrent hemorrhage and erosion and is believed to result from the regurgitation of bile salts, lysolecithin, and pancreatic enzymes into the stomach. Aluminum-containing antacids have been used to precipitate bile salts with some success, and the anion exchange resin, cholestyramine, which binds bile salts, has had limited benefits. The cytoprotective benefits of cimetidine may also provide some relief from this annoying problem. It is not certain that this form of gastritis is the cause of the gastric cancer seen often in patients who have had partial resections years before, but such an association has been made.

Postoperative Peptic Ulcers. We have seen that recurrent ulceration in the stomach or at the anastomosis is a recognized problem after most types of gastric surgery (Figure 6–10), but is quite infrequently seen after selective vagotomy and antrectomy. Before contemplating further surgery in patients with recurrences, it is highly important to measure serum gastrin and calcium levels, and particularly to determine the serum gastrin following the administration of calcium, secretin, or both, as previously described. The possibility of an associated gastrinoma or hyperparathyroidism as precipitating causes for the ulcer must be kept in mind. In the absence of these conditions, recurrent ulcerations should be treated medically first, further surgery being left for those which do not heal under that treatment. Ci-

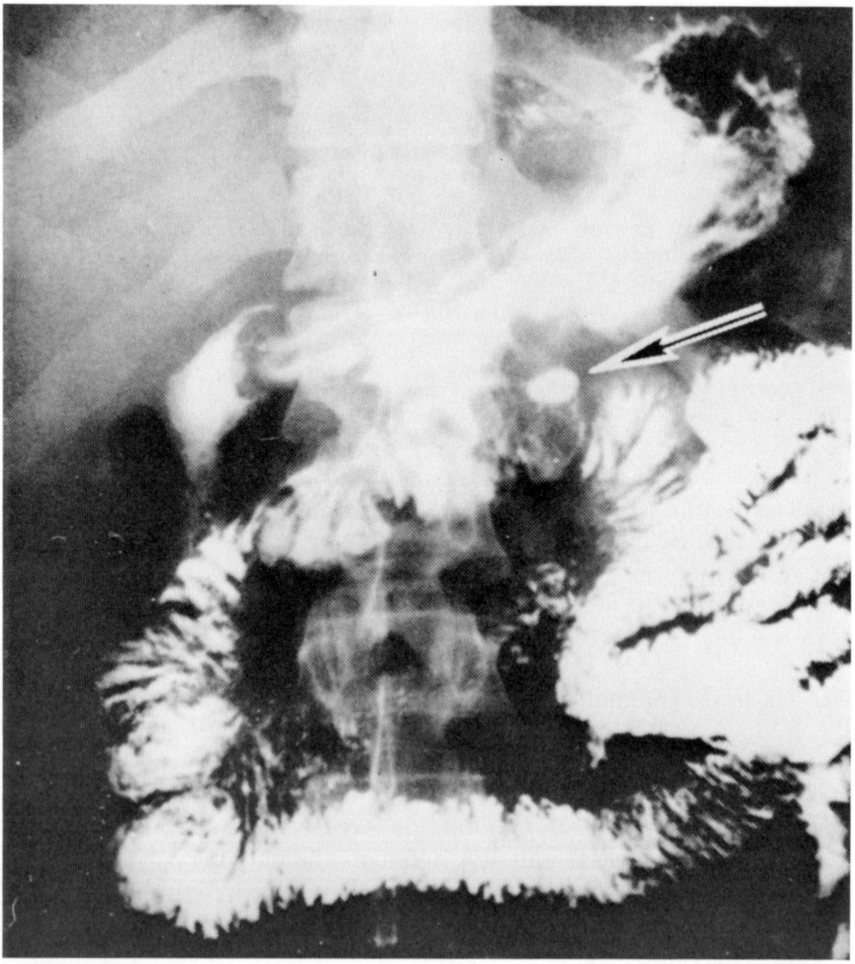

Figure 6–10. The arrow points to a marginal ulcer on the jejunal side of a gastrojejunostomy. From Haubrich WS. In: Bockus HL, ed. Gastroenterology, vol 1, 3rd ed. Philadelphia: WB Saunders, 1974. Reprinted by permission.

metidine in ordinary doses is highly effective in treating stomal ulcers (Gugler et al 1979).

In summary, newer surgical techniques show promise of being effective in reducing the incidence of recurrent ulcer and in avoiding serious chronic complications. Their mere existence should, however, make obvious the fact that a decision to operate upon a patient for peptic ulcer disease should not be made lightly, and should be reached only after other treatment has proved ineffective, and the patient has a full understanding of its necessity.

HISTORICAL DIGRESSION

Personages mentioned without further reference in this chapter include: Christian Albert Theodor BILLROTH (1829–1894), Swiss surgeon, Zurich and Vienna, described I gastric resection 1881, II gastric resection 1885; Johann Conrad BRUNNER (1653–1727), German anatomist, Mannheim, Heidelberg; Wenzel TREITZ (1819–1872), Polish pathologist, Cracow, defined ligament at duodenal-jejunal junction.

SELECTED REFERENCES

Baron JH, Sullivan FM, eds. Carbenoxylone sodium. London: Butterworths, 1970.

Binder HJ, Cocco A, Crossley RJ, et al. Cimetidine in the treatment of duodenal ulcer. A multicenter double blind study. Gastroenterology 74: 380–88, 1978.

Brodie, DA. Experimental peptic ulcer. Gastroenterology 55:125–34, 1968.

Buchman E, Kaung DT, Dolan K. Unrestricted diet in the treatment of duodenal ulcer. Gastroenterology 56:1016–20, 1969.

Dawson IMP. The endocrine cells of the gastrointestinal tract and the neoplasms which arise from them. In: Morson BC, ed. Pathology of the Gastrointestinal Tract. Berlin: Springer-Verlag, 1976:221–58.

Earlham R. A computerized questionnaire analysis of duodenal ulcer symptoms. Gastroenterology 71:314–17, 1976.

Elashoff JD, Grossman MI. Trends in hospital admissions and death rates for peptic ulcer in the United States from 1970 to 1978. Gastroenterology 78:280–85, 1980.

Engel GL. Memorial lecture: The psychosomatic approach to individual susceptibility to disease. Gastroenterology 67:1085–93, 1974.

Feldman M, Richardson CT. Histamine H_2-receptor antagonists. Adv Int Med 23:1–24, 1978.

Freston JW. Cimetidine in the treatment of gastric ulcer. Review and commentary. Gastroenterology 74:426–30, 1978.

Freston JW. Cimetidine and granulocytopenia. Ann Int Med 90:264–65, 1979.

Gugler R, Lindstaedt H, Miederer S, et al. Cimetidine for anastomatic ulcers after partial gastrectomy. N Engl J Med 301:1077–80, 1979.

Gugler R, Somogyi A. Reduced cimetidine clearance with age. N Engl J Med 301:435, 1979.

Guth PH, Aures D, Paulsen G: Topical aspirin plus HCl gastric lesions in the rat. Cytoprotective effect of prostaglandin, cimetidine, and probanthine. Gastroenterology 76:88–93, 1979.

Guth PH, Paulson G, Lynn D, et al. Mechanisms of prevention of aspirin-induced gastric lesions by bile duct ligation in the rat. Gastroenterology 71:750–53, 1976.

Gwyn Morfam A, McAdam WAF, Pacsoo C, et al. Cimetidine: an advance in gastric ulcer treatment? Br Med J 2:1323–26, 1978.

Hetzel DJ, Hansky J, Shearman DJC et al. Cimetidine treatment of duodenal ulceration. Short term clinical trial and maintenance study. Gastroenterology 74:389–92, 1978.

Ippoliti AF, Sturdevant RAL, Isenberg JL, et al. Cimetidine vs. intensive antacid therapy for duodenal ulcer. A multicenter trial. Gastroenterology 74:393–95, 1978.

Ivy KH. Anticholinergics: Do they work in peptic ulcer? Gastroenterology 68: 154–66, 1975.

Johansen AA. Early gastric cancer. In: Morson BC, ed. Pathology of the Gastrointestinal Tract. Berlin: Springer-Verlag, 1976:1–47.

Kruss DM, Littman A. Safety of cimetidine. Gastroenterology 74:478–83, 1978.

Levant JA, Walsh JH, Isenberg JI. Stimulation of gastric secretion and gastrin release by single oral doses of calcium carbonate in man. N Engl J Med 289:555–58, 1973.

Lohrmann A, Hotz J, Exbelein V, et al. Effects of intraduodenal administration of ranitidine and cimetidine on secretion of gastric acid, pepsin, gastrin and pancreatic polypeptide in man. Gastroenterology 78:1210, 1980.

Mann FC, Williamson CS. The experimental production of peptic ulcer. Ann Surg 77:409–22, 1923.

Mendeloff AI. What has been happening to duodenal ulcer? Gastroenterology 67:1020–22, 1974.

Mendeloff AI, Dunn JP. Digestive Diseases. Cambridge: Harvard University Press, 1971:7–36.

Nelson SW. The discovery of gastric ulcers and the differential diagnosis between benignancy and malignancy. Radiologic Clin North America 7:5–26, (April) 1969.

Peterson WL, Sturdevant RAL, Frankel HD, et al. Healing of duodenal ulcer with an antacid regimen. N Engl J Med 294:341–45, 1977.

Polish E, Brady JV, Mason JW, et al. Gastric contents and the occurrence of duodenal lesions in the Rhesus monkey during avoidance behavior. Gastroenterology 43:193–201, 1962.

Richardson CT, Feldman M, Brater C, et al. Tiotidine, a new long-acting histamine H2-receptor antagonism: Comparison with cimetidine. Gastroenterology 80:301–6, 1981.

Robert A. Prostaglandins: Their effect on the digestive system. Viewpoints Dig Dis 11:1–4, (Jan) 1979.

Robert A, Schultz JR, Nezamis JE, et al. Gastric antisecretory and antiulcer properties of PGE_2, 15-methyl PGE_2, and 16,16-dimethyl PGE_2. Intravenous, oral and intrajejunal administration. Gastroenterology 70:359–70, 1976.

Rotter JI, Rimoin DL, Gursky JM, et al. HLA-B5 associated with duodenal ulcer. Gastroenterology 73:438–40, 1977.

Rotter JI, Sones JQ, Samloff IM, et al. Duodenal ulcer disease associated with elevated serum pepsinogen I. An inhibitory autosomal dominant disorder. N Engl J Med 300:63–66, 1979.

Samloff IM, Liebman WM, Panitch NM. Serum group I pepsinogens by radioimmunoassay in control subjects and patients with peptic ulcer. Gastroenterology 69:83–90, 1975.

Schentag JJ, Calleri G, Rose JQ, et al. Pharmacokinetic and clinical studies in patients with cimetidine-associated mental confusion. Lancet 1:177–81, 1979.

Scheurer U, Witzel L, Halter H, et al. Gastric and duodenal ulcer healing under placebo treatment. Gastroenterology 72:838–41, 1977.

Sekine T, Woodward ER, McGuigan JE. Effects of taurocholic acid on gastric acid secretion and gastrin release. Gastroenterology 78:57–61, 1970.

Silver BA, Bell WR. Cimetidine potentiation of the hypoprothrombinemia effect of warfarin. Ann Int Med 90:348–49, 1979.

Steinberg WM, Lewis JH. Mylanta II inhibits the absorption of cimetidine. Gastroenterology 78:1269, 1980.

Takeuchi K, Johnson LR. Pentagastrin protects against stress ulcers. Gastroenterology 76:327–34, 1979.

Taylor RH, Menzies-Gow N, Lovell D, et al. Apparent healing of malignant gastric ulcers with cimetidine. Gut 19:A442, 1978.

Thompson JC, Swierczek JS. Acid and endocrine responses to meals varying in pH in normal and duodenal ulcer subjects. Ann Surg 186:541–48, 1977.

van Thiel BH, Gavaler JS, Smith WI Jr. Hypothalamic-pituitary-gonadal dysfunction in men using cimetidine. N Engl J Med 300:1012–15, 1979.

Villeneuve JP, Warner HA. Cimetidine hepatitis. Gastroenterology 77:143–44, 1979.

Walsh JH, Richardson CT, Fordtran JS. pH dependence of acid secretion and gastrin release in normal and ulcer subjects. J Clin Invest 55:462–68, 1975.

Welch CE, Malt RA. Abdominal surgery. N Engl J Med 300:648–53, 1979.
Winters SJ, Banks JL, Loriaux DL. Cimetidine is an antiandrogen in the rat. Gastroenterology 76:504–8, 1979.

CLINICAL CONFERENCE 3

This 51-year-old male construction worker was admitted to the hospital because of abdominal pain, loss of weight, exertional dyspnea, and weakness which had become progressively worse since starting three months earlier. The pain felt like a "knotting up in the stomach" and was most prominent in the epigastrium. It was continuous, aggravated by eating and alcohol, and was generally relieved within 30 minutes after the ingestion of Alka-Seltzer. The pain often woke him at night and was occasionally associated with, but not relieved by, vomiting a clear yellow liquid. Appetite was poor, and the patient had lost about 20 pounds with the illness. The color of his stools was normal. Shortness of breath and weakness started two months prior to admission.

In the past his health had been excellent. About two and one-half years before admission he had become despondent because of lack of work and mounting bills and began to consume up to a pint of whiskey daily. Shortly thereafter he began to vomit several times a day and also lost a small amount of weight. He consulted a physician who advised abstinence from alcohol, a "light diet" and a "white liquid medicine in a blue bottle" four times a day. On this regimen he became asymptomatic, gained weight, and after a few weeks he found a job. He remained well until the episode leading to the present admission. Review of systems was completely negative. There had been no previous hospitalizations, and the patient denied taking any medications other than those mentioned above.

On admission he was a well-developed thin man, blood pressure was 140/72, pulse 64, temperature 37°C, and weight 129 pounds. Physical findings were normal except for slight dryness of the mucous membranes, a grade 2 harsh systolic ejection murmur at the cardiac apex, moderate tenderness to epigastric pressure, and two large prolapsed hemorrhoids. Liver and spleen were not palpable.

Hematocrit on admission was 16 percent, while cell count 5,300, and urinalysis normal. On smear, the red cells appeared to be microcytic and hypochromic, and the differential count was normal. Blood type was AB, Rh positive. The serum iron was 10 μg with a total iron-binding capacity of 416 μg per dl. One stool specimen was negative for occult blood, and a morning gastric aspiration produced 25 ml of colorless gastric juice, which was also negative for occult blood. A one-hour basal gastric analysis produced 1.98 mEq of HCl. In 30 to 90 minutes after stimulation with 360 μg of pentagastrin, 53 mEq of acid was obtained from the stomach. Fasting serum gastrin level was 115 pg per ml, rising to 250 after lunch. Representative films from his upper gastrointestinal X rays are reproduced in the accompanying photograph (Figure 6–11).

1. What are the possible diagnoses in this case? Select the one that is most likely and defend it by citing reasons from the protocol and from your reading.
2. What further studies would be useful in substantiating the dianosis? Why?
3. What mechanisms are involved in producing the disorder in this patient?
4. What complications have appeared and what others may occur if the disease is untreated?
5. What types of treatment are available? What is the rationale for these treatments? Which treatment would you choose? Why?

CLINICAL CONFERENCE 4

A 71-year-old man was hospitalized after 10 days of copious vomiting that were followed by 2 days of generalized weakness and spasms in his hands and forearms. Emesis occurred only once or twice daily and was preceded by dull epigastric distress, which subsided after the vomiting ceased. The vomitus usually contained food that had been ingested as long as 12 hours before, and it was sour to taste. The patient had been in excellent health until 15 years earlier, when he noted the appearance of mild upper abdominal distress occurring a few hours after meals and relieved quickly by the ingestion of baking soda. This had never been treated medically, since the symptoms were readily controlled and the attacks lasted for only two to three weeks at a time.

During the half-year prior to admission, pain had become more severe and less responsive to baking soda. One month earlier the discomfort had begun to appear shortly after meals and was no longer relieved by antacids. He felt full much of the time, ate little, and lost about 25 pounds. He did not become alarmed about his symptoms until the vomiting began. Weakness and muscular spasms were completely new symptoms. The patient lived alone, worked as a janitor, consumed little alcohol, but drank an average of 10 cups of coffee per day.

On examination, he was a thin well-developed man whose skin showed poor turgor. Blood pressure was 90/40, pulse 102, temperature 38°C, and respiration 18. He became quite weak on standing, and his pulse rate increased to 120. He was well oriented. Pertinent physical findings included dryness of the oral mucosa, an emphysematous chest and marked epigastric tenderness. The upper abdomen was slightly distended and a succussion splash was identified in this area. The remainder of the abdomen and the rectum were normal. Stool showed a 3-plus guaiac response. Gentle tapping

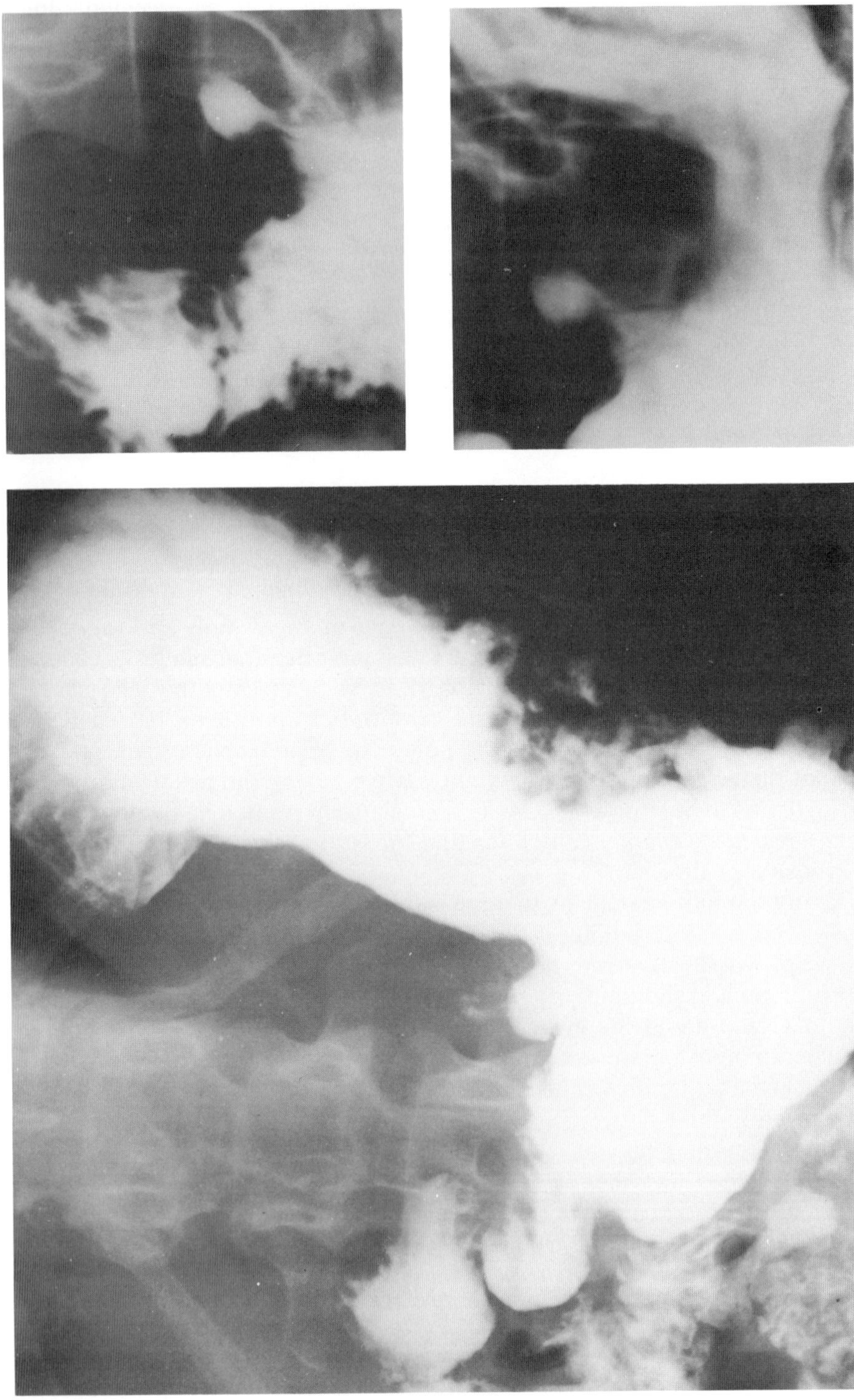

Figure 6–11. X rays of stomach and duodenum, Clinical Conference 3. The two smaller pictures on the right are spot films of the distal lesser curve of the stomach.

of the left zygomatic arch caused the facial muscles on the left to go into a short period of spasm.

Urinalysis on admission showed specific gravity, 1.026; pH 7.8; albumin and sugar, negative; sediment, normal. The hematocrit was 50 percent, and the white cell count 12,200 with 78 percent neutrophils. A nasogastric tube was passed into the stomach and 2 liters of a clear watery fluid containing small particles of partially digested food were aspirated. Gastric contents were guaiac negative, and Töpfer's solution turned bright red when added to a small aliquot. On the following morning, an X ray film (Figure 6–12) was taken after the patient had ingested a few ounces of barium.

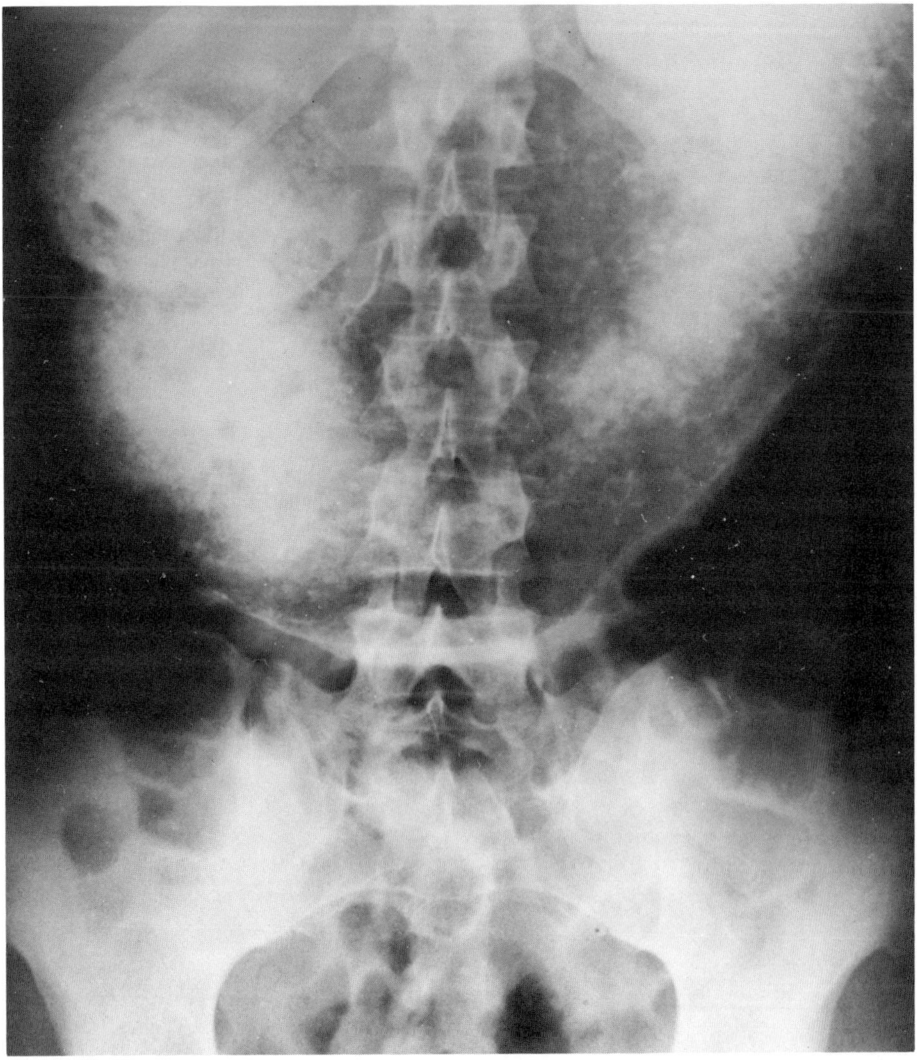

Figure 6–12. X ray of stomach, Clinical Conference 4.

The urea nitrogen was 46 mg, creatinine 0.4 mg, glucose 96 mg, calcium 10.2 mg, and phosphorus 3.6 mg per dl. The sodium was 128 mEq, the potassium 3.2 mEq, the chloride 78 mEq, and the carbon dioxide 38 mEq per liter. Serum amylase was 80 Somogyi units, the arterial pH 7.58, and serum gastrin 125 pg per ml.

1. Reconstruct the pathogenesis of this illness and suggest what diseases may be responsible.
2. Describe the mechanisms of this patient's fluid and electrolyte derangements.
3. List the elements of a therapeutic program for this patient and state your reason for each measure. Would there be any reason for operating on this patient? Why?

CHAPTER 7

The Liver: Structure and Function

A glance at the title of this chapter may cause the reader to wonder why our downward progression through the gastrointestinal tract is being interrupted by a diversionary movement to the liver, biliary tract, and pancreas. Actually, this is not an interruption, being instead an important element of the progression. Small intestinal physiology and pathophysiology cannot be understood without a clear knowledge of the role which the liver, biliary tree, and pancreas play in their actions. Similarly, one cannot consider the significance of intestinal complaints in patients without giving close consideration to possible hepatobiliary-pancareatic causes. This close interrelationship makes one wonder at efforts being made presently to distinguish between liver-bound and enteric-bound gastroenterologists. Such distinctions should not be made. Hepatology is a part of gastroenterology!

Dr. George Gabuzda enjoyed referring to the liver as "the dean of the viscera," and in the sense that it presides over a "faculty" of many and diverse organs, supplies them with the essential wherewithal for their function, removes much of their wastes, and insofar as possible pardons their sins, this is an extremely apt analogy. For the liver is in a unique position at the head of the portal circulation where it is the prime recipient of nutrients and other constituents absorbed from the intestinal tract, and is responsible for metabolizing those while simultaneously subserving a number of other specialized functions. When all of its responsibilities are considered, it is indeed surprising that this 1,400 to 1,800 g organ, sitting so quietly in the upper right quadrant of the abdomen, and subject to so many onslaughts from the various foods, drugs, and poisons prudently or ill-advisedly ingested by its possessor, functions so well and so long in most people. Clearly, the liver is an admirable and complex organ, and the following summary can only touch on the variety of activities that it subsumes every day.

ANATOMICAL CONSIDERATIONS

Gross Description

In shape somewhat like Gibraltar, in color variable from tannish brown to deep red, the liver has the singular feature among abdominal viscera of a dual blood supply, receiving its major proportion of blood, poorly oxygenated, from the stomach and intestines by way of the portal vein, and its fully oxygenated blood from the aorta by way of the celiac axis and the hepatic artery. In total, the liver receives an average of 1.5 liters of blood per minute, 80 percent through the portal vein, the amount increasing after meals and decreasing during exercise. Portal vein flow is slow and at low pressure, splenic vein blood passing largely to the left lobe of the liver, and superior and inferior mesenteric venous blood to the right.

The liver is divided into four lobes, the large right and left lobes lying anteriorly, while the small caudate and underlying quadrate lobes are posterior. The right and left lobes are separated from one another by the dense falciform ligament, and the right lobe is two to three times larger than the left. Frequently, the right lobe is pulled downward, like a broad tail, by a fibrous connection to the mesocolon; the resulting deformity is called a *Riedel lobe.* Save for an area beneath the diaphragm extending to the posterior aspect of the organ, the entire liver, including the portal vein, is invested by a tough layer of transparent fibrous tissue, called the *Glisson capsule,* strands of which continue into the parenchyma as the fibrous supporting structure of the liver. The posterior surface and free margins of the caudate and quadrate lobes, where they are not adherent to the posterior portion of the right lobe, are also covered by Glisson capsule.

External Vascular and Ductular Anatomy. Portal vein and hepatic artery enter the undersurface of the liver at the porta hepatis, the portal vein, about 7.5 cm long, having been formed by the juncture of the splenic and inferior mesenteric veins. Later in its rightward ascending course in the lesser omentum, the portal vein is joined successively by the superior mesenteric and left gastric (coronary) veins before entering the liver. Two large ducts, the right and left hepatic ducts, emerge also from the porta hepatis, one from each of the two main lobes of the liver. Just below the liver, these ducts converge into a single larger trunk, the common hepatic duct, which proceeds for another 2 to 3 cm and is joined by the cholecystic duct leading from the gall bladder. The resulting common bile duct progresses downward through the head of the pancreas where it is usually joined by the main pancreatic duct of Wirsung at a slightly dilated area called the ampulla of Vater, which actually lies in the wall of the inner curve of the descending duodenum, and terminates in the lumen of the duodenum in a 2- to 3-mm elevation called the papilla of Vater. Control of biliary and pancreatic flow into the duodenum is maintained by a two-part complicated muscular ring, the sphincter of Oddi. Total daily flow of bile is from 600 to 800 ml.

The liver almost completely envelopes the uppermost portion of the inferior vena cava for a distance of 5 to 6 cm below the diaphragm. Blood slowly emerging from the liver empties into the vena cava at this level through two to five short, large, veins, called the hepatic veins, the largest of which come from the right and left lobes. Flow through the hepatic veins is under very low pressure (3–4 mm Hg).

Hepatic Regeneration. The hepatocytes of a normal liver show very little mitotic activity, but any sort of injury leads to a marked increase in DNA synthesis and increase in cell and nuclear size, unless the liver has been massively damaged. Similarly, surgical removal of a portion of the liver leads to a rapid regrowth of lost mass, at a rate of 50 to 100 g per day. In both instances, it appears that certain factors are responsible for maintaining a critical mass of functioning hepatic tissue. It is not at all clear what these factors are, although work reported by Starzl et al (1978) indicates that insulin is probably an important hepatotrophic factor. They have shown that in dogs who have been operated upon so that one lobe of the liver receives portal blood from only the intestines, while the other lobe receives blood from the pancreas, stomach, duodenum, and spleen, the lobe receiving intestinal blood atrophies, while the other lobe shows cellular hypertrophy and hyperplasia. Pancreatectomy and chemically induced (alloxan) diabetes wipes out the benefits noted in the lobe receiving pancreatic blood, and insulin tends to neutralize the changes. Junge and Creutzfeldt (1978) suggest that glucagon and somatostatin may also be trophic factors in addition to insulin, and that gastrin, cholecystokinin, and secretin are not. While this work is not conclusive in itself, there is a definite implication that the stimulus for regeneration of hepatic mass after resection or after cellular injury comes from extrahepatic sources. This may also have some relevancy to the appearance of hepatocellular carcinomas in chronically regenerating liver tissue.

HISTOLOGY

The Hepatic Lobule. The rather monotonous histology of the liver does not begin to suggest the multiplicity of its functions, nor does it truly define its circulatory network. It does, however, describe a lobular structure (Figure 7–1) which is a convenient base for the description of pathologic changes. What one sees on light microscopy is a series of discrete, lozenge-shaped lobules, each consisting of a thin-walled central vein from which cords of rectangular hepatocytes radiate toward the lobular periphery. The cords appear to be one cell layer in thickness, with a thin bile canaliculus running between the layers. Each cord is separated from the next by a sinusoid lined with Kupffer cells and other phagocytes and containing small amounts of blood flowing toward the central vein. At the periphery of each lobule, one or more portal areas are seen, the margins of which are clearly set apart from adjacent lobular tissue by a limiting plate of hepatocytes. Each portal area contains three vessels, a terminal arteriole, a terminal branch of the portal vein, and a small bile duct lined with cuboidal epithelium, surrounded by loose fibrous stroma. A few histiocytes and round cells, but not polymorphonuclear leukocytes, are located in the portal areas surrounding the major vessels.

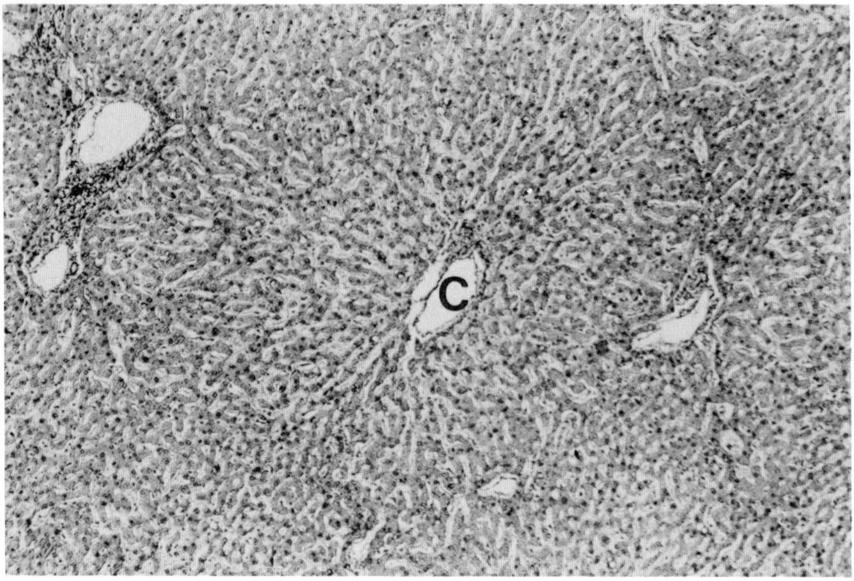

Figure 7-1. Normal liver. Section shows a hexagonal-shaped hepatic lobule with prominent central vein (C) and several portal tracts in the periphery. Original magnification x70.

It would appear from this microscopic picture that each lobule is supplied with its own artery and portal venule, that blood flows through them toward the central vein by way of the sinusoids, and that biliary constituents flow in the other direction from hepatocytes to canaliculi to portal biliary ductule. However, this is not the case. Rappaport (1975) has shown by injection studies that single portal vessels supply adjacent portions of two or more lobules, that each lobule is supplied by several portal areas, and that venous drainage of blood from one portal area may be through more than a single central vein. He thus describes an acinus rather than the lobule as the basic functioning unit of the liver (Figure 7-2). Acini may interdigitate with one another, but do not conform to the lobular pattern. Neither do liver cells proliferate in cords; they lie mainly in closely apposed plates. This three-dimensional concept of a functioning liver unit conforms much better to patterns of hepatic disease than does the two-dimensional lobular concept.

Parenchymal Circulation. Arterial blood supply to the liver terminates in three different capillary beds: that in the portal tract itself, from which branches enter the sinusoids; that around the bile ductules, which also give branches to collateral arteries and peripheral sinusoids; and that which flows directly to the sinusoids without more proximal branching. There are also anastomoses in the portal areas and beyond with branches of the portal vein. This complex system provides for several different types of blood flow, directly to hepatocytes, partially to supporting hepatic structures, or completely bypassing hepatocytes. Flow is regulated by an intricate system of sphincters. The portal venous channels terminate both in portal areas and in sinusoids, providing for hepatocytic bypasses in this system as well. Because of anastomoses, sinusoidal blood contains elements of portal and arterial blood at all levels.

The sinusoids of the hepatic parenchyma are extremely thin walled and are lined by fenestrated endothelial cells and phagocytic Kupffer cells. The area underlying the sinusoidal endothelium, the space of Disse, is penetrated by hepatocytic microvilli, which penetrate endothelial fenestrae into the sinusoidal lumen (Figure 7–3) (Jones and Schmucker 1977). Kupffer cells are large, stellate phagocytes laden with lysosomes. Spaces of Disse probably represent the source of hepatic lymphatic drainage. Sinusoids empty into small collecting venules at their distal ends, and thence flow into central veins (terminal hepatic venules of Rappaport).

The Hepatocyte. The isolated hepatocyte has been shown to be spherical in shape, and to be covered with a multitude of microvilli (Figure 7–4). In the liver, stresses induced by the reticular stroma and compression from adjacent cells alter this shape to a 12-sided solid that tends to appear hexagonal on cross-section. The cytosol of the hepatocyte includes a large double-membraned nucleus containing a nucleolus which synthesizes messenger, transfer, and ribosomal RNA. The nuclear membrane has pores on its surface that allow the egress of nucleic acids into the cytosol. Cytoplasmic organelles include numerous egg-shaped mitochondria with cristae; linear collections of rough and smooth endoplasmic reticulum; special organelles probably arising from endoplasmic reticulum, called microbodies; lysosomes; and the lamellated Golgi apparatus. Rough endoplasmic reticulum is the site of protein formation, while smooth endoplasmic reticulum subserves the processes of conjugation of endogenous and exogenous chemicals, and other detoxifying functions. Both forms of endoplasmic reticulum produce glucose-6-phosphatase, which is essential in the metabolism of glycogen.

Schaffner and Popper (1975) describe three distinct regions in the hepatocytic border: the greatest length is in apposition to neighboring hepatocytes, and consists of both loose and tight, sometimes peg-in-groove junctions; the second region borders a hepatic sinusoid, and is cast into irregularly shaped microvilli which penetrate either into the sinusoid directly, or into spaces of Disse when the sinusoid is separated from the hepatocyte by overlying Kuppfer cells; the remaining border region of the hepatocyte, about 6 percent of the entire perimeter, comprises the microvillous border of a bile canaliculus.

Origins of the Biliary System. The Golgi apparatus of the hepatocyte appears to control the flow of hepatocytic secretions into biliary canaliculi. The lu-

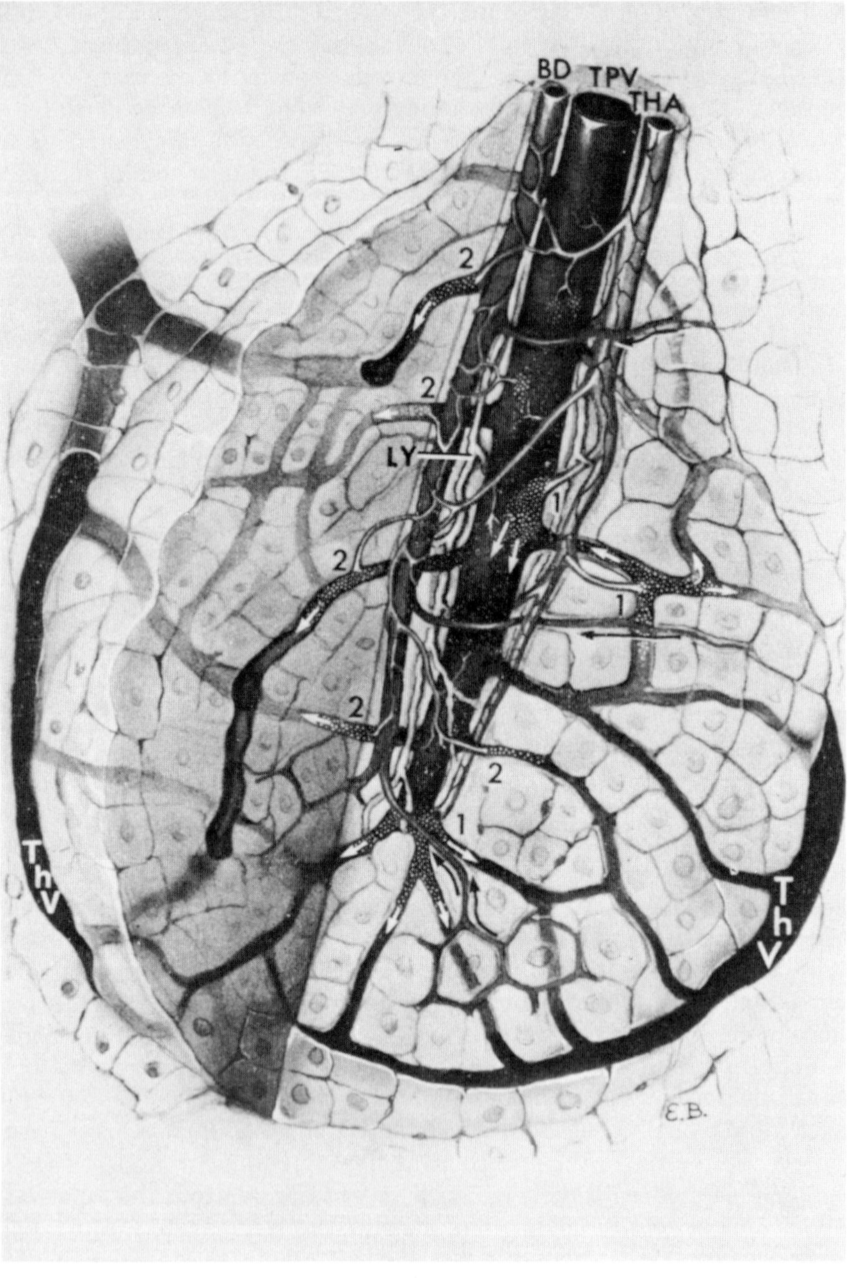
BD
TPV
THA
2
2
LY
1
2
1
2
2
1
ThV
ThV
E.B.

men of the canaliculus is tightly sealed by dense tight junctions which bind one hepatocyte to its neighbors. Canaliculi flow into biliary ductules lined by cells containing few organelles. Ductular channels, the canals of Hering, pass in close apposition to hepatic sinusoids in their flow toward portal bile ducts. This proximity of biliary to blood flow probably allows for fluid and electrolytic interchanges to occur. From acinar ductules, bile passes into portal bile ducts.

HEPATIC FUNCTION

While the liver subserves a myriad of important functions in humans, consideration is given here primarily to those functions which, when altered by disease, can provide measurements of the cause and severity of the underlying pathophysiology. Among these functions are the elaboration of plasma proteins, the production of cholesterol, bile acids, and phospholipids, the transport of bilirubin, the formation and secretion of bile, and the release of enzymes synthesized at hepatocytic canalicular borders and in the hepatocyte. Some of these activities are subserved solely by the liver, while others are shared with other organs in the body. Chapter 8 considers ways in which these functions are altered by disease.

Plasma Proteins

Except for the gamma globulins, which are also produced by B-lymphocytes throughout the body, the liver is the major site for the formation of all serum proteins. There is a great variety of hepatocytic proteins: albumin; various factors essential to blood coagulation; the protease inhibitor, α-1 antitrypsin; α and β lipoproteins; haptoglobin; thyroid-binding globulin; and the metal-containing proteins, ceruloplasmin (copper), transferrin (iron), and transcobalamin (vitamin B_{12}). Production of some of these proteins is under genetic control, including the lipoproteins, α-1 antitrypsin, and ceruloplasmin, their excess or deficiency having been associated with distinctive diseases of a hereditary nature. The stability of hepatocytic proteins is quite

Figure 7–2. A microcirculatory hepatic unit. The unit consists of the terminal portal venule (TPV) with the sinusoids branching off it and forming a glomus; the hepatic arteriole (THA) lacing with its branches, and forming a plexus around the terminal bile ductule (BD). Arterioles empty either directly (1) or via the peribiliary plexus (2) into the TPV and sinusoids. The sinusoids run along the outside of cell plates and cords, inside which are the capillaries of the hepatic secretory and excretory system. The glomus of sinusoids is drained by at least two terminal hepatic venules (ThV). LY = lymphatics. From Rappaport AM. Microvasc Res 6:212–228, 1973. Reprinted by permission.

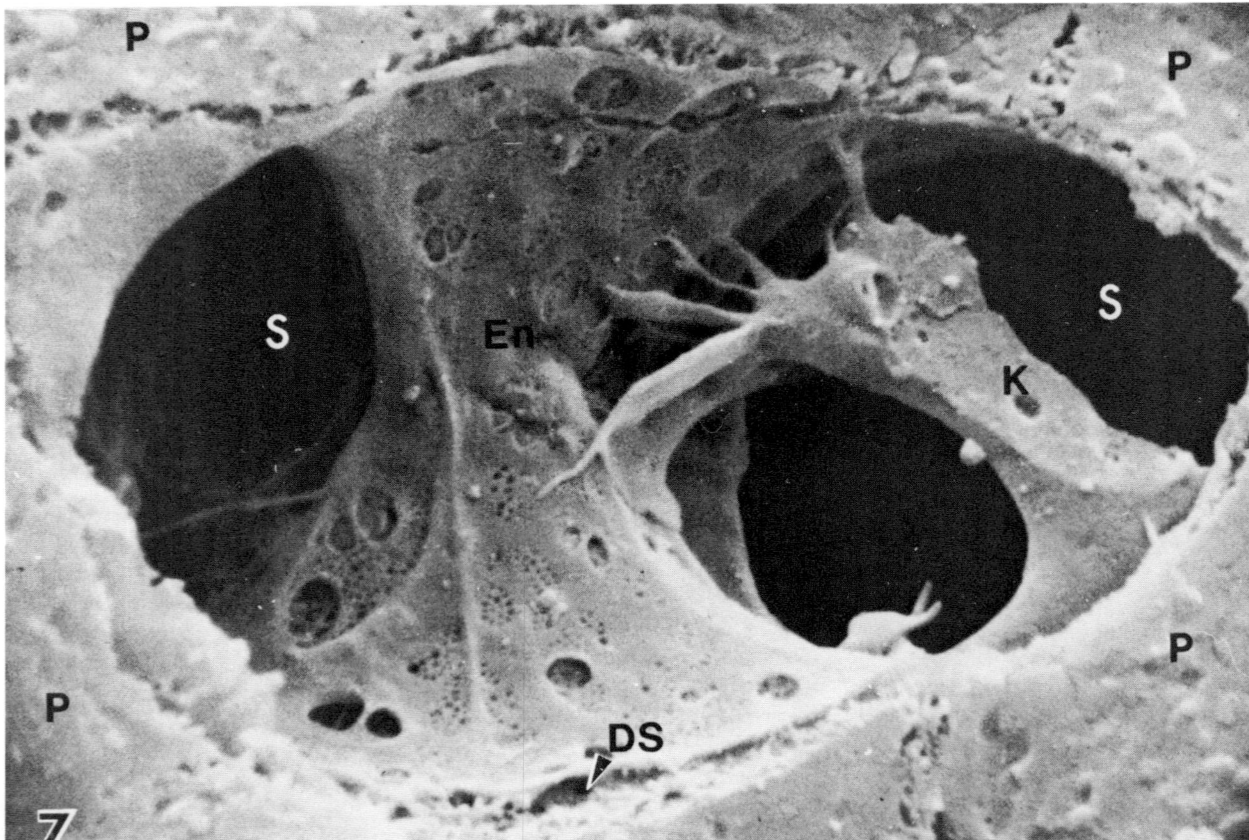

Figure 7–3. Scanning electron photomicrogram showing bifurcation of a liver sinusoid (S) and demonstrating the relationship of Kupffer cell (K) to the endothelium (EN) and surrounding parenchyma (P). The surface pits noted in the Kupffer cell may represent an area of endocytic or exocytic activity. DS = space of Disse. Approximate magnification x7500. Reprinted by permission of the publisher by Jones AL, Schmucker DL. Gastroenterology 73:833–51. Copyright 1977 by the American Gastroenterological

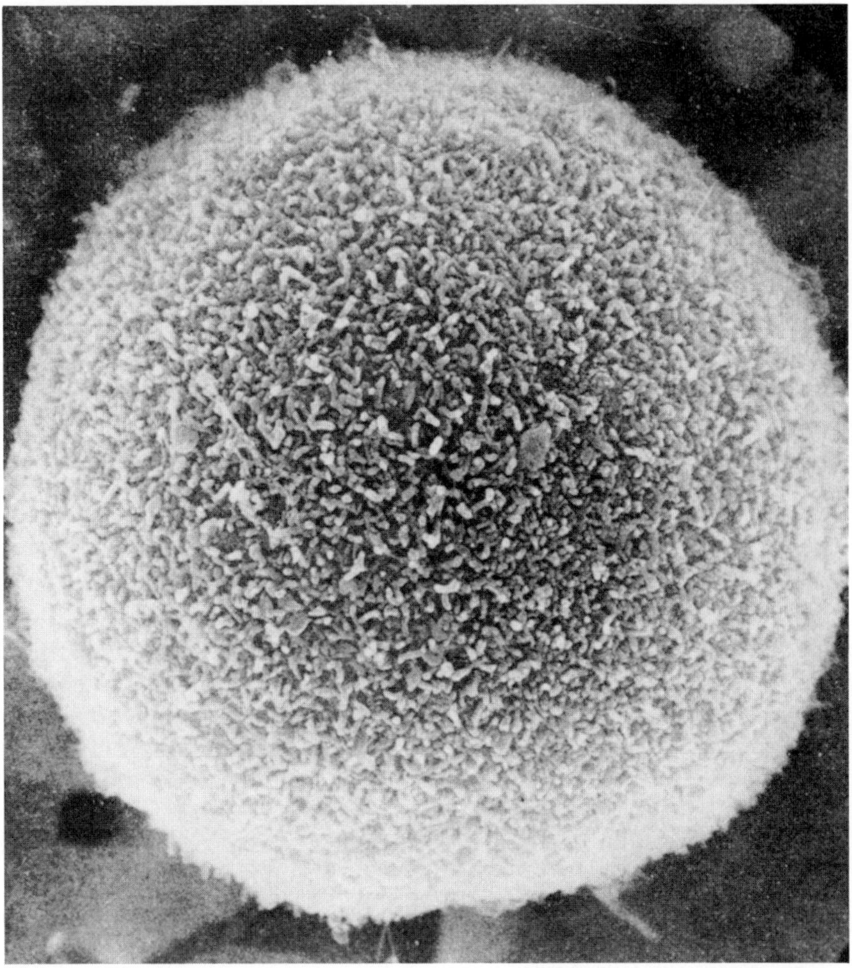

Figure 7–4. Scanning electron micrograph of an isolated hepatocyte. The cell surface is covered with microvilli. Magnification x6200. Reprinted by permission of the publisher from Drochmans P, Wanson JC, May C, et al. In: *Hepatotrophic Factors*, Ciba Foundation Symposium 55 (ns). Amsterdam: Elsevier, Excerpta Medica, North-Holland, 1978:7–29.

variable, and ranges from a half-life of 15 days for albumin, to half-lives of 12 hours for α-1 antitrypsin and 7 hours for serum prothrombin conversion accelerator (factor VII). At least four of the clotting factors require vitamin K for their synthesis, including factor II (prothrombin), factor VII, factor IX (Christmas factor), and factor X. Vitamin K adds gamma carboxy groups to glutamate complexes at the *N*-terminal of these polypeptide factors, thereby enabling them to bind calcium and phospholipids. This markedly hastens the conversion of prothrombin to thrombin by factor X (Jackson 1978). Vitamin K is not needed for the initial synthesis of these factors. Fibrinogen (factor I) and proaccelerin (factor V) are also produced in the liver, but their activation does not require vitamin K.

Alpha Fetoprotein. Alpha fetoprotein is a globulin of medium half-life, produced in large quantities by fetal liver, and only in small amounts by normal adult livers. Its clinical importance resides in the fact that rapidly regenerating hepatic tissue and rapidly multiplying malignant hepatocellular carcinomas produce alpha fetoprotein in large amounts, and it thus becomes a marker of serious disease.

Carcinoembryonic Antigens. Carcinoembryonic antigens are a mixture of glycoproteins produced in neoplastic and fetal tissues. The healthy liver degrades carcinoembryonic antigen, and levels increase in patients with alcoholic liver disease. Serum elevations are nonspecific, however, because they are also noted with cancer and inflammations of the colon, pancreas, and lungs, and in smokers.

Antibody Markers. Aberrations of immunity appear in many patients with chronic inflammatory disease of the liver. While the resultant antibodies are not hepatocytic, they are probably formed from mononuclear infiltrates in the liver and are thus considered to be abnormal proteins of hepatic origin. Among these are: antinuclear antibodies to deoxyribonucleoprotein and polymorphonuclear leukocytes seen in certain patients with chronic active hepatitis; smooth muscle antibodies to hepatocytic membranes, also seen in patients with chronic hepatitis; and antibodies to kidney or salivary mitochondria, a protein usually present in one type of chronic cholangitis, chronic nonsuppurative cholangitis or primary biliary cirrhosis.

Cholesterol and Bile Acids

Production of Cholesterol. While cholesterol is produced endogenously in a variety of tissues, synthesis in the liver and the mucosa of the gastrointestinal tract, especially the ileum, accounts for 97 percent of the total. Production is controlled by several variables. Synthesis in the liver, but not in intestinal mucosa, varies inversely with the amount of dietary cholesterol, ingestion causing a block primarily at step four in the accompanying diagram (Figure 7–5), the conversion of hydroxymethyl glutaryl CoA to mevalonate (Dietschy and Wilson 1970). To achieve this effect, cholesterol must be absorbed into intestinal lymphatics, a step for which a critical micellar concentration of bile salts is necessary to solubilize the cholesterol. In the absence of bile salts, cholesterol absorption is reduced and hepatic synthesis is stimulated. Fasting also reduces the synthesis of cholesterol in the

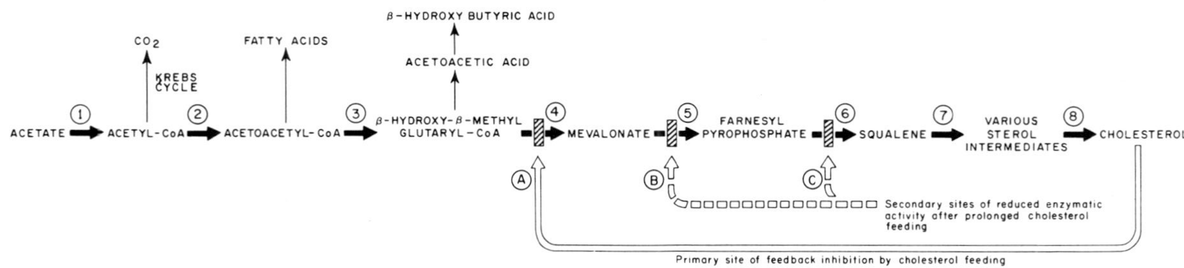

Figure 7–5. Diagrammatic representation of the major steps in the synthesis of cholesterol and the biochemical steps where metabolic control takes place. The three sites where feedback control is thought to be mediate are shown by the hatched blocks—step 4, the primary site of feedback inhibition, and steps 5 and 6, the sites of secondary control. From Dietschy JM, Wilson, JD. N Engl J Med, 282:113, 1970.

liver at step four, without affecting intestinal production. Synthesis of cholesterol in the intestine is controlled at least in part by intestinal concentrations of bile acids, production varying inversely with bile acid levels. Thus, when the bile acid pool is reduced in size, intestinal production of cholesterol increases. Bile acids are also required for the transfer of cholesterol and cholesterol esters into mesenteric lymphatics.

Removal of Cholesterol. A number of coprostanols are present in stool, having been converted from cholesterol and other sterols by intestinal bacteria. In the case of cholesterol, most of this contribution probably comes from sloughed intestinal mucosa. Very little if any fecal cholesterol appears to derive from dietary or biliary sources, since most of this has been absorbed in the upper small intestine. The major mechanism of cholesterol removal is by conversion to bile acids. A large proportion of cholesterol is hydroxylated in the hepatocyte, forming two primary bile acids, a 3,7,α-dihydroxy form (chenodeoxycholic acid) and a 3,7,12α-trihydroxy form (cholic acid). Total body pool size of chenodeoxycholate ranges from about 1 to 2.5 g, and for cholate from 0.7 to 1.2 g. These are rapidly conjugated with either taurine or glycine in hepatic lysosomes and are found in bile as glyco or tauro-cholates or chenodeoxycholates, glycoconjugates comprising about 70 to 80 percent of the total (Figure 7–6)) Javitt 1975).

Formation of Secondary Bile Acids. Bile acid conjugates reach the small intestine by way of the biliary tree and participate in forming micelles with ingested fats, aiding thereby in absorption of lipids from the upper small intestine. A small proportion of conjugated bile acids is reabsorbed by diffusion from the upper small bowel, but most is reabsorbed actively from the ileum. Roughly 1 to 2 percent of the 30 to 40 g of conjugated bile salts entering the intestine daily are lost in the stool, the remainder being retained by this enterohepatic circulatory mechanism. Deconjugation of bile salts occur through the action of bacterial (enterococcal, bacteriodal, clostridial) hydrolases, and further bacterial action dehydroxylates primary bile acids at the 7 alpha position, forming secondary bile acids, deoxycholic from cholic, and lithocholic from chenodeoxycholic. Deoxycholate is absorbed readily from the ileum and appears as a regular constituent in normal bile, even though it is a secondary bile acid. Lithocholate is absorbed poorly, and while small amounts do appear in normal bile, almost all is excreted in the feces. Concentrated gall bladder bile contains the following amounts of bile acids: cholate 18.3; chenodeoxycholate 11.5; deoxycholate 5.7; and lithocholate 1.5 mg per ml (Nakayama 1967).

Bile Acid Pool. Measurements of total bile acids in normal humans by radioactive indicator dilution techniques show a pool size averaging 3.0 to 4.0 g. While fasting, almost the entire pool remains in the gall bladder. The pool is be-

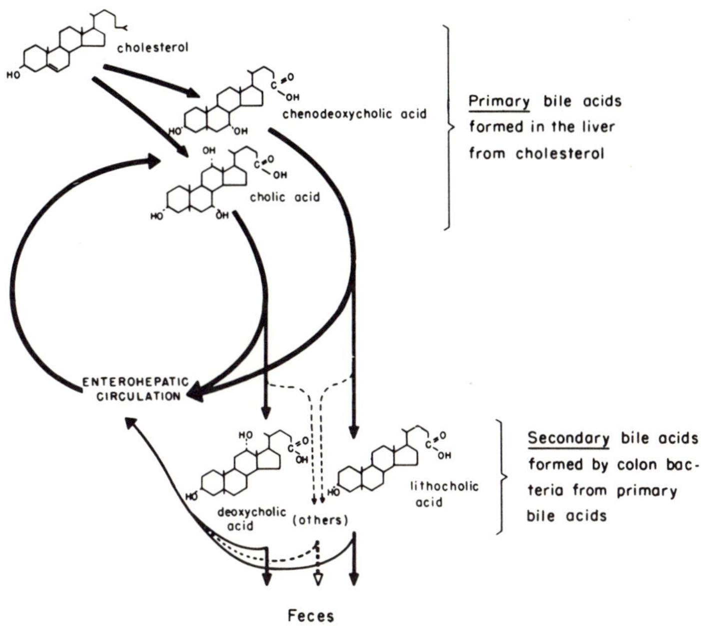

Figure 7–6. Formation of primary and secondary bile acids from cholesterol and the enterohepatic circulation of bile salts. From Javitt NB. In: Schiff L, ed. *Diseases of the Liver*, 4th ed. Philadelphia: J.B. Lippincott, 1975. Reprinted by permission.

lieved to circulate approximately twice with each meal, an average of 7 to 10 times daily. The small loss of bile salts into the stool is readily made up by formation of new bile acids from cholesterol in the liver. Since the maximal hepatic capacity to replace bile acids is about two to three times the normal daily loss, any disease which causes more than an 8 to 10 percent loss of bile acids daily, or which reduces hepatic production of bile salts, can result in significant decreases in pool size.

Measurement of Serum Bile Acids in Humans. Tiny amounts of bile acids, up to 1 or 2 μg per ml, are present normally in the blood, and concentrations of trihydroxy (cholic) and dihydroxy (chenodeoxycholic) acids are about equal. With diseases causing intrahepatic or extrahepatic obstruction, however, these levels of serum bile acids rise substantially, often up to 100 times normal. Where hepatocellular function is not heavily compromised and obstruction is the major component, elevations are greater in the trihydroxy fraction, and the trihydroxy to dihydroxy ratio may rise to as high as 6 or 7. In cirrhosis of the liver due to alcohol, total bile acid levels may be normal or increased, but the increases are greater in the dihydroxy fraction, and the ratio tends to fall well below unity.

Production of Phospholipids

Lecithin (phosphatidylcholine) is, along with cholesterol and bile acids, the third major lipid constituent in bile. It is formed in the hepatocyte from phosphatidyl ethanolamine and three methyl groups borrowed from s-adenosylmethionine, and is the major endogenous source of choline in the body. Its concentration in hepatic bile ranges from 1 to 6 g per liter. Lecithin is an amphiphilic compound whose head groups are hydrophilic and water soluble and whose nonpolar tail groups are hydrophobic and fat soluble. It is thus capable of forming soluble micelles with cholesterol which is, by itself, essentially insoluble in water. Lecithin-cholesterol micelles are believed to reside in the hepatocytic canalicular membrane. The flow of these membrane micelles into bile canaliculi is probably dependent upon the simultaneous excretion of bile acids, since cholesterol and lecithin secretion is very low when no bile salts are being transported. It is felt that bile acids allow the transition of lecithin cholesterol micelles into mixed bile-salt-lecithin-cholesterol micelles which are much more water soluble. Not all cholesterol is secreted in company with lecithin; a small amount is solubilized into micelles by bile acids alone (Wheeler and King 1972). The increased efficacy of the mixed micelle as a solubilizer of cholesterol is demonstrated by the fact that whereas 20 to 30 moles of bile acids are required to micellarize a single mole of cholesterol, a second mole is solubilized by the addition of as little as 3 moles of lecithin.

Transport of Bilirubin (Figure 7–7)

Bilirubin is a yellow tetrapyrrole formed in the reticulendothelial system from the protoporphyrin ring of heme, the iron-containing component of hemoglobin. Eighty-five percent of heme comes from the hemoglobin released from aging red blood cells at the termination of their 100- to 140-day life span, and a small amount comes from hemoglobin released during early, ineffective erythropoiesis. The remainder of this unconjugated or free bilirubin is derived from cytochromes in the liver and elsewhere, and from myoglobin.

Conversion of heme to bilirubin occurs in two steps. In the first step, which is rate limiting, the methene bridge which closes the protoporphyrin ring of heme is broken and iron is released, forming biliverdin. This compound is reduced to free bilirubin by the addition of two hydrogen ions. Each of the two enzymes involved in this process, heme oxygenase and biliverdin reductase, are dependent upon NADPH. The former enzyme is inducible by increased release of hemoglobin, epinephrine, glucagon, and starvation.

Schmid (1978) points out that the free bilirubin formed in humans (bilirubin IXα) is insoluble in water by virtue of the fact that its structure is folded in upon itself due to linkage of the propionic acid groups of its two

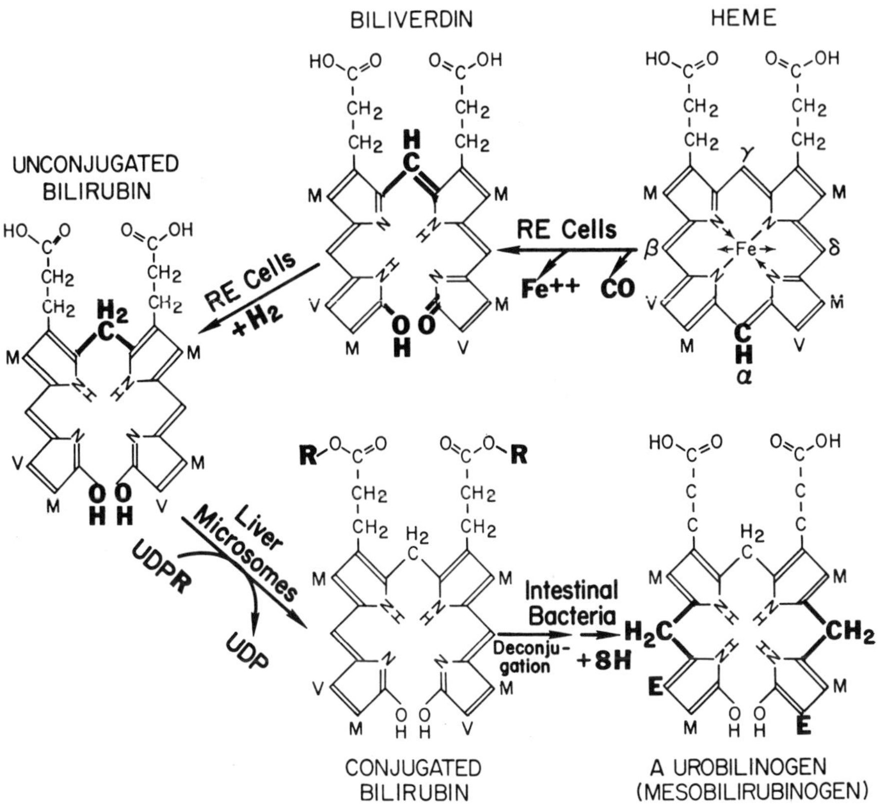

Figure 7-7. Biochemical steps in the catabolism of heme and bilirubin. M = methyl, V = vinyl, E = ethyl, UDP = uridine diphosphate, R = monosaccharide or oligosaccharide group. Two other urobilinogens are formed by further reduction of the two end pyrrole rings. From Ostrow JD. Viewpoints Dig Dis 4:1–4, (Sept) 1971. Reprinted by permission.

inner pyrrole rings with the nitrogen atoms of the two outer rings (Figure 7-8). This bilirubin molecule is transported in blood bound to albumin and, because of its insolubility, is not secreted into the urine.

Hepatic Uptake and Conjugation of Bilirubin. Bilirubin is released from albumin at the hepatocytic sinusoidal membrane and traverses that membrane and attaches to an intracellular protein called ligandin. Thus bound, it is transported to the smooth endoplasmic reticulum where conjugation of its propionic side groups occurs with one or two glucuronic acid molecules. This process is dependent on the presence of two enzymes, uridine diphosphoglucose (UDPG) dehydrogenase, which catalzyes the dehydrogenation of UDPG to the acid form (UDGPA), and glucuronyl transferase, which accel-

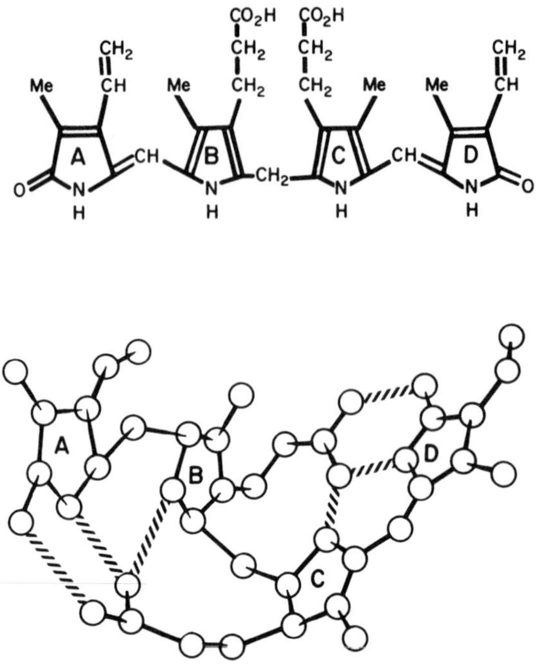

Figure 7-8. Structure of bilirubin IX: conventionally written structure (*top*) and involuted hydrogen-bonded structure (*bottom*). In the latter, the propionic acid groups of pyrrole rings B and C are linked to the nitrogens of the opposite pyrrole rings (broken lines). From Schmid R. Gastroenterology 74:1307–12, 1978. Reprinted by permission.

erates the conjugation of one or two molecules of UDGPA to one molecule of free bilirubin (Figure 7–9). Most of the bilirubin in bile is a diglucuronide, a small amount is in the monoglucuronide form, and some is conjugated to glucose and xylose. Glucuronidation opens the in-folded structure of bilirubin, making it a polar, water-soluble compound. A minor fraction of the glucuronide is also deconjugated in the hepatocyte (Gollan et al 1979). The details of the excretion of bilirubin glucuronide across the canalicular membrane into the biliary system are not known.

Both glucuronyl transferase and ligandin are lacking or present in reduced amounts in newborns, and this might account for the presence of physiologic jaundice in many infants. The process is usually self-limited since the production of these substances usually reaches normal levels within 7 to 10 days. If jaundice rises rapidly, an inducing agent, such as phenobarbital, may hasten the production of ligandin and glucuronyl transferase. In actual clinical practice, however, treatment is usually with ultraviolet light, which converts bilirubin to colorless dipyrroles and possibly also allows the patients to excrete unconjugated bilirubin owing to changes in its isomeric structure induced by ultraviolet light.

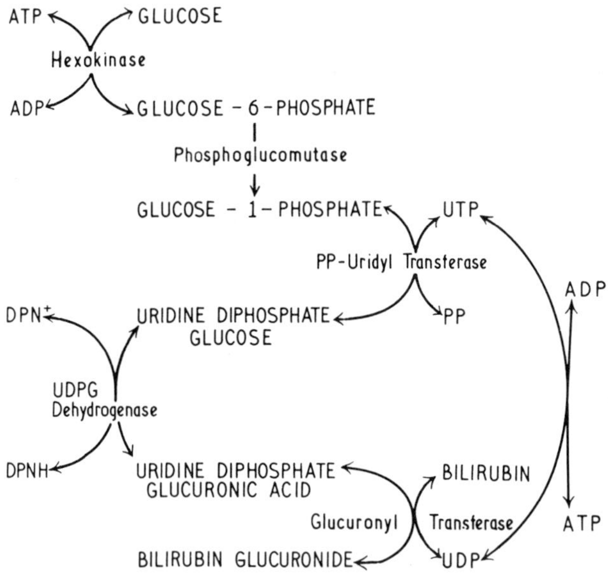

Figure 7–9. Probably mechanism for conjugation of bilirubin with glucuronic acid. (From Billing BH, Lathe GH. Am J Med 24:111, 1958. Reprinted by permission.)

Secretion of Bilirubin into the Biliary Tract and Intestine. Bilirubin is, of course, a constituent in bile, and is present in concentrations of from 10 to 70 mg per dl. It is responsible for the golden yellow color of bile in the hepatic ducts and, when concentrated in the gall bladder, imparts a black (melancholy) color to the bile. Being in a water-soluble form it rarely precipitates from bile, although it may do so if glucuronidases are present in the gall bladder.

Upon exposure to anaerobic bacterial glucuronidases in the lower small intestine and colon, bilirubin becomes deconjugated, and all of it is eventually reduced to one of a variety of urobilinogens, which are colorless tetrapyrroles. Some of these are oxidized to dipyrroles, one of which, mesobilifucsin, appears to account for the brown color of normal stool.

A large amount of urobilinogen remains in the stool, and the remainder is absorbed in the small intestine where it recirculates to liver and is reconverted there to bilirubin. Excess urobilinogen, beyond the liver's capacity to metabolize, circulates to the kidney and is excreted as urinary urobilinogen. Urinary urobilinogen levels increase after meals when large amounts of bile enter the small bowel, and when, because of disease, the liver is not able to metabolize the urobilinogen presented to it. Urobilinogen imparts no color to the urine. Its presence is detected by the addition of Ehrlich aldehyde reagent which alters it to a deep red chromogen. Porphobilinogen undergoes a similar change when treated with Ehrlich reagent, but the resultant chromogen, unlike that from urobilinogen, is insoluble in chloroform or butyl alcohol.

The Formation and Secretion of Bile

Cholesterol, bile acids, lecithin, and bilirubin are the major organic constituents of bile. Other organic compounds including drugs and dyes, such as sulfobromophthalein (BSP) and indocyanine green (ICG), are also excreted in bile following their exogenous administration. Both BSP and ICG have been used heavily in the past as tests of liver function, since the rapidity of their disappearance from the blood parallels the ability of the liver to excrete them. The use of these agents as testing compounds depends on proper intravenous injection, adequate circulation of blood to the liver, uptake by the hepatocyte and transfer to an intracellular acceptor, and secretion into bile canaliculi. The excretion of BSP additionally requires conjugation, primarily to glutathione, as part of the transfer process. These tests have lost popularity because of the numerous variables that enter into their interpretation, the increasing incidence of serious hypersensitivity reactions to BSP, their ineffectuality because of competition for acceptors with bilirubin and drugs in patients with jaundice or taking certain therapeutic agents cleared by the liver, and the availability of other less demanding and more accurate hepatic function tests.

The lipids in bile are in a clear solution as mixed micelles, bilirubin is present as a mono or diglucuronide, and other organic substances are conjugated to glucuronic acid, glucose, glutathione, sulfate, or other anions. Inorganic constituents in canalicular bile are present in concentrations approximating those in plasma, except that sodium concentrations are higher and potassium lower.

Canalicular Secretion. Canalicular secretion of bile is an active process which has two major components, that which is dependent on the simultaneous secretion of bile acids, and that which is independent of bile acid secretion. Bile acids are highly ionized at prevailing canalicular pH levels, and their active secretion carries obligate amounts of water along with it. This active process requires energy and differs from the process of glomerular filtration that is determined by pressure differentials. Those bile acids which form micelles, such as taurocholate, cause less bile flow (choleresis) at the canalicular level than do bile acids which do not form micelles, such as the synthetic dehydrocholic acid, presumably because micelles are larger and thus less osmotically potent than are ionized bile acids themselves. This type of canalicular bile secretion is referred to as bile acid dependent flow.

Certain compounds, such as theophylline, a phosphodiesterase inhibitor, and glucagon, which stimulates cyclic AMP, produce increases in canalicular bile flow without increasing bile acid excretion. Hydrocortisone causes similar effects. This bile acid independent flow comprises approximately 40 to 50 percent of canalicular secretion in humans, and may result from cyclic AMP induction in the cell with increased $Na^{+}K^{+}$ ATPase-mediated transport of sodium from the cell in exchange for potassium. Phenobarbital also increases bile acid independent flow, but the mechanism does not appear to be related to this sodium pump (Figure 7-10) (Javitt 1976; Forker 1977; Boyer 1978; Jones and Meyers 1979).

Ductular Secretion. Ductular secretion also contributes to bile flow. The gastrointestinal hormone, secretin, has been shown to stimulate the secretion from isolated canine bile ducts of a watery bile rich in bicarbonate. The administration of secretin does not increase the flow of agents, such as erythritol, which are secreted in bile canaliculi. Cholecystokinin and gastrin also stimulate ductal secretion, but in much smaller volumes than does secretin, so their physiologic importance is questionable. Insulin causes increased ductular secretion, possibly through vagal stimulation, the effect appearing to be weakened by vagotomy and the administration of anticholinergics. The physiologic role of insulin also is uncertain, but the importance of secretin appears to be established.

Absorption of electrolytes and water occurs in bile ductules, without causing changes in the osmolarity of the bile. Organic compounds become more concentrated, but total osmotic activity is kept unchanged by the simultaneous absorption of electrolytes.

Role of the Gall Bladder. This organ has the capacity to reduce the volume of hepatic bile by 80 to 90 percent, largely through the active absorption of water. The kinetics of this process are not clear but appear to be dependent on the presence of bicarbonate, chloride, and sodium. Absorption from the gall bladder ceases when bicarbonate and chloride concentrations in bile

	Canalicular Flow		Liver	Plasma	Membrane
	BDS**	BAIS*	Na^+, K^+ -ATPase	Adenyl Cyclase	Permeability
CHOLERETICS					
Taurocholate	↑				
Phenobarbital		↑	↑		
Thyroid Hormone	↑	↑	↑		
Glucagon		↑		↑	
Theophylline		↑		↑	
CHOLESTATIC AGENTS					
Ethynyl Estradiol	↓	↓	↓		↑
Sodium Taurolithocholate	↓	↓			↑
Chlorpromazine	↓	↓	↓		

Note: ↑- Increase; ↓- Decrease

Figure 7-10. Chemical modifiers of canalicular bile formation. Bile acid dependent -BDS** and independent secretion-BAIS*. From Boyer JL. Viewpoints Dig Dis 10:1-4, (Jan) 1978. Reprinted by permission.

and cholecystic mucosa are similar. The mucosa is normally impermeable to bilirubin and lipids, and even concentrated gall bladder bile is isotonic with plasma. Sodium and calcium levels are higher than in plasma, 200 and 25 mEq per liter, respectively, while chloride and bicarbonate levels are lower. Bile acid, lecithin, and cholesterol constitute 90 percent of the solutes in cholecystic bile.

The gall bladder fills passively at pressures above 8 to 10 cm of water. These pressures are induced by the force of biliary ductular secretion acting against the closed sphincter of Oddi. Cholecystic emptying is under hormonal control, primarily through the release of cholecystokinin from the duodenum in response to a fatty meal. Emptying is accomplished by relaxation at the sphincter of Oddi and sustained contraction of the musculature of the gall bladder.

Enzymes Produced at Hepatocytic Canalicular Membranes

Alkaline Phosphatases. Alkaline phosphatases are a family of enzymes which catalyze the hydrolysis of phosphate esters, releasing inorganic phosphate, at alkaline pH levels. In addition to their production in the liver, alkaline phosphatase isoenzymes are formed in the bone, intestine, and placenta. Serum alkaline phosphatase in normal blood is mainly osseous, since the hepatic enzyme is readily secreted into bile. The importance of hepatic alkaline phosphatase resides in its use as a blood test of hepatic function. Any disorder that causes a degree of stasis of bile flow leads to elevations of serum levels of this enzyme. The problem in interpretation is due to the uncertainty after determination of serum phosphatase activity regarding the site of enzyme formation. Fortunately, the isoenzymes have different degrees of stability after heating to 56°C for 15 minutes, the placental variety being extremely stable, the osseous fraction being markedly unstable to heat, and the hepatic isoenzyme having a moderate degree of stability. The isoenzyme from bone loses about 85 percent of its activity after heating, while hepatic alkaline phosphatase is degraded by around 60 percent. This differential allows for proper clinical conclusions to be drawn in most cases. Where a clear distinction cannot be made, it is possible to separate the isoenzymes by electrophoresis, but this expensive test is usually not necessary.

5′-Nucleotidase. 5′-nucleotidase is a phosphatase which hydrolyzes phosphate ester bonds of nucleotides joined to the fifth carbon atom on pentoses. The enzyme is produced only at hepatocytic canalicular membranes, and its elevation in blood is caused by stasis of bile flow, as is the case with alkaline phosphatase. Because it is not produced in bone, elevations of 5′-nucleotidase levels are more specific indicators of liver disease than are elevations of alkaline phosphatase. Since alkaline phosphatases also hydrolyze phosphate pentose bonds, their activity must be suppressed before 5′-nucleotidase levels are measured.

Leucine Aminopeptidase. Leucine aminopeptidase hydrolyzes amino acids from the N-terminal of proteins, and is a bile canalicular enzyme produced solely in that location, except during the later stages of pregnancy. Thus, in almost all cases, its elevations are most specific for hepatic disorders than are elevations of alkaline phosphatase.

Enzymes Produced in the Hepatocyte

Aspartate Aminotransferase. Aspartate aminotransferase (AsAT) (formerly called glutamic oxaloacetic transaminase, GOT) catalyzes the reversible reaction between glutamate and oxaloacetate resulting in aspartic acid and alpha-ketoglutarate. This enzyme appears in all tissues, particularly heart, muscle, liver, and kidneys, and is released into the blood after cellular damage in these organs. While estimations of AsAT in blood are not specific for hepatocellular damage in themselves, they are very useful measures of injury when considered as a part of the entire clinical picture.

L-Alanine aminotransferase. L-Alanine aminotransferase (formerly called glutamic pyruvic transaminase, GPT) catalyzes the reversible reaction between glutamate and pyruvate which results in alpha-ketoglutarate and alanine. This enzyme occurs in hepatic cells primarily, and is somewhat more specific for hepatocellular injury than is AsAT, tending to rise to higher levels with acute disease. However, from a practical point of view, there is little to choose between the two enzyme measurements in the evaluation of patients with liver disease, and AsAT measurements are more commonly available because of their wider applicability.

Microsomal Demethylation. Microsomal demethylation occurs in hepatocytes, and can be measured by the release of a tagged label in the breath after the oral administration of the isotope. In practice, ^{14}C aminopyrine is ingested, and the release of radioactivity in the breath is measured two hours later (Galizzi et al 1978). Normal individuals excrete 4 to 6 percent (mean 5.2 percent) of the label per hour, while patients with advanced hepatocellular disease (cirrhosis, hepatitis) excrete much less. There is very little overlap between normals and abnormals, and the test is considered to be a good measure of hepatocellular function, although probably not better than measurements of prothrombin activity or aminotransferase levels.

Lactic Dehydrogenase. Lactic dehydrogenase (LDH) occurs in five isoenzymes, fraction 5 being confined to the liver cell and fraction 1 being cardiac in origin. The isoenzymes can be separated by electrophoresis or by their heat stability, the hepatic fraction being less heat stable than the cardiac. LDH determinations in hepatocellular disease are useful because the elevations continue for longer periods than do elevations of the aminotransferases after acute injury and more likely to persist in patients with chronic disease.

Gamma-Glutamyl Transpeptidase. Gamma-glutamyl transpeptidase (GGTP) catalyzes the removal of glutamyl groups of aromatic amines to other amine receptors on peptides or amino acids. Largest amounts of this enzyme are found in the kidney, with smaller accumulations in the liver and heart. It is a microsomal enzyme, but levels are frequently elevated in patients with liver disease characterized by stasis of bile flow. GGTP is also elevated in patients with acute hepatocellular injury and in alcoholics; it is not elevated during pregnancy. A major value of this test is in confirmation of the significance of elevated levels of alkaline phosphatase.

THE AGING LIVER

While healthy subjects over the age of 60 have been shown to have normal liver function (Kampman et al 1975), they do demonstrate decreased weight of the liver and an increase in the size of hepatocytes (Watanabe et al 1978). Decreases with aging have been demonstrated in both hepatic blood flow and in first-pass clearance of drugs, such as propranalol (Castelden and George 1979). As for the metabolism of other drugs, there is evidence that agents which require microsomal oxidation for processing are handled less well in the healthy aged than in younger subjects, while drugs such as isoniazid, which require acetylation, are handled normally (Farah et al 1977). It has been suggested that reduced capacity to handle certain pharmacologic agents may be the result of a decreased concentration of membrane receptors with aging (Cafurny 1979). The ability of the liver to undertake 25 hydroxylation of vitamin D is reduced with aging, and this may partially explain the increased incidence of chronic bone disease among the elderly. It is clear that one should administer drugs with great care in the elderly and be acutely conscious of indications of intolerance or overdosage.

Table 7-1. Clinical Chemical Values

Aminotransferases		
aspartate, GOT	serum	10–40 U/ml
L-alanine, GPT	serum	6–35 U/ml
Ammonia	blood	80–110 μg/dl
Amylase	serum	4–25 U/ml
Ascorbic acid	blood	0.4–1.5 mg/dl
Bilirubin	serum	
Total		up to 1.0 mg/dl
Direct (conjugated)		up to 0.4 mg/dl
Calcium	serum	8.5–10.5 mg/dl
Carbon dioxide content	serum	24–30 mEq/1
Carotenoids	serum	0.8–4.0 μg/ml
Ceruloplasmin	serum	27–37 mg/dl
Chloride	serum	100–106 mEq/l

Table 7–1. Clinical Chemical Values (Continued)

Copper	serum	100–200 μg/dl
Creatinine	serum	0.6–1.5 mg/dl
Ethanol	blood	
Marked intoxication		0.3–0.4%
Stupor		0.4–0.5%
Coma		over 0.5%
Gamma glutamyl trans-peptidase	serum	5–35 U/ml
Glucose, fasting	plasma	70–110 mg/dl
Iron	serum	50–150 μg/dl
Iron-binding capacity	serum	250–410 μg/dl
Lactic acid	blood	0.6–1.8 mEq/l
Lactic dehydrogenase	serum	60–120 U/ml
Leucine aminopeptidase	serum	50–200 U/ml
Lipase	serum	2 U/ml or less
Lipids		
Cholesterol	serum	120–220 mg/dl
Cholesterol esters	serum	60–75% of total
Phospholipids	serum	9–16 mg/dl
Total lipids	serum	450–1,000 mg/dl
Triglycerides	serum	40–150 mg/dl
Magnesium	serum	1.5–2.0 mEq/l
5′-Nucleotidase	serum	0.3–3.2 Bodansky U
Osmolality	serum	285–295 mOsm/kg water
Oxygen saturation (art)	blood	96–100%
P_{CO_2}	blood	35–45 mm Hg
pH	blood	7.35–7.45
p_{O_2}	blood	75–100 mm Hg
Phosphatase (alkaline)	serum	13–39 IU/l; up to 130 u/l
Phosphorus	serum	3.0–4.5 mg/dl
Potassium	serum	3.5–5.0 mEq/l
Protein: total	serum	6.0–8.4 g/dl
Albumin	serum	3.5–5.0 g/dl
Globulin	serum	2.3–3.5 g/dl
Electrophoresis	serum	
Albumin		52–68%
Globulin		
Alpha 1		4.2–7.2%
Alpha 2		6.8–12%
Beta		9.3–15%
Gamma		13–23%
Pyruvic acid	blood	0–0.11 mmol/l
Sodium	serum	135–145 mEq/l
Sulfobromophthalein (BSP)	serum	5% or less retention in 45 min
Urea nitrogen	blood	8–25 mg/dl

Table 7-1. Clinical Chemical Values (Continued)

Uric acid	serum	3.0–7.0 mg/dl
Vitamin A	serum	0.15–0.6 μg/ml
Amylase	urine	24–76 U/ml
Copper	urine	0–100 μg/day
Coproporphyrin	urine	50–250 μg/day
Porphobilinogen	urine	0
Urobilinogen	urine	up to 1.0 unit per 2 hr (postprandial)
	Hematologic Values	
Coagulation factors		
Factor I (fibrinogen)	plasma	0.15–0.35 g/dl
Factor II (prothrombin)	plasma	60–140%
Factor V (accelerator globulin)	plasma	60–140%
Factor VIII (antihemophilic globulin)	plasma	50–200%
Factor IX (plasma thromboplastic co-factor)	plasma	60–140%
Factor X (Stuart factor)	plasma	70–130%
Factor XI (plasma thromboplastic antecedent)	plasma	60–140%
Factor XII (Hageman factor)	plasma	60–140%
Coagulation screening tests		
Bleeding time		3–9 min
Partial thromboplastin time	plasma	25–37 sec
Prothrombin time		Less than 2-sec deviation from control
Fibrinogen split products	serum	negative at greater than 1:4 dilution
Blood counts		
Hematocrit	blood	male: 45–52% female: 37–48%
Hemoglobin	blood	male: 13–18 g/dl female: 12–16 g/dl
Leukocyte count	blood	4,300–10,800/mm^3
Red cell count	blood	4.2–5.9 x 10^6/mm^3
Mean corpuscular volume	blood	89–94 Mm^3
Mean corpuscular hemoglobin	blood	27–32 pg

Table 7-1. Clinical Chemical Values (Continued)

Mean corpuscular hemoglobin concentration	blood	32–36%
Erythrocyte sedimentation rate	blood	male: 1–13 mm/hr; female: 1–20 mm/hr
Ferritin	serum	20–300 ng/ml
Folic acid	serum	Above 1.9 ng/ml
Haptoglobin	serum	100–300 mg/dl
Platelet count	blood	150–350 x $10^3/mm^3$
Reticulocyte count	blood	0.5–1.5% of red cells
Vitamin B_{12}	serum	90–280 pg/ml
	Miscellaneous Values	
Alpha-fetoprotein	serum	abnormal if present
Autoantibodies		
Antinuclear	serum	negative at 1:10 dilution
Mitochrondrial	serum	negative
Parietal cell	serum	negative
Smooth muscle	serum	negative
Carcinoembryonic antigen	plasma	0.25 ng/ml (non-smokers)
Gastrin	serum	30–200 pg/ml
Immunoglobulins		
IgA	blood	66–344 mg/dl
IgG	blood	540–1663 mg/dl
IgM	blood	39–290 mg/dl
Immunologic tests		
Alpha 1-antitrypsin	blood	200–400 mg/dl
Complement, total hemolytic	blood	150–250 U/ml
Stool fat	stool	less than 5 g/day or 4% of ingested fat in 3days
Thyroxine-binding globulin capacity	serum	15–25 $\mu g/T_4/dl$
D-Xylose		
Absorption	blood	40 mg/dl 24 hr after ingestion of 25 g orally
Excretion	urine	5–8 g in 5 hr after ingestion 25 g

Note: dl = deciliter = 100 ml.

Adapted from Case Records of the Massachusetts General Hospital, N Engl J Med 302:37–48, 1980.

HISTORICAL DIGRESSION

Names mentioned in this chapter refer to the following personages in medical history: CHRISTMAS factor, named after child with factor IX deficiency; see Biggs R, Douglas AS, MacFarlane RG et al. Christmas Disease: A condition previously mistaken for haemophilia. Br Med J 2:1378–82, 1952; Joseph D. DISSE (1852–1912), anatomist of Gottingen, Halle, and Marburg, described space between hepatic sinusoids and liver cell plates; Paul EHRLICH (1854–1915), German hematologist and immunologist, Gottingen, Berlin, Frankfurt A/M, Nobel Laureate, 1908, described diazo reaction, 1883; George J. GABUZDA, Jr. (1920–1975), American hepatologist and nutritionist, Boston, Cleveland; Francis GLISSON (1597–1677), Regius professor of physic, Cambridge University, described hepatic capsule in 1654; Camillo GOLGI (1843–1926), pathologist of Pavia, described complex structure in cytoplasm near nucleus, Nobel laureate in medicine, 1906; Carl Ewald Konstantin HERING (1834–1918), physiologist of Vienna, Prague, Leipzig, described hepatic cholangioles; Karl Wilhelm von KUPFFER (1829–1902), anatomist of Kiel and Munich, described phagocytic star cell of hepatic sinusoids; Ruggero ODDI (1864–1913), surgeon of Bologna, described ampullary sphincter; Bernhard Moritz Carl Ludwig RIEDEL (1846–1916), surgeon of Jena, described hepatic anomaly in 1888, also described form of thyroiditis which bears his name; Abraham VATER (1684–1751), anatomist of Wittenberg, described common duct ampulla and papilla in 1720; and Johann Georg WIRSUNG (1600–1643), prosector to Vesalius of Padua, described main pancreatic duct in 1642.

SELECTED REFERENCES

Boyer JL. Bile secretion and the pathogenesis of cholestasis. Viewpoints Dig Dis 10:1–4, (Jan) 1978.

Cafurny EJ. Pharmacology and aging. Fed Proc 38:1899, 1979.

Castelden CM, George CF. The effect of aging on the hepatic clearance of propranalol. Br J Clin Pharmacol 7:49–54, 1979.

Dietschy JM, Wilson JD. Regulation of cholesterol metabolism. N Engl J Med 282:1128–38, 1179–83, 1241–49, 1970.

Farah F, Taylor W, Rawlins MD, et al. Hepatic drug acetylation and oxidation: Effects of aging in man. Br Med J 2:155–56, 1977.

Forker EL. Mechanisms of hepatic bile formation. Ann Rev Physiol 39: 323–47, 1977.

Galizzi J, Long RG, Billing BH, et al. Assessment of the (^{14}C) aminopyrine breath test in liver disease. Gut 19:40–45, 1978.

Gollan J, Hammaker L, Licko V, et al. Hepatic deconjugation of bilirubin glucuronides: A normal metabolic pathway. Gastroenterology 77:A14, (Nov) 1979.

Jackson CM. The biochemistry of prothrombin activation. Br J Haematol 39: 1–8, 1978.

Javitt NB. Bile acids and hepatobiliary disease. In: Schiff L, ed. Diseases of the Liver, 4th ed. Philadelphia: J.B. Lippincott 1975:111–45.

Javitt NB. Hepatic bile formation. N Engl J Med 295:1464–69, 1511–16, 1976.

Jones AL, Schmucker DL. Current concepts of liver structure as related to function. Gastroenterology 73:833–51, 1977.

Jones RS, Meyers WC. Regulation of hepatic biliary secretion. Ann Rev Physiol 41:67–82, 1979.

Junge U, Creutzfeldt W. Hepatotrophic effects of pancreatic and gastrointestinal hormones in the rat *in vivo* and *in vitro*. In: Ciba Foundation Symposium 55 (ns), Hepatotrophic factors. Amsterdam: Elsevier-Excerpta Medica-North Holland, 1978:269–83.

Kampmann JP, Sinding J, Moller-Joregenson I. Effect of age on liver function. Geriatrics 30:91–95 (Aug) 1975.

Nakayama F. Quantitative microanalysis of bile. J Lab Clin Med 69:594–609, 1967.

Rappaport AM. Anatomic considerations. In: Schiff L, ed. Diseases of the liver, 4th ed. Philadelphia: JB Lippincott, 1975:1–50.

Schaffner F, Popper H. Electron microscopy of the liver. In: Schiff L, Diseases of the liver, 4th ed. Philadelphia: JB Lippincott, 1975:51–87.

Schmid R. Bilirubin metabolism. State-of-the-art. Gastroenterology 74:1307–12, 1978.

Starzl TE, Porter KA, Francaville JA, et al. A hundred years of the hepatotrophic controversy. In: Ciba Foundation Symposium 55 (ns), Hepatotrophic factors. Amsterdam: Elsevier-Excerpta Medica-North-Holland, 1978:111–29.

Watanabe T, Shimada H, Tanaka Y. Human hepatocytes and aging: A cytophotometrical analysis in 35 sudden-death cases. Virchows Arch B Cell Path 27:307–16, 1978.

Wheeler HO, King KK. Biliary excretion of lecithin and cholesterol in the dog. J Clin Invest 51:1337–50, 1972.

DISCUSSION QUESTIONS

1. Following sudden massive hepatocellular destruction, which hepatocytic proteins would become most rapidly depleted? How would this depletion be most easily measured? How might it be manifested?
2. What hepatocytic enzyme levels rise most precipitously in common bile duct obstruction? Which are most significant for this condition?

CHAPTER 8

Mechanisms and Diagnosis of Hepatic Disease

There is a multitude of causes of liver injury and a variety of ways in which the liver may react to them. Recognition of the nature of any hepatic disease rests on a thorough understanding of the effects of the various etiological agents, the multiple ways in which these agents can react in different patients, and the specific tests which can aid in their recognition. Without attempting to concentrate on any specific hepatic diseases, save for the congenital disorders of bilirubin metabolism, this chapter attempts to identify the major pathways that hepatic injury may follow, the various effects of injury on hepatic morphology, and the tests and procedures that can help to clarify the cause of the clinical picture.

MECHANISMS OF ACUTE LIVER DISEASE (Table 8–1)

The liver can be considered to have three functional components: the hepatocytes and Kupffer cells, the biliary system, and the vascular system. Most disease, at least in its early stages, tends to predominate in one or another of these components, and it is frequently possible to deduce this by careful clinical appraisal.

Hepatocellular Disease

Clinical Picture. Acute damage to hepatocytes and reticuloendothelial cells (Figure 8–1), as in viral hepatitis or in hepatitis due to alcohol or other hepatocellular toxins, results in ill-defined symptoms of malaise, anorexia, nausea, and fever of slight to moderate degree. Premonitory symptoms such as arthritis, urticaria, or other rash, believed due to circulating immune complexes, may have preceded or accompanied these symptoms where hepatitis B virus or drug hypersensitivity is the causative agent. Since the liver often becomes edematous and enlarges suddenly in patients with acute hepato-

Table 8-1. Clinical and Pathological Pictures in Prototype Liver Diseases

Symptoms, Signs, Findings	*Hepatocellular*	*Cholestatic*	*Congestive*
Upper right quadrant pain	occasional	occasional	frequent
Pruritus	occasional	common	rare
Jaundice	frequent	frequent	occasional
Bilirubinuria	yes	yes	yes
Stool color	normal to acholic	tends toward acholic	normal
Urobilinogen	present	reduce to absent	present
Elevations of			
Aminotransferases	marked	moderate	moderate-marked
Alkaline phosphatase	moderate	marked	moderate
Bile salts	moderate	marked	moderate
^{14}C breath test	reduced	normal	reduced
Prothrombin time	normal to prolonged	normal to prolonged	normal to prolonged
Response to vitamin K	no, partial	complete	no, partial
Liver biopsy	1. focal or confluent necrosis 2. lobular infiltrates 3. centrilobular cholestasis 4. portal infiltrates 5. piecemeal necrosis at times 6. hypertrophy of Kupffer cells	1. minimal necrosis 2. feathery degeneration 3. central and periportal cholestasis 4. variable portal infiltrates 5. bile pigment in Kupffer cells	1. centrilobular nonsinusoidal dilatation and hemorrhage 2. atrophy of liver cell plates 3. centrilobular necrosis 4. hypertrophy of Kupffer cells

cellular disease with distention of the capsule of Glisson, patients may complain of mild upper right quadrant discomfort and note pain when pressure is exerted on the liver. Jaundice may be present at onset, but usually appears after prodromal symptoms, and often does not occur at all.

Laboratory Findings. Cytoplasmic enzymes are released in large quantities into the general circulation as a result of damage to hepatocytic membranes and may be detected as extreme elevations of aminotransferases and lactic dehydrogenase. Since transport of bilirubin through hepatocytes to bile

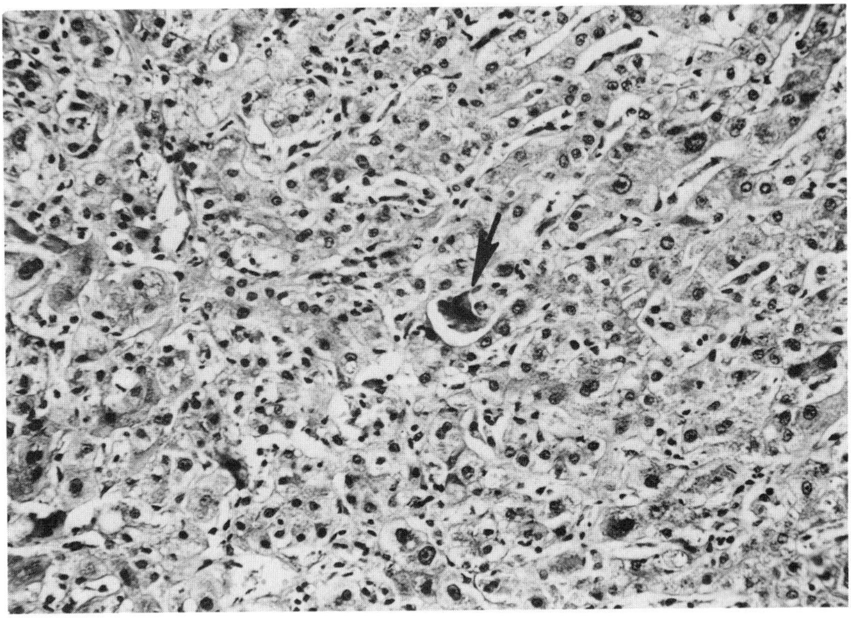

Figure 8–1. Acute viral hepatitis. The normal cordlike arrangement of hepatocytes is in disarray, and many hepatocytes themselves exhibit ballooning degeneration and necrosis. The arrow points to a Councilman body, which is a necrotic hepatocyte with eosinophilic cytoplasm and a pyknotic nucleus, lying loosely in a sinusoid. Kupffer cells are prominent and a degree of neutrophilic infiltration is present. Original magnification x200.

canaliculi is generally disturbed to varying degrees, the pigment regurgitates into hepatic sinusoids and appears in the circulating blood, primarily in the conjugated form. Since conjugated bilirubin is soluble in water, the pigment also appears in the patient's urine, and causes it to become deeply amber in color. Despite the fact that the injured hepatocyte continues to conjugate bilirubin, the rate of conjugation is slowed enough to cause an elevation of unconjugated bilirubin levels in the blood as well. Thus, the hyperbilirubinemia of patients with hepatocytic disease consists of both conjugated and unconjugated elevations, the former usually being slightly higher than the latter.

While bile flow is often reduced considerably in patients with acute hepatocellular disease and may even be completely suppressed in the earliest stages, enough bile pigment enters the intestinal tract to maintain normal stool color during most of the period of jaundice. During periods of complete suppression of bile flow, stool color becomes light yellow and is commonly referred to as a clay-colored stool. Reduction of bilirubin to urobilinogens in the lower intestinal tract continues at a normal rate, and much of the absorbed urobilinogen appears promptly in the urine, often in increased amounts because the acutely damaged liver is unable to reconvert urobilinogen to bilirubin at the normal rate. Of course, when decreased amounts of bile pigment reach the intestine in acute hepatocellular disease, decreased amounts of urobilinogen are formed. This fact, plus reduced hepatic uptake, may result in normal levels of urine urobilinogen. Thus urinary urobilinogen may be absent in patients with acute hepatitis while they are in a complete cholestatic phase, it may be increased when normal production is accompanied by decreased hepatic uptake, and it may be decreased when intestinal production is low and hepatic uptake, while low, is adequate to metabolize the amount of urobilinogen circulated from the intestine. Thus, while the absence of urobilinogen from the urine is suggestive of complete cholestasis, its presence in reduced, normal, or increased amounts does not give any solid information about the severity of the underlying hepatic disease.

Alkaline phosphatase and 5′-nucleotidase levels may be elevated in patients with acute hepatitis, paralleling the degree of associated cholestasis. However, it is characteristic of patients with hepatocellular disease that elevations of alkaline phosphatase, if present, are proportionately much less than are elevations of intracellular enzymes, such as the aminotransferases, which may rise to 20 to 40 times the normal serum values. Alkaline phosphatase elevations are rarely more than thrice the upper limit of normal in such patients.

Serum proteins with long half-lives, such as albumin, are usually normal in patients with acute hepatitis. Prothrombin times, however, are excellent measurements of the severity of the disease. Since many of the coagulation components are short-lived, their levels fall quickly in the presence of acute, severe damage, and the one-stage prothrombin time is prolonged. Patients may also note prolonged bleeding times after receiving small cutaneous injuries. The only precaution to be taken in interpreting the one-stage prothrombin result is to be assured that an excess of vitamin K is present at the time the study is made. Since some patients with acute hepatitis pass through periods of cholestasis and consequent malabsorption of fat and fat-soluble vitamins, like vitamin K, and since vitamin K is essential to the formation of factors II, III, IX, and X, prolongation of the one-stage test may simply be the result of depleted vitamin K stores. If the time remains prolonged following administration of parenteral vitamin K, it is clear that the hepatic injury is quite severe. If it reverts to a normal level, the prognosis is much better, since the causative cholestasis in acute hepatitis is usually a self-limited process.

Bile acid concentrations, while not commonly performed in clinical laboratories, have been found (Javitt 1975) to rise considerably in acute hepatocellular diseases, their concentrations paralleling the degree of cholestasis. The ratio of trihydroxy (cholic) to dihydroxy (chenodeoxycholic) acids is usually well above unity. When this ratio falls below that level for more than several days, the prognosis for the underlying disease is worsened.

Pathologic Changes. Changes appear throughout the liver, although the intensity may vary from place to place. Hepatic lobules, especially in centrilobular and periportal areas, biliary canaliculi, and portal areas are involved, the vasculature generally being spared. A spectrum of disease is defined, from the most mild to the very severe.

Hepatocytes in acute hepatitis are markedly affected; the damage is called *confluent* if it affects a large group of neighboring cells and particularly if it affects neighboring acini, or *focal* if neighboring acini are not involved. Individual hepatocytes enlarge and their cytoplasm becomes granular as they degenerate, a process called *ballooning necrosis*. Later on, cytoplasm condenses, nuclei shrink, and deeply eosinophilic residues, called *Councilman* or *acidophilic bodies*, are seen attached to sinusoids. In the same areas, regeneration is also seen, manifested by large, multinucleate hepatocytes, as a response to the surrounding necrosis. This combination of necrosis and regeneration distorts the architecture of the usually regular plates of liver cells, but the architecture of the lobule itself is well preserved. Kupffer cells become swollen and often contain iron granules derived from necrotic hepatocytes. Infiltration with mononuclear cells occurs throughout the lobule to varying degrees, in response to hepatocytic necrosis. Complete regeneration of the liver can occur as long as the reticulin framework is not distorted by the inflammatory process. If the reticulin structure is damaged, healing occurs only with a scar.

In more severe cases of hepatitis, areas of confluent lobular necrosis occur, resulting in portal to central *bridging, or submassive necrosis*, a process which renders a poor prognosis and always results in scarring. *Massive necrosis* is the most severe form of acute hepatitis. No hepatocytes or Kupffer cells remain, there being only large areas of amorphous, fibrillar eosinophilic material containing iron particles. Portal tracts are seen, but they are often in varying stages of degeneration and tend to fall closer to one another because of loss of the supporting reticulin framework of the liver. Massive hepatic necrosis is rarely, if ever, compatible with survival.

Ultrastructurally, hepatocytic necrosis reveals distortion of the smooth and rough endoplasmic reticulum, decreased amounts of cytoplasmic glycogen, mitochondrial swelling, and increased numbers of lysosomes. Loss of cytoplasmic fluid and collapse of organelles probably give rise to the acidophilic bodies seen on light microscopy. Nuclear changes occur late and are manifested by clumping of chromosomes and finally by nucleolar degeneration.

Bile canaliculi, especially in the centrilobular area, may contain bile thrombi in patients with acute hepatocellular disease. The intensity of this process is generally proportional to the degree of jaundice. There is nothing distinctive about this *centrilobular cholestasis*, and the diagnosis of acute hepatocytic disease rests on the findings already described of hepatocellular change and mononuclear infiltrates. By electron microscopy, bile canaliculi appear to be dilated and distorted, and their lumens may be filled by swollen microvilli. Hepatocytes may also show intracellular cholestasis, with bile deposits appearing as fibrillar and vesicular elements aggregated at the sites of partially depleted glycogen bodies.

Portal areas show moderate amounts of inflammatory infiltrate in acute hepatocellular disease, the portal areas being distended largely by accumulations of mononuclear cells, and also by occasional plasma cells and rare eosinophils. There is usually little evidence of damage or proliferation of bile ducts, but some ductular cells may swell and undergo necrosis in places where inflammatory infiltrates are heavy. Portal infiltrates, in severe hepatitis, may extend directly into adjacent hepatic lobules and blur the usually sharp outlines of the limiting plate. This process may appear to be exactly like the significant *piecemeal necrosis* characteristic of active chronic hepatitis, but may be distinguished by the shorter duration of the disease and by the fact that chronic hepatitis is usually not associated with as much diffuse hepatocellular necrosis as is encountered in acute hepatitis.

In alcoholic hepatitis (Figure 8–2), the diagnosis is usually established by seeing areas of focal necrosis of hepatocytes surrounded or infiltrated by neutrophils. While not requisite to the diagnosis, necrotic or swollen cells commonly also contain cytoplasmic inclusions of a reddish pink material called *Mallory hyalin bodies.* This material may also be found in patients with Wilson disease and in primary biliary cirrhosis, but is most common in

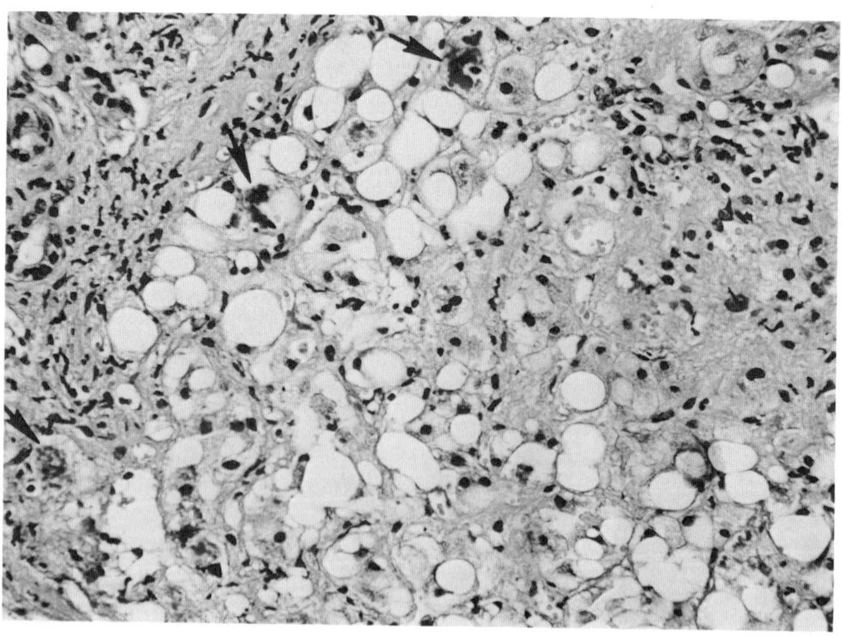

Figure 8–2. Alcoholic hepatitis. Focal necrosis and neutrophilic infiltration on the right of the picture are typical of this condition. The presence of hydropic hepatocytes containing Mallory bodies (arrows) and the fatty changes are also distinctive. Original magnification x225.

alcoholic liver disease, and appears to result from an increase of microfilaments probably arising from the hepatocytic cytoskeleton (Denk et al 1981). Many hepatocytes may also contain fat, especially in centrilobular areas, in patients with alcoholic hepatitis. Fat tends to accumulate first in the dilated channels of a partially disorganized smooth endoplasmic reticulum, and later fuses into large globules which push the nucleus to the side of the cell.

Drugs may also cause acute hepatocytic necrosis, but the changes are rarely specific, and the diagnosis usually rests on the patient's history. Fatty change is also a common result of drug reaction. Scheuer (1974) points out that centrilobular necrosis and fatty change are typical of reactions to carbon tetrachloride and paracetamol (acetominophen). Fatty change alone occurs in patients receiving large doses of tetracycline intravenously. Halothane, alpha methyldopa, isoniazid, and methotrexate, among many other drugs, are capable of causing limited to extensive hepatocytic necrosis.

Granulomatous hepatitis (Figure 8-3) is also caused by a variety of agencies. Granulomas are defined "as compact, rounded collections of histiocytes (usually epithelioid cells) not necessarily accompanied by other features such as necrosis" (Poulsen and Christoffersen 1979). Giant cells commonly result from coalesence of epithelioid cells. The granulomas appear most commonly in periportal areas, and are frequently infiltrated by lymphocytes, plasma cells, and fibroblasts. Hepatocytic necrosis around

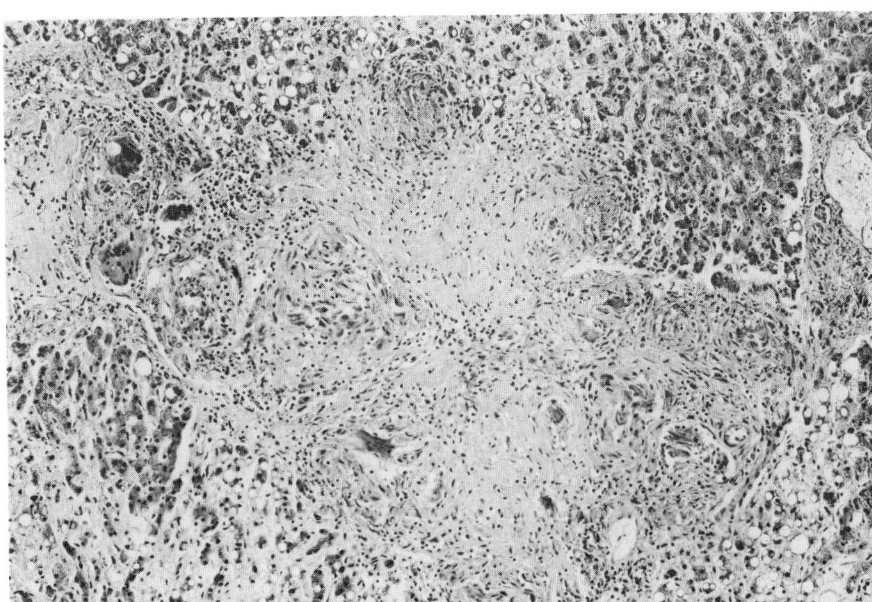

Figure 8-3. Granulomatous hepatitis in a patient with sarcoidosis. This granuloma system involves a portal tract and contains epitheliod cells, lymphocytes, and giant cells. Original magnification x80.

granulomas is variable and may be absent. This form of inflammation is seen in many disorders including: tuberculosis, sarcoidosis, schistosomiasis, primary biliary cirrhosis, talc injection, and as a response to a variety of drugs, including halothane, phenylbutazone, and allopurinol.

Cholestatic Liver Disease

Diseases of the biliary ductal system, whether intrahepatic or extrahepatic, are obstructive to the flow of bile constituents and are grouped under the general heading of cholestatic disorders. They are manifested primarily by the appearance in the blood of those products which the liver normally secretes into the biliary tract, and usually are unassociated, until late in their course, with significant degrees of hepatocellular dysfunction. When obstruction is confined to bile canaliculi, it must be quite extensive before clinical or laboratory signs appear. But when sudden obstruction occurs in a large extrahepatic bile duct, especially the common bile duct, a lesion of small size and quite localized may promptly cause marked clinical abnormalities. The symptoms of obstructive disease may be quite insidious, and a patient might not be aware of illness until jaundice occurs. There are many causes of *intrahepatic cholestasis*, including drugs, hormones, viruses and endotoxins. Genetic predisposition also plays a part in some cases. Popper (1981) points out that the mechanisms of intrahepatic cholestasis are also multiple, and include dysfunction of the $Na^+ K^+$-ATPase ion pump on the basal lateral surface of the hepatocyte, disturbances in the physico-chemical characteristics of the hepatocytic canalicular membrane, alterations in the cytoskeleton, and changes in flow through hepatocytic tight junctions.

Clinical Picture. Jaundice in cholestasis results from the inability of bilirubin to bypass the obstructed biliary passages and its consequent detour into the bloodstream. Since hepatocellular function is good, most of the bilirubin is conjugated and water soluble and appears in the urine. If obstruction is complete, bile fails to enter the intestinal tract, stool becomes clay-colored, and urobilinogen disappears from the urine. Failure of bile acids to enter the intestinal tract results in reduced micellarization of ingested lipids and the appearance of increased amounts of fat in the stool (steatorrhea). Patients may note that stool not only becomes light in hue, but bulky, foul smelling, and oily as result of bile diversion. Itching is also a common complaint and is related to elevations in serum bile acid levels.

Biliary obstruction, or stasis, at the canalicular level may be caused by drugs such as chlorpromazine or methyl testosterone, granulomatous hepatitis, or viral hepatitis. Larger bile ducts, particularly those beyond the liver, may become obstructed by calculi, strictures, or ductal neoplasms, as well as by extrabiliary diseases such as pancreatic carcinoma, pancreatitis, or carcinoma of the ampulla of Vater. When biliary tract infection supervenes, especially when common duct obstruction is partial, as is often the case with biliary calculi and pancreatitis, microabscesses and macroabscesses may appear in the liver, causing chills, fever, and frequently, septicemia.

Laboratory Findings. Cytoplasmic enzymes tend to rise slightly in patients with cholestasis, due probably to mild membrane damage caused by obstruction. The elevations may be two to three times the upper limit of normal but do not approach the massive increases seen in acute hepatocytic disease.

Alkaline phosphatase and 5′-nucleotidase levels rise massively in cholestatic syndromes and are indeed the laboratory hallmark of this disease category. Obstruction actually induces the formation of these enzymes at hepatocytic canalicular microvillous membranes, so that levels are even higher than what might be expected from obstruction alone. They may rise to five or six times the upper normal limits. Serum levels of cholesterol also rise, but not to the same extent as the alkaline phosphatase. Increased production presumably results from the reduced access of bile salts to the intestine.

Total serum protein levels are usually unaffected by early cholestasis. Prothrombin times may be increased because of reduced absorption of fat-soluble vitamins but revert promptly to normal after the parenteral administration of vitamin K. This response indicates that hepatocellular function is intact.

Bile acid concentrations in the blood are elevated, almost by definition, in patients with cholestatic disorders, and often to very high levels. While the rise occurs in both trihydroxy and dihydroxy bile acids, the elevation is usually proportionately higher in the trihydroxy fraction, with a resultant increase in their normal ratio of unity. The ratio in cholestasis may occasionally rise to as high as seven, and does not fall below unity unless considerable hepatocellular disease is also present. Bile acid concentrations may be elevated in patients who do not have pruritus and are always elevated in those who do.

Pathologic Changes. As might well be expected, microscopic changes in cholestasis (Figure 8–4) are most prominent in the biliary system. They are seen earliest in centrilobular areas and consist of bile thrombi in dilated canaliculi and bile pigment granules in hepatocytes and Kupffer cells. The lobular architecture is preserved and hepatocytic necrosis is minimal or absent in pure acute disease, although centrilobular hepatocytes may show enlargement and variation in nuclear size in patients with drug-induced cholestasis. Periportal cholestasis, consisting of bile clumps in liver cells but not canalicular thrombi, is characteristic of chronic disorders. In drug-induced cholestasis, portal areas are often infiltrated with eosinophils.

In large bile duct obstruction, cholestasis is more likely to cause spotty damage to hepatocytes. Cells become swollen, and the cytoplasm stretched into thin bands, a picture called *feathery degeneration*, which probably re-

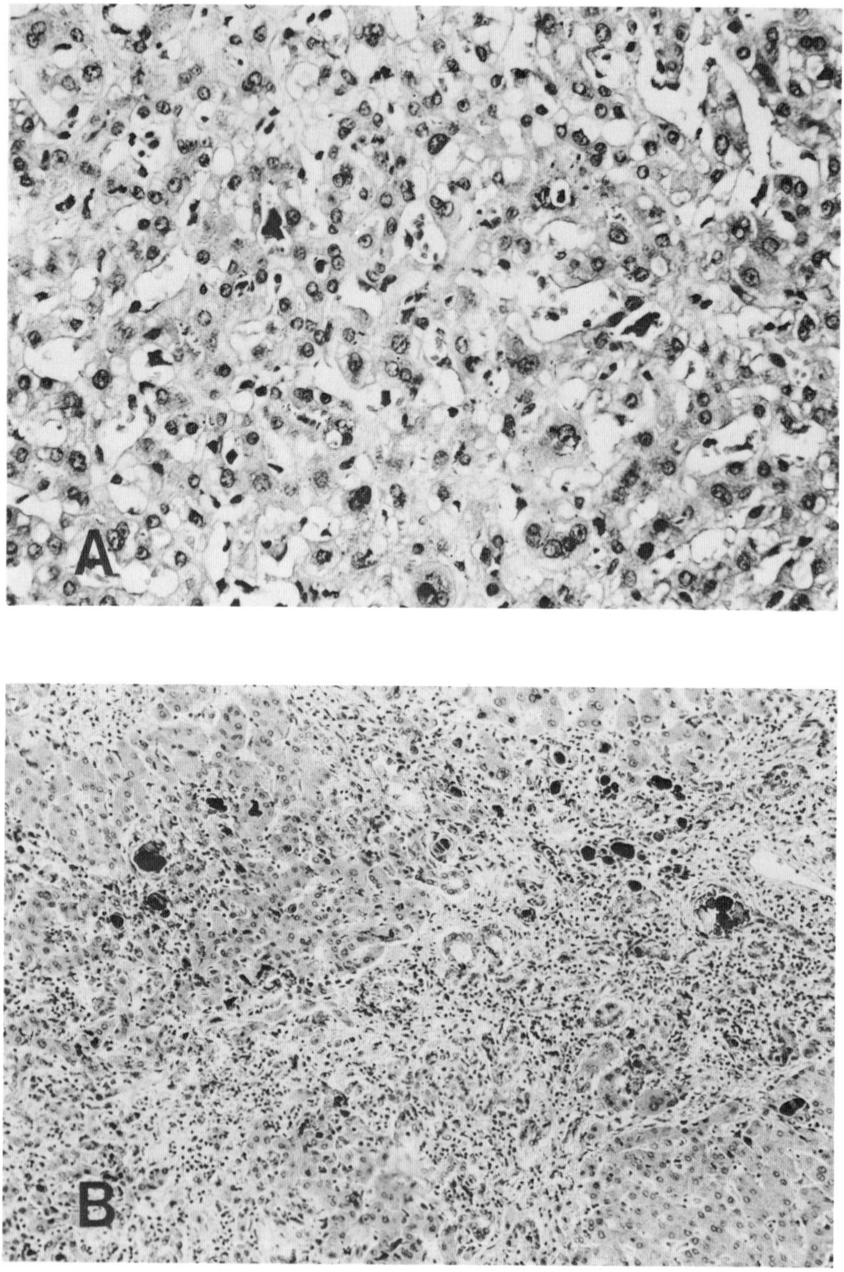

Figure 8–4. Cholestasis. *A*, drug-induced intrahepatic cholestasis. Bile thrombi are seen in dilated canaliculi, and bile pigment is present in adjacent hepatocytes and Kupffer cells. Original magnification x250. *B*, extrahepatic cholestasis due to choledocholithiasis. Bile thrombi are again present in ducts and canaliculi, but there is also marked acute and chronic inflammation in the portal tracts. Original magnification x80.

sults from cytoplasmic damage by bile acids. Groups of these cells clumped together, usually around a portal area, are called *bile infarcts*. Small amounts of inflammatory infiltrate eventually appears around these areas. Large ductal obstruction leads to swelling of portal tracts and appearance of a mixed inflammatory infiltrate, containing neutrophils. A classical change, the appearance of proliferating bile ductules, occurs at the margins of portal areas, the ductal nuclei varying in size and shape. Bile leakage from ducts occurs occasionally and may form *bile lakes* in the periportal parenchyma. While diagnostic of large bile duct obstruction, both bile infarcts and bile lakes occur rarely in this condition and should not be considered as being essential to the diagnosis. With prolonged obstruction to large bile ducts, periportal fibrosis occurs and, with ascending cholangitis, intraductal neutrophils and periportal abscesses may be seen.

Primary biliary cirrhosis presents in its earliest stages as an irregular necrosis of the epithelium of larger intrahepatic bile ducts, surrounded by a heavy infiltrate of lymphocytes and plasma cells, and by small numbers of eosinophils. Granulomas may also be present, but the diagnostic lesion is the bile duct damage. The portal infiltrates may overrun the limiting plates of adjacent liver lobules and show a picture of piecemeal necrosis. In later stages of the disease, ductular proliferation occurs and, still later, scarring and cirrhosis.

Hepatic Disease of Vascular Origin

Circulatory diseases of the liver may involve either the afferent (hepatic arterial or portal vein) or efferent (hepatic vein) channels. Thrombosis of the portal vein (pylethrombosis) may occur as a result of infiltration with pancreatic, biliary, or other cancers, as a result of cirrhosis of the liver, or as a consequence of pylephebitis secondary to an untreated pelvic or appendiceal abscess. Save for ascending septic phlebitis in the liver, resulting from the latter cause, portal venous obstruction in itself causes very little damage to the liver because obstruction occurs gradually and collateral flow is rich. Ligation of the hepatic artery may lead to prompt ischemic necrosis of the liver, infarction, and death. Fortunately, this disorder is seen very rarely, as a surgical misadventure.

Major hepatic circulatory disorders involve obstruction to hepatic vein flow (Budd-Chiari syndrome) by thrombi, as in polycythemia rubra vera, or by tumor, or increased hepatic vein pressures induced by chronic right-sided heart failure or constrictive pericarditis. Patients taking herbal medicines containing senecio or crotalaria or some patients with bone marrow transplants may develop serious veno-occlusive disease of the liver characterized by endothelial damage and narrowing of hepatic sinusoids and small hepatic veins.

Clinical Picture. Hepatic congestion usually has a slow onset and is often associated with deep upper right quadrant pain resulting from distention of the hepatic capsule. Ascites occurs commonly as a result of increased intrahepatic pressure, followed by rupture of hepatic lymphatics and weeping from the surface of the liver. A mild degree of jaundice may also be seen.

Physical examination shows that the liver is distended and tender, and that patients with congestive right heart failure show a pronounced hepatojugular reflex. Ascites may also be demonstrated.

Laboratory Findings. No diagnostic laboratory changes are found in patients with hepatic congestion, but conjugated bilirubin levels are commonly elevated to a moderate degree. Aminotransferase levels may be extremely high if there is a great deal of acute hepatic necrosis.

Pathologic Changes. Centrilobular dilatation of sinusoids and atrophy of liver cell plates with preservation of lobular architecture are the constant features of venous congestion of the liver (Figure 8–5). Confluent necrosis in the centrilobular areas and hemorrhage with separation of liver cords is also commonly seen, the degree depending on the severity of the obstruction. Hypertrophy and hyperplasia of Kupffer cells occurs in response to the necrosis.

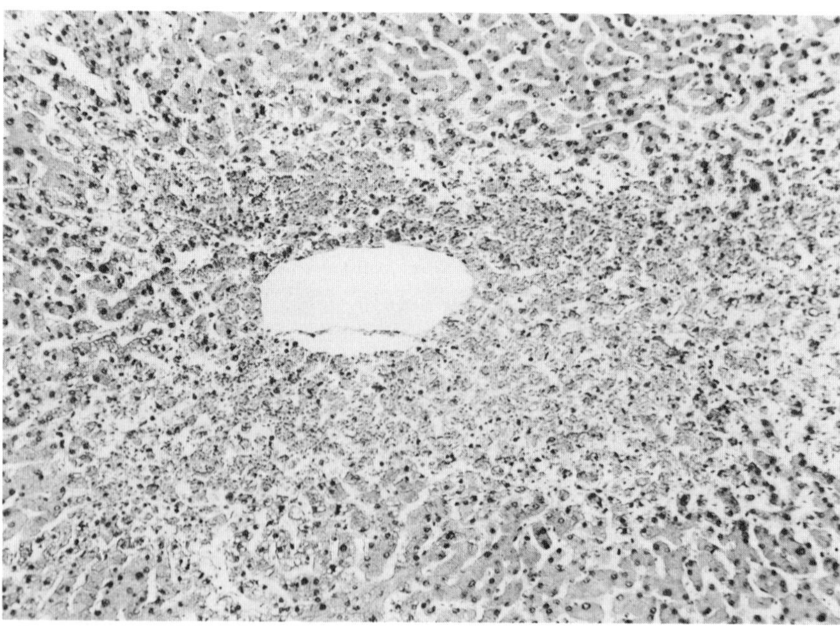

Figure 8–5. Acute hepatic congestion. The sinusoidal spaces in the centrilobular region are distended with red blood cells and the central vein is enlarged. Original magnification x115.

MECHANISMS OF CHRONIC HEPATIC DISEASE

Most acute diseases of the liver heal spontaneously when the causative agent, such as hepatitis virus, toxic medications, alcohol, biliary ductal obstruction, and congestive heart failure, is removed or controlled. In a number of instances, however, resolution is not complete and the liver disease enters a chronic phase. This change to a chronic process is often insidious and may result from a patient's inability to be rid of hepatitis virus, the initiation of destructive autoimmune processes, the unknowing continued exposure to toxic agents, the continued exposure to known toxins such as alcohol, lack of availability of effective therapy, as in sarcoidosis, primary biliary cirrhosis and certain extrahepatic cancers, and not infrequently, the patient's inability to recognize the existence of hepatic disease. A number of stages have been identified pathologically in this process of chronicity and have led to a clearer understanding of the pathogenesis of chronic liver disease than was the case in the past. While these stages have been most closely related to the progression of viral hepatitis, especially type B and type C (non-A, non-B), they may also apply to toxic and alcoholic hepatitis as well, and possibly to acute hepatitis from other cause. These stages are slowly resolving hepatitis, persistent chronic hepatitis, active chronic hepatitis, lobular chronic hepatitis, cirrhosis of the liver, and hepatocellular carcinoma. These stages are not necessarily successive and do not always change from one to another. They are merely various stations along the way at which chronic hepatitis can lodge temporarily or permanently (Popper and Schaffner 1971).

Slowly Resolving Hepatitis

This designation is merely a term of convenience to describe those patients with acute hepatitis whose symptoms and abnormal hepatic function tests continue beyond six to eight weeks after onset. Slowly resolving hepatitis may continue for up to three months and is not necessarily associated with a poor prognosis. Patients in this category may have no symptoms or may notice continued weakness, fatigability, and possibly persistent mild icterus (jaundice). In more severe forms, patients may notice some signs of hepatic insufficiency, such as the presence of spider angiomata in the skin and easy bruisability due to depletion of blood clotting factors. More extreme symptoms, such as deepening jaundice, onset of edema, and hepatic encephalopathy suggest another diagnosis, such as submassive hepatic necrosis.

Laboratory Findings. Liver function studies may show sustained mild elevations of prothrombin time, up to 2 to 3 sec above control levels, and of aminotransferases up to 200 to 300 units per ml. Mild elevations of bilirubin to 3 to 4 mg per dl, mainly in the conjugated (direct reacting) fraction, are also common. Longer lived serum proteins, such as albumin, should remain within normal ranges. The ^{14}C aminopyrine breath test may also be mildly abnormal.

Pathology. The liver biopsy is characterized by changes similar to those of acute hepatitis. Many hepatocytes are swollen and often multinucleate. Spotty necrosis, consisting of a few degenerating cells and Councilman bodies, is common, and Kupffer cells show hyperplasia and increased presence of cytoplasmic iron pigment. Bile plugs may be seen in centrilobular canaliculi, and infiltrates of round cells or plasma cells are present spottily in parenchyma and in portal areas. The lobular architecture of the liver is preserved, and no fibrosis is apparent in lobular and periportal areas. Piecemeal necrosis, if present, is only minimal, and bile duct hyperplasia is not seen. Bridging necrosis from portal to centrilobular areas is a poor prognostic sign, if present, and is not compatible with the diagnosis.

Treatment. Slowly resolving hepatitis requires no specific treatment other than patience and careful observation with regular appraisal of hepatic function studies. Worsening of symptoms or of laboratory tests suggests a more severe diagnosis and probably calls for a trial of therapy with small doses of glucocorticoids, especially if the patient shows evidence of autoimmune changes, such as positive tests for DNA and nuclear or smooth muscle antibodies.

Persistent Chronic Hepatatis

This is primarily a pathologic diagnosis but does relate to a group of patients who continue, with or without an identifiable preceding attack of acute hepatitis, to have mild chronic lassitude, occasional upper right quadrant discomfort of hepatic origin and mild aberrations in hepatic function tests. They have none of the stigmata of chronic liver disease discussed below, require no treatment aside from infrequent reassessment of hepatic function tests, and enjoy a very good prognosis. Rarely may persistent chronic hepatitis progress into a more severe stage of hepatic disease.

Findings. On examination, the liver may be slightly enlarged, but the edge is smooth and rarely tender. Hepatic function tests are characterized by slight elevations of aminotransferase levels to two to three times normal, and usually no or very slight elevations in alkaline phosphatase and bilirubin. Prothrombin content and serum albumin are normal. Hepatitis B antigenemia may be present.

Pathology. Persistent chronic hepatitis on liver biopsy (Figure 8-6) is typified by the mildness of its changes, which are confined almost exclusively to

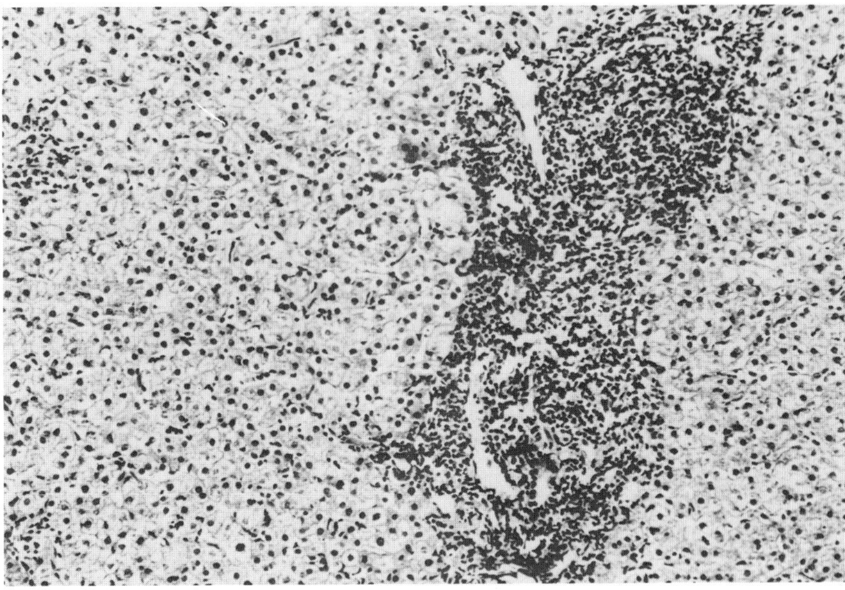

Figure 8–6. Chronic persistent hepatitis. The portal tract is abundantly infiltrated with lymphocytes, but the outline of the portal tract is distinct and shows no evidence of piecemeal necrosis. A small focus of lobular infiltration is seen in the left upper corner of the picture. Hepatocytes are intact. Original magnification x150.

portal tracts. In these, there is a modest mononuclear infiltrate with occasional plasma cells, and only very minimal piecemeal necrosis, if any. Occasional hepatocytic necrosis may be seen, and there may be small amounts of mononuclear infiltrate in the lobules.

Lobular Chronic Hepatitis

If persistent chronic hepatitis can be considered to be synonymous with portal chronic hepatitis, then there must also be a rubric for lobular chronic hepatitis, for a small number of such cases have been defined clinically and pathologically (Wilkinson et al 1978).

Findings. The clinical picture is one of successive attacks resembling acute hepatitis, often extending over a period of many years. Individual attacks are often prolonged and may require the use of glucocorticoids to induce a remission. The disease, unlike active chronic hepatitis, does not progress to cirrhosis and is not associated with hepatitis B virus infections. While evidences of autoimmunity, such as smooth muscle and nuclear and mitochondrial antibodies, are usually present, the fact that the disease appears acute on successive biopsies often months or years apart suggests that attacks probably represent reactivation of a single virus strain harbored by the patient, rather than continuous disease. At least one fatality has been reported, associated with deepening jaundice and septicemia.

Individual attacks closely resemble acute hepatitis, with malaise, nausea, and deep conjugated jaundice being invariably found. During remissions, whether induced or maintained by glucocorticoids or occurring spontaneously, symptoms and icterus disappear, and patients are clinically well. Function tests are similar to those seen in acute hepatitis with marked elevations of bilirubin and aminotransferases. They differ from tests in acute hepatitis, however, by showing hyperglobulinemia, which may be persistent, in most cases, and by the presence of autoantibodies.

Pathology. Biopsy changes durng relapses are indistinguishable from those of acute hepatitis, with spotty necrosis, mononuclear infiltrates and Kupffer cell hyperplasia in hepatic lobules, and mild portal infiltrates. Occasionally, confluent necrosis is seen. In remissions, residual changes in portal areas may be similar to those of persistent chronic hepatitis, but with evidence of lobular infiltrates and mild centrilobular necrosis as well.

Active Chronic Hepatitis

The alternative name for this disorder, aggressive chronic hepatitis, expresses the serious, progressive nature of this form of chronic disease. That name was coined, however, by pathologists to describe the advanced picture of hepatic necrosis and fibrosis seen not only in patients with active hepatitis, but also in patients with severe toxic hepatitis, autoimmune hepatitis, and Wilson disease.

Findings. Symptoms vary from being almost entirely absent to marked fatigability and moderate jaundice. Abdominal discomfort, anorexia, and increased bleeding tendency are common associated symptoms. Other than jaundice, patients exhibit hepatomegaly in most cases, splenomegaly in about one-half the cases, spider nevi and palmar erythema frequently, and ascites and hepatic encephalopathy occasionally. The disorder is most common in women, who make up around 80 percent of patients in most series, and is usually identified in the second and third decades of life, although its occurrence in children and in patients over age 50 is not rare. In something like half the patients, the disease eventually becomes inactive, but many of these have already developed cirrhosis. Esophageal varices, the result of portal hypertension, and gastrointestinal hemorrhage are common complications. Bleeding may be from peptic ulcers or gastric erosions rather than from varices, and is often aggravated by coexistent reductions in coagulation factors due to hepatocellular necrosis, and platelets due to hypersplenism. In one series of 82 patients (Mistilis 1970), survival rates were

76 percent in treated and 55 percent in untreated patients after six years, 58 percent and 55 percent after 10 years, although the groups were small in later years. Death is due to progressive hepatic failure, often associated with gastrointestinal bleeding and septicemia.

Laboratory studies in patients with active chronic hepatitis frequently shows a moderate anemia, leukopenia, and thrombocytopenia due to hypersplenism, although some of the anemia may result from iron deficiency as well. Bilirubin levels are almost always elevated, but usually at levels below 10 mg per dl, and aminotransferase levels are similarly always increased, but not massively so. Prothrombin times are often increased by several seconds over controls, albumin levels are often reduced, and serum globlin levels are typically increased due to broad elevations of gamma fractions. Nuclear, smooth muscle and DNA antibodies are common, and some patients form lupus erythematosus rosettes as well.

Pathology. Changes in the liver biopsy are often not uniform and can range from mild to severe in different parts of the same organ. Piecemeal necrosis (Figure 8-7), or spillage of portal infiltrates beyond the limiting plate and

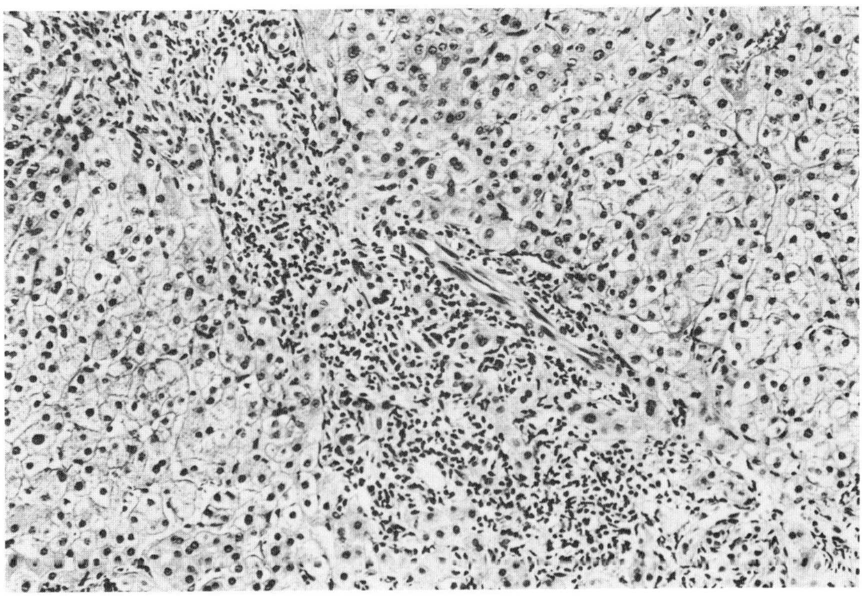

Figure 8-7. Chronic active hepatitis. The limiting plate, which is the junction between the portal tract and hepatocytes, is ragged and irregular showing clusters of degenerated hepatocytes completely surrounded by inflammatory cells. This erosion of periportal hepatocytes by inflammatory exudate is known as piecemeal necrosis and is the most important histologic feature of this disease. Original magnification x150.

into the lobular parenchyma, is the hallmark of active chronic hepatitis. Often small groups of perilobular hepatocytes are cut off from the remainder of the lobule by the exudate. Portal areas themselves show a heavy mononuclear exudate and proliferation of bile ducts. Fibrous tissue strands often develop around periportal hepatocytes and proliferated biliary ductules. If bridging necrosis (Figure 8–8) from portal to central areas is present, which is uncommon, the collapsed reticulin framework may be seen as a fibrous septum. Balloon cells are marked in perilobular areas, and occasional Councilman bodies may be seen. Rosettes, or tubules formed by the apposition of three or more hepatocytes arranged around a central focus, may be seen adjacent to areas of necrosis. They are separated by sinusoids and inflammatory cells and may represent areas of adenomatous regeneration. Hepatocytes in midzonal and pericentral portions of the lobule are often quite normal in milder cases of active chronic hepatitis. In advanced cases, lobular architecture may be markedly distorted, and early evidence of cirrhosis (Figure 8–9) (regenerative nodules) may be seen.

Cirrhosis of the Liver

Scheuer (1974) defines cirrhosis "as widespread fibrosis of the liver, nodular hyperplasia and portal-systemic shunting resulting from liver in-

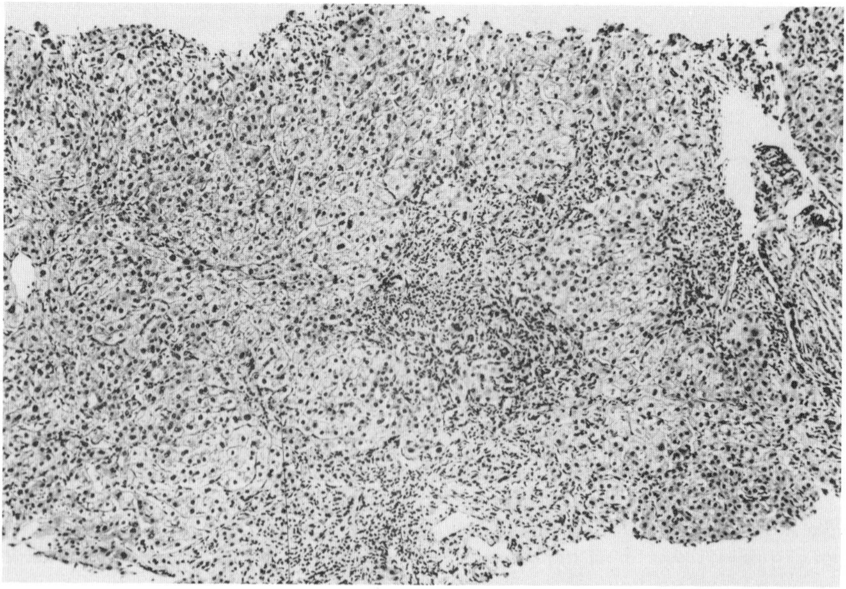

Figure 8–8. Bridging necrosis. The lobular structure is altered by extensive chronic inflammation and fibrosis in the portal tracts, a process which eventually spreads to involve adjacent portal and centrilobular areas in bridges of necrosis. Original magnification x80.

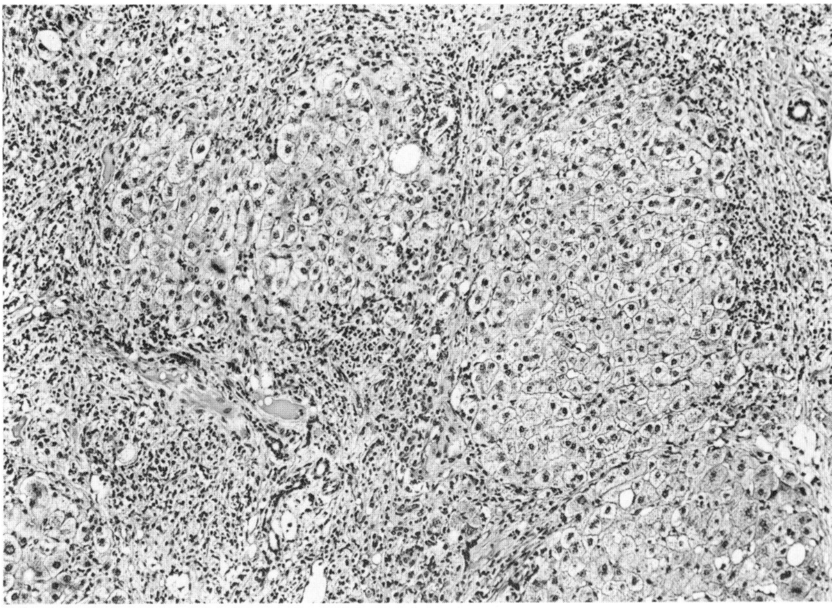

Figure 8–9. Regenerating nodules. The normal lobular architecture is lost and replaced by regenerating hepatocytic nodules completely surrounded by fibrous septa and inflammatory exudate. Central veins are not present in these nodules. Original magnification x100.

jury." The presence of bile duct proliferation would be an added criterion of many pathologists.

Clinical Picture. Cirrhosis of the liver commences when a continuing etiologic agent of hepatocytic necrosis produces enough damage to the reticulin framework that regeneration of liver tissue along normal lines is no longer possible. The causes of cirrhosis of the liver are multiple; in the Western world, alcohol, continued infection or autoimmune responses to hepatitis viruses B and C, and certain toxic agents appear to be the major ones. Biliary cirrhosis appears not infrequently, especially among middle-aged women, as the result of a primary destructive cholangitis of unknown cause. and occasionally occurs secondarily to long-standing obstruction of large bile ducts. In children, biliary cirrhosis is a common outcome of congenital atresias of the large bile ducts. While uncommon, cirrhosis is a recognized and serious consequence of certain genetically transmitted diseases. These may lead to accumulations of nonmetabolizable endogenous precursors, or of certain metals, in the hepatocyte. Alpha 1 antitrypsin deficiency is an example of the first group; hemochromatosis and Wilson disease (hepatolenticular degeneration), the second. Retention of copper has been implicated in the genesis of both Wilson disease and primary biliary cirrhosis, but the case is most clear in the former.

There are no distinctive symptoms that herald the transition from mere ongoing hepatocellular damage to cirrhosis. Often, the patients are not aware that anything is amiss, unless chronic symptoms of malaise are present, as in chronic hepatitis. Ankle edema due to hypoalbuminemia or ascites (accumulation of intraperitoneal fluid) due to hypoalbuminemia and portal hypertension may be initial symptoms. Gastrointestinal hemorrhage from coagulation disorders, with or without esophageal varices, may be an early complaint. Other symptoms may be jaundice, malaise, increased bleeding tendency, loss of weight, or confusion, the last being an indication of hepatic encephalopathy. Early complaints in patients with bile duct obstruction, especially those with primary biliary cirrhosis, are pruritus and the occurrence of subcutaneous fatty infiltrates in the eyelids (xanthelasma), on elbows, or over extensor tendons of hands (xanthomata). Cirrhosis, then, is an insidious disease that develops over a long period of time, gradually saps hepatic function, and often presents suddenly when a single or several hepatic functions are reduced to the point where their loss can no longer be compensated.

Physical findings are also variable. Cutaneous signs of hepatic insufficiency are common. Palmar erythema presents as an unusual degree of reddening of the thenar and hypothenar eminences, the ridge overlying the metacarpophalangeal joints and the skin over the distal phlanges of the fingers, with whitening of the central palmer areas, all resulting from presumed arteriovenous anastomoses in the hand. Spider nevi are small cutaneous arteriovenous communications in the skin which occur on the face, neck, and upper shoulders. Telangiectases may also occur, especially over the cheeks. These cutaneous signs are not solely the result of liver disease, may occur also with aging and during pregnancy, and appear to result from heightened estradiol levels. Gynecomastia also occurs frequently, and has been related to decreased hepatic extraction of adrenal androstenedione which is converted peripherally to estrogens. Testicular atrophy is a common result of androgenic deficiency. The appearance of subcutaneous hemorrhages parallels deficiencies of blood coagulation factors or platelets.

Jaundice is a common symptom of cirrhosis, usually associated with active hepatocytic necrosis. Stool color may be lighter than normal but is usually not acholic (clay-colored), except in those rare instances where biliary obstruction is complete.

Mental confusion, especially disorientation and decreased attention to personal care, is found in many cirrhotics as an early manifestation of hepatic encephalopathy. Muscular atrophy, especially in the neck, shoulder girdles, arms, and chest, results from decreased nutrition in advanced cirrhotics. Mild to marked ascites and edema of ankles, legs, and thighs is common. Inspection of the upper abdomen and periumbilical areas often shows prominent cutaneous veins, representing enlarged collateral channels of venous return from the lower trunk which bypass the liver and indicate the presence of portal hypertension.

If hepatomegaly is present, the surface of the liver is firm and occasionally nodular, and the edge is blunt and inflexible. Often one lobe is more prominent than the other. The spleen is usually very large if portal hypertension is present, and its surface is also firm. Occasionally ascites is so massive that the enlarged liver and spleen cannot be palpated, except occasionally by ballotment.

Laboratory findings can usually be predicted from the physical findings. Anemia due to iron deficiency, hypersplenism, and chronic disease is common. Leukocytes and platelets are often decreased in patients with splenomegaly, but leukocytosis is often seen in patients with alcoholic hepatitis and cirrhosis. Urine contains urobilinogen and bilirubin in most icteric patients, unless complete obstruction leads to the absence of urobilinogen production. Serum albumin is usually reduced below normal levels, especially when edema and ascites are present. Hyperglobulinemia is also common in cirrhotics, being most pronounced in patients with chronic hepatitis and cirrhosis. Hyperlipidemia occurs frequently in patients with primary, and occasionally in patients with secondary, biliary cirrhosis. Prothrombin times are usually prolonged, sometimes to extreme degrees, and do not improve completely after administration of vitamin K. Aminotransferase levels are mildly to moderately increased depending on the degree of hepatocytic necrosis present, and alkaline phosphatase levels are only mildly elevated, unless the cirrhosis is primarily obstructive in nature. Abnormalities in the ^{14}C amino pyrine breath test are in line with prothrombin abnormalities. Bile acid levels are raised in cirrhosis, elevations being much higher in biliary than in other types. Patients with alcoholic cirrhosis commonly show a trihydroxy to dihydroxy ratio of less than unity, while in patients with biliary cirrhosis the ratio may rise to two or above.

Pathology. The pathologic picture of cirrhosis (Figure 8–10) appears when preceding hepatocytic necrosis is associated with degeneration of the reticulin framework, and hepatocytic regeneration occurs but is no longer in a regular pattern because of the stromal damage. Completely necrotic areas of the liver lobule are replaced by strands of fibrous tissue, while less damaged or normal hepatocytes regenerate in irregular patterns because of the loss of stroma. Regenerating hepatocytes grow in a nodular fashion, and the size of the "regenerating nodules" is limited by the density of the fibrosis. Irregular sinusoidal and canalicular growth also occurs, and nodules may outgrow their blood supply and canalicular drainage with the result that necrosis may occur at the center of nodules. Nodular hepatocytes are found often to contain bile pigments. Nodules may occasionally look at first glance like hepatic lobules, but central veins cannot be identified. Similarly, liver cell cords are commonly two or three or more cells instead of one cell in width. Because adjacent hepatic lobules have collapsed and become fibrotic due to necrosis, surrounding portal areas may appear to have fallen together, so that several portal areas may be seen closely apposed to one

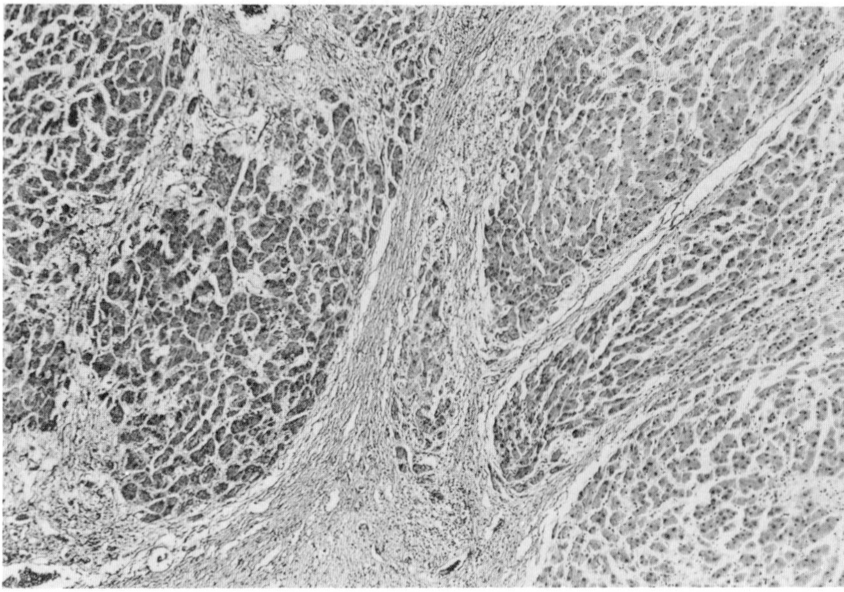

Figure 8–10. Macronodular cirrhosis. Regenerating nodules of variable size are separated by dense fibrous septa-containing proliferating bile ducts. Original magnification x50.

another. Similarly, vascular injury in the liver leads to the development of an irregular supply of sinusoidal blood to nodules, and numerous intrahepatic shunts develop in the damaged liver between hepatic arterioles and portal venules, and between these and hepatic venules. Thus, considerable amounts of blood may flow through the cirrhotic liver without having come into contact with hepatocytes.

Cirrhosis occurs descriptively in two major forms: *micronodular,* in which nodular size is 1.0 cm or less in diameter and the liver is involved homogeneously by the process; and *macronodular,* in which nodules are usually much larger than 1 cm, and the size of nodules may be quite variable in different portions of the liver. There is evidence that micronodular disease may, in time, be transformed into macronodular cirrhosis by increases in the size of micronodules. Micronodular cirrhosis is seen commonly as a consequence of alcoholic liver disease, and also in early stages of the cirrhosis following active chronic hepatitis, biliary obstruction (primary and secondary), passive congestion of the liver, and hemochromatosis. Macronodular cirrhosis tends to occur either after submassive necrosis of the liver, or secondarily, after long-standing micronodular cirrhosis of any cause. An intermediate stage between these two types in which both micronodules and macronodules are present, is seen occasionally. A posthepatitis form of macronodular cirrhosis has been described, in which abnormal but thin strands of fibrous tissue surround each liver nodule, while portal areas and central veins are fairly well preserved. This is distinguished from the postnecrotic form, in which nodules lack portal areas and central veins, and fibrous septa are broad and irregularly distributed throughout the liver. The broad areas of fibrosis have resulted from large areas of previous hepatic necrosis with collapse of the reticulin framework of the liver.

Micronodular cirrhosis is characterized on biopsy (Figure 8-11) by the regularity of nodular size and the presence of slender strands of fibrous tissue surrounding and entering into the nodules. While the severity of the process may vary in different parts of the liver, it is usually present to some degree throughout. Proliferating bile ducts are noted characteristically in the fibrous strands, and vascular areas are also usually increased. Hepatocytes in the nodules show variable degrees of necrosis and regeneration. In alcoholic cirrhosis, necrosis and fibrosis begin in centrilobular areas and extend later to portal areas. In the cirrhosis accompanying chronic hepatitis, inflammatory infiltrates are usually heavy in active disease, and piecemeal necrosis and lobular exudates are common. Plasma cells are prominent in the exudate, and neutrophils may also be present. Central

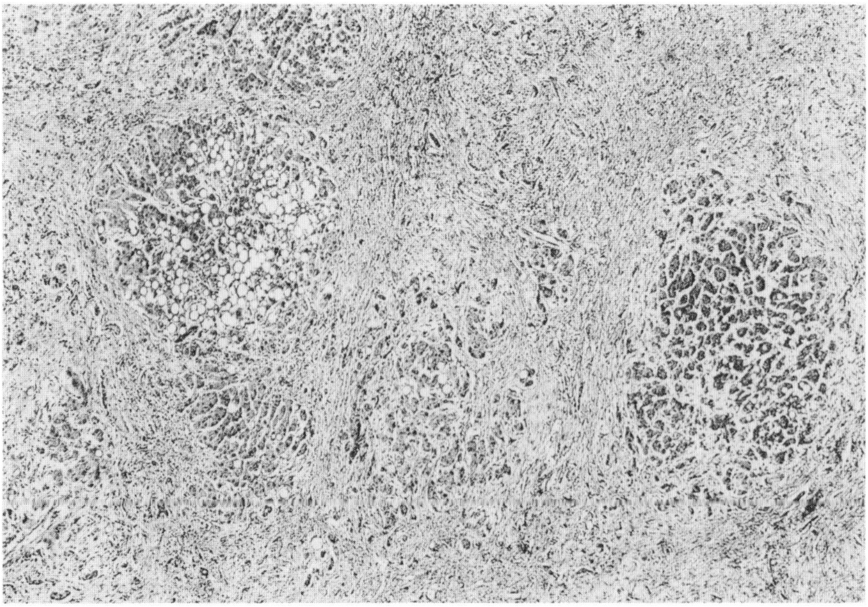

Figure 8-11. Micronodular cirrhosis. Regenerating nodules, small and uniform in size, are surrounded by broad fibrous septa. Original magnification x50.

veins are usually not visible in the nodules, indicating that these are indeed regenerative nodules rather than damaged hepatic lobules.

Specific etiologies of the cirrhosis may be identifiable. Hepatocytes whose nucleus is pushed to one side and whose walls are distended by a homogeneous ground-glass-appearing cytoplasm are characteristic of hepatitis virus type B infections. These cells may also appear in cases of persistent or active chronic hepatitis due to hepatitis B virus. Reduction in the number of bile ductules and necrosis of those seen is characteristic of late stages of primary biliary cirrhosis, especially when inflammatory exudate is heavy and granulomas are also present. Hyaline sclerosis of centrilobular areas, focal necrosis of hepatocytes with neutrophilic infiltrates, and often cytoplasmic Mallory bodies and fat strongly suggest the presence of alcoholic cirrhosis. In secondary biliary cirrhosis, that due to large bile duct obstruction, the fibrosis and nodularity of the liver are accompanied by marked proliferation of bile ducts with cholestasis and edema of portal tracts with infiltration by neutrophils. So-called cardiac cirrhosis in response to prolonged passive congestion of the liver is rare but may be identified by the continued presenoe of sinusoidal swelling near central veins and by fibrous septa from portal to central vein areas.

Macronodular cirrhosis has essentially the same basic pathologic picture as micronodular cirrhosis and differs only by the facts that nodules are larger and more variable in size and that fibrosis, while widely distributed, is laid down in bands of varying width. Proliferation of bile ducts is always present, and the amount and type of hepatocellular necrosis varies with the type and activity of the cirrhosis. Macronodular cirrhosis without exudate and necrosis is referred to as *inactive cirrhosis*.

Hepatocellular Carcinoma

While this disease may appear spontaneously in otherwise normal livers, it is seen most commonly in the West in company with preexisting macronodular cirrhosis and has been considered to be part of a continuum from hepatocytic regeneration to atypia to cancer. As many as 70 percent of cases of hepatocellular carcinoma occur in cirrhotics, and about 15 percent of patients dying with cirrhosis have the associated malignancy. Patients with hepatitis B antigenemia and cirrhosis, hemochromatosis, and macronodular alcoholic cirrhosis, in descending order, seem to be at greatest risk. Both exogenous natural products and chemicals appear to be important in causing hepatocellular carcinomas in humans without cirrhosis and may also increase the risks of patients with cirrhosis. Among causes that have been implicated are aflatoxins produced by naturally occurring fungi, certain plant toxins, synthetic agents with occupational exposures, such as chloroform, carbon terachloride, and DDT, and substances used medically, such as isonicotinic acid and methotrexate. All these agents have been shown to be capable in animals of altering cellular DNA and promoting regeneration of mutated forms at the expense of normal strains (Zimmerman 1978). A clear connection has been made in humans between exposure to vinyl chloride and development of angiosarcoma, rather than hepatocellular carcinoma.

Clinical Picture. Unfortunately, there is no clearly identifiable change in a patient's clinical situation which predicts the subsequent occurrence of carcinoma of the liver. In groups of patients at high risk, such as those with chronic hepatitis due to hepatitis B virus infections and with inadequately treated hemochromatosis, it is well to perform regular examinations aimed at monitoring hepatic size and function. This program is likely to identify hepatocellular carcinomas relatively early in their course, at times when they may be most amenable to chemotherapy or lobar resection of the liver.

Whenever a patient known to have a stable or moderately active form of cirrhosis develops anorexia, loss of weight, or weakness without obvious anemia or deterioration in hepatocellular function, hepatic cancer should be suspected. Pain, fever, and changes in hepatic configuration on physical examination should also alert physicians to this possibility. Beyond these symptoms and findings, the clinical picture of hepatocellular carcinoma blends so closely into the picture of deteriorating hepatic function due to progressive liver failure that distinctions cannot be made readily.

Laboratory findings in hepatocellular carcinoma are highlighted by marked increases in alkaline phosphatase and 5′-nucleotidase levels, out of proportion to alterations in hepatocellular function tests. This is due to obtrusion of the intrahepatic mass on canalicular bile flow. When these measurements of cholestasis appear, further study with radionuclide hepatic scans and sonograms is clearly indicated. Numerous patients with hepatocellular carcinomas also develop elevated hematocrits, the erythrocytosis resulting from autonomous production of erythropoietin by the tumor. The appearance of alpha fetoprotein in the serum is almost a diagnostic marker of hepatocellular carcinoma.

Pathology. The histological picture (Figure 8–12) is variable and ranges from nodules of fairly normal-appearing hepatocytes to a tumor growing in a ductular pattern to advanced anaplasia. Most commonly seen is nonlobular proliferation of hepatocytes in liver cell plates more than two cells thick. Cytological changes consist of prominent and often multiple nucleoli, increased mitoses, hyperchromasia of nuclei, and pleomorphism. Tumor hepatocytes typically secrete bile into canaliculi, and Kupffer cells are reduced in number. Vascular invasion is occasionally seen. In well-differentiated carcinomas one must look carefully for these changes at times, and they are often most clearly adduced when the tumor area is compared with normal or cirrhotic portions of the same liver.

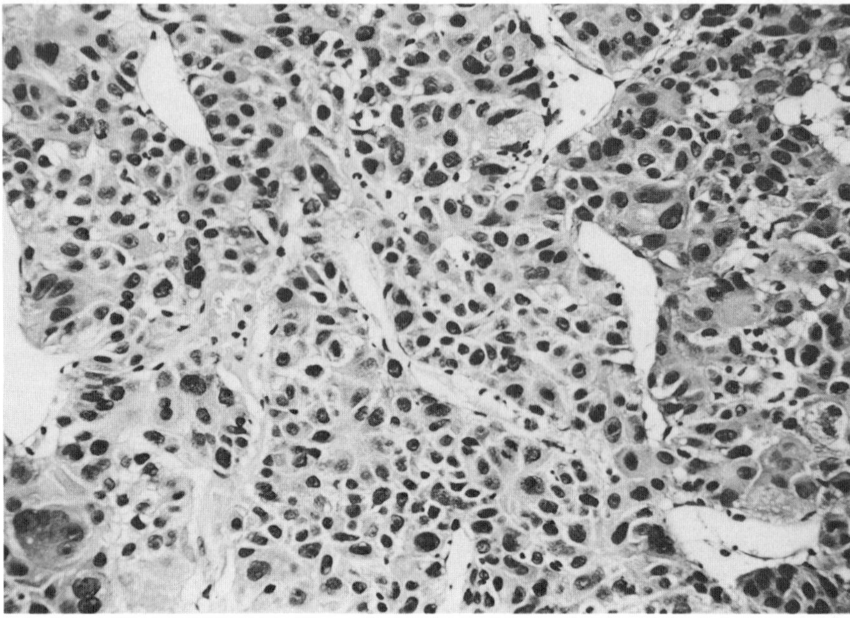

Figure 8-12. Hepatocellular carcinoma. The malignant cells are surrounded by capillaries resembling the sinusoidal pattern seen in normal liver. But cell strands contain several rows of hepatocytes, nuclei are hyperchromatic and large, and their cytoplasm is eosinophilic and abundant. Prominent nucleoli can be seen in some of the malignant cells. Original magnification x200.

DIFFERENTIAL DIAGNOSIS OF HYPERBILIRUBINEMIA

The tireless and attentive reader should, at this point, be able to distinguish between at least two of the three major types of hyperbilirubinemia (jaundice) seen in clinical practice, that due primarily to hepatocellular disease and that due primarily to cholestasis or ductal obstruction. It should also be recognized that in many diseases of the liver, one encounters combinations of these two types of hyperbilirubinemia and that the diagnostic conclusions made in each patient depend mainly on which form is more prominent.

Pure hepatocellular hyperbilirubinemia is characterized by elevations of both conjugated and unconjugated bilirubin in the blood, the former fraction being larger than the latter. The conjugated elevation results from inability of bilirubin to pass out of the hepatocyte at normal rates due to postconjugative damage to the hepatocyte, while the unconjugated levels are raised because the delay in excretion slows the entire process of conjugation and consequently delays the uptake of prehepatocytic (unconjugated) bilirubin. Bilirubinuria is always presents because of the solubility in water of bilirubin glucuronide, and stool color is normal because bile pigments do enter the intestinal tract, even though the rate of entry may be reduced. Finally, the presence of bilirubin in the lower intestine means that bacterial reduction to urobilinogens will take place and that urobilinogenuria will be associated with this type of hyperbilirubinemia. The only exception to this last attribute of hepatocellular jaundice occurs in those uncommon situations where bacterial flora in the intestine are reduced because of concomitant administration of antibiotics, or in newborns who develop this picture before bacterial flora have fully appeared. In these situations, urobilinogenuria may be absent in association with hepatocellular jaundice.

Pure cholestatic or obstructive hyperbilirubinemia is also associated with elevations of both conjugated and unconjugated blood levels of bilirubin, and usually levels of the former are greater. The mechanism is the same for hepatocellular jaundice, although the obstruction is beyond, rather than in, the hepatocyte. Accordingly, bilirubinuria is also present. The major clinical aspect of complete cholestasis that allows the resultant jaundice to be distinguished from pure hepatocellular hyperbilirubinemia is the presence of acholic (clay-colored) stools and the absence of urobilinogenuria. Both of these findings are, of course, direct results of failure of bile pigments to enter the intestine.

Pure hemolytic hyperbilirubinemia usually occurs as a result of increased red cell destruction in patients with normal hepatobiliary systems. The resulting jaundice is simply caused by overproduction of bilirubin in the spleen and other portions of the reticuloendothelial system, exceeding the capacity of the liver to conjugate and excrete it. Thus, the bilirubin found in the blood is almost entirely prehepatocytic or unconjugated and it does not appear in the urine because it is not soluble in water, and circulates in the blood bound to albumin. Urine color thus remains normal in pure hemolytic hyperbilirubinemia. Stool color is also normal and urobilinogenuria is present because there is no obstruction to the biliary flow or intestinal treatment of conjugated bilirubin. Quantitative measurements of urobilinogen indicate increased production in hemolytic states.

Extrahepatic Causes of Unconjugated Hyperbilirubinemia

There is a very long list of disorders that can result in the transient or permanent overproduction of bilirubin and jaundice of the "hemolytic" type. That list is summarized here in order that one may become alert to the various possibilities.

Ineffective Erythropoiesis. In the presence of disorders such as pernicious anemia and thalassemia minor, heme production is abnormal, and a portion of it is never incorporated into erythrocytes. This is rapidly converted to bilirubin and is carried off in the blood. Similarly, a group of patients with dyserythropoietic jaundice (shunt hyperbilirubinemia) has been identified, in which heme turnover is rapid, erythroid hyperplasia exists in the bone marrow, but red cell life span is normal. This disorder is not primarily hemolytic, being principally a defect of hemoglobin synthesis. The resultant hyperbilirubinemia is unconjugated and the cause is unknown, although it may be the result of agents interfering with nucleic acid synthesis. In the DiGuglielmo syndrome and in other forms of ineffective erythropoiesis, cytoplasmic development of red cell precursors seems normal, while nuclear maturation is defective.

Hemolytic Anemias. In addition to unconjugated hyperbilirubinemia, patients with hemolytic anemias also show diminished red blood cell survival times, increases in urinary and plasma hemoglobin and iron when hemolysis is intravascular, often a decrease in serum haptoglobins, and increased presence of reticulocytes in peripheral blood. Hemolytic disorders are either congenital or acquired.

Congenital hemolytic anemias can be subdivided into three categories: abnormalities of hemoglobin structure, abnormalities of the erythrocytic membrane, and abnormalities of red cell enzymes. Some 300 varieties of abnormal hemoglobin have been described and many lead to premature destruction of erythrocytes. Sickle cell disease is prominent among those which cause aggregates of deoxygenated hemoglobin, leading to deformity and early destruction of the erythrocyte. Unstable hemoglobins show molecular lability, which leads to hemolysis (hemoglobin Zeurich, for example). The reaction may be precipitated by sulfonamides or other drugs. Mutations in hemoglobin may interfere with the uptake or release of oxygen, causing cyanosis on the one hand, and erythrocytosis on the other. Thalassemia is an example of hemolytic disorders resulting from imbalances in the synthesis of hemoglobin polypeptide chains. Heinz bodies are accumulations of condensed abnormal hemoglobins which are identifiable in erythrocytes of patients with this type of hemolysis.

Hereditary spherocytosis is the prime example of hemolytic disorders resulting from membrane abnormalities. The abnormal shape of the erythrocytes may be due to defective production of intracellular spectrin and is responsible for early destruction of erythrocytes in the spleen. Enzymic abnormalities leading to hemolysis are deficiencies of enzymes essential to developing energy from glycolysis, such as pyruvate kinase, and deficiency of hexose monophosphate shunt enzymes, such as glucose-6-phosphate dehydrogenase.

Acquired hemolytic states include dysplasia of red cells leading to increased fixation of the third component of complement to membranes and early hemolysis. Paroxysmal nocturnal hemoglobinuria is an example of this defect. Immune hemolytic anemias result from the development of antibodies to the patient's own cells, to substances, such as drugs, adherent to erythrocytes, or to transfused cells. Antibodies may be non-complement-fixing IgG (Rh antibodies, penicillin), complement-fixing IgG (systemic lupus erythematosus, chronic lymphocytic leukemia), or complement alone (rheumatoid arthritis). Fragmentation of erythrocytes is another acquired cause of hemolysis and is seen in patients with prosthetic heart valves and with injury to red cells by intravascular fibrin strands, as in disseminated intravascular coagulation. Splenomegaly is the final cause of acquired hemolysis. Enlargment of the spleen appears to lead to increased tortuosity and complexity of the splenic circulation, which leads to entrapment and destruction of otherwise normal erythrocytes.

Familial Uptake and Conjugative Disorders of Bilirubin Metabolism (Table 8–2)

Physiologic Jaundice of the Newborn. While this disorder is common among newborn infants and is usually mild, there appear to be certain kindreds in which the manifestations of unconjugated hyperbilirubinemia are more marked than usual. Jaundice begins early in the first week of life and tends to disappear by 10 to 14 days of age. It is believed to be due to immaturity in one or more of three systems: uptake of unconjugated bilirubin by hepatocytes, conjugation of bilirubin, and reduction of bilirubin in the intestine to urobilinogen and dipyrroles. These multiple etiologies are supported by knowledge that concentration of the uptake protein, ligandin, are reduced in the newborn, as are concentrations of the glucuronidative enzymes, uridine diphospho-glucose dehydrogenase, and glucuronyl transferase. It has also been shown that bilirubin-reducing intestinal microflora are not fully established until late in the first week of extrauterine life. Efforts to trap free bilirubin in the gut by the administration of oral agar, and thus prevent its absorption, distinctly reduce the level of icterus in infants with physiologic jaundice (Poland and Odell 1971). Ligandin levels reach normal at 10 days, but glucuronyl transferase may not reach adult concentrations until infants near one month of age.

Infants with unconjugated hyperbilirubinemia due to physiologic jaundice probably require no treatment until bilirubin levels exceed 10 to 12 mg per dl. At that point, the use of ultraviolet light is indicated.

Gilbert Syndrome (Constitutional Hepatic Dysfunction). This benign disorder is apparently inherited as an autosomal dominant characteristic, and may exist in either heterozygous or homozygous forms. Liver function and biopsy are normal. In this benign conjugative disease patients have a mild, fluctuating, unconjugated bilirubinemia which is associated with decreased hepatic levels of both ligandin and glucuronyl transferase. The disorder may not be detected until adulthood. Exercise, alcohol ingestion, infections, and fasting aggravate the hyperbilirubinemia. Fasting increases the activity of heme oxygenase and may hasten the breakdown of hemoglobin. It also in-

Table 8–2. Distinctive Features of Types of Hyperbilirubinemia Seen in Infancy and Childhood

Feature / *Disorder*	*Bilirubin* *Total*	*Bilirubin* *Conjugated*	*Urobilin-ogen*	*Stool Color*	*Alkaline Phosphatase*	*Liver Biopsy*	*Response to Phenobarbital*	*Glucuronyl Transferase*	*Kernicterus*	*Hereditary*
Hemolysis	+ + - + + +	0	Yes	N	N	N	No	N	Yes	Some types
Physiologic jaundice	+ - + +	0	Slight	Light	N	N	Yes	Low	Possibly	Dominant
Crigler-Najaar Type I	+ + +	0	No	Clay	N	Abnormal SER	No	Absent	Yes	Recessive
Type II	+ - + +	0	Slight	Light	N	"	Yes	Low	No	Dominant
Breast Milk	+ +	0	Slight	Light	N	"	Yes	Inhibited	Possibly	Possibly
Gilbert	+ - + +	±	Yes	N	N	N	Yes	Low	No	Prob dominant
Dubin-Johnson	+ +	Yes	Yes	N	+	Pigment	No	N	No	Recessive
Rotor	+ +	Yes	Yes	N	+	N	No	N	No	Recessive
Neonatal Hepatitis	+ + - + + +	Yes	0-slight	N-clay	+ – + +	Giant cell necrosis	No	N	No	No
Benign cholestasis	+ - + +	Yes	No	Clay	+ - + +	Cholestasis; focal necrosis	No	N	No	Poss recessive
Byler disease	+ + - + + +	Yes	0-slight	Clay	+ + +	Distended canaliculi	Slight	? low	No	Recessive
Biliary atresia	+ + - + + +	Yes	0-slight	N-clay	+ + +	Marked cholestasis, portal inflammation	No	N	No	No

N = Normal; O = Absent
\+ = Slightly increased; + + = Moderately increased; + + + = Markedly increased

creases the breakdown of fatty tissue stores. The effect of fasting on unconjugated bilirubin levels is blocked by the administration of nicotinic acid, which is an antilipolytic agent, and by fat feeding. Phenobarbital reduces bilirubin levels promptly, probably by inducing production of ligandin. Glucuronyl transferase levels do not appear to rise.

Mild cases of Gilbert syndrome are identified frequently in programs which routinely perform multiple blood analyses. It is of no clinical significance and, in practice, is diagnosed by finding unconjugated hyperbilirubinemia on more than one occasion, no other abnormality in liver function, and no evidence of hemolysis, such as reticulocytosis or anemia. Biopsies of the liver are unnecessary.

Crigler-Najjar Syndromes. Homozygous members of the Gunn strain of Wistar rats exhibit permanent unconjugated hyperbilirubinemia of advanced degree, absence of glucuronyl transferase from the liver, inability to induce glucuronyl transferase activity with phenobarbital, and hepatic function which is otherwise normal. They are unable to conjugate bilirubin and develop severe degrees of brain disease (kernicterus, see below). Heterozygous Gunn rats also become jaundiced but are able to conjugate bilirubin partially and experience a rapid decline of serum bilirubin levels to normal when glucuronyl transferase activity is induced by phenobarbital.

Crigler-Najjar syndrome, type I is a rare recessive characteristic in infants, and is the exact counterpart of the disorder seen in homozygous Gunn rats. Kernicterus is a serious and common complication, and the bile of these infants contains no conjugated bilirubin. Foreign substances, such as menthol and cholecystographic agents, cannot be conjugated either, and phenobarbital is ineffective in correcting the defect. Ultraviolet light can keep bilirubin concentrations at safe levels.

Crigler-Najjar syndrome, type II is the counterpart of the hyperbilirubinemia seen in the heterozygous Gunn rat, with the singular exception that it does not occur in families of patients with the type I syndrome and is probably not genetically related to it. It appears to be transmitted as an autosomal dominant, shows lesser degrees of hyperbilirubinemia than type I, and is associated with little or no brain damage. Phenobarbital induces glucuronyl transferase and reduces bilirubin levels in type II patients.

Breast Milk Jaundice. This disorder was found by Israel and Arias (1976) to occurr in breast-fed infants of mothers who secrete pregnane 3-alpha, 20-beta diol in their milk. This isomer of pregnanediol inhibits glucuronyl transferase activity but is not associated with levels of jaundice causing kernicterus. The unconjugated jaundice continues until infants are withdrawn from the breast and is probably not a reason for discontinuing this form of feeding.

Kernicterus (Unconjugated Bilirubin Encephalopathy). Unconjugated bilirubin is nonpolar and lipid soluble. In its free (unconjugated) form, bilirubin promptly crosses such biological membranes as the placenta, the small intestine, and the "barrier" which separates the hemic compartment from brain and spinal cord fluids. Normally, such migration of free bilirubin from the blood is prevented by tight binding to receptors on the albumin molecule. However, when the concentration of free bilirubin in the blood is greater than the albumin receptor capacity, because of hypoalbuminemia or increased bilirubin levels, or because bilirubin has been displaced from albumin receptors by other anions, such as salicylates, sulfasoxazole, or free fatty acids, the proportion of unbound and unconjugated bilirubin in the circulation increases, and large amounts may enter the brain compartment. Acidosis also favors the unbinding of free bilirubin from albumin. Thus, at any given level of unconjugated hyperbilirubinemia, hypoalbuminemia, acidosis, starvation, and the presence of certain drugs will increase the likelihood of bilirubin crossing the blood brain barrier. This is a reversible process which moves in the opposite direction when these factors are absent (Diamond 1966).

Pathology and symptoms.

Although the blood brain barrier appears to be permeable to free bilirubin throughout life, it is probably more permeable in infancy. While free bilirubin causes cerebal neurotoxicity at low concentrations, the precise nature of the damage is not clear. Bilirubin pigmentation involves all parts of the brain, but appears to concentrate in the basal ganglia and cerebellum. Chronic changes consist of gliosis and loss of ganglion cells. Functional changes of unconjugated bilirubin encephalopathy consist initially of hypotonia, lethargy, and diminished suck reflex.

Prevention and treatment.

Bilirubin encephalopathy should be considered to be a wholly preventable condition. It occurs most commonly in association with hemolytic diseases of infancy, especially erythroblastosis fetalis, although Crigler-Najjar syndrome and even severe cases of physiologic jaundice certainly account for some cases. Erythroblastosis fetalis is now almost completely preventable by several measures, including administration of antiRhD antibodies (RhoGAM) to Rh negative mothers following pregnancy or miscarriage, and by monitoring elevations in antiD levels by intrapartum amniocentesis in Rh negative mothers with Rh positive mates. Intrauterine indications of Rh incompatibility are managed by fetal transfusions and early delivery, followed by exchange transfusions, as indicated. Ultraviolet light treatment, prompt feeding, correction of acidosis by respiratory toilet, and occasionally the administration of albumin to infants with unconjugated hyperbilirubinemia, can reduce the incidence of serious bilirubin encephalopathy. In infants with normal levels of serum albumin, 20 mg per dl is taken as the point at which corrective measures for hyperbilirubinemia must be instituted. It is important to remember, however, that mild degrees of brain damage leading to mental retardation can occur at lower levels. Thus, in practice, one should institute ultraviolet therapy at the 15-mg level, especially if bilirubin concentrations are rising rapidly.

Familial Disorders of Bilirubin Excretion (Table 8–2)

Dubin Johnson Syndrome. This is a benign autosomal recessive characteristic in which heterozygotes display the trait but never become icteric. Patients develop conjugated hyperbilirubinemia, especially in the second to third decades of life and display no other hepatic abnormality but the inability to excrete conjugated bilirubin and exogenous conjugates, such as sulfobromophthalein and cholecystographic agents. Biopsies of the liver show completely normal structure, save for the appearance of a black pigment in centrilobular hepatocytes (Figure 8–13). A similar disorder has been detected in a mutant strain of Corriedale sheep, and the pigment has been found to be metanephrine glucuronide, which is a metabolite of epinephrine and a precursor of melanin. Patients excrete reduced amounts of coproporphyrin III and increased amounts of coproporphyrin I in their urine, and heterozygote relatives exhibit this same tendency to a lesser degree.

Other than for hyperbilirubinemia, which may rise to more than 20 mg per dl and is largely conjugated, patients have few complaints. They may notice vague abdominal pain, weakness, and anorexia, and symptoms tend to worsen after stress, alcohol, and surgery, during pregnancy, and while taking oral contraceptives.

Rotor Syndrome. This disorder is similar clinically to Dubin Johnson syndrome in most respects. Jaundice is conjugated, prognosis is good, and the process appears to be inherited as an autosomal recessive characteristic. However, no pigment is demonstrable in the liver, and excretion of coproporphyrin as isomer I is midway (60 percent) between that seen in Dubin Johnson syndrome (90 percent) and in normals (25 percent). Thus, Dubin Johnson and Rotor syndrome, although similar clinically, are probably not genetically related.

Benign Recurrent Intrahepatic Cholestasis. This is a rare condition in which repeated attacks of obstructive jaundice, pruritus, nausea, and loss of weight occur over a period of many years. Each attack is self-limited and is followed by a period in which hepatic function tests and liver biopsies return to normal. During an attack, the biopsy shows centrilobular cholestasis, focal hepatic necrosis, and nonspecific portal infiltration with mononuclear cells. Bile canaliculi are dilated during an attack, canalicular microvilli are

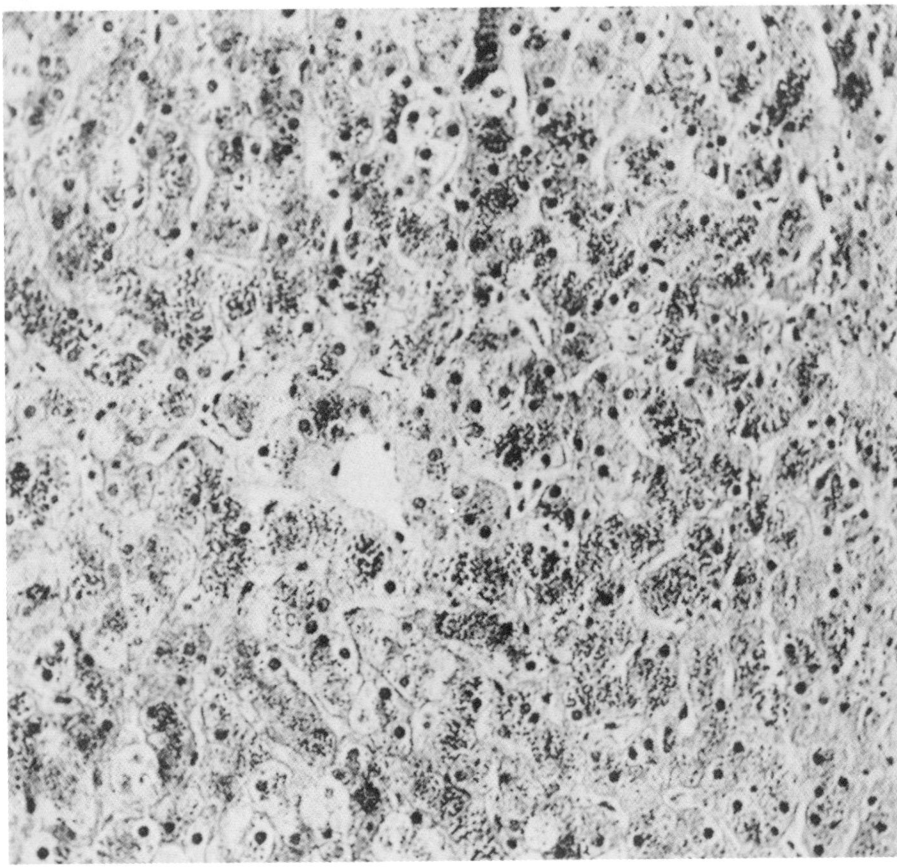

Figure 8–13. Dubin Johnson syndrome. The centrilobular distribution of the pigment and the normal hepatic architecture are typical. From Dubin IN, Johnson FB. Medicine 33:155–97, 1954. Reprinted by permission. Original magnification x50.

reduced in number, and the canalicular membrane expands in places to obstruct the lumen (Biempica et al 1967). Bile pigment is found in Kupffer cells and hepatocytes. Between attacks, these findings regress nearly to normal. There is no clear genetic inheritance of this syndrome, although it has been described in one pair of cousins. Since it usually commences in childhood, it is doubtless a congenital disorder.

Fatal Familial Intrahepatic Cholestasis (Byler Disease). This is clearly a familial recessive disorder in which there is a defect of excretion of conjugated bile acids across the canalicular membrane (Linarelli et al 1972). It was first identified in two consanguineous families and was named after them. Obstructive conjugated hyperbilirubinemia appears early in childhood and is preceded often for some months by steatorrhea, loss of weight, and failure to develop. Hepatosplenomegaly occurs early, and death from chronic hepatic failure and cirrhosis occurs within eight years. Laboratory data consist of hyperbilirubinemia, elevated alkaline phosphatase levels, normal serum cholesterol, and hypoprothrombinemia responsive early on to vitamin K (Clayton et al 1969). Treatment with a bile acid chelating agent (cholestyramine), ultraviolet light, phenobarbital, and triglycerides which do not require bile salts for absorption (medium chain length), often relieves symptoms and improves nutrition. Blood levels of lithocolic acid are increased, and this may be responsible for the hepatic injury. Parents of patients (heterozygotes) may show a reduced tendency to excrete loads of sulfobromophthalein but are otherwise quite well.

Other Neonatal Disorders of Bilirubin Excretion

Giant Cell Hepatitis (Neonatal Hepatitis Syndrome). This is a syndrome with many etiologies, drawn together under one heading because of the characteristic appearance in most cases of numerous multinucleated giant cells (Figure 8–14). Other signs of inflammation include varying degrees of distorted lobular structure, hepatocytic necrosis, inflammatory infiltrate, cholestasis, and extramedullary hematopoiesis. Jaundice is mild to marked, hepatomegaly is common, obstruction is variable. Cholestasis is present in

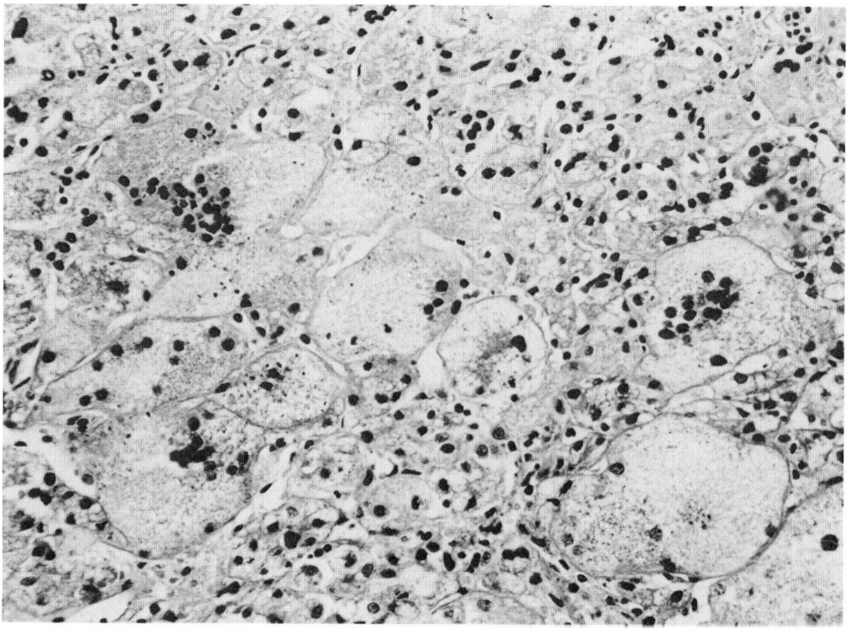

Figure 8–14. Neonatal giant cell hepatitis. Multinucleated giant hepatocytes are infiltrated by mononuclear cells. Original magnification x250.

almost all cases and might be quite marked in some. Chronic cholestasis might follow and, in some cases, lead to cirrhosis after many years (Heathcote et al 1976).

The multiple causes of this syndrome include: toxoplasmosis; viral disorders, such as rubella, hepatitis B, cytomegalic inclusion disease, herpes, and ECHO; and metabolic disorders, such as alpha-1 antitrypsin deficiency (Hirschberger and Stickler 1977). Each of these etiologies must be considered whenever cholestatic hepatocellular jaundice appears in the newborn period.

Extrahepatic Biliary Atresia. The cause of imperfect formation of the extrahepatic biliary tree with resultant obstruction of bile flow from the liver to the intestine is not known. In some cases it may be the result of intrauterine maternal infections with rubella or cytomegalic virus, but in most cases no clear infection or inheritance can be defined. Jaundice usually commences in the first few weeks of extrauterine life. Hyperbilirubinemia is conjugated, stools are clay colored, and urobilinogen is absent. Hyperlipidemia and xanthomata often develop in untreated cases. The liver biopsy is characterized by cholestasis, although giant cells and focal hepatic necrosis may be present. Biliary cirrhosis is a later consequence. Diagnosis depends on visualization of the biliary tree by percutaneous cholangiography. Some types of biliary atresia can be corrected surgically.

Congenital Dilatation of Intrahepatic Bile Ducts. Caroli and Corcos (1964) have described a primary condition in which ectasias may occur throughout the extrahepatic and intrahepatic biliary tree. While marked obstruction to bile flow does not occur, mild degrees may be present. Liver function is usually quite good early on, but the course of the disease is punctuated by recurrent attacks of biliary sepsis and ascending cholangitis. It is believed that bacteria populate the bile because the ducts themselves cannot move them along. Their means of access to the biliary tract is unknown. The disorder does not appear to be inheritable. Treatment is primarily with antibiotics for attacks of cholangitis.

Death occurs in a large proportion of affected infants. Spasticity, opisthotonos, and fever occur late in the course. Seizures, choreoathetosis, and deafness are characteristic of the chronic residual state of the disease. Mild kernicterus has been implicated as a cause of the cerebral palsy and mental deficiency.

DIAGNOSTIC PROCEDURES IN HEPATOBILIARY DISEASE

Plain Abdominal Radiography

Because they are simple, convenient, harmless, cheap, and capable of providing diagnostic information, plain abdominal radiographs should be taken in all patients with suspected disease of the liver, biliary tract, or pancreas. Both anteroposterior and lateral views should be obtained. The main abnormalities that can be detected relative to diseases in these areas are enlargements of the liver and spleen, calcifications of or in the gall bladder, liver, and pancreas, the presence of air in the biliary tree or liver, the presence of ascites, and occasionally anterior displacements of the gastric air bubble, suggesting a retroperitoneal mass. Calcification in the wall suggests a porcelain gall bladder, the presence of opaque homogeneous content in the gall bladder suggests chronic infection and milk of calcium bile, calcification of gallstones occurs in certain tumors and in echinococcal cysts, pancreatic calcifications occur in around 20% of all patients with cholelithiasis, hepatic calcification occurs in some patients with chronic pancreatitis, and air in the biliary tree may result from previous ampullary surgery, the formation of spontaneous communications between the upper intestine and the duodenum, or infections with gas-forming bacteria. While none of these disorders is common, the ease with which they can be detected by this straightforward procedure mandates that it be performed routinely.

Percutaneous Liver Biopsy

Although it is an invasive procedure, percutaneous needle biopsy of the liver is associated with a very low incidence of serious morbidity and a high level of diagnostic accuracy. Almost any of the tissue manifestations of hepatobiliary disease described earlier can be clearly demonstrated on a liver biopsy of adequate size. A long, 18-gauge (Menghini) needle is quickly inserted into the liver under suction, and the resulting tubular specimen is fixed in formalin or Bouin solution, then stained with hematoxylin and eosin to reveal cellular structure and architecture, and with a trichrome stain for collagen and fibrin staining. Special stains that can be used additionally are: periodic-acid Schiff staining for glycogen and other carbohydrate moieties; silver impregnation for reticulin staining; Prussian blue staining for iron; and rubeanic acid stain for copper. Portions of the biopsy can also be used for bacterial and fungal cultures, and for electron microscopic examination, prior to routine fixation.

Before performing a biopsy of the liver, care must be taken to determine that the patient's blood coagulates in a satisfactory manner. A biopsy should not be undertaken if the prothrombin time is greater than 3 seconds above the control, if the partial thromboplastin time is greater than 1 minute, or if the platelet count is less than 75,000 per cu mm, for bleeding is the most serious complication of percutaneous biopsies. Patients should be cooperative and able to hold their breath for a second or two, and they must understand the purpose of the procedure. In the suspected presence of complete extrahepatic biliary tree obstructions, some physicians hesitate to perform biopsies because of possible postoperative biliary-peritoneal leakage; there is also considerable hesitancy in performing biopsies in patients with suspected abscesses of the liver. These are reasonable precautions, especially since other procedures can document these disorders better than can a biopsy. With proper preoperative care, complications of percutaneous liver biopsy should be reducible to the vanishing point.

Radionuclide Scanning of the Liver

A gamma-emitting agent, ^{99m} technetium sulfur colloid, is rapidly taken up by hepatic Kupffer cells after injection, and the resultant radiation, when exposed to a gamma camera, can give an accurate outline of the size, shape, position, and homogeneity of the liver (Figure 8–15). These liver scans are widely used and can detect mass lesions (such as tumors and abscesses) in the liver and processes associated with extensive fibrosis. The scanning compounds are well tolerated by patients and have short half-lives, so that

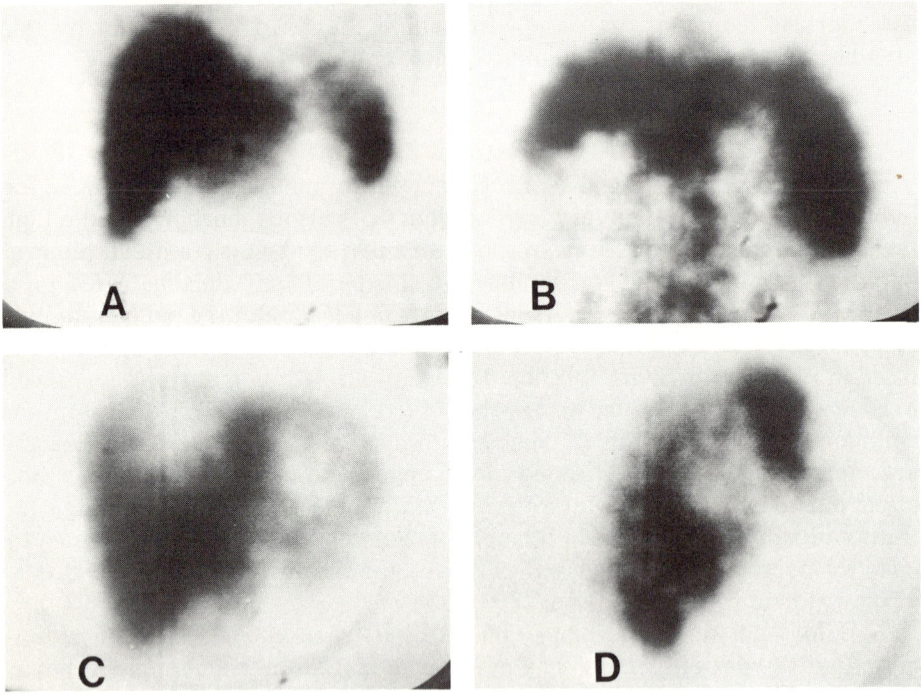

Figure 8–15. Isotopic hepatosplenic scanning. Using ^{99m}technetium, an emitter of gamma rays (half-life, six hours), and scanning with a gamma camera, good opacification of the liver and spleen is obtained. Compare normal anteroposterior view of liver and spleen, *A*, with cirrhosis of the liver, *B*. Note the small liver and enlarged spleen in *B*, and the uptake of the isotope by the vertebral bone marrow, an indication of portal hypertension. Two large intrahepatic defects (metastatic cancer) are visible in *C*, and at least one defect is seen in a lateral view of the liver in the same patient, *D*. Courtesy of Dr. Abbas Rejali.

no radiation danger exists. There are no contraindications to hepatic scanning, and satisfactory studies can be obtained in patients with any stage of hepatic disease.

Most scanning agents in use today are also taken up by other reticuloendothelial tissues, and thus also delineate the spleen, but not so well as the liver. Splenomegaly, plus uptake in vertebral brone marrow, is a reliable indicator of the existence of portal hypertension in radionuclide scans.

While radionuclide scans are relatively inexpensive to perform, trouble-free to patients, and continue to be the primary scanning technique for screening purposes, their interpretation is subject to inaccuracies. Small hepatic masses lying more than 2 to 3 cm below the surface of the liver are often undetected by nuclide scans, it is often difficult to differentiate between cysts and solid tumors in the liver, and irregular uptake of the isotope may lead to false positive interpretations. The accuracy is between 75 to 80 percent overall. In equivocal cases, gray scale ultrasonography will frequently resolve confusing diagnostic problems.

Oral Cholecystography

Iodinated, un-ionized, fat-soluble compounds, such as iopanoic acid, are micellarized by intestinal bile salts, then diffuse across the intestinal mucosa, and are carried to the liver via the portal circulation rather than by lymphatics. Hepatic excretion requires release from albumin at hepatocytic membranes, transfer to ligandin, and conjugation with glucuronide prior to excretion into bile canaliculi. Some iopanoic acid is excreted into the urine, but most enters the biliary system and is eventually concentrated in the normal gall bladder within 12 to 14 hours after ingestion.

Concentrated iopanoic acid in the gall bladder is radiopaque and outlines the organ very well on radiographs. Radiolucent calculi are outlined by the opaque dye, and abnormalities of the gall bladder wall can also be detected. Timely appearance of iopanoic acid in the gall bladder is also a good test of hepatic function. An injection of cholecystokinin, or the ingestion of a fatty meal, causes the gall bladder to empty, and occasionally the iopanoic acid may outline the cystic and common bile ducts during this process. Since iopanoic acid is reabsorbed from the intestine after excretion, it may appear more concentrated after 36 hours than it was at 14 hours.

Oral cholecystography is a useful test in detecting gallstones in those patients whose gall bladders retain their ability to concentrate bile (Figure 8–16). Often, however, patients with cholelithiasis also have chronic cholecystitis, cannot concentrate iopanoic acid, and are found on cholecystography to show no filling of the gall bladder. Nonfilling by itself is a fairly good indication of gall bladder disease provided that (1) the patient has taken the iopanoic acid the night before the examination, (2) no fat has been

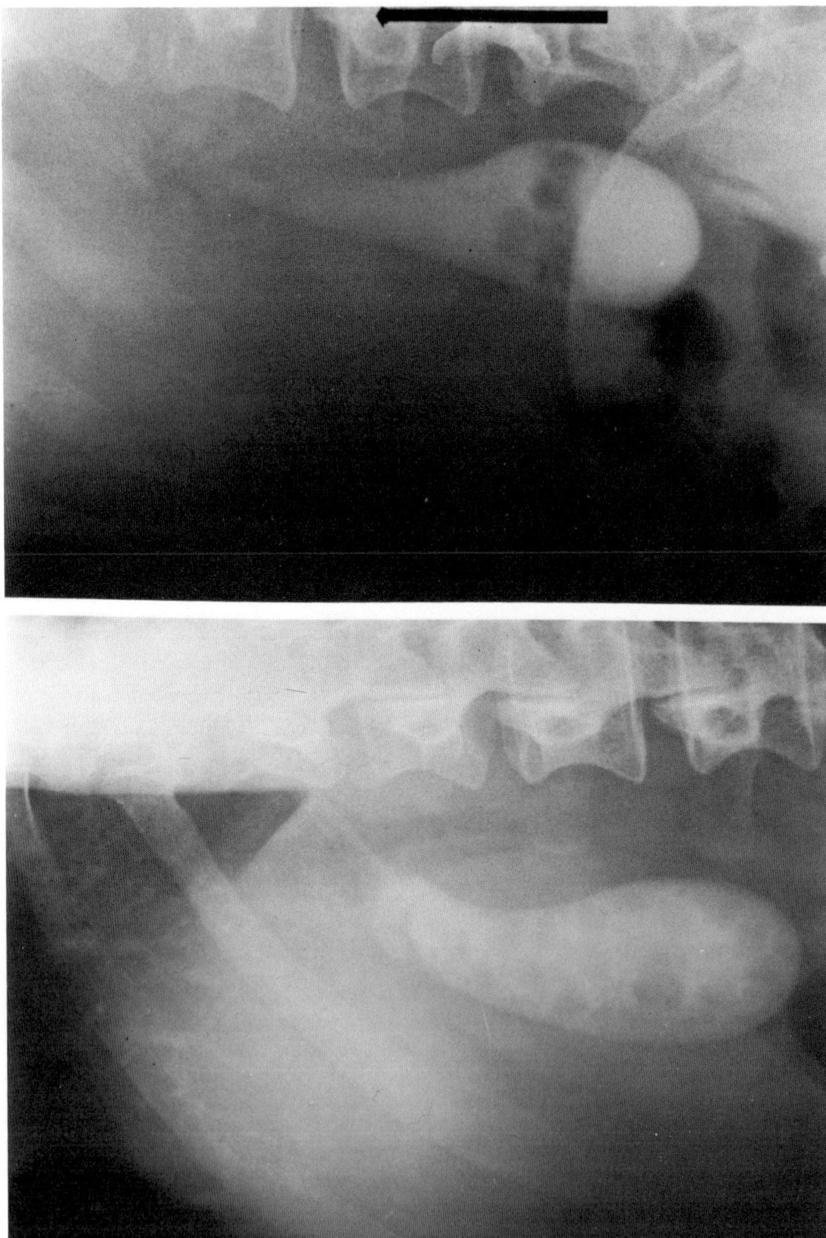

Figure 8–16. Cholecystograms taken with patients recumbent (*left*) and standing (*right*). The numerous radiolucent densities in the gall bladder represent gallstones. When the patient is upright, the gallstones layer above the more dense contrast medium. Courtesy of Dr. Harold P. Roth.

ingested since the contrast medium was taken, (3) severe diarrhea did not result from taking it, and (4) there is no coexisting hepatocytic or cholestatic liver disease severe enough to interfere with the biliary excretion of the medium. If the gall bladder has been removed surgically, iopanoic acid will not concentrate well enough to visualize the remaining extrahepatic ductal system. Oral cholecystograms should not be undertaken when serum bilirubin levels are greater than 3 mg per dl, since the contrast medium is unlikely to be excreted normally.

Linear tomography of the gall bladder can be used immediately after conventional cholcystograms if that study is inconclusive regarding possible gallstones or nonfilling. Tomography allows the X ray beam to focus on the plane of the gall bladder and extrahepatic biliary tree, which is about two-thirds of the distance from the patient's back to anterior wall (Stephens et al 1976). Occasionally, poorly visualized calculi and gall bladders can be more clearly outlined by this added technique.

Intravenous Cholangiography

In patients who are suspected of having recurrent stones or other disease of the extrahepatic biliary tract after a cholecystectomy, or in patients whose previous oral cholecystograms have shown nonfilling, it is often desirable to attempt to visualize the biliary tree by other means. One such approach is to inject an iodinated compound, methylglucamine iodipamide, intravenously (Figure 8–17). This substance is taken up by hepatocytes, but much that survives the first pass through the liver is excreted by the kidneys. Iodipamide is not conjugated and appears rapidly in the biliary tree. Since it stimulates bile acid independent bile secretion, its contrast effects are often attenuated. It is ineffective in the presence of advanced liver disease or if bilirubin levels are greater than 2 to 3 mg per dl. In most cases, however, it provides a fair outline of the extrahepatic biliary tree below the junction of the right and left hepatic ducts, especially when focused by linear tomography. The presence of calculi in, or stricture and dilatations of, the ductal system is usually quite well detected by intravenous cholangiography (Schoenfield 1977).

The fact that reactions to iodipamide are not infrequent (1 in 700), and the emergence of other accurate and noninvasive techniques for appraising the biliary tree have reduced the value of intravenous cholangiography in modern practice.

Gray Scale Ultrasonagraphy of the Liver, Gall Bladder, Bile Ducts, and Pancreas

Ultrasound frequences range from 1 to 20 MHz, are generated from piezoelectric transducers, and range through the body at different rates

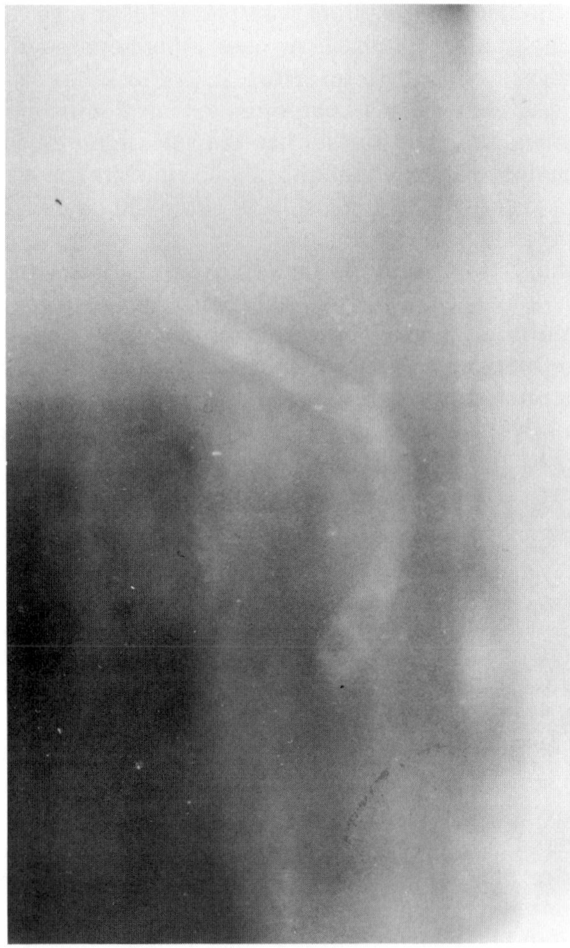

Figure 8–17. Intravenous cholangiogram, using linear tomography, in a previously cholecystectomized patient. The right and left hepatic ducts are seen to be merging at the top of the film, to form the common hepatic duct. There are two radiolucent densities, biliary calculi, in the distal common bile duct, and the duct is not dilated. Courtesy of Dr. Harold P. Roth.

depending on impedences in collagen tissue, which is the main source of internal echoes (Ferrucci 1979). Wide-dynamic-range (gray scale) displays allow the mapping of differential tissue "textures" based on these echoes. Gray scale units permit shading of echoes on television video scan converters in 8 to 16 shades of gray, thus allowing considerable distinction between and in organs (Figure 8–18).

In the liver, ultrasonic examinations can detect diffuse diseases such as cirrhosis and fatty infiltration. Alterations in the size of the liver, regen-

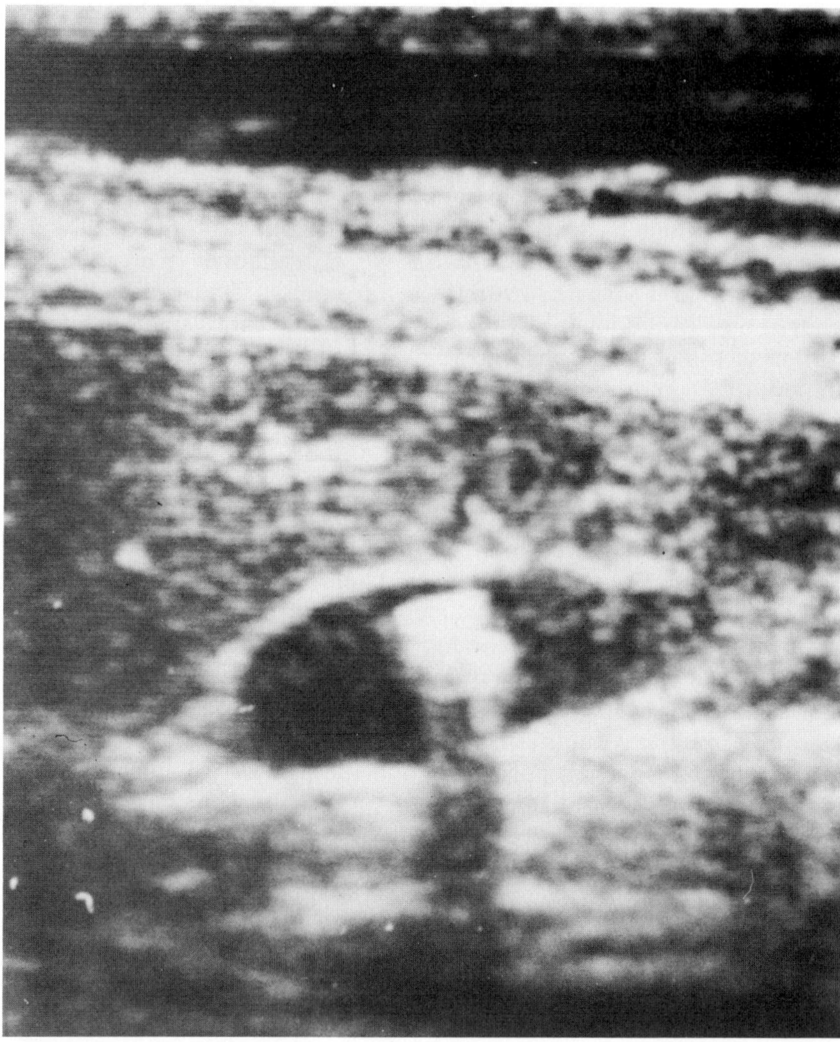

Figure 8-18. Gray scale ultrasonogram of a gall bladder containing a large gall stone. Note the cystic gall bladder containing an echogenic gallstone, and the anechoic shadow beyond the stone. Courtesy of Dr. Renate Duchesneau.

erating lobes, dilatations of portal vein branches, ascites, and splenomegaly are easily shown. Fibrosis accompanying cirrhosis produces increased echogenicity. Focal lesions are readily detected, and distinctions can be made between cystic and solid masses. Metastatic tumors can usually be distinguished from primary tumors of the liver by their distribution and number, but tumor histology can rarely be identified by sonographic patterns.

Overall accuracy of hepatic ultrasonography is probably greater than 90 percent. It is also an excellent tool for directing a biopsy needle toward specific intrahepatic lesions.

Cholelithiasis is detectable in almost all cases by ultrasound, through the demonstration of echogenic areas in the gall bladder, movement of these areas with changes in position of the body, and anechoic shadows behind the echogenic areas. Accuracy falls slightly if all of these features are not present. Calculi as small as 3 mm in diameter can be identified, and sludging of bile or collections of smaller calculi are identified by diffuse low amplitude echoes in the gall bladder, which move with changes in position. Identification of calculi is less accurate if they are not surrounded by liquid bile, as when the gall bladder is shrunken or if calculi rest in smaller bile ducts. Dilatation of the gall bladder and thickening of its wall can usually be detected by ultrasonic examination. Overall, false negative rates for ultrasonography of the gall bladder have ranged from 3 to 5 percent, and false positive rates from 5 to 14 percent. Most authorities agree that oral cholecystography should remain the primary screening procedure because of its relatively low cost and its considerable accuracy.

Sonography has proved to be an excellent technique for distinguishing between intrahepatic and extrahepatic cholestasis. Dilated bile ducts are demonstrated nearly all the time when extrahepatic obstruction is complete, and less often with partial obstruction. Dilated intrahepatic ducts can be detected when the caliber is 4 mm or larger; ducts obstructed due to sclerosis cannot usually be detected. The accuracy of sonography and computed tomography in biliary ductal diseases are about equal.

Ultrasonography has perhaps made its greatest diagnostic contributions in connection with diseases of the pancreas, an organ which can be imaged well only by this technique or by computed tomography. Gray scale techniques have allowed delineation of the size, contour, and parenchymal texture, as well as identification of vascular landmarks of the organ. The normal pancreatic surface is coarsely echogenic and can be readily distinguished from the less echogenic surface of the liver. Diffuse edema and swelling of the pancreas, with blurring of its margins, are hallmarks of pancreatitis; pseudocysts complicating pancreatitis are variable in shape and contain anechoic fluid. Localized tumors are commonly identified, but there is some difficulty in distinguishing between cancers of the pancreas and areas of localized chronic pancreatitis. Overall, the procedure is 87 percent accurate in detecting pancreatic disease, and the detection of pancreatic carcinoma ranges between 75 and 95 percent. The pancreas can be identified in 70 percent of normal subjects, the chief reason for failure being the presence of gas in the intestine, particularly those portions overlying the body and tail of the pancreas. In these areas, computed tomography is more accurate.

Computed Tomography of the Upper Abdomen

Rather than sound waves as a source, this procedure uses ionizing radiation and oral contrast materials to obtain computed "pictures" based on differential attenuations of electron flow resulting from differences in the mass density of organs. Computed tomography thus distinguishes between tissues with different atomic composition. Ultrasonic images, in contrast, are based more on tissue or macromolecular structure and are thus more organ specific. Thousands of density readings are taken with each pass of the X ray tube across the body in computed tomography, and the data stored on tapes or disks from which analog pictures can be produced. Contrast between tissues can be altered and recorded ranges of densities can be changed, so that resulting pictures can be specialized to show the area of interest most clearly. (See Figures 13-3 and 13-4.)

Since the biliary tract is quite well evaluated by sonography, the special attributes of computed tomography have been used most beneficially in evaluation of the liver and, especially, of the pancreas. In the latter organ, tomography has effectively distinguished solid tumors, cystic tumors, and chronic pancreatitis, especially in the body and tail where sonography is least accurate. In the liver, computed tomography has been able to distinguish normal liver, fatty liver, and hemosiderosis, because of its ability to distinguish differences in electron structure. It also reveals intrahepatic tumors well, but possibly not in a way superior to sonography.

The major drawbacks to computed tomography in hepatobiliary and pancreatic disorders are its expense, availability, and the radiation exposure involved. It cannot, for example, be used repeatedly, as sonography can, in monitoring the course of pancreatitis. It is, however, a powerful and valuable diagnostic tool at the tertiary level, after conventional radiography and sonography, and its images are often easier to interpret than are abdominal sonograms.

Percutaneous Transhepatic Cholangiography

In cases where obstruction of large bile ducts is high on the list of diagnostic possibilities and where other procedures fail to provide accurate localization, it is presently possible to inject iodinated contrast material directly into the intrahepatic ductal system and thereby visualize the entire extrahepatic biliary tract down to the obstruction, and a large part of the intrahepatic tract as well. This procedure can be used in patients who are icteric, and needs to be avoided only in cases where blood coagulation is abnormal or where cooperation cannot be obtained from the patient. It has been made possible by the development of a small-bore, flexible, needle

(Chiba University) which does not tear the capsule of the liver during respiratory excursions. There is usually no difficulty in passing the tip of the needle into an intrahepatic bile duct, especially when the ducts are dilated by obstruction downstream.

Endoscopic Retrograde Cholangiopancreatography

This procedure involves passing an endoscope perorally into the descending duodenum, slipping a catheter into the ampulla of Vater, injecting contrast material, and taking radiographs of the upper abdomen immediately afterward. With skill, admixed with a certain amount of luck, it is possible to obtain excellent retrograde filling of the extrahepatic biliary tree and the main pancreatic duct. In regard to delineation of the extrahepatic biliary system, it is probably no more effective, and considerably more expensive and time-consuming, than transhepatic cholangiography. It may be useful, however, in difficult cases of suspected ductal obstruction where transhepatic cholangiograms could not be obtained, either because of technical problems or because abnormalities of blood clotting were not responsive to vitamin K administration.

Endoscopic pancreatography (Figure 8–19) is a helpful procedure in distinguishing between cancer of the pancreas and pancreatitis, and in localizing psuedocysts. It is not clear whether the procedure is in any way preferable to sonography or computed tomography of the pancreas. Patient discomfort and expense are far greater than with sonography and tomography.

Peritoneoscopy

The anterior peritoneal cavity, liver, gall bladder, and spleen can be examined quite well by passing a rigid endoscope into the peritoneal cavity through a small 1-cm supraumbilical incision. Direct visualization of the surface of the liver allows photographs and biopsies to be taken. Patient discomfort is modest, but careful observation is required for at least 12 hours after completion of the procedure. This is an older procedure, and its current position as a diagnostic measure in the evaluation of patients with hepatic diseases is not clear. My guess is that it will never become popular.

HISTORICAL DIGRESSION

Proper names used in this chapter include the following: Paul B. BOUIN (1870–1962), French histologist, Algiers, Nancy, Strasbourg; George B. BUDD (1808–1882), British internist, London, described hepatic vein throm-

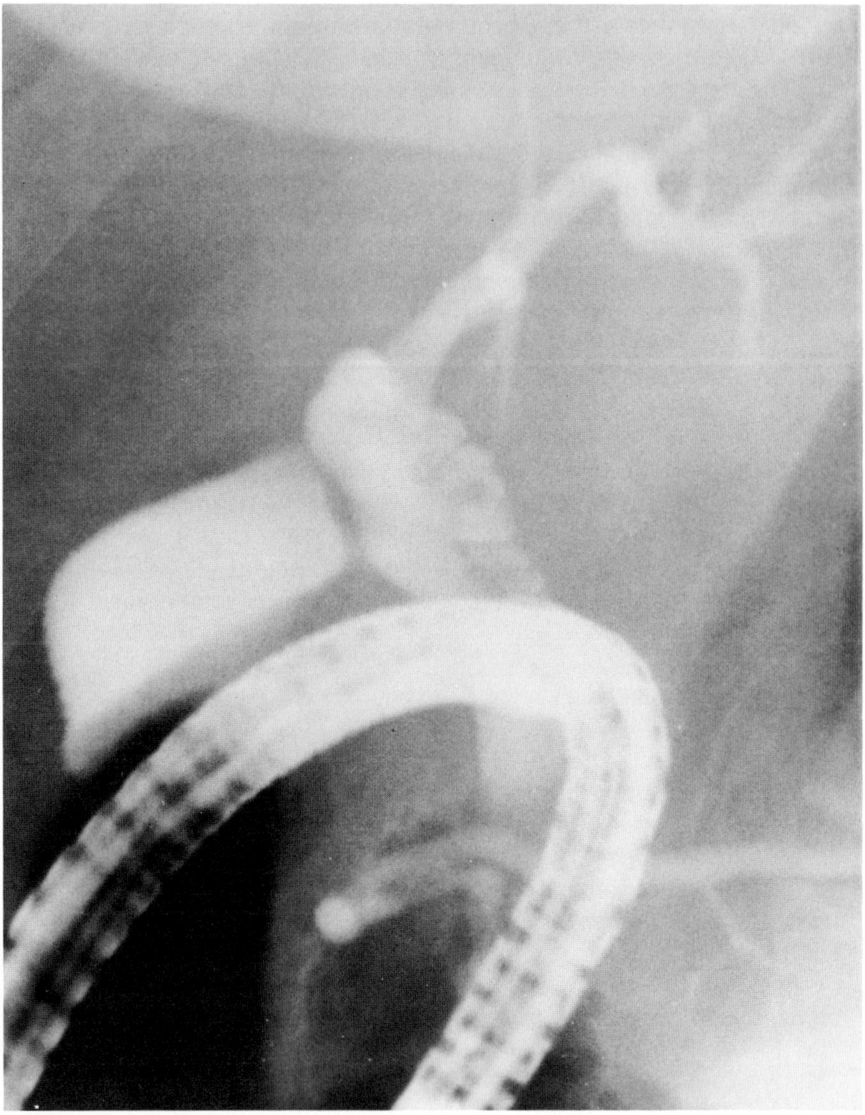

Figure 8–19. Normal endoscopic retrograde cholangiopancreatogram. The common bile duct, gall bladder, hepatic ducts, and pancreatic ducts are clearly visible. The endoscope is seen in the lower right corner of the film. Courtesy of Dr. Renate Duchesneau.

bosis 1845; Hans CHIARI (1851–1916), Austrian pathologist, Vienna, Prague, described hepatic vein thrombosis 1899; William Thomas COUNCILMAN (1854–1933), American pathologist, Baltimore, Boston; John Fielding CRIGLER, JR (1919–), American pediatrician, Baltimore, Boston, described congenital familial nonhemolytic jaundice with kernicterus 1952; Giovanni DIGUGLIELMO, contemporary Italian hematologist, Rome, described acute erythremic disorders 1917; Isadore Nathan DUBIN (1913–), Canadian-American pathologist, Washington, Philadelphia, described chronic idiopathic jaundice 1954; Nicolas Augustin GILBERT (1858–1927), French internist, Paris, described nonhemolytic jaundice 1907; Frank Bacchus JOHNSON (1919–), American pathologist, Washington, with Dubin; Frank Burr MALLORY (1862–1941), American pathologist, Boston, described "alcoholic" hyaline 1911; Giorgio M. MENGHINI, contemporary Italian physician, Perugia, described biopsy needle 1957; Victor Assad NAJJAR (1914–), Lebanese-American, Baltimore, Boston, with Crigler; Arturo B.R. ROTOR, contemporary Filipino internist, Manila, described idiopathic jaundice without pigment in liver 1948; Hugo SCHIFF (1834–1915), German biochemist in Florence; Samuel Alexander Kinnier WILSON (1877–1937), British internist and pathologist, London, described hepatolenticular degeneration 1912; WISTAR INSTITUTE, Philadelphia, anatomical research center.

SELECTED REFERENCES

Biempica L, Gutstein S, Arias IM. Morphological and biochemical studies of benign recurrent cholestasis. Gastroenterology 52:521–35, 1967.

Caroli J, Corcos V. La dilitation congénitale des voies biliares intrahépatique. Rev Medicochir Mal Foie 39:1–70, 1964.

Clayton RJ, Iber FL, Ruebner BH, et al. Byler's disease. Fatal familial intrahepatic cholestasis. Amer J Dis Child 117:112–24, 1969.

Denk H, Franke WW, Dragosics B, et al. Pathology of cytoskeleton of liver cells: Demonstration of Mallory bodies (alcoholic hyalin) in murine and human hepatocytes by immunofluoresence microscopy using antibodies to cytokeratin polypeptides from hepatocytes Hepatology 1:9–20, 1981.

Diamond I. Kernicterus: Revised concepts of pathogenesis and management. Pediatrics 38:539–46, 1966.

Ferrucci JT Jr. Body ultrasonography. N Engl J Med 300:538–42; 590–602, 1979.

Heathcote J, Deodhar KP, Scheuer PJ, et al. Intrahepatic cholestasis in childhood. N Engl J Med 295:801–5, 1976.

Hirschberger M, Stickler GB. Neonatal hepatitis and alpha-1-antitrypsin deficiency. The prognosis in five patients. Mayo Clin Proc 52:241–45, 1977.

Israel JB, Arias IM. Inheritable disorders of bilirubin metabolism. Adv Int Med 21:77–96, 1976.

Linarelli LG, Williams CN, Phillips MJ. Byler's disease: Fatal intrahepatic cholestasis. J Pediatr 81:484–92, 1972.
Mistilis SP, Blackburn CRB. Active chronic hepatitis. Am J Med 48:484–95, 1970.
Poland RL, Odell GB. Physiologic jaundice: The enterohepatic circulation of bilirubin. N Engl J Med 284:1–6, 1971.
Popper H. Cholestasis: the future of a past and present riddle. Hepatology 1:187–91, 1981.
Popper H, Schaffner F. The vocabulary of chronic hepatitis. N Engl J Med 284:1154–56, 1971.
Poulsen HE, Christofferson P. Atlas of liver biopsies. Copenhagen, Munksgaard (Lippincott), 1979.
Scheuer PJ. Liver biopsy interpretation 2nd ed. Baltimore, The Williams & Wilkins Company, 1974.
Schoenfield LJ. Diseases of the gallbladder and biliary system. New York, John Wiley & Sons, 1977.
Stephens DH, Carlson HC, Gisvold JJ: Tomography in problem cholecystograms. Radiol Clin North Am 14:15–22, (April) 1976.
Wilkinson SP, Portmann B, Cochrane AMG et al. Clinical course of chronic lobular hepatitis. Report of five cases. Q J Med 47:421–29, 1978.
Zimmerman HJ: Hepatotoxicity. New York, Appleton-Century-Crofts, 1978.

DISCUSSION QUESTIONS

1. What type of hyperbilirubinemia is commonly associated with hepatocytic jaundice, and how is this type easily identified?
2. Can the jaundice that results when the common bile duct is blocked be distinguished from the jaundice of viral hepatitis by determining the concentrations of "direct" (conjugated with glucuronic acid) and "indirect" (unconjugated) bilirubin in the serum? Explain your answer.
3. Patients with jaundice secondary to hepatocytic disease may excrete increased, normal, or decreased quantities of urobilinogen into the urine. Explain this fact using your knowledge of the metabolism of bilirubin and urobilinogen.
4. A 20-year-old man was rejected for military service because of a palpable liver. He felt completely well, had never been jaundiced, and had no gastrointestinal complaints. He denied the use of drugs and alcohol, nor had he been exposed to jaundiced persons or received any injections. Physical examination was normal, except for a sharp, smooth nontender liver edge palpable 2 cm below the right costal margin in the midclavicular line. The lateral edge of the liver was 3 cm medial to the lateral margin of the abdominal wall. Spider nevi, palmar erythema, ascites, jaundice, and splenomegaly were absent. Hematocrit was 45 percent, white

blood count 6,700, differential count normal. Aspartate aminotransferase was 30 units per ml, and alkaline phosphatase was 24 IU per liter. What is the differential diagnosis in this case? How would you arrive at the single most likely diagnosis?

5. A 28-year-old woman complains of the recent onset of malaise and pruritus. Just prior to consulting you, the color of her urine changed from normal to dark amber. What would be the sequence of your evaluation in this case?

In the following four problems, discuss the possible causes of jaundice, studies which would clarify the diagnosis, and potential methods of treatment:

6. A 2,550 g baby girl, born of a 25-year-old primiparous woman, was first noted to be jaundiced 12 hours after birth. Total serum bilirubin was 8.3 mg per dl at 18 hours, and had risen to 15.6 mg per dl at 30 hours when the infant developed lethargy and a poor suck reflex. Direct reacting bilirubin was 0.9 mg per dl, urine color was normal, and urobilinogen was absent from the urine. A two-volume exchange transfusion was performed.

   The mother had a healthy previous history, and denied prior blood transfusions or drug intake. Her blood type was O, Rh positive. The pregnancy had been uneventful until a urinary tract infection developed in the 35th week. This was treated with sulfasoxazole (Gantrisin), 4 g daily. Two weeks later, the mother was admitted in labor, and her hematocrit was found to be 29 percent. Urinalysis was normal. The 8-hour labor was uneventful and was performed under meperidine analgesia and caudal block. The membranes ruptured 20 minutes before delivery, which was by low forceps. Presentation was cephalic. The baby cried immediately and lustily, and was normal to physical examination at birth.

7. A 5-day-old infant was noted to be icteric during an examination conducted because of lethargy and decreased interest in feeding. Delivery had been normal after an uneventful full-term pregnancy. Examination at birth was normal, and hematocrit was 54 percent. Breast feeding commenced on the third day of life. Mother and infant received no medication during labor, which was conducted by the Lamaze procedure. Neither parent had had any recent illnesses or contact with jaundiced persons. At five days, the infant's serum bilirubin was 18 mg per dl, urinary bilirubin was positive, serum direct-reacting (conjugated) bilirubin was 3.5 mg per dl, and urinary urobilinogen was negative.

8. A 25-year-old man was seen in consultation for evaluation of jaundice and fatigue during the previous five months. Jaundice first

appeared during an acute upper respiratory infection, which was otherwise typical of a head cold. He is not sure whether there was ever any associated change in the color of his urine or stools. The jaundice subsided shortly after the cold disappeared, but it reoccurred on three subsequent occasions, lasting for five to seven days at a time. It was usually associated with periods of fatigue and inadequate rest; on one occasion it appeared shortly after he began a Weight Watchers diet. He denied loss of weight, abdominal pain, indigestion, anorexia, chills, or fever. There was no family history of jaundice, and he denied excessive use of alcohol. He took secobarbital at times for sleep.

Examination revealed slight scleral icterus but no other abnormalities. The liver was not enlarged. Hematocrit was 43 percent, white blood count 8,000, urine and stools normal. Serum bilirubin was 4.6 mg per dl.

9. A 40-year-old woman was seen for evaluation of episodic jaundice since age 15. The initial episode had occurred during an acute febrile illness, which lasted 10 days and was associated with a slightly enlarged liver and dark urine, but no splenomegaly. The next episode occurred at age 22, during her first pregnancy. It lasted 6 weeks and subsided weeks before delivery. That episode was accompanied by dark urine, light stools, and vague upper abdominal pain, but no itching, fever, or indigestion. Serum bilirubin was 1.6 mg per dl 10 weeks postpartum, and two successive cholecystograms failed to visualize the gall bladder. A cholecystectomy was performed, and the pathologist reported a normal gall bladder without stones. The surgeon reported that the liver looked "odd" at surgery, but a biopsy was not taken.

Several similar attacks of jaundice have occurred subsequent to the operation, especially following periods of increased physical activity or during upper respiratory infections. Bilirubin levels range from 6.8 mg per dl during attacks to 1.2 mg between spells. She feels quite well between attacks.

Examination is normal, save for mild jaundice. Hematocrit is 44 percent, white blood count 6,800. Urine is amber in color, but otherwise normal. Serum bilirubin is 4.4 mg per dl, alkaline phosphatase 42 IU per liter.

CHAPTER 9

Complications of Advanced Liver Disease

We come now to consider a number of conditions closely related to acute and chronic diseases of the liver, each of which can and often does adversely affect the outcome of these diseases. The conditions to be discussed are hepatic encephalopathy, the hepatorenal syndrome, the syndrome of fulminant hepatic failure, portal hypertension, and ascites. The first three of these complications occur both in acute and chronic hepatic injury, while the final two are almost solely confined to patients with either cirrhosis of the liver, or advanced hepatic space-occupying lesions, usually neoplasms. A degree of uncertainty exists in our understanding of each of these complications, in some more than others. But considerable information is available, attesting again to the importance of normal hepatic function in bodily homeostasis.

HEPATIC ENCEPHALOPATHY

"If your appendix goes wrong, we can take it out and have you back on duty in almost no time at all. But come to us with a liver complaint and you can fool us for weeks. The liver, you see, is a large, ugly mystery to us. If you've ever eaten liver you know what I mean. We're pretty sure today that the liver exists, and we have a fairly good idea of what it does whenever it's doing what it's supposed to be doing. Beyond that, we're really in the dark. After all, what is a liver?"* This comment is an uncomfortably apt description of much of our present understanding of the mechanisms of hepatic encephalopathy. While many observations have been made and effective methods of treatment have been devised, large gaps in our knowledge are all too obvious.

---

*Heller J. Catch 22. New York: Simon and Schuster, 1955.

Pathophysiology

Cerebral dysfunction in liver disease occurs as a consequence of hepatocellular damage, or from the shunting of blood around functioning hepatocytes, or from both factors operating simultaneously. Shunts may occur as intrahepatic pathways from portal arteries and veins to hepatic venules formed as a result of preceding hepatic injury, or as extrahepatic portasystemic pathways either formed spontaneously as a result of portal thrombosis or created surgically for the relief of portal hypertension. Whenever blood is not regularly exposed to functioning hepatocytes, severe changes in cerebral function are likely to occur. These changes result from varying combinations of alterations of neuronal membranes, derangements of intracellular oxidative metabolic processes, or defects in neurotransmission. The uptake of oxygen by the brain is also decreased.

Substances that have been implicated in the pathogenesis of hepatic encephalopathy are: ammonia, glucagon, mercaptans, short chain (C5, 6, 8) free fatty acids, amino acids, and biogenic neurotransmitters. Increased permeability of the blood brain barrier has also been assigned a role in the process. One is left with the distinct impression that hepatic encephalopathy may be the direct result of a variety of metabolic abnormalities, each of which is contributed to by the diseased or underperfused liver.

Ammonia. Ammonia excess clearly affects cerebral metabolism adversely, probably by fixing adenosine triphosphate and increasing the production of lactate (Schenker et al 1967). Ammonia also adversely affects the neuronal membrane, causing decreased frequency of spike potentials and alteration of electron and water movement across the membrane (Hoyumpa et al 1979). Elevations of arterial, venous, and cerebrospinal ammonia have been found repeatedly in patients with hepatic encephalopathy, but the level does not always correlate well with the degree of consciousness, and some patients appear to develop a degree of tolerance to ammonia (Zieve and Nicoleff 1975). Excessive levels of ammonia in the blood may accumulate for a variety of reasons, each of which depends either on exceeding the capacity of the liver to form urea or on portahepatic bypasses of the liver. Ammonia is produced in the wall of the jejunum and ileum from glutamine, in the wall of the colon from glutamine and urea, in the lumen of the lower bowel by bacterial ureases, and in the brain from urea, proteins, and various amino acids (Schlam and van der Mey 1979; Weber and Veach 1979). It is also produced in the kidney. In patients with classical or distal renal tubular acidosis, the kidney is unable to maintain a steep hydrogen ion gradient in the distal tubule, potassium is exchanged for sodium, and ammonia is formed from glutamine and passes into the renal vein (Shear et al 1969). Azotemia also leads to increased production of ammonia from urea by mucosal and bacterial ureases.

Colonic and lower small intestinal bacterial ureases are a major source of ammonia production from ingested proteins. Meat proteins appear to generate more ammonia than milk protein. The presence of blood in the intestinal tract greatly adds to levels of ammonia entering the portal vein. Absorption of ammonia from the colon is mainly by nonionic (ph dependent) diffusion, but a small amount of passive ionic diffusion probably also occurs (Wolpert et al 1970).

Upon entering the liver, ammonia is normally converted into urea by way of the urea cycle, which is dependent on five hepatocytic enzymes. Two of these enzymes, carbamyl phosphate synthetase and ornithine transcarbamylase, are mitochondrial and have been shown to be deficient in the acute hepatic damage occurring in Reye syndrome (Snodgrass and DeLong 1976; Brown et al 1967). Reductions in urea cycle enzymes may be responsible for the hyperammonemia seen in other instances of acute hepatocytic damage.

Glucagon. Increased nitrogen loading may result in hyperammonemia by overwhelming the capacity of the liver to form urea. Elevation of plasma glucagon levels may, in part, be responsible for nitrogen loading because this hormone releases aromatic amino acids from hepatic protein in the process of promoting gluconeogenesis. Glucagon levels correlate well with levels of ammonia, aromatic amino acids, and tryptophan in hepatic encephalopathy (Marchesini et al 1979); glucagon may also be hypersecreted or hypometabolized in patients with liver disease, especially when portasystemic shunts are present (Sherwin et al 1974). By promoting deposition of amino acids into muscular protein, insulin tends to counteract this effect. While blood levels of insulin are also increased in hepatic failure, the ratio of insulin to glucagon is lower than normal, because glucagon levels are proportionately greater. Increasing the levels of insulin by oral feedings supplemented with glucose has been reported to reduce glucagon levels and to prevent elevations of blood ammonia after meals in patients with portasystemic shunts (Walker et al 1974).

Mercaptans. Mercaptans and their metabolites, especially methanethiol, have been shown to cause coma in rats, possibly by inhibitng the activity of cerebral Na^+, K^+, ATPase. Mercaptans are derived from methionine which, in turn, has been shown to be elevated in the spinal fluid of patients in acute hepatic coma (Zieve 1979). Mercaptans also inhibit the conversion of ammonia to urea and are believed to be responsible for the sweet breath odor, or *fetor hepaticus*, noted so often in patients with hepatic failure or portasystemic shunts.

Short Chain Fatty Acid Levels. These are often elevated in patients with hepatic encephalopathy, and administration has been found to cause coma in experimental animals. Short chain fatty acids appear to inhibit the metabolism of ammonia and also to damage neuronal membranes.

Defects in the Metabolism of Amino Acids. These occur regularly in patients with hepatic encephalopathy, although the pattern is somewhat different in the type accompanying acute hepatic failure than in that associated with chronic disease of the liver (Rosen et al 1977). Plasma aromatic amino acids (phenylalanine, tryptophan) are elevated in both acute and chronic encephalopathy, but levels of branched chain amino acids (leucine, isoleucine, valine) are either normal or slightly reduced in acute disease and markedly reduced to half of normal in chronic encephalopathy. The explanation of these changes is not clear, but elevation of aromatic amino acids could result from reduced hepatic metabolism, while decreased branched amino acids could be secondary to alterations in the insulin to glucagon ratio. Tryptophan and phenylalanine cause coma in dogs when administered together but not when given separately. This coma can be prevented or reversed by the administration of solutions rich in branched amino acids (James et al 1979). Excessive levels of tryptophan in blood may affect the balance of neurotransmitters in the brain, since tryptophan competes with tyrosine for receptor sites. In one study (Ono et al 1978), tryptophan was the only amino acid found to be significantly increased in the spinal fluid of patients in coma compared to cirrhotic controls.

Neurotransmitters. Neurotransmitters have been studied increasingly in patients with hepatic encephalopathy in recent years. Conclusions have been difficult to reach because outcomes have differed in various studies, questions arise about the relationship of blood to brain levels of various metabolites, and observed alterations in the blood or spinal fluid levels of a single neurotransmitter or its metabolites do not usually pinpoint the reason for the alteration. Certain observations, however, are of interest.

In several studies of patients with liver failure, plasma levels of aspartate and glutamate, which are important neurotransmitters themselves, and also of tyrosine, have been found to be elevated. Of the biogenic amines which are neurotransmitters, serotinin is derived from tryptophan, dopamine and norepinephrine from tyrosine, and acetylcholine from choline. Numerous studies indicate that cerebrospinal levels of serotonin and its metabolite 5-hydroxy indolacetic acid are elevated in patients with encephalopathy. A tyrosine metabolite, tyramine, is elevated in the plasma of cirrhotic patients with encephalopathy (Faraj et al 1976). Normally, tyramine is rapidly metabolized by monoamine oxidase in the liver to 4-hydroxyphenylacetic acid (Figure 9–1). In the presence of portasystemic shunts or hepatocytic disease, excess tyramine is presented to the brain where it is converted to octopamine, a weak or false neurotransmitter, by the action of dopamine-beta-hydroxylase, which is the same enzyme used for conversion of dopamine to norepinephrine, both of which are true neurotransmitters.

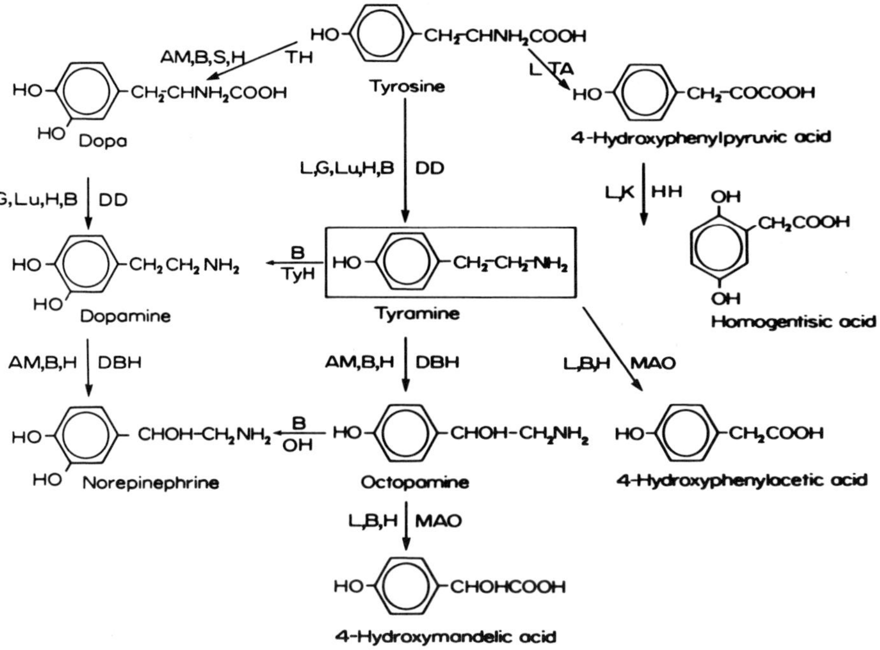

Figure 9–1. Biosynthesis and metabolism of tyramine. In the organ system, AM denotes adrenal medulla; B, brain; S, spleen; H, heart; L, liver; G, gut; and Lu, lung. In the enzyme system, TH denotes tyrosine hydroxylase; DD, dopa decarboxylase; DBH, dopamine-beta-hydroxylase; TyH, tyramine hydroxylase; MAO, monoamine oxidase; TA, tyrosine aminotransferase; and HH, *p*-hydroxyphenylpyruvate hydroxylase. After Faraj BA, Bowen PA, Isaacs JW, et al. N Engl J Med 294:360–64, 1976. Reprinted by permission.

This displacement is believed to reduce norepinephrine production. At the same time, excess tyrosine is converted to tyramine in liver, gut, and brain by dopa decarboxylase, thereby reducing the producing of dopamine from dopa, which depends on the same enzyme. Excess tyrosine is available for the conversion to tyramine because the hepatic enzyme which converts most of it normally to 4-hydroxy phenylpyruvic acid, and the brain enzyme, tyrosine hydroxylase, which converts some tyrosine to dopa, are both reduced. The net result is increased production of octopamine at the expense of dopamine and norepinephrine. This derangement of neurotransmitter synthesis could plausibly interfere with cerebral metabolism, although it has not been shown that reduction of true transmitter levels, or increasing octopamine levels, will alter consciousness in normal animals. Treatment of hepatic encephalopathy with L-dopa has not been successful (Michel et al 1977). However, in at least one patient (Morgan et al 1977), the dopamine receptor agonist, bromocriptine, was found to be beneficial for treating a form of hepatic encephalopathy resistant to more standard measures.

Alterations in the Blood Brain Barrier. Normally, cerebral capillaries are impermeable to many substances which distribute widely in other parts of the body. This barrier effect has been ascribed to tight junctions between endothelial cells of cerebral capillaries, which serve both to exclude many substances from the brain and to retain certain essential substances, such as neurotransmitters. Acute hepatic coma after hepatectomy in the rat (Livingstone et al 1977) has been shown to damage cerebral capillaries and to disrupt the blood brain barrier, allowing certain substances usually excluded (such as inulin, *d*-sucrose, trypan blue), to enter the brain. Phenylalanine was taken into the brain in larger quantities than normal, and may explain why levels of other amino acids in the brain are elevated in hepatic coma.

Pathology

Cerebral edema is seen frequently in fulminant hepatic failure, and is often associated with herniation of the cerebellar tonsils and compression of the medulla. Livingstone et al describe edema of cerebral white matter and astrocytic foot processes in acute encephalopathy. In chronic encephalopathy, astrocytic changes are prominent, showing both hypertrophy of cytoplasmic organelles and hyperplasia. This may reflect a reaction to prolonged hyperammonemia (Victor et al 1965). Cortical and subcortical white matter shows neuronal loss and demyelinization, especially in the parietal and occipital region. A similar process may also appear in the basal ganglia, and less commonly in the cerebellum and spinal cord. Certainly the acute changes are reversible with treatment, and so also is the hyperplasia of astrocytes. Actual neuronal loss, however, is probably irreversible.

Clinical Picture

It is important to know that the signs and symptoms of hepatic encephalopathy are often completely reversible, and do not necessarily suggest the presence of permanent brain damage. Their onset is usually associated with either advancing hepatocytic necrosis or the intervention of an acute stress, such as the administration of certain drugs or the onset of gastrointestinal bleeding, which temporarily increases the load of ammonia entering the brain. Designing a therapeutic program with full understanding of these stress factors will often go a long way in preventing and treating this serious complication of hepatic disease.

Stages of Hepatic Encephalopathy. Four levels have been described: the prodome, the confusional state, the stuporous state, and deep coma (Schenker et al 1974).

1. *Prodomal symptoms* include inappropriate behavior, restlessness, untidiness, irritability, and irresponsibility. Because symptoms frequently develop in an insidious fashion, this is the most difficult stage of encephalopathy to identify. It is recognizable only if friends, family, and medical advisers are alert to the possibility of its occurrence. Candidates are patients with either chronic or severe acute disease. A formerly quiet patient becomes loquacious. A formerly neat patient becomes unkempt. A formerly precise patient becomes forgetful. A patient who usually sleeps well develops sudden insomnia. Any of these subtle changes in behavior should suggest the onset of encephalopathy in candidate subjects.

Physical findings may show appearance of an intention tremor. Axterixis, the inability to keep outstretched hands hyperextended steadily for more than a few seconds, produces a flapping tremor and is an important early sign of encephalopathy. While asterixis is not confined to patients with disease of the liver, and may appear in patients with uremia, hypercapnia, and hypokalemia, its onset in candidate patients is highly significant. The process involves the inability of patients to sustain muscular contraction in any part of the body, and it probably results from defective transmission at neuromuscular junctions, and reduced proprioception.

Handwriting is often affected to the point where signatures show decreasing legibility, and the patient's ability to draw a straight line connecting successive numbers written randomly on a sheet of paper becomes markedly impaired. Fetor hepaticus may be present occasionally; seizures are rare.

2. The confusional state may be the first indication of encephalopathy and presents with varying degrees of disorientation, often associated with signs and symptoms of stage 1 disease. Confabulation and mental impairment may be present, suggesting Korsakoff psychosis, but this may occur with hepatic diseases other than those resulting from ethanol. Visual or auditory hallucinations may be present as well.

3. Stupor may appear rapidly, especially in patients with encephalopathy resulting from acute or fulminant hepatic necrosis. The patient, while rousable, responds poorly, is usually disoriented, and may be incontinent. Asterixis is not demonstrable since the patient is usually unable to contract muscles on request.

4. Deep hepatic coma is an extremely poor prognostic sign in patients with fulminant acute liver disease, 70 to 80 percent expire, and many of these have cerebral edema, occasionally with herniation of the cerebellar tonsils through the foramen magnum (Ware et al 1971). In patients with chronic disease of the liver and stage 4 encephalopathy, the prognosis for reversal is somewhat better because the complication is more likely due to exogenous factors that can be controlled. Where this complication is the direct result of hepatocytic necrosis, it is much less subject to therapeutic manipulation.

Laboratory Findings

Liver function tests do not necessarily deteriorate in proportion to the severity of the encephalopathy, especially in patients with chronic liver disease where the cause of the coma is often exogenous. In patients with fulminant hepatic necrosis, progressive worsening of blood coagulation often does herald or accompany the onset of encephalopathy. Aminotransferase levels commonly remain unchanged or improve, suggesting that a stage of maximal necrosis has already been reached.

Electrolyte disturbances are common, particularly alkalosis and hypokalemia, both of which may aggravate the neurologic state. Alkalosis results from hyperventilation or from diuretics, while hypokalemia may result from diarrhea, diuresis or distal renal tubular acidosis. Hypoglycemia is a rare finding, and probably results from depleted glycogen stores in the liver and decreased gluconeogenesis.

Blood ammonia levels are commonly elevated in hepatic excephalopathy of any stage, but venous levels do not correlate well with the stage of encephalopathy. Correlation with arterial levels of ammonia is better, but since the course of the condition can be followed well by clinical signs, it is usually inadvisable, because of bleeding tendencies, to obtain arterial ammonia determinations regularly.

Electroencephalography shows increased slow or delta wave activity in any or all leads, and is a very useful way to follow the course of encephalopathy. Since uremia, hypercapnia, and hypoglycemia can cause similar changes, the electroencephalogram has to be interpreted in the light of these other possibilities.

Management

Detection of Iatrogenic or Extrinsic Causes of Encephalopathy. The cardinal measure in the treatment of hepatic encephalopathy is a review of therapeutic and other exogenous agents which the patient has recently received, looking particularly for those which may lead to increments in ammonia levels. Among these are: a high protein meal; diuretics; laxatives and intravenous fluids capable of causing hypokalemia; aspirin or other nonsteroidal anti-inflammatory agents that might cause gastrointestinal bleeding; anticoagulants; sedatives; and analgesics. All too often, for example, patients in early stages of encephalopathy are given sedatives because they cannot sleep, and they quickly pass into a deeper stage. Anorectic patients with hepatic disease may become comatose while receiving protein hydrolysates or fluids low in potassium intravenously, and patients with ascites may develop prerenal azotemia and encephalopathy from an overly large paracentesis or diuresis.

Detection of Bleeding into the Castrointestinal Tract. Alimentary bleeding is one of the major causes of worsening encephalopathy in patients with either acute or chronic hepatic failure. Blood clotting is often abnormal for a variety of reasons, including deficiency of liver-dependent factors, thrombocytopenia from splenic congestion, and consumption coagulapathies. In addition, the incidence of lesions with a high propensity toward bleeding, such as esophageal varices, gastric erosions, and peptic ulcer, increases with the severity and duration of the hepatic disorder. When bleeding is massive, detection presents no problem, although therapy commonly does. In patients without gross bleeding, stools should be promptly examined for occult blood, since the extra nitrogen load from blood in the lower intestine can lead to prompt hyperammonemia.

Detection of Occult Infections. Pulmonary, urinary tract, and peritoneal infections are often followed by increasing encephalopathy, probably by causing increased protein catabolism, and occasionally by causing hypovolemia and azotemia. Chest X ray and cultures of urine, sputum, and peritoneal fluid, if present, will often reveal the site of infection and suggest appropriate treatment. When such cultures are negative and the suspicion of infection is high, lumbar puncture in indicated to detect a possible meningeal site.

Cleansing of the Alimentary Canal. This cleansing particularly of blood and stool, is an important measure in reducing nitrogenous loading. Enemas, sodium-free osmotic laxatives (citrate or milk of magnesia), and lactulose, a nonabsorbable synthetic disaccharide, are useful for this purpose. The control of bleeding may be difficult and includes such measures as antacids, vasopressin, and esophageal tamponade, preceded by endoscopy. The management of massive upper gastrointestinal bleeding was discussed in Chapter 5, and measures for controlling variceal bleeding will be discussed later in this chapter. Cimetidine should be used with care, for it has been shown to cause confusion in some patients with liver disease.

Reduction of the Population of Urease-producing Bacteria in the Bowel. Neomycin, a poorly absorbed aminoglycoside, has been shown to be capable of eliminating the aerobic bacterial flora of the intestine and reducing the gram-positive anaerobic flora. It has also been found to be effective in treating all stages of hepatic encephalopathy, presumably because it effectively reduces the population of enteric bacteria which produces ureases, particularly the nonsporing anaerobes. It may also reduce the population of bacteria capable of forming ammonia in the bowel. Neomycin is effective when given by either the oral or rectal route, in divided doses of 4 to 6 g per day. Its short-term use in the treatment of hepatic encephalopathy is established. It should be commenced only after the bowel has been rid of stool, and is most effective in treating encephalopathy not primarily due to hepatocytic damage.

The efficacy of neomycin is limited to short-term use because of its tendency to cause nephrotoxicity and ototoxicity, even though only 1 percent of the ingested drug is absorbed. It may also lead to diarrhea by altering the gut flora, and occasionally causes malabsorption resulting from intraluminal precipitation of bile salts. At times, the presence of neomycin-resistant, urease-producing bacteria (*Klebsiella, Proteus*) renders the drug useless. Absorbable antibiotics, such as ampicillin, are also effective in the treatment of encephalopathy, but the emergence of resistant bacteria is a deterrent to their continued use.

Alteration of Intracolonic pH Levels. Lactulose (1,4-galactosidofructose) is not absorbed or hydrolyzed in the upper intestine and is metabolized by lower intestinal flora to acetic, lactic, and formic acids. It produces an osmotic diarrhea because it is unabsorbed, and its metabolites effectively change the pH of stool from a normal of 7.0 to as low as 5.0 to 5.5, without producing obvious changes in bowel flora. This fall in pH is effective in reducing the nonionic diffusion of ammonia from the colon into the portal system, and is probably the main beneficial effect of lactulose. When given in divided doses to a total of 25 to 75 g daily, enough to produce two to three stools per day, lactulose is as effective as neomycin (about 90 percent) in controlling encephalopathy (Conn et al 1977). Except that it causes diarrhea and abdominal cramps at times, lactulose is essentially nontoxic. There is little reason to prefer it over neomycin in most cases of acute encephalopathy, although it is the drug of choice in patients with chronic encephalopathy and with renal disease. Occasionally patients who are not helped by neomycin or lactulose alone may be benefited by the simultaneous use of both drugs.

Correction of Electrolyte Disorders. Where hypokalemia or alkalosis coexist with hepatic encephalopathy, their correction by electrolyte replacement is often associated with marked improvement. Patients with chronic hypokalemia, or patients who require diuretics regularly for the management of ascites, may require regular potassium supplementation.

Control of Protein Intake. The fact that increased protein ingestion aggravates hepatic encephalopathy has been known for years, ever since Eck first described meat intoxication in dogs with end-to-side portacaval shunts. This presumably results from the increased production of ammonia from protein substrates, and from increased absorption of aromatic amino acids. Meat protein appears to be more "toxic" than isocaloric amounts of vegetable and dairy protein. Patients with all degrees of hepatic encephalopathy are improved by protein restriction, and in some this may be the only therapeutic measure required. Generally, protein intake is reduced to 10–20 g per day for a short time, then increased while the patient's condition is followed with handwriting, behavioral, and electroencephalographic monitoring. If adequate amounts of protein (40 to 50 g daily) cannot be reintroduced without exacerbating encephalopathic symptoms, the addition of neomycin or lactulose should be made.

Branched Chain Amino Acids. These have been used with some success (James et al 1979) in certain patients resistant to all other forms of therapy for hepatic encephalopathy. The solutions are administered intravenously and are well tolerated. Solutions are not presently available for general use, but studies on them are being done at various centers. Their future in therapy is uncertain. So also is therapy with dopamine precursors, such as l-dopa and bromocriptine, although limited success has been reported with these agents.

THE HEPATORENAL SYNDROME

This general term has been used to describe various types of renal dysfunction occurring in patients with hepatic disease, which are directly related to that disease and may also be a consequence of either inadequate or overly intensive therapy. While the term was originally applied to azotemia associated with complete obstruction of the extrehepatic biliary tree (Stein and Fadem 1978), renal dysfunction can clearly occur as a complication of any severe disease of the liver, acute or chronic.

All renal disorders associated with diseases of the liver are circulatory in nature. One of the best descriptions of the three varieties has been given by Shear et al (1965), who identified acute tubular necrosis, prerenal azotemia, or an oliguric, hyponaturic state in a series of 15 patients with cirrhosis who died with renal failure. Subsequently it has been shown that any of these types, but especially the first two, can also occur in patients with acute hepatic necrosis.

Acute Tubular Necrosis

This condition is typified by azotemia associated with the production of moderate volumes of urine nearly isotonic with plasma and containing large amounts of sodium. It commonly occurs in association with the hypotension of advanced hepatic failure, and with the decreased renal blood flow consequent to massive hemorrhage. Without taking proper safeguards, overly zealous treatment of ascites with diuretics and of hepatic encephalopathy with lactulose may also lead to a hypovolemic, hypokalemic state resulting in acute tubular necrosis. Thus, this condition may result either directly from the hepatic disease itself, or indirectly from improper treatment. Patients may recover, particularly if careful attention is given to volume and electrolyte replacement, and if renal dialysis is used as indicated, especially in those patients whose tubular necrosis was iatrogenic in origin. Where it occurs in association with advancing hepatic necrosis, the prognosis is much poorer, although the longer that patients can be supported, the greater the possibility that hepatic regeneration will commence.

Prerenal Azotemia

This complication occurs less commonly than the other two renal circulatory disorders of hepatic disease and is almost always consequent to reduced blood flow from either heart failure or volume depletion. It is characterized by decreased urinary volume, good urinary concentration because of normal tubular function, and low urine sodium levels due to aldosterone release. Treatment, of course, differs according to the cause. Congestive heart failure may occur from volume overloading of an already damaged heart and should be treated with digitalization and cautious diuresis. Volume depletion is a common complication of bleeding or overdiuresis and should be treated with expansion of volume, whole blood, packed red cells, or plasma, as needed. At times, urinalysis alone cannot clearly distinguish between early acute tubular necrosis and prerenal azotemia; a short-term trial of volume expansion is often helpful in distinguishing between the two problems.

Oliguric, Hyponaturic Azotemia

This is a common problem among patients with chronic liver disease, especially when ascites is also present. While its onset may be precipitated by diuresis, bleeding, or an overly large paracentesis, many patients enter this state spontaneously. Characteristically, a rising blood urea nitrogen and creatinine level is associated with production of scanty, dilute urine containing tiny amounts (less than 10 mEq per liter) of sodium. Hypoalbuminemia and jaundice are also frequently associated.

The renal state causing this complication is clearly reversible, since kidneys from patients dying from this form of azotemia show no clear abnormalities at autopsy and have been used successfully as transplants for patients with end-stage renal disease (Koppel et al 1969). Arteriography shows that cirrhotic patients with oliguric, hyponaturic azotemia demonstrate marked constriction, beading, and toruosity of renal cortical vessels, which is replaced by a normal vascular pattern after death (Epstein et al 1970). This decrease in renal cortical flow is believed to result from a circulating vasoconstrictive agent, such as a false neurotransmitter, bacterial endotoxins, or angiotensin II. The exact cause is not clear, and treatment is quite ineffective. Volume expansion is without value, and may even be dangerous, sodium administration worsens the condition, prednisone has no effect, the angiotensin II blocking agent, saralasin, induces extreme hypotension, and beta blocking agents are not beneficial. Sugarman et al (1971) were able to benefit some patients with metaraminol, a weak alpha adrenergic agent, and occasional benefit has been found from the use of L-dopa. Whatever improvement is found with these agents is almost invariably transitory, and the mortality rate from hyponaturic, oliguric azotemia is nearly total.

FULMINANT HEPATIC FAILURE

This state, which results from acute, severe hepatic necrosis, carries a mortality rate of 60 to 95 percent in various series. It is seen most commonly as a consequence of extensive acute viral or toxic hepatitis, and also with fatty liver of late stage pregnancy. An occasional patient with sudden acute hepatic congestion from heart failure may also show its features. Fulminant hepatic failure occurs as well in some patients with chronic liver disease, especially when hepatic function deteriorates rapidly following a sudden insult, such as massive gastrointestinal bleeding. This complication occurs in less than 1 percent of patients with hepatitis due to virus A, in 2 percent or more of patients with hepatitis B, and in higher percentages of patients with certain types of drug-induced hepatitis, such as that due to the anesthetic agent, halothane. A degree of hepatic encephalopathy accompanies all cases of fulminant failure, and the survival rates are poorest in patients with the deepest levels of coma. One large study of patients in deep coma (Trey 1972) from viral or drug hepatitis showed survival rates to be 34 percent in patients under age 15, 22 percent in patients from 15 to 44 years old, and only 5 percent in patients over age 44.

A recent study of fulminant hepatic failure and encephalopathy of variable degrees (Rakela 1979) found that in 188 cases, 2 percent were due to type A virus, 2 percent to type A and B combined, 56 percent to type B, 34 percent to non-A, non-B (?C) virus, and 6 percent to drug-induced hepatitis. Survival rates were 33 percent in A and B virus infections, 13 percent in non-A, non-B, and 8 percent in the drug group. In the 15- to 44-year-old patients, survival rates were significantly higher among type B hepatitis patients than in non-A, non-B cases. Survival rates between these two types of infection were not significantly different among patients aged 45 and over. Other studies indicate that the quality of supportive care during the episode of fulminant hepatic failure correlates with the outcome.

Pathology

Histologic changes compare very closely with the clinical picture. Boyer and Klatskin (1970) showed that subacute hepatic necrosis (confluent necrosis, bridging of necrosis from lobular central vein to portal area, or from portal area to adjacent portal area) (Figure 9–2) was present in 52 of 170 patients with acute hepatitis, while only "classic necrosis" (spotty necrosis, small irregular areas of necrosis without bridging) was present in the remaining 118 patients. Patients with classic necrosis developed no acute or chronic problems during a follow-up period of four months to nearly 16 years, while 20 percent of patients with bridging necrosis developed fulminant failure and all but 1 (10 percent) died within four months of the onset of their illness. Furthermore, 19 patients with bridging (36 percent) developed chronic hepatitis with cirrhosis (active in 10, inactive in 9). Only 21 (42 percent) of the original 52 patients with bridging necrosis recovered completely. While 11 patients with bridging developed hepatitis presumably from virus A infection, none of these died or developed chronic disease, thus confirming a general impression that fulminant hepatic failure and chronic hepatitis result mainly from type B or type C (non-A, non-B) viral infections. Horney and Galambos (1977) biopsied the livers of 14 patients with fulminant failure and found bridging necrosis in 9, a more severe multilobular necrosis in 4, and portal inflammation only in 1 patient. Five of 10 patients who were biopsied again showed normal livers, while 3 showed chronic active hepatitis, 1 with associated cirrhosis. Autopsies on patients

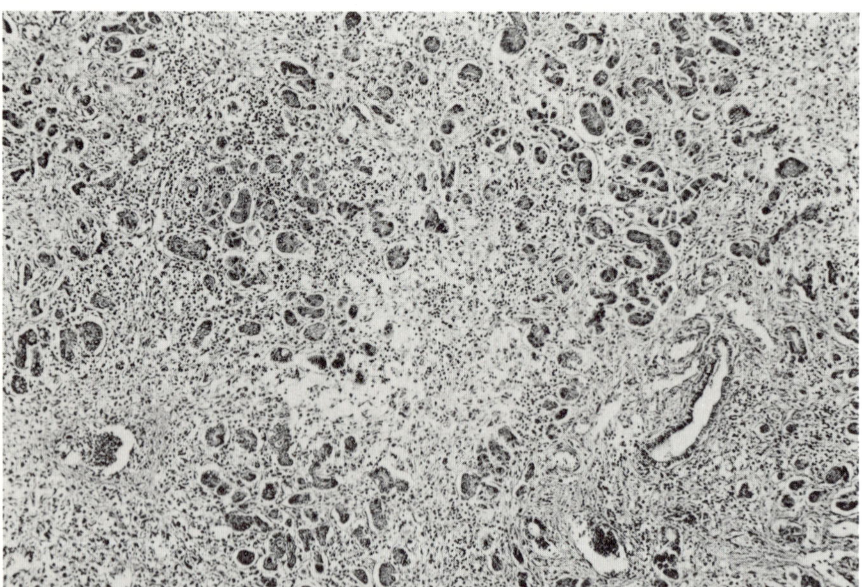

Figure 9–2. Confluent necrosis. Extensive necrosis and loss of hepatocytes results in collapse of the reticulin framework and a marked inflammatory reaction. Islands of surviving hepatocytes are arranged in acinar groups, especially in the periportal areas. Original magnification x80.

dying with fulminant hepatic failure usually show massive or submassive hepatic necrosis.

Clinical Picture

Hepatic Encephalopathy. Occasionally unassociated with hyperammonemia, hepatic encephalopathy is the hallmark of fulminant hepatic failure. Deepening jaundice may be present, but occasional patients have no, or slight, hyperbilirubinemia. In the early stages, encephalopathy may be manifested only by bizarre behavior of the patient or inappropriate affect. Hallucinations or convulsions may occur, especially in children. The progress from stage 1 to stage 4 encephalopathy may be very rapid.

On examination, disorientation and asterixis are common findings. The inability to palpate a recently enlarged liver is an ominous sign, suggesting extensive necrosis. An increased tendency to bleed is found in about half of the patients. Edema and ascites may also appear in those most severely ill. In stage 4 or deep coma, hyperventilation and respiratory alkalosis are common. Oliguria, cardiac arrhythmias, and gastrointestinal hemorrhage are ominous signs. The likelihood of aspiration and respiratory arrest is great. Death is usually the direct result of cardiac arrest.

Hemostatic Disorders. While hepatic encephalopathy is the basis for grading fulminant hepatic failure clinically, more severe cases also develop the hepatorenal syndrome and various disorders of hemostasis. Disorderly blood clotting may arise from a simple lack of production of essential factors by the diseased liver but is more commonly due to a consumption coagulapathy, and rarely to increases in platelet destruction or in fibrinolysis. Hemostatic disorders are manifested commonly by spontaneous hemorrhage into or beneath the skin, bleeding from the nose or gastrointestinal tract, or oozing of blood from needle puncture sites. Gastrointestinal bleeding aggravates encephalopathy. Spontaneous intracranial hemorrhage is rare but may occur if patients receive even slight cranial injuries.

1. Reduction of coagulation factors produced in the liver is a direct result of hepatocytic damage. While most clotting factors produced by the liver are dependent on vitamin K as well, levels of factor V (proaccelerin) and fibrinogen, which do not require this vitamin for synthesis, may also be low. The resultant defects can be monitored by the one-stage prothrombin and the thrombin times.

2. Disseminated intravascular coagulation may be present to a slight extent in patients with cirrhosis of the liver but is much more severe in fulminant hepatic failure. Without treatment, the mortality rate is probably total (Rake et al 1970). The thrombin time is prolonged, fibrinogen levels and platelet counts are low, and fibrinogen degradation products are elevated. In vitro, partial thromboplastin and one-stage prothrombin times are cor-

rected by normal plasma, but the administration of fresh frozen plasma to patients provides only transient relief because of rapid consumption of the added clotting factors. The major site of intravascular coagulation appears to be in the liver itself, where fibrin sinusoidal clots are often seen on tissue specimens taken at autopsy. It appears to be the result of damage to sinusoidal endothelium by degenerating hepatocytes and the release of cellular thromboplastin and blood clotting factors. The clots themselves may lead to further hepatic damage by causing ischemia.

3. Platelet abnormalities may be encountered in patients with chronic liver disease, and in some patients with fulminant failure who have congestive splenomegaly. Platelet production is usually normal, but there is increased trapping in splenic capillaries, due to slowing of blood flow and increased tortuosity of the vascular channels. Most reduction of platelet counts in fulminant failure, however, is a probable result of accelerated aggregation by intravascular fibrin degradation products.

4. Increased fibrinolysis has been demonstrated in some patients with fulminant failure and in patients with cirrhosis of the liver. It is commonly associated with intravascular coagulation. Fibrinolysis may be due to one or more of several factors: increased production or reduced excretion of activators of plasminogen or depression of inhibitors (Ratnoff 1975). It does not appear to be a major problem in fulminant hepatic failure due to acute hepatocellular necrosis. Fibrinolytic inhibitors should not be given to patients with intravascular coagulation because they may worsen the coagulapathy.

Principles of Treatment

The management of fulminant hepatic failure is largely supportive. The hope is that the patient may be kept alive long enough to allow hepatic regeneration to occur. Accordingly, great attention must be given to fluid and electrolytic balance, to pulmonary toilet, and to prevention or treatment of infection. Catheters should be avoided, needle punctures kept to a minimum, and oral feeding should not be given to patients in moderate or deep coma, for fear of aspiration. Sedative drugs should be given as little as possible, or not at all, and hepatic encephalopathy and the hepatorenal syndrome should be treated intensively. Expert nursing care is essential.

Reduction of coagulation factors can be transiently treated by the administration of fresh frozen plasma, although the life of most of these factors is very short, and transfusions may have to be frequent. Unless the underlying disease of the liver is primarily cholestatic, the administration of vitamin K is almost always ineffectual, though it should be tried because of occasional benefit.

Treatment of disseminated intravascular coagulation in hepatic necrosis is mainly supportive and usually ineffective. Early optimistic results of treatment with heparin have not been substantiated in later trials.

Other supportive measures have been tried or suggested in the treatment of fulminant hepatic failure, but each has been found to be either too complex for regular use, ineffectual, or of unproved benefit. In controlled studies, glucocorticoids have proved to be without value, and may perhaps aggravate bleeding tendencies. Exchange transfusions, extracorporeal perfusion of hog liver with patient's blood, and total body perfusion with balanced electrolyte solutions during hypothermia have all been attempted in the treatment of fulminant failure, but none have been found to be persuasively beneficial in controlled studies. Furthermore, the complex nature of these procedures prohibits their use on a large scale. Farivar et al (1976) found that the administration of a mixture of insulin and glucagon to mice at the time of infection with a lethal dose of murine hepatitis virus reduced the severity of the resultant fulminant hepatic failure and increased survival rates from zero in controls to 40 percent in treated animals. Survival was associated with increased labeling of hepatocytic nuclei with ^{3}H-thymidine, supposedly the result of increased cellular regeneration induced by the hormones. This treatment has not, as yet, been employed in humans.

PORTAL HYPERTENSION AND ESOPHAGEAL VARICES

The portal venous system is a vascular network which drains blood into the liver from the stomach, small intestine, and colon, from the spleen, pancreas, and gallbladder, and from the greater and lesser omentum. Normal pressure in the system ranges between 8 and 12 cm of water. The absence of valves in any of the participating veins permits the reversal of blood flow whenever a blockage to outflow exists, either in the liver, the portal vein itself, or in one of its major tributaries. The anatomy of the portal system is variable from person to person, but its normal features have been outlined quite well by Douglass et al (1950) (Figure 9–3). All physicians should be familiar with this anatomy, since the portal system participates in one of the major catastrophic consequences of chronic hepatic disease (hemorrhage from esophageal varices), and since it may occasionally become obstructed (pylethrombosis) from other causes as well.

The Splenic Vein

Blood enters the spleen from two sources, the splenic artery and the short gastric veins. The splenic artery is a major branch of the celiac axis, and the short gastric veins, which number from three to five, carry blood from the greater curve of the upper stomach into the upper portion of the spleen. An average of three (two to six) separate venous trunks emerge from the hilus of the spleen and join within a short distance to form a single splenic vein, 4.5 mm in diameter, which then passes posterior to and some-

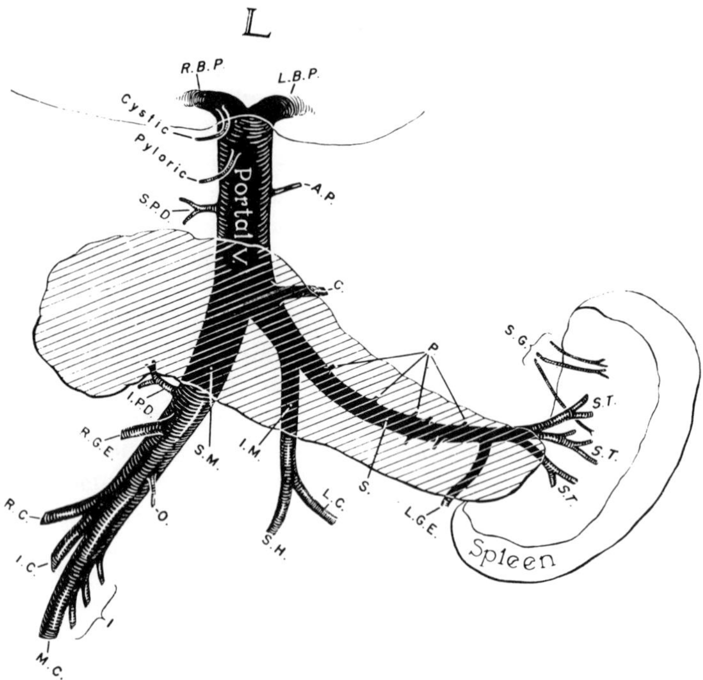

Figure 9–3. The extrahepatic system of veins, anterior aspect. The pancreas is represented by the shaded area. AP, accessory pancreatic vein; C, coronary vein; I, intestinal veins; IC, ileocolic vein; IM, inferior mesenteric vein; IPD, inferior pancreaticoduodenal vein; L, liver; LBP, left branch of portal vein; LC, left colic vein; LGE, left gastroepiploic vein; MC, middle colic vein; O, omental vein; P, pancreatic veins; RC, right colic vein; RGE, right gastroepiploic vein; RBP, right branch of portal vein; S, splenic vein; SG, short gastric veins; SH, superior hemorrhoidal vein; SM, superior mesenteric vein; SPD, superior pancreaticoduodenal vein; ST, splenic trunks. From Douglass BE, Bagenstoss AH, Hollinshead WH. Surg Gynecol Obstet 91:562–76, 1950. Reprinted by permission.

times through the tail and distal body of the pancreas for a length of 15 cm. The splenic vein receives blood from the greater curve of the stomach; the greater omentum, through the left gastroepiploic vein, which joins the splenic vein near its origin; and the pancreas, through a number (3 to 13) of short veins draining the posterior portion of that organ. It is usually joined at right angles, 3 to 4 cm from its termination, by the inferior mesenteric vein. This vessel averages 3 mm in diameter and drains the superior hemorrhoidal, sigmoidal, and left colic veins. Commonly, the inferior mesenteric vein terminates either by directly joining the superior mesenteric vein or by connecting at the junction of the splenic and superior mesenteric veins.

The Superior Mesenteric Vein

This major vessel is 8 mm in diameter and receives the ileocolic, right colic, middle colic, intestinal, right gastroepiploic, inferior pancreatoduodenal, and omental veins. It passes anterior to the third (transverse) portion of the duodenum and posterior to the head of the pancreas, where it joins the splenic vein at right angles to form the portal vein.

The Portal Vein

This large (9-mm diameter) vessel flows behind the pancreas and duodenum and into the hilus of the liver, where it divides into two major trunks, one each for the right and left lobes of the liver. In its course rightward and upward, the portal vein usually receives the following tributaries in order: the coronary (left gastric), the superior pancreatoduodenal, the accessory pancreatic, the pyloric (right gastric), and the cholecystic veins. The coronary vein (2.5 mm diameter) passes from right to left along the lesser curve of the stomach and receives tributaries from the stomach and the greater omentum. Just below the esophagastric junction, the coronary vein turns rightward and shortly joins the portal system, either the portal vein itself near its origin, the junction of the splenic and superior mesenteric veins, or the splenic vein. At this turning point, the coronary vein receives several esophageal tributaries. Its normal length is about 7 cm.

Hyperdynamic Inflow of Arterial Blood

In addition to obstruction of portal outflow in the bed of the liver, patients with cirrhosis also show increased flow of aterial blood into the portal system (Witte et al 1978). Mesenteric venous blood is well oxygenated, blood volume is increased, and cardiac output is often elevated, all of which suggest a hyperdynamic state. It is known that arteriovenous fistulas exist in the cirrhotic liver as well as in the skin, as demonstrated by palmar erythema and vascular spider nevi. Similar arteriovenous bypasses probably exist in the mesentery as well, and contribute heavily to this increased flow state. Thus the degree of portal hypertension obtaining at any one time is the product of the degree of portal venous obstruction and the amount of arteriovenous shunting, and both play a part in its complications and therapy.

Consequences of Portal Hypertension

With the anatomical picture in mind, it is possible to comprehend the consequences of obstruction at various levels of the portal system. Almost all such obstructions are gradual in onset and are associated proximal to the blockade with increased venous pressure, passive congestion of organs, and the opening of collateral venous channels seeking to bypass the block. McIndoe (1928) has divided the collateral pathways that form consequent to portal hypertension into three categories: those which result from reversal of flow in established venous pathways at the esophagogastric junction and in the rectum; those which open residual fetal pathways in partially obliterated embryological vessels in the falciform ligament of the liver; and those occurring where the alimentary organs are retroperitoneal, such as at the base of the mesentery, the ascending and descending colon, the pancreas and the spleen, and the dome of the liver. Channels described by Retzius connect the mesenteric vessels with the inferior vena cava in the rectum and at the base of the mesentery, while the veins of Sappey communicate with systemic diaphragmatic veins over the dome of the liver. In patients with postoperative omental adhesions, collaterals also develop to veins in the abdominal wall (Figure 9-4). Collaterals develop and enlarge because increased venous pressure proximal to the blockage causes endothelial proliferation.

Congestive splenomegaly is a hallmark of hypertension in the splenic vein, and is caused both by portal hypertension and arteriovenous intrasplenic shunts. Distention of the short gastric veins and passive congestion of the greater curve of the stomach and of the distal pancreas are often associated. Enlargment of the spleen is followed by intrasplenic vascular proliferation and tortuosity with resultant increased destruction of red and white blood cells and platelets. The resultant hemolytic anemia, leukopenia, and thrombocytopenia are associated with hyperactivity of the bone marrow, a condition called hypersplenism. It is a common finding in patients with portal hypertension due to chronic disease of the liver, a condition often referred to as Banti syndrome.

Internal hemorrhoids develop when portal obstruction is distal to the junction of the inferior mesenteric with the splenic vein. Pressure rises in the superior hemorrhoidal veins and collaterals open into the inferior hemorrhoidal veins which drain eventually into the inferior vena cava. Since hemorrhoidal veins are just beneath the anorectal epithelium, their enlargement causes protrusions into the lumen of the bowel, which bleed profusely if they are injured, especially by straining at stool.

Esophageal varices are, in a manner of speaking, the counterpart of hemorrhoids located in the upper stomach and lower esophagus. Increased pressure in the coronary (left gastric) vein leads to engorgement of esophageal tributaries and proliferation of vascular channels in the lower esophagus to the azygous vein. These vessels are also close to the luminal surface of the esophagus (Figures 9-5 and 9-6) and may bleed vigorously and massively when they rupture into the esophagus. Bleeding from esophageal varices, however, is much more difficult to manage than is bleeding from hemorrhoids: (1) esophageal varices are usually more extensive and larger than internal hemorrhoids and bleed more rapidly; (2) access to varices is much

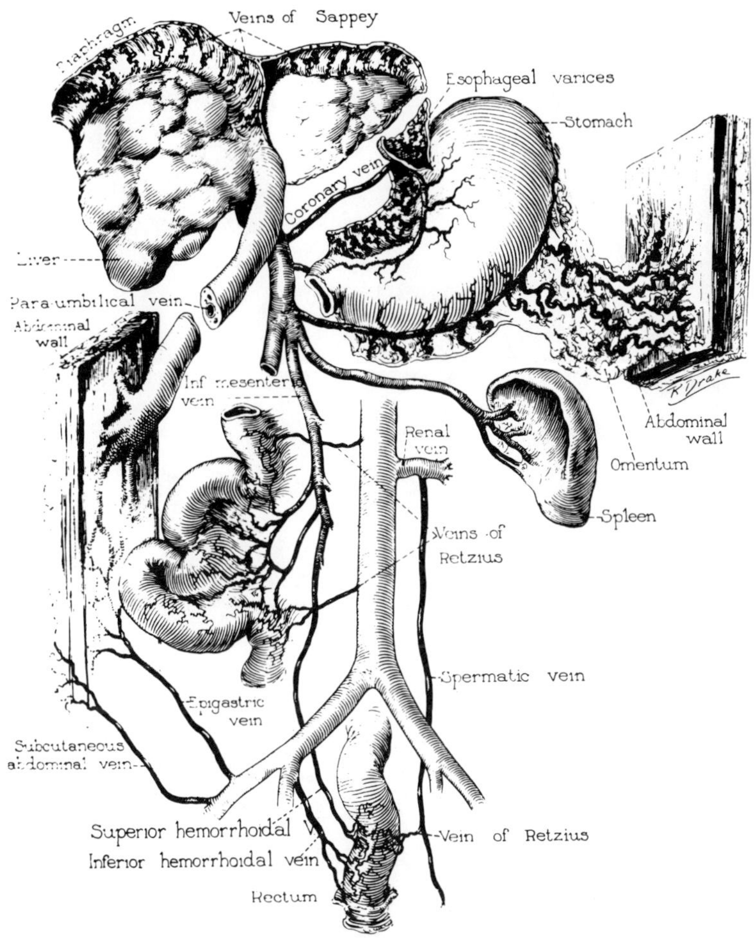

Figure 9–4. Schematic representation of the collateral circulation in portal hypertension. From McIndoe AH. Arch Path 5:23–42, 1928. Copyright 1928, American Medical Association.

more difficult, and bleeding is consequently harder to control; (3) hepatic encephalopathy is much greater after esophageal variceal bleeding, because of the high protein load passed suddenly into the upper intestine.

Intestinal varices may also develop, especially in the jejunum and ileum, in response to portal hypertension among patients who have had previous abdominal surgery. They are usually associated with omental or other adhesions to the anterior abdominal wall, and may bleed excessively if they are close to the mucosal surface.

Dilated abdominal veins are commonly seen in patients with portal hypertension due to a block distal to the superior mesenteric vein and to

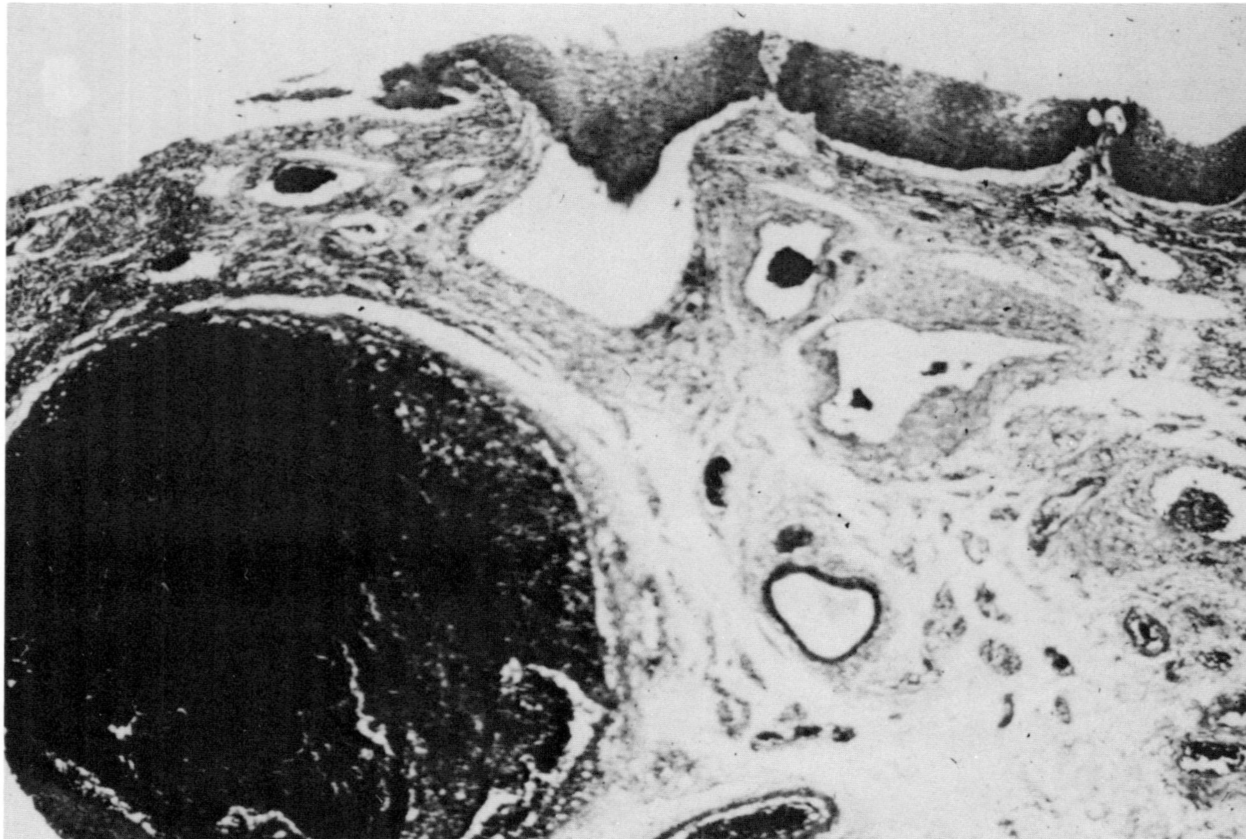

Figure 9–5. Esophageal varix. Note the proximity of the large varix to the lumen of the esophagus, and the erosion of the mucosa. Original magnification x10.

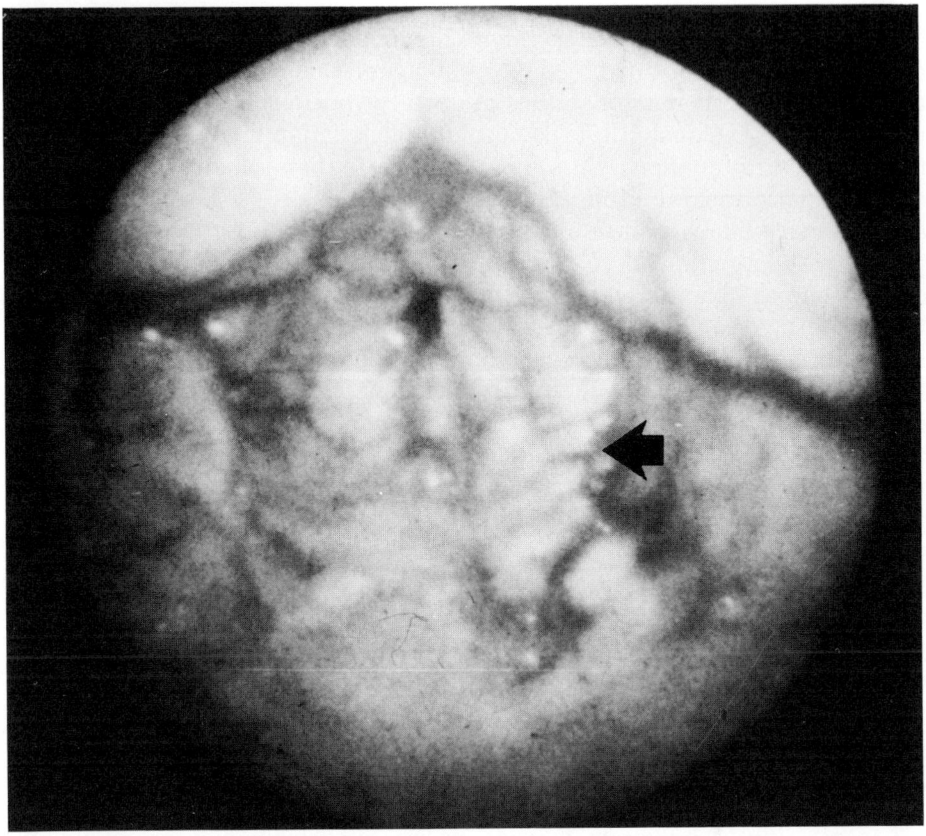

Figure 9–6. Esophageal varices in a patient with cirrhosis of the liver. The varices are represented by the vermiform swellings in the submucosa of the distal esophagus.

liver blockade. They represent collaterals through hypogastric veins and through fetal venous channels remaining in the falciform ligament. If the umbilical vein is still patent at the time portal hypertension develops, marked distention of paraumbilical veins may occur, the *caput medusae* (Cruveilhier-Baumgarten syndrome). Because of the rapid and turbulent flow of blood through a caput medusae, a palpable thrill and an audible bruit are often present on examination.

Classification of Portal Hypertension

Increased portal venous pressure may be caused by lesions in the system proximal to the liver, in the liver itself, or in the hepatic veins. The hepatic lesions can be further classified into those which cause obstruction in the portal tracts, proximal to the hepatic lobule (presinusoidal), those which obstruct sinusoidal flow primarily, and those which obstruct hepatic vein flow (postsinusoidal). This classification is important to keep in mind when considering treatment of bleeding esophageal varices and ascites, which are the major serious implications of portal hypertension. Patients with intrahepatic or extrahepatic presinusoidal obstruction usually have good to normal hepatic function, while those with more distal obstruction have reduced hepatic reserve. The latter patients are much poorer surgical risks and are more likely to pass into fulminant hepatic failure postoperatively.

Extrahepatic portal vein obstructions are usually the result of partial or complete obstructions of the portal vein, secondary to thrombosis or infiltration with tumor. Portal vein thrombosis (pylethrombosis) was commonly seen in the past in children consequent to exchange transfusions in infancy by way of the umbilical vein, and is occasionally seen today as a result of peritonitis from a ruptured appendix or pelvic inflammatory disease, and in patients with thrombocytosis. Such patients may develop esophageal varices and bleeding, but not ascites.

Intrahepatic presinusoidal obstruction occurs in patients with liver diseases confined to the bile ducts and portal areas. Among these are: schistosomiasis, where deposition of ova leads to portal fibrosis; early stages of primary biliary cirrhosis, where the inflammatory process is confined to portal areas; sarcoidosis and other disorders causing granulomas in portal areas; and metastatic carcinoma of the liver, where tumor masses partially block portal venular flow.

Wedged hepatic vein pressure is normal in patients with presinusoidal portal hypertension and elevated in patients whose obstruction is more distal, because this technique records pressure at sinusoidal levels only.

Sinusoidal obstruction causing portal hypertension is primarily the result of cirrhosis of the liver, which by the process of necrosis, destruction of reticulin framework of the liver, and nodular regeneration shrinks and compresses the intrahepatic circulation at all levels. The portal hypertension of cirrhosis is then most likely a consequence of varying degrees of blockade at presinusoidal, sinusoidal, and postsinusoidal levels (Sherlock 1978). In addition, increased hepatic arterial flow and intrahepatic arteriovenous anastomoses contribute to the portal hypertension associated with cirrhosis.

Postsinusoidal obstruction occurs primarily as a consequence of hepatic vein thrombosis (the Budd-Chiari syndrome). It may also be seen in patients with prolonged passive congestion of the liver from cardiac failure, but this disorder is rarely associated with significant portal hypertension.

Hemorrhage from Esophageal Varices

There is no clear answer to questions regarding the direct cause of bleeding from esophageal varices. Suffice it to say that bleeding does occur, often massively, when portal pressures achieve levels high enough and are sustained long enough to cause rupture. Sudden increases in mesenteric arteriovenous shunting may also contribute or bleeding may come as a consequence of vomiting, administration of aspirin or other prostaglandin inhibitors, and occasionally of reflux esophagitis. Most often, the hemorrhage starts spontaneously, without obvious precipitating factors. In patients with hepatic disease, the severity of the hemorrhage is aggravated by lack of coagulation factors normally produced in the liver. The tendency for variceal hemorrhage to recur after it once discontinues is very high indeed and is almost invariable. Thus, treatment must include consideration both of efforts to stop the instant hemorrhage and of procedures to prevent further episodes.

Morbidity. Most patients with cirrhosis of the liver develop esophageal varices, but not all of them bleed. The use of prophylactic surgical shunting procedures to prevent hemorrhage is clearly effective in its primary objective but does not reduce the overall mortality rate in chronic liver disease (Conn et al 1972). Forty to over 90 percent of patients with cirrhosis of the liver die from their disease or its complications within 10 years of diagnosis. These widely discrepant rates are doubtless reflections of the severity of the disease at the start of the observation period, and may also relate to the quality of care provided. In one study of 146 patients with alcoholic cirrhosis and portal hypertension (Soterakis et al 1973), 61 percent survived for 10 years, and the rate of survival was only slightly improved among patients who abstained from further alcohol. In a larger study of 467 patients with cirrhosis and varices, 84 percent due to alcohol ingestion (Garceau and Chalmers 1963), 253 (54 percent) died during the follow-up period. Thirty-four percent of deaths were due to gastrointestinal hemorrhage, 32 percent to hepatic failure, 11 percent to anuria, and 9 percent to infection. Nearly 80 percent of the deaths occurred during the first year of study. In evaluating these data, it is important to know that these patients were very ill at the outset of the study. Not only did all subjects have esophageal varices, but 81 percent had ascites, 78 percent were jaundiced, and 61 percent were encephalopathic.

Patients with esophageal varices from nonalcoholic macronodular cirrhosis probably fare as badly as do those with alcoholic disease. However, the prognosis of patients whose varices result from extrahepatic or intrahepatic presinusoidal blockade is much better, primarily because liver function is good.

Management of Variceal Hemorrhage

Nonsurgical Management. The general principles of treating upper gastrointestinal hemorrhage apply equally to patients who are bleeding from esophageal varices. Associated liver disease and the high probability that hepatic failure, encephalopathy, and the hepatorenal syndrome will occur as complications of the bleeding place variceal bleeders, or indeed any patient with severe liver disease and gastrointestinal bleeding, at a high risk of mortality. Supportive care must include rapid cleansing of blood from the intestinal tract, careful attention to urinary output, and prompt replacement of deficiencies in blood clotting factors, as well as the usual measures for circulatory support and replacement of electrolytes. Because so many patients with variceal bleeding also have sodium retention and ascites, special care must be taken in these patients to avoid overloading their circulation with additional sodium, which will increase their fluid retention. Since the incidence of respiratory and urinary tract infections is so high among cirrhotics, a strong case can also be made for the preventative use of antibiotics, such as ampicillin, in their acute care.

Gastric lavage and endoscopy should be performed promptly. Approximately one-half of all patients with chronic liver disease, esophageal varices and upper gastrointestinal hemorrhage are found to be bleeding from peptic ulcers, Mallory-Weiss tears, or hemorrhagic gastritis, rather than varices. If varices are indeed found to be the cause, further special measures, such as the use of vasopressin and esophageal tamponade, should be considered.

Vasopressin has been clearly shown to cause spasm in the superior and inferior mesenteric arteries and the celiac axis, to reduce splanchnic blood flow and portal venous pressure, and to slow variceal bleeding in over 90 percent of patients. It is most readily administered into a peripheral vein either as a bolus of 20 units in 20 min every two to four hours as required, or continuously at the rate of 0.25 to 0.5 units per minutes. Blood pressure and electrocardiogram should be carefully monitored, since hypertension and myocardial ischemia may complicate the treatment. Urinary output should also be watched for signs of anuria and sodium retention. The rate of administration of vasopressin is decreased as bleeding slows.

Esophageal tamponade with an elongated rubber balloon mounted on a nasogastric tube may stop bleeding temporarily by compression of varices. This tube must be placed carefully with radiographic monitoring, and the assembly should be anchored in the stomach with a smaller balloon. A single (Sengstaken-Blakemore) tube has been devised for this purpose, and has been found useful in managing some patients with acute variceal hemorrhage. The use of vasopressin in recent years has greatly reduced the need for esophageal tamponade. This is fortunate because the tube itself and the assembly needed to keep it in place cause a great deal of discomfort to patients. Esophageal tamponade has not been shown to reduce the mortality from variceal hemorrhage; its main benefit has been in affording more time to ready patients for more definitive therapy.

Other nonsurgical methods have been devised to control intractable variceal bleeding in patients whose liver disease makes them too ill to withstand the risk of surgery. Although direct injection of varices with sclerosing agents during esophagoscopy has proved to be effective at times, a new method for thrombosing portal collateral vessels has been devised and shows some promise of being better. This method involves passage of a flexible needle through the liver and into the porta hepatis percutaneously. With continuous fluoroscopic guidance, a catheter is passed through the needle into the portal vein, and thence to the coronary vein. Individual varices are then thrombosed with thrombin and gelfoam, thus reducing variceal flow. This method may stop bleeding enough to permit improvement in hepatic function. Bleeding from the procedure itself can usually be controlled by administration of fresh frozen plasma.

Surgical Management. There are few things more certain in medicine than the probability that patients with portal hypertension who have once bled from esophageal varices will do so again, usually within a very short period of time. It is almost certain that hepatic function will be poorer after subsequent hemorrhages than it was after the first. The five-year mortality rate in patients who have once bled from varices is between 60 and 85 percent and is highest in those with poorest hepatic function. The aim of acute treatment is to stop bleeding long enough to allow time for hepatic function to improve to the point where the risk of surgery is acceptable. This is not always possible, however, because bleeding often fails to stop during medical therapy, or may recur promptly after a short time.

The objective of surgery is to reduce pressure in the portal system by deviating some portal blood into the systemic circulation without, at the same time, worsening hepatic function. Direct portacaval shunts reduce pressure well and prevent further bleeding, but are accompanied by a high rate of recurrent or chronic hepatic encephalopathy and hepatic failure postoperatively. This is true whether the shunt is made side-to-side between the portal vein and the vena cava, or whether the portal vein is transected and the proximal end implanted, end-to-side, into the vena cava. Another popular method has been to anastomose the proximal splenic vein to the renal vein after splenectomy, but reduction of portal pressure is less than in portacaval shunts and there is a tendency for the shunt to thrombose postoperatively. The frequency of encephalopathy is reduced with this operation. Recently, a "distal" splenorenal shunt has been tried with some success, the splenic vein being divided at its junction with the superior mesenteric and the splenic end of the vein joined to the left renal vein. The coronary and right gastroepiploic veins are also ligated (Warren and Galambos 1973). Blood from the small and large intestine and the head of the pancreas continues to flow into the portal vein, so that hepatotrophic factors (possibly insulin and glucagon) continue to enter the liver. Variceal bleeding is distinctly reduced although varices do not regularly disappear; hypersplenism is also improved (Welch and Malt 1979). A simpler portasystemic anastomosis has also been used with some success in high risk patients and in cases where a portacaval shunt is not technically feasible. This involves placing a synthetic graft between the superior mesenteric and inferior caval veins, but graft thrombosis and hepatic encephalopathy are significant postoperative complications.

The risk of portasystemic shunt surgery is related directly to the severity of hepatic disease at the time of the operation. Child and Turcotte (1964) classified their patients with cirrhosis into three groups, based on the severity of their hepatic disease: Minimal (group A), moderate (group B), and advanced (group C) (Table 9–1). When end-to-side portacaval shunts were done on a series of 128 patients so classified, mortality rate was zero in group A, 9 percent in group B, and 53 percent in group C. Overall operative mortality was 17 percent. Furthermore, among group C patients surviving surgery, 80 percent were dead from liver failure within three years, and many of these patients had been encephalopathic. The incidence of these complications among patients in groups A and B was much less, and at seven years postoperatively, group A survival was over 90 percent; group B, about 55 percent. The long-term mortality rates are, of course, due to the cirrhosis itself, since patients with patent shunts do not usually suffer recurrent gastrointestinal hemorrhage. However, there is clear evidence that total shunting (end-to-side) of portal blood to the systemic circulation does predispose patients with advanced liver disease to hepatic failure and encephalopathy shortly after the operation.

The most beneficial surgical shunt has not been identified. Conn et al (1981) performed a randomized comparison of portasystemic and distal splenorenal shunts in 53 patients with moderately severe liver disease followed for a mean period of 21 months after surgery. Twenty-five percent died in the distal shunt group, as against 41 percent with portacaval shunts. Encephalopathy occurred among 32 percent of the former group, and among 23 percent of the latter. No significant difference of results was noted between the two procedures. Survival rates among patients over 60 years of age are not noticeably different from those in younger patients after distal splenorenal shunting (Livingstone et al 1979).

Table 9–1. Classification of Patients with Cirrhosis in Terms of Hepatic Functional Reserve

Group	*A* *Minimal*	*B* *Moderate*	*C* *Severe*
Serum bilirubin (mg per dl)	below 2.0	2.0-3.0	over 3.0
Serum albumin (g per dl)	over 3.5	3.0-3.5	under 3.0
Ascites	none	easily controlled	poorly controlled
Neurological disorder	none	minimal	advanced
Nutrition	excellent	good	poor

After Child and Turcotte (1964).

There appears to be no benefit of end-to-side portacaval shunts over proximal splenorenal shunts, and the portacaval shunt is technically easier to perform. The side-to-side portacaval shunt is the preferred operation in patients with hepatic vein thrombosis, since it is clearly associated with a reduced rate of hepatic failure when compared with end-to-side shunts (Malt et al 1979).

Deciding when to perform a portasystemic shunt on patients with variceal bleeding is still not agreed on. Most experts would recommend surgery in the group A or B patient with repeated episodes of bleeding, and many would recommend the operation after only one hemorrhage in view of the 90 percent likelihood of recurrence. Those who do not agree with prompt surgery point to the high incidence of encephalopathy and increased days of hospitalization associated with the operation. Reynolds et al (1978) have performed a decade-long study of 89 group A patients with alcoholic cirrhosis and a single variceal hemorrhage, randomized to medical or surgical groups. While 23 of the 44 medical patients died from recurrent hemorrhage compared to none of the patients with surgery, 34 percent of the surgical patients developed encephalopathy, 7 percent died from surgery, and 41 percent died from hepatic failure. Sixteen percent of the "medical" patients had to be operated on for subsequent bleeding. There was no significant difference in survival rates between the two groups when plotted by the life table method.

Disheartened by the high recurrence rate of variceal bleeding, Orloff et al (1975) undertook surgery in 138 consecutive patients with alcoholic cirrhosis, regardless of their state of hepatic function. Portacaval shunting was performed after a few hours, during which bleeding was controlled with vasopressin, transfusions were commenced, and various diagnostic procedures were performed. Survival was adversely affected to a significant degree by the presence of ascites, advanced muscular atrophy, a small liver, bilirubin greater than 5.5 mg per dl, and prothrombin content less than 20 percent of normal. Forty-nine percent of the patients died within one month, but 43 percent of the group survived for seven years, and two-thirds of those remained in good to excellent condition. When one considers that 35 percent of the patients were in Child's Group C at the time of surgery, this survival rate is not terribly bad, and lends some support to the position of Orloff.

While no studies currently available favor one approach clearly over any other in the management of variceal bleeding, certain conclusions may be drawn. A patient in group A or B who has suffered more than one hemorrhage from esophageal varices should doubtless have a shunting procedure performed. If there has only been a single hemorrhage, data indicate that the trade-off of probable hepatic encephalopathy for future freedom from bleeding may not be worth the risk, although the encephalopathy can usually be treated. If bleeding cannot be stopped medically, there is no choice, of course. For the group C patient, all means short of surgery should be tried. These include vasopressin, tamponade, and attempts to embolize varices with transhepatic catheterization of the left gastric vein. While the latter procedure has not been shown to be free of danger, the risk is less than that of surgery in patients with advanced hepatic failure, and thus appears to be acceptable. Finally, in patients who are untrustworthy and may continue to drink alcohol after hospitalization, consideration should be given to the use of immediate surgery for variceal bleeding.

ASCITES

Ascites, esophageal varices, and congestive splenomegaly are the three major complications of portal hypertension. The ascitic fluid is more often a "transudate" (specific gravity 1.020 or less) than an "exudate." But it must be kept in mind that cirrhotic ascites may occasionally have a fairly high protein content. Wilson et al (1979), for example, found that the specific gravity of the ascitic fluid in their patients was above 1.020 in 22 percent, the protein content was 3 g or greater per dl in 24 percent, and the white cell count was over 500 per cu ml in 22 percent.

Mechanism of Ascites Formation

Portal hypertension is the essential ingredient for the formation of ascites in patients with cirrhosis of the liver. The ascites which accumulates rapidly in the presence of hepatic vein obstruction (Budd-Chiari syndrome) is believed to result directly from postsinusoidal blockade of venous flow, distention of spaces of Disse, and hepatic lymphatics, with resultant seepage of lymph containing large amounts of sinusoidal protein from the surface of the liver. Such weeping of ascitic fluid from the hepatic surface has been demonstrated in patients with hepatic vein obstruction and probably also occurs in some patients with chronic congestive heart failure. It occurs only to a small extent in patients with cirrhosis of the liver.

The origin of ascites in patients with portal hypertension due to presinusoidal and sinusoidal block, as in cirrhosis, is different. It is the result of increased formation of hepatic lymph, plus a limited capacity of larger lymphatic channels to convey lymph to the general venous circulation.

Increased Splanchnic Lymph Flow. Ascitic fluid is usually low in protein and, in common with splanchnic lymph, may be chylous at times. Splanchnic lymph flow has been found to be greatly increased in patients with cirrhosis of the liver, and thoracic duct flow may be over twice its usual volume of 8 to 9 liters per day (Witte et al 1971). Since this increased flow of lymph probably results directly from the blockade to venous runoff, the transudate usually contains much less protein than does normal splanchnic lymph. Since portal hypertension and increased splanchnic lymph flow often exist in the absence of ascites, another element appears to be required before ascites appears.

Limited Capacity for Conveyance of Lymph. A good case can be made for the assumption that ascites appears in cirrhotics only when the production of lymph exceeds the capacity of the thoracic ductal system to convey that lymph to the subclavian vein. This may be the result of exceeding the compliance of the thoracic duct, functional narrowings in the thoracic duct, or increased central venous pressure. Surgical widening of the junction of the thoracic duct with the subclavian vein has been shown to relieve ascites in some patients.

Reduced Excretion of Salt and Water. This commonly occurs in patients with ascites, will clearly aggravate ascites formation and may indeed be a primary cause. Salt retention is commonly associated with increased renin levels in the blood, resulting possibly from increased production due to cortical shunting of blood flow, or decreased catabolism in the liver, due to decreased production of renin substrate (angiotensinogen) (Barnardo et al 1970). Elaboration of renin leads to release of aldosterone by the kidney, and this hormone increases the reabsorption of sodium in the distal tubule in exchange for hydrogen and potassium. This mechanism accounts for the hyponaturic, oliguric, hypokalemic alkalosis commonly seen in patients with cirrhosis and ascites. However, sodium retention may occur without the increased release of aldosterone (Chonko et al 1977).

Hypoalbuminemia. Because of decreased production of albumin in the liver and possibly to increased loss in the intestine consequent to portal hypertension, hypoalbuminemia may contribute to the formation of ascites in cirrhotics by lowering of plasma colloid oncotic pressure. It is probably a direct cause of the peripheral edema of cirrhosis. Hypoalbuminemia is invariably seen in cirrhotic patients with peripheral edema but is not always associated with ascites. The contribution of hypoalbuminemia to ascites formation is small, probably because the colloid oncotic pressure of plasma even moderately deficient in albumin is still greater than the oncotic pressure of the splanchnic lymph produced by the stimulus of portal hypertension. The use of intravenous albumin in patients with cirrhosis does not usually reduce the volume of ascites.

Consequences of Ascites

Ascites causes adverse effects largely through mechanical alterations related directly to the volume and mass of the accumulated fluid. Ascitic volume may approach as much as 20 liters at times, and often the process is well along before patients recognize what is happening. In early days, they will often think that the increased weight and enlarging abdominal girth is simply the result of overeating; but the continued increase in weight despite reduced intake and the occasional later onset of ankle edema quickly deny that notion. In some patients, particularly alcoholics, the enlarged abdomen is worn like a merit badge of masculinity, and help is not sought until reduced hepatic function, encephalopathy, or a direct complication of the ascites makes it mandatory.

The major consequences of ascites are: cosmetic aberrations, changes in the truncal center of gravity, aggravation of incipient hernias, reduced capacity for food, respiratory embarrassment, and masking of other intra-abdominal pathology.

Cosmetic aberrations refer principally to the concern, particularly of women with cirrhosis, that their bodily contours are changing unfavorably. This is a fortunate observation, because it usually leads to early recognition and treatment of the underlying hepatic disorder. The major danger of this complaint is that it might lead to overly zealous treatment with diuretics, and consequent iatrogenically aggravated renal dysfunction. Patients should be encouraged to be content with slower methods of treatment.

Changes in the center of gravity caused by ascites will often force patients to lean backward as they walk, thereby placing added stress on the vertebral column. It is not a serious problem, but recognition of the unusual posture will occasionally lead to early diagnosis of ascites.

Incipient hernias in the inguinal and umbilical areas are commonly enlarged by the increased abdominal pressure from ascites. Scrotal and penile edema are common concomitants. Umbilical hernias may become massive and resemble the contours of an elephant's trunk. Tight stretching of the skin overlying umbilical hernias may lead to pressure necrosis and to spontaneous tearing of the skin, with sudden external drainage of ascites. Hiatal hernias are also worsened frequently by ascites, but adverse consequences are rare.

Reduction in food capacity is a serious complication and may lead to the superficially paradoxical clinical picture of a person who, while eating little, continues to gain weight. One notes marked decreases in muscle mass, particularly in the upper extremities, shoulder girdles, neck, face, and chest. The patient looks cachectic above the diaphragm and massively obese below. Muscular weakness is prominent, and the situation is self-perpetuating. Prompt treatment of the ascites can, if successful, lead to increasing caloric intake and improvement in muscle mass.

Respiratory embarrassment is a direct result of diaphragmatic elevation from ascites, with lowered lung compliance, decreased vital capacity, hyperventilation, and occasionally respiratory alkalosis. Where the problem is severe, early paracentesis, with removal of no more than a liter or two of ascitic fluid, is indicated.

Masking of other intra-abdominal pathology, such as acute appendicitis or pancreatitis, is an occasional consequence of ascites. The parietal peritoneum, being separated from the inflamed abdominal viscus, does not become inflamed promptly, and localizing symptoms and signs do not develop. One has to rely often on the appearance of fever and leukocytosis to confirm clinical impressions. Patients with ascites are also subject to a form of *primary peritonitis* due to bacteria, such as pneumococci and enterococci. The cause of this entity is not certain, but it is believed to be due in part to the presence of bacteria in portal blood which then bypass the liver. Organisms thus become free to contaminate the ascitic fluid, which is a good culture medium.

Treatment of Ascites

Once the diagnosis of ascites has been made, it is important to determine its etiology. Most often, patients with liver disease have other clear signs, such as jaundice, subcutaneous collateral veins, spider nevi, and palmar erythema, to point to that etiology. Where the etiology is not clear, and perhaps in any case, a small-volume diagnostic paracentesis should be performed. This involves aspirating up to 300 ml of ascitic fluid from either flank with a syringe and small-bore needle. The fluid sample is cultured, checked for specific gravity, white blood count, cytology, and amylase. In this way, infections, pancreatitis, and malignant effusions can be rather reliably excluded from further consideration. The problem then becomes one of reducing the ascites as completely and as permanently as possible. For this purpose, salt exclusion, careful diuresis and peritoneovenous shunting are very powerful therapeutic tools. Large paracenteses should never be used, except in the most dire respiratory emergencies after all other measures have failed. Since paracentesis does nothing to remove the primary or secondary causes of ascites formation, the procedure is followed rapidly by sudden shifts of fluid from the vascular to the ascitic compartment, and the liability toward hypovolemia, shock, azotemia and reduced hepatic function is very great indeed.

Sodium Exclusion. Sodium exclusion has been shown by Gabuzda (1970) to be a very effective means for reducing fluid retention in many cirrhotic patients, particularly those who are excreting more than 10 mEq sodium per liter in their urine. In some patients with lesser amounts of urine sodium, spontaneous diuresis may also occur. The diet should contain no more than 10 to 12 mEq (230–275 mg) sodium daily, and if serum sodium levels are low, fluid restriction to about 1 to 1.2 liters per day should be added. Diuresis may not be immediate, but can be effective in over half of the patients, particularly those whose ascites is of recent onset.

Diuretics. Diuretics in small doses are added when the response to simple sodium exclusion is delayed. It is my custom to use them after three to four days of ineffectual dietary management. An aldosterone inhibitor (spironolactone) and a tubular diuretic are used, one of the better programs consisting of 100 mg aldactone daily, followed after two to three days by 40 to 80 mg furosemide daily (Fuller et al 1977). Large amounts of fluid can be mobilized, upward of 1 liter daily, and the incidence of complications is very small. Patients should be observed daily for signs of prerenal azotemia, hypokalemia, and reduced blood volume. It has been shown that diuresis of more than 1.0 to 1.2 liters per day in patients with ascites and edema, or of 0.3 to 0.4 liters per day in patients with ascites alone, may lead to hypovolemia (Shear et al 1970).

Peritoneovenous Shunting. Peritoneovenous shunting (LeVeen and Wapnick 1978) by means of a long plastic tube connecting the peritoneal cavity with the right internal jugular vein has been found to be extremely effective in reducing the ascites of patients who are refractory to other means of treatment. The tube drains the upper abdomen and is passed subcutaneously up the right anterior chest wall, thus bypassing the thoracic duct route without slowing the production of ascitic fluid. Urine flow is markedly increased, and cortical renal perfusion is improved in many patients. Diuretics may have to be continued in those patients who exhibit continued retention of sodium. The reduction of ascites is commonly associated with a marked improvement of appetite, especially in those patients with stable liver disease, and the return of muscle mass is extremely gratifying. This procedure should not be used in patients with progressive hepatic failure, because the tube may aggravate coagulapathies and, more important, because ascites is never as important a problem as is hepatic failure when the two conditions coexist.

Placement of the peritoneovenous shunt is not without a number of possible complications. In a series of 23 patients so treated, Greig et al (1980) encountered early complications in 17 (74 percent) including 4 technical problems, 6 infections, 2 patients with cardiorespiratory and 2 with hepatic difficulties, and 9 patients with coagulopathies, 4 of whom developed disseminated intravascular coagulation. The shunt had to be revised or removed in 10 patients, and 6 deaths (26 percent) occurred during the early postoperative period. Fifty-eight percent of patients survived for six months. Despite this bad news, the same authors (Greig et al 1981) do report that patients freed of ascites by shunting do exhibit normalization of renin and aldosterone levels, improved sodium excretion, improved creatinine clearance, and a significant decrease in wedged hepatic vein pressures. However, they continue to retain a moderate amount of sodium, and they are not entirely freed of the risk of variceal hemorrhage. Clearly, peritoneovenous shunting has distinct dangers and limitations. It should be reserved only for those patients whose ascites cannot be mobilized with diuretics.

HISTORICAL DIGRESSION

Proper names used in this chapter include the following: Guido BANTI (1852–1925), Italian pathologist, Florence; Paul Clemens von BAUMGARTEN (1848–1928), German pathologist, Tubingen; Arthur Hendley BLAKEMORE (1897–1969), American surgeon, New York, described tube for esophageal tamponade, 1950; Jean CRUVEILHIER (1791–1874), French pathologist, Paris; Nikolai Waldimirowitsch von ECK (1847–1908), Russian physiologist, Moscow; Sergei Sergewitsch KORSAKOFF (1854–1900), Russian psychiatrist, Moscow, described alcoholic disorientation syndrome, 1887; Anders Adolf RETZIUS (1796–1860). Swedish anatomist, Lund; Marie Philibert Constant SAPPEY (1810–?), French anatomist, Paris, published Atlas of Descriptive Anatomy, 1879; and Robert William SENGSTAKEN (1923–1978), American neurosurgeon, New York.

SELECTED REFERENCES

Barnardo DE, Summerskill WHJ, Strong CG, et al. Renal function, renin activity and endogenous vasoactive substances in cirrhosis. Am J Dig Dis 15:419, 1970.

Boyer JL, Klatskin G. Pattern of necrosis in acute viral hepatitis. Prognostic value of bridging (subacute hepatic necrosis). N Engl J Med 283:1063–71, 1970.

Brown T, Hug G, Lansky L. Transiently reduced activity of carbamyl phosphate synthetase and ornithine transcarbamylase in liver of children with Reye's syndrome. N Engl J Med 294:861–67, 1967.

Child CG, III, Turcotte JG. Surgery and portal hypertension. In: Child CG, III ed. The Liver and Portal Hypertension. Philadelphia: WB Saunders, 1964:185.

Chonko AM, Bay WH, Stein JH, et al. The role of renin and aldosterone in the salt retention of edema. Am J Med 63:881–89, 1977.

Conn HO, Leevy CM, Vlahcevic ZR, et al. Comparison of lactulose and neomycin in the treatment of chronic portal-systemic encephalopathy: a double-blind controlled trial. Gastroenterology 72:573–83, 1977.

Conn HO, Lindenmuth WW, May CJ, et al. Prophylactic portocaval shunt. A tale of two studies. Medicine 51:27–40, 1972.

Conn HO, Resnick RH, Grace ND, et al. Distal splenorenal shunt vs. portal-systemic shunt: current status of a controlled trial. Hepatology 1:151–160, 1981.

Davis M, Peters R, Redeker A, et al. Appraisal of the mortality in acute fulminant viral hepatitis. N Engl J Med 278:1248–53, 1968.

Douglass BE, Bagenstoss AH, Hollinshead WH. The anatomy of the portal vein and its tributaries. Surg Gynecol Obstet 91:562–76, 1950.

Epstein M, Berk D, Hollenberg NK, et al. Renal failure in the patient with cirrhosis: the role of active vasoconstriction. Am J Med 49:175–85, 1970.

Faraj BA, Bowen PA, Isaacs JW. Hypertyraminemia in cirrhotic patients. N Engl J Med 294:1360–64, 1976.

Farivar M, Wands JR, Isselbacher KJ, et al. Effect of insulin and glucagon on fulminant murine hepatitis. N Engl J Med 295:1517–19, 1976.

Fuller RK, Khambatta PB, Gobezie GC. An optimal diuretic regimen for cirrhotic ascites. A controlled trial evaluating safety and efficacy of spironolactone and furosemide. JAMA 237:972–75, 1977.

Gabuzda GJ. Cirrhosis, ascites, and edema. Clinical course related to management. Gastroenterology 58:546–53, 1970.

Garceau AJ, Chalmers TC. The natural history of cirrhosis. I. Survival with esophageal varices. N Engl J Med 268:469–73, 1963.

Greig PD, Blendis LM, Langer B, et al. Renal and hemodynamic effects of the peritoneovenous shunt. II. Long term effects. Gastroenterology 80:119–25, 1981.

Greig PD, Langer B, Blendis LM, et al. Complications after peritoneovenous shunting for ascites. Am J Surg 139:125–28, 1980.

Horney JT, Galambos JT. The liver during and after fulminant hepatitis. Gastroenterology 73:639–45, 1977.

Hoyumpa Jr AM, Desmond PV, Avant GR. Hepatic encephalopathy. Gastroenterology 76:184–95, 1979.

James JH, Freund H, Fischer JE. Amino acids in hepatic encephalopathy (letter). Gastroenterology 77:421–22, 1979.

Koppel MH, Coburn JW, Mims MM, et al. Transplantation of cadaveric kidneys from patients with the hepatorenal syndrome: Evidence for functional nature of renal failure in advanced liver disease. N Engl J Med 280:1367–71, 1969.

LeVeen HH, Wapnick S. Peritoneo-venous shunt for ascites. Surg Ann 10: 191–214, 1978.

Livingstone AS, Potvin M, Goresky CA, et al. Changes in the blood-brain barrier in hepatic coma after hepatectomy in the rat. Gastroenterology 73:697–704, 1977.

Livingstone A, Zeppa R, Hutson D, et al. Selective portasystemic shunts in the elderly. Gastroenterology 77:A24 (Nov), 1979.

McIndoe AH. Vascular lesions of portal cirrhosis. Arch Path 5:23–42, 1928.

Malt RA, Nabseth DC, Orloff MJ, et al. Portal hypertension, 1979. N Engl J Med 301:617–18, 1979.

Marchesini G, Forlani G, Zoli M, et al. Insulin and glucagon levels in liver cirrhosis. Relationship with plasma amino acid imbalance of chronic hepatic encephalopathy. Dig Dis Sci 24:594–601, 1979.

Michel H, Cauvet G, Granier PM, et al. Treatment of cirrhotic hepatic encephalopathy by l-dopa. A double-blind study of 58 patients. Digestion 15:232–33, 1977.

Morgan MY, Jakobovits A, Elithorn A, et al. Successful use of bromocriptine in the treatment of a patient with chronic portasystemic encephalopathy. N Engl J Med 296:793–94, 1977.

Ono J, Hutson DG, Dombro RS, et al. Tryptophan and hepatic coma. Gastroenterology 74:196–200, 1978.

Orloff MJ, Charters AC, III, Chandler JG, et al. Portacaval shunt as emergency procedure in unselected patients with alcoholic cirrhosis. Surg Gynecol Obstet 141:59–68, 1975.

Rake MO, Flute PT, Pannell G. Intravascular coagulation in acute hepatic necrosis. Lancet 1:535–37, 1970.

Rakela J. Etiology and prognosis in fulminant hepatitis. Gastroenterology 77:A33 (Nov), 1979.

Ratnoff OD. Disordered hemostasis in hepatic disease. In: Schiff L, ed. Diseases of the Liver, 4th ed. Philadelphia: JB Lippincott, 1975, pp 184–201.

Reynolds T. Donovan A, Mikkelsen W, et al. Results of an 11-year randomized trial of end-to-side portacaval shunt in patients with alcoholic liver disease. Gastroenterology 75:982, 1978.

Ritt, DJ, Whelan G, Werner DJ, et al. Acute hepatic necrosis with stupor or coma. Medicine 48:151–72, 1969.

Rosen HM, Yoshimura N, Hodgman JM, et al. Plasma amino acid patterns in hepatic encephalopathy of differing etiology. Gastroenterology 72: 483–87, 1977.

Schenker S, Breen KJ, Hoyumpa AM, Jr. Hepatic encephalopathy: current status. Gastroenterology 66:121–51, 1974.

Schenker S, McCandless DW, Brophy E, et al. Studies on the intracerebral toxicity of ammonia. J Clin Invest 46:838–48, 1967.

Schlam SW, van der Mey T. Hyperammonemic coma after hepatectomy in germ-free rats. Gastroenterology 77:231–34, 1979.

Shear L, Bonkowsky HL, Gabuzda GJ. Renal tubular acidosis in cirrhosis. A determinant of susceptibility to recurrent hepatic precoma. N Engl J Med 280:1–7, 1969.

Shear L, Ching S, Gabuzda GJ. Compartmentalization of ascites and edema in patients with hepatic cirrhosis. N Engl J Med 282:1391–96, 1970.

Shear L, Kleinerman, J, Gabuzda GJ. Renal failure in patients with cirrhosis of the liver. I. Clinical and pathological characteristics. Am J Med 39: 184–98, 1965.

Sherlock S. Progress report. Portal circulation and portal hypertension. Gut 19:70–83, 1978.

Sherwin R, Joshi P, Hendler R, et al. Hyperglucagonemia in Laennec's cirrhosis. The role of portal-systemic shunting. N Engl J Med 290:239–42, 1974.

Snodgrass PJ, DeLong GR. Urea-cycle enzyme deficiencies and an increased nitrogen load producing hyperammonemia in Reye's syndrome. N Engl J Med 294:855–60, 1976.
Soterakis J, Resnick RH, Iber FL. Effect of alcohol abstinence on survival in cirrhotic portal hypertension. Lancet 2:65–67, 1973.
Stein JH, Fadem SZ. The renal circulation. JAMA 239:1308–12, 1978.
Sugarman HJ, Berkowitz HD, Miller LD. Metaraminol in "hepatorenal syndrome" (letter). N Engl J Med 285:180–81, 1971.
Trey C. The fulminant hepatic failure surveillance study. Brief review of the effects of presumed etiology and age on survival. Can Med Assoc J 106: 525–26, 1972.
Victor M, Adams RD, Cole M. The acquired (non-Wilsonian) type of chronic hepatocerebral degeneration. Medicine 44:345–96, 1965.
Walker C, Peterson Jr W, Unger R. Blood ammonia levels in advanced cirrhosis during therapeutic elevation of the insulin:glucagon ratio. N Engl J Med 291:168–71, 1974.
Ware AJ, D'Agostino AN, Combes B. Cerebral edema: a major complication of massive hepatic necrosis. Gastroenterology 61:877–84, 1971.
Warren WD, Galambos JT. Distal splenorenal shunt for portal hypertension. Hosp Pract 8:77–86 (Sept), 1973.
Weber Jr FL, Veach GL. The importance of the small intestine in gut ammonium production in the fasting dog. Gastroenterology 77:235–40, 1979.
Welch CE, Malt RA. Abdominal surgery. N Engl J Med 300:705–12, 1979.
Wilson JAP, Suguitan EA, Cassiday WA, et al. Characteristics of ascitic fluid in the alcoholic cirrhotic. Dig Dis Sci 24:645–48, 1979.
Witte CL, Witte MH, Dumont AE. The portal triad in hepatic cirrhosis. Surg Gynecol Obstet 146:965–74, 1978.
Witte MH, Witte CL, Dumont AE. Progress in liver disease: physiological factors involved in the causation of cirrhotic ascites. Gastroenterology 61:742–50, 1971.
Wolpert E, Phillips SF, Summerskill WHJ. Ammonia production in the human colon. Effects of cleansing, neomycin and acetohydroxamic acid. N Engl J Med 283:159–64, 1970.
Zieve L. Amino acids in liver failure. Gastroenterology 76:219–21, 1979.
Zieve L, Nicolett DM. Pathogenesis of hepatic coma. Ann Rev Med 26:143–57, 1975.

DISCUSSION QUESTION

Relate briefly and in order the diagnostic and therapeutic measures which should be undertaken when a patient with established cirrhosis of the liver develops hepatic encephalopathy. Do the same for upper gastrointestinal bleeding and for ascites.

CHAPTER 10

Agents Causing Acute Hepatitis

VIRUSES

History 1

Thunder reverberated along Michigan Avenue in the summer of 1942. "How," asked the indignant editors of the *Chicago Tribune,* "did it happen that wholesale vaccinations were undertaken with a vaccine which quite obviously had not been thoroughly tested in advance?" As a reaction to the occurrence of nearly 50,000 cases of hepatitis, and ultimately 84 deaths, among the nearly 3.25 million personnel in the armed forces who had received immunizations against yellow fever, the editorial pique was certainly justifiable. And the response of the *Journal of the American Medical Association* (1942, 119:1110) to the effect that this result was "far less serious than would be an epidemic of virulent yellow fever among soldiers sent to the tropical areas in which our army is now engaging the enemy," seemed weak, albeit patriotic. For in truth, a great, though understandable, error had been made. Owing to a deep fear that morbidity from yellow fever would be high among American troops, and because there was no way of determining in advance which units would eventually serve in endemic parts of Africa and southwest Asia, immunization was ordered for all. Previous use of the virus vaccine had proved its effectiveness. Small amounts of human serum were added to the vaccine to improve its stability, and sterility was achieved by heating each batch to 56°C for 30 minutes. It was not tested further, because there appeared to be nothing else to do. A costly lesson was about to be learned.

It was eventually shown that some batches of vaccine caused hepatitis, while others did not. The causative agent appeared to be something in the donor serum, and it was remarkably resistant to heating. And the resulting disease appeared different from the usual catarrhal jaundice or epidemic hepatitis seen in the United States; it had a very long incubation period (8 to 23 weeks), and the onset of jaundice was more insidious, without as many prodromal symptoms.

Earlier medical literature had documented outbreaks of jaundice in patients vaccinated with human serum components (Lurman 1885), or injected with poorly sterilized lancets or with sterilized needles attached to unsterilized syringes (Flaum et al 1926), but these accounts were not well known, and there was considerable pressure to perform the immunizations quickly in 1942. By the fall of that year, although yellow fever immunizations were continued, human serum was no longer being added to the vaccine, and the incidence of what came to be known as *homologous serum hepatitis*, an apparently viral disease, declined markedly. The ironic conclusion of this significant episode is that yellow fever never became a problem among American troops. An Army historian comments laconically, "No cases of yellow fever occurred. Neither was there appreciable exposure to the disease."*

History 2

The American wartime experience with hepatitis did not end after the yellow fever vaccine problem was corrected, not by a long shot. Shortly after the landings in North Africa late in 1942, and then more heavily with the actions in Sicily and Italy, icteric hepatitis appeared in even larger outbreaks. This disease was more like what was seen sporadically at home: five to seven days of prodrome including fairly high fever, occasional chills, nausea, anorexia, and headache, followed by darkening of the urine and progressive jaundice for the next week and then, surprisingly, sudden marked symptomatic improvement at times when the jaundice was its deepest. The liver was usually enlarged and tender for a time, the white blood count often fell to below 5,000 per cu mm, and atypical lymphocytes would often appear as the count rose during convalescence. An increasing prothrombin time, unresponsive to vitamin K administration, was a poor prognostic sign, and the overall mortality rate was 0.4 percent. Patients who died with fulminant hepatic failure in less than 10 days showed massive necrosis of the liver without regeneration, while patients who died subacutely within three to eight weeks showed confluent necrosis with areas of regeneration. Recovery was slow, and most patients were unable to return to duty for two to three months after an attack of what came to be called *infectious hepatitis*. Unlike homologous serum hepatitis, this disease appeared to be spread by direct contact, and appeared to be worse when sanitation was poorest and flies were heaviest, particularly in late summer and early fall. Numerous outbreaks occurred in the Mediterranean and Near East zones from 1943 to 1945. Infectious hepatitis did not occur among American troops in northern Europe until after they had linked up physically with Seventh Army troops coming north overland from Italy. Other epidemics occurred in the Pacific in 1945. Altogether 182,400 cases of hepatitis, approximately 70 percent of

*Long AP. The Army immunization program. In: Preventive medicine in World War II, vol 3. Washington, DC: Government Printing Office, 1955:311.

which were infectious, occurred among the 25 million Americans under arms during 1942 to 1945 (Havens 1968).

A good bit more was learned about infectious hepatitis during and immediately after the war. While patients who had acquired the disease once were immune to further infections, they were not immune to homologous serum hepatitis, and vice versa. Tests with volunteers showed that fecal suspensions and duodenal secretions from patients in the acute phase of disease could transfer infectious hepatitis but not homologous serum hepatitis to healthy persons. Furthermore, many patients, perhaps more than half, developed prodromal symptoms without becoming icteric, although in some, transient mild bilirubinemia might have occurred. Patients with *anicteric hepatitis* tended to have less hepatomegaly than did those with jaundice and were ill for shorter periods. Finally, evidence was accumulating at the end of the war that injections of pooled human gamma globulin (0.14 to 0.28 ml per Kg of body weight) would prevent or attenuate attacks of infectious hepatitis for periods of six months but had no benefit against homologous serum hepatitis.

There was less excuse for military authorities to be unaware of the likelihood that American troops would encounter infectious hepatitis during World War II than there was for them to suspect the possible occurrence of homologous serum hepatitis. While it is true that hepatitis is uncommon and usually sporadic in civilian life, its epidemic occurrence in wartime was well known, literally throughout history. Among Union troops during the first year of the American Civil War, nearly 11,000 cases of epidemic jaundice and 40 deaths occurred, the attack rate reaching 80 per 1,000 in General Grant's army (Woodward 1863). At Gallipoli in 1915 during the First World War, some British and Empire units experienced attack rates of "epidemic jaundice of campaigns" approaching 250 cases per 1,000, and attention was called to the importance of controlling flies and dust, of covering latrines, and of avoiding contamination of water (Willcox 1916; Martin 1917). The disease was clearly distinguished from the rat-borne spirochetosis (Weil disease) which was reported among troops engaging in trench warfare, in that hemorrhagic phenomena, nephritis, and death were extremely rare in epidemic hepatitis. Neither did the disease appear to be related to typhoid or paratyphoid fevers, since cultures were usually negative, and true cases of typhoid were rarely associated with jaundice. Even the British and German experiences with massive attacks rates of infectious hepatitis earlier in World War II at El Alamein and eastern North Africa, where sanitary facilities were egregious, should have prepared American medical authorities for the possibility of epidemics. But such was not the case.

The only excuse for the failure of American military physicians to anticipate infectious hepatitis among their troops in World War II was their own experience during the First War. In that campaign, hepatitis was a minor problem, although many other infectious diseases occurred. The low attack rate was probably due to the fact that American troops were engaged only in northern Europe, where the endemic occurrence rate of hepatitis is slight, and did not come into contact with Mediterranean troops. Thus, the good fortune, in this respect, of World War I probably accounts for the sad experiences in World War II. As Havens (1968) writes, "The story of hepatitis in World War II will not soon be forgotten."

THE VIRUSES OF HEPATITIS

There are at least three important hepatitis viruses other than cytomegalovirus and herpes simplex virus. These latter agents have been discussed earlier as causes of giant cell hepatitis among newborns and children. The Epstein Barr virus should also be mentioned since it causes a usually mild, though transient, hepatitis in almost every patient with infectious mononucleosis. The three hepatitis viruses are distinctive, cause somewhat different diseases, exhibit no cross immunity, and carry differing long-term implications. They are presently called viruses A, B, and C. Virus A (MS-1) is the cause of infectious hepatitis, virus B (MS-2) causes serum hepatitis, and virus C causes non-A, non-B hepatitis. The differences between the names of the viruses and the diseases that they cause is, of course, purely historical, since the diseases were described long before their etiological agents were identified. Actually, prior to World War II, all nonbacterial hepatitis was assumed to be due to a single agent. Today, it would be no surprise to discover that there are still other viruses, from D onward, which plague mankind.

Virus A

This agent was discovered long after virus B, following careful examination by electron microscopy of stools from patients with active disease (Feinstone et al 1973). Antibodies to the viral antigen were shortly found in sera from patients with active hepatitis, commencing either acutely or within three to four weeks of onset, depending on the immunological test employed (Koff 1978). Anti-A can now be readily demonstrated in patients by immune adherence hemagglutination and remains in the blood indefinitely as a permanent marker of previous infection, and a homologous protective agent against reinfection. The virus has not been cultured. It is a uniform, 27-nm round, gearlike particle (Figure 10–1) containing RNA, and having the characteristics of either a picorna type enterovirus or a parvovirus. The virus has been shown to induce hepatitis in simians and appears in the stool within 14 days of ingestion, about two to three weeks before the onset of the symptoms, and about one week before viremia appears. Stool continues to be infectious for about 10 days after the onset of prodromal symptoms. Both stool and blood are thus infectious to unprotected subjects during this time. In one study (Szmuness et al 1976), less than 5 percent of patients with anti-A could recall having had an attack of acute hepatitis. Chronic antigenemia

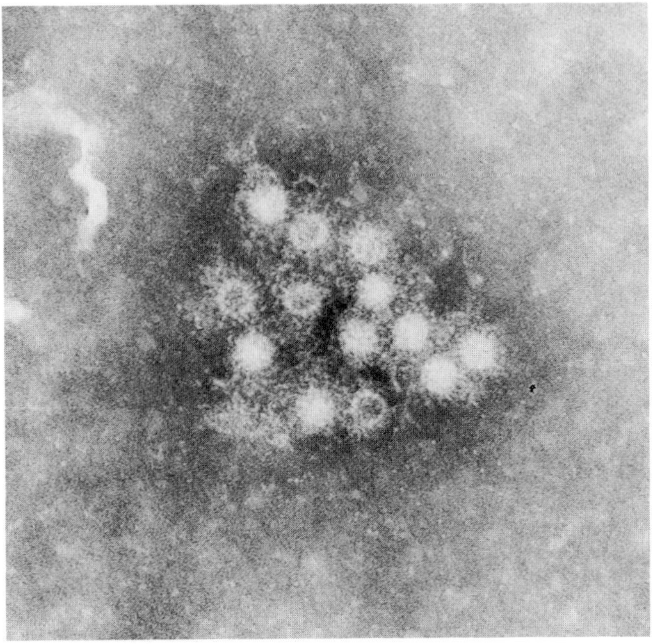

Figure 10–1. Hepatitis A virus immune aggregate, after incubation of a stool filtrate with serum from a convalescent patient. The aggregate is composed of "full" particles, and "empty" particles coated with antibody. Magnification x150,000. (Courtesy of Drs. Stephen M. Feinstone and Robert H. Purcell).

and a carrier state for this agent have not been demonstrated, so the disease is probably transmitted largely by patients with active infections who are unaware of being ill (Barker et al 1978).

The presence of anti-A tends to correlate with lower economic levels and with increasing age. There is also a rough correlation with remote hepatitis B infections. Thus, 54 percent of middle-class whites who had serological evidence of previous infections with hepatitis B, also showed anti-A activity, while only 31 percent were B negative and A positive. Seventy-seven percent of subjects with less than 9 years of education showed anti-A activity, compared with 31 percent of subjects having 17 years or more of education. These differences are believed to be largely based upon the poorer sanitary facilities available to lower income groups. An annual incidence rate for hepatitis A of 22 percent has been found among homosexual men engaging in oral–anal sexual activity (Corey and Holmes 1980).

The following conclusions may be drawn about hepatitis A from these and other observations:

1. Hepatitis A is apparently caused worldwide by the same single agent, a 27-nm RNA enterovirus.

2. The virus is transmitted from person to person through the direct or indirect ingestion of infected feces. Transmission by oral anal contact, infected food handlers, infected food (e.g., oysters), and poor sanitation have been documented. Flies are also a probable vector. Blood and stools of patients are infectious for a period of about two weeks, partly before and partly after the onset of symptoms.
3. Most patients acquire infections with hepatitis A virus without ever becoming aware of illness, and probably constitute an ever-changing but ongoing reservoir for the disease. There is no known host for the virus other than humans. Volunteer studies indicate that the appearance of clinical disease after exposure to hepatitis A virus is probably dependent on the amount of virus ingested.
4. Lifelong immunity, marked by the appearance of anti-A antibodies, is conferred by either clinical or subclinical infections.
5. The active disease appears after an incubation period of 20 to 40 days, and is usually mild. Fulminant hepatitis is rare, and case fatality rate is less than 0.2 percent.
6. Chronic hepatitis does not appear to occur from hepatitis A infections.
7. The virus is apparently not transmissible during pregnancy from mother to fetus (Tong et al 1978).
8. Immune serum globulin, especially that processed from subjects with high anti-A levels, confers temporary passive immunity.

Virus B

The virus of hepatitis B was identified and described well before the hepatitis A virus was identified, the quest for the former and the development of increasingly sensitive immunologic techniques helped immeasurably to facilitate the discovery of the latter. The detection process for hepatitis A was, in fact, the reverse of the process followed in hepatitis B. Hepatitis B markers were almost inadvertently found during immunologic studies on a variety of serum samples. The viral particles on which these markers were attached were then found, and finally the complete virion was described. Hepatitis A virus was demonstrated in stool before immunologic testing was commenced. Viral particles were used as antigen to detect antibody in patients, and later the antibody was used to detect antigen.

Surface Antigen and Antibody. In the 1960s, two separate lines of inquiry discovered what is known presently as the surface antigen of the hepatitis B virus (HBsAg) and its antibody (antiHBs). Blumberg et al (1965) were using immunodiffusion techniques to study the occurrence of precipitins to human lipoproteins among patients with hemophilia who had received multiple transfusions of blood and blood products in previous years. Two of these hemophilic sera formed a nonlipid precipitin with a normal serum taken from an Australian. This unusual protein was determined to be an alpha globulin, and was named the "Australia antigen." This antigen was later found frequently among patients with Down syndrome and leukemia, patients who had received multiple blood transfusions, and healthy inhabitants of the Mediterranean area and the Orient. It was not found among healthy Americans and was originally thought to be a possibly genetic marker of susceptibility to certain diseases. Later (Blumberg et al 1969), the Australia antigen came to be recognized as a marker of acute and chronic hepatitis, even though it was only transiently present in most cases of acute hepatitis and might, in some cases, appear without clinical evidence of hepatitis.

At about the same time, less than 100 miles away from Blumberg's laboratory, Alfred Prince was working on a separate, but converging, line of inquiry into possible immunologic markers of homologous serum hepatitis. Prince (1968) diffused the serum of patients with hepatitis against the serum of a single hemophiliac donor who, having received over 10,000 units of blood and blood products during the course of the disease, was presumed to possess circulating antibodies to serum hepatitis virus. Sera from patients with serum hepatitis, especially in the early stages of disease, did indeed form precipitin lines with the donor serum and were deemed to contain serum hepatitis (SH) antigen. The donor substance appeared to be a gamma globulin antibody, and the antigen, on electron microscopy, appeared to be viral particles 22 to 25 nm in diameter. Later, it was determined that the SH and Australia antigens were identical, and their association with many cases of serum hepatitis was widely confirmed.

It remained for Dane et al (1970) to point out that the lipoprotein particles found by Prince, sometimes round, sometimes elongated, were less dense and less regular than known viruses of similar size and were often present in much larger numbers (1 million per ml) than was customary in other viral illnesses. They went on to demonstrate in several patients the presence of a few unique 42-nm particles of complex structure, after clumping with antiserum followed by centrifugation (Figure 10–2). The surface of these structures was covered by the material described by Prince (hence the term "surface antigen"), while the inner body was 28 nm in diameter, had a 2-nm shell and an inner delicate lacelike structure (the core antigen). Some of the core elements were free of coating; others were complete. The latter complete structure was, for a time, referred to as the Dane particle, but is now believed to be the hepatitis B virion. The surface antigen alone is not infectious; the core antigen probably is.

The surface antigen has been found to have one member each of two families of genetic determinants, *d* or *y* and *w* or *r*, making it possible for the antigen to occur in one of four separate phenotypes (Robinson and Lutwick, 1976). These subtypes breed true in transmission studies, and certain types

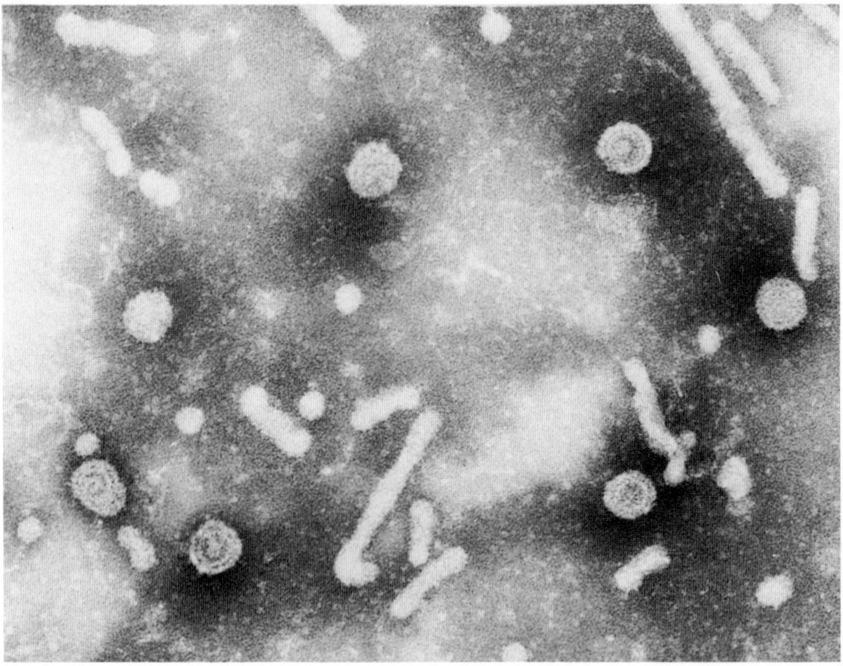

Figure 10–2. Complete hepatitis B virions (Dane particles) showing inner bodies and outer coats. The numerous rod-like particles probably represent surface antigen residues. Magnification x150,000. (Courtesy of Drs. John L. Gerin and Robert H. Purcell)

appear to predominate in certain geographic areas, but they are probably not of great significance otherwise. Mixed infections with more than one subtype of surface antigen may occur, and occasional patients may develop surface antibodies to just one subtype, and thereby making the patient infectious for the remaining subtype.

Core Antigen and Antibody. When the surface antigen of Dane particles is removed by detergent action, the remaining, or core, antigen may be aggregated by convalescent sera from patients with serum hepatitis who do not show anti-HBs activity (Almeida et al 1971). This, and other similar observations led to the discovery that hepatitis B virus contains a distinctive core antigen (HBcAg) and that patients may respond with a distinct antibody (anti-HBc) to that antigen. Anti-HBc has turned out to be a significant marker of infectivity, since it has been shown that blood with this antibody may transmit hepatitis to recipients even though the donor blood is negative for surface antigen (Hoofnagle et al 1978).

DNA polymerase activity has been found in association with the core, but not the surface, antigen of some patients with hepatitis B. Circular double-stranded DNA molecules have also been recovered from the core of the virus, and are believed to function as a replicative template for the polymerase reaction. This action appears to take place in the core of the virus and is not inhibited by sera containing anti-HBs or anti-HBc. While DNA replication does occur in the core, it has been suggested that the circular molecules identified to date do not appear to be large enough to encode all of the genetic information necessary for viral replication.

e Specificity. The e specificity was first described by Magnius and Espmark in 1972, and has since been determined to have at least three subtypes (Trepo et al 1978). *e* antigen is located in the core of some, but not all, hepatitis B virions, and antibodies occur frequently. The presence of *e* correlates well with the presence of DNA polymerase and infectivity of blood (Alter et al 1976). Mothers with *e* antigenemia are highly likely to transmit hepatitis B to their infants during pregnancy, while the presence of anti-*e* appears to be protective (Okada et al 1976). *e* antigen correlates well also with the presence of HBcAg and Dane particles in the blood of carriers. HBsAg mothers who were HBcAg negative and positive for anti-*e* did not transmit HBs antigen activity to their infants and were presumably not infectious. In regard to subtypes, all patients with *e* antigenemia show e_1 activity, while 44 percent of symptomatic *e* carriers also show subtype e_3, which may be a further marker of infectivity. Anti-*e* has been shown to be capable of aggregating the virion of hepatitis B and to form complexes with it which are then removed from the circulation by macrophages. Anti-*e* is probably thus protective against hepatitis B transmission.

Nielsen et al (1974) found *e* antigenemia in 19 of 182 patients with acute hepatitis B, only 1 of whom went on to complete resolution of the hepatitis. In 11 of the 19 patients who developed chronic hepatitis or cirrhosis after the acute infection, *e* antigen was demonstrated during the acute illness. There have been a number of instances where the administration of HBsAg-positive, anti-e blood transfusions has not been followed by the development of hepatitis in the recipient. When neither *e* nor anti-*e* are present, HBsAg positive blood may be infectious to recipients.

Immune Complexes. These may be formed when HBAg binds to immunoglobulins, with or without complement. These complexes depress antibody-dependent cell-mediated cytotoxicity and are found in association with hepatitis B infections occasionally, before the onset of hepatitis symptoms. Deposition of such complexes in the cutaneous blood vessels is believed to cause the prodromal urticaria occasionally seen in type B hepatitis, while hepatitis B-immunoglobulin-complement complexes have been found deposited in synovia of patients with arthritis preceding hepatitis attacks. *e* antigen-antibody complexes with complement have been found deposited in glomerular capillaries of patients with membranous glomerulonephritis preceding hepatitis B (Takekoshi et al 1979), and immune complexes of HBc and gamma globulin have been found in hepatocytic nuclei of patients with chronic active hepatitis and hepatitis B viremia. The immunoglobulin probably represents anti-HBc and may account for the hepatic necrosis typical of this condition (Gerber et al 1976).

Usual Immune Response to Hepatitis B Infection. The incubation period of hepatitis B varies from as short a time as two to three weeks to as long as six months, and appears to depend on both the virulence of the infection and the immune status of the host. Serum DNA polymerase activity rises as the hepatic function tests become abnormal and is followed shortly by detectable HBsAg. Anti-HBc appears in the blood toward the latter portion of the acute illness and may remain permanently (Kaufman et al 1979). Anti-HBs does not rise until the convalescent period. Its appearance signals the end of the illness and the appearance of permanent immunity. HBc is not usually detected in the blood unless it is released from the core of circulating Dane particles by previous treatment with detergents. HBe antigen may appear as the disease reaches its peak, and anti-e is found during convalesence in some cases. Anti-HBs may appear during recovery of some patients who were not found to have HBs antigenemia during the acute illness. This would indicate that the original infection had been mild, and that HBsAg levels had been too low to measure at that time.

Anti-HBs and anti-e are signs of immunity and noninfectivity. Persistence of HBs indicates continuing replication of surface antigen, and the onset of a carrier state. Such patients may be infectious if they are producing complete virions as well as surface antigen. If they also show anti-e, they are probably not infectious; if they carry anti-HBc, they probably are. Persistence of DNA polymerase activity signals ongoing disease and infectivity, but its absence does not imply that chronic disease and infectivity have also disappeared. Persistence of e antigen in HBsAg carriers is an almost certain sign of infectivity.

HBsAg is detectable in from 0.1 to 0.5 percent of American adults, the levels being highest in institutionalized patients, narcotic addicts, homosexual men, prostitutes, and patients with reduced immunity. Anti-HBs, an index of past infection, is found in 4 to 14 percent of the general population.

Among 1,192 randomly selected physicians attending medical conventions, 18.5 percent were found to be positive for anti-HBs (Denes et al 1978). This evidence of previous infection with HB increased with the length of medical career, and was higher in physicians with urban practices. Surgeons and pathologists showed the highest incidences of past infections, and only 69 of 220 antibody-positive subjects recalled having had acute hepatitis. While HBsAg has been found in almost all human secretions, including breast milk, saliva, semen, and urine, the disease is spread largely by direct contamination with infected blood, injected intravenously or spread on open lacerations. Transmission may also be by the oral route, as in medical laboratory workers, by sexual intercourse, and by direct transmission from mother to child either during pregnancy or, following birth, through breast milk. Fecal oral spread, which is the main route of hepatitis A transmission, appears to play only a small part, if any, in the propagation of hepatitis B.

Importance of the Host Reaction to Hepatitis B Infection. Courouce et al (1979) stress that the immunologic response of the host to hepatitis B virus plays an essential role in the clinical consequences of the illness. The host response is believed to be the key that determines why some patients with B virus infection demonstrate total latency, while others undergo the typical acute diseases, and still others experience devastating acute reactions, such as fulminant hepatitis, or prolonged problems, such as chronic active hepatitis, cirrhosis, and even hepatocellular carcinoma.

Viral replication in the host may be of two types, complete and incomplete. Replication of virus in hepatocytes does not appear to harm the cells (Edgington and Chisari 1975). Complete replication occurs in all patients with hepatitis for a time, during which they have surface antigen, DNA polymerase, Dane particles (complete virions), and often *e*-antigen in their blood, and cytoplasmic surface antigen and nuclear core antigen in hepatocytes. As immunity builds and convalesence begins, replication of cellular HBcAg, circulating DNA polymerase, and *e* disappear, but incomplete replication of surface antigen continues for a short time. Blood may show persisting HBsAg and anti-*e*. Finally, anti-HBs appears, and the infection terminates. Patients with chronic hepatitis remain at the stage of complete replication, probably because of altered immunity, while many carriers of HBsAg remain at the stage of incomplete viral replication and continue to show numerous 22-nm spheres and some surface rods in their blood. Disappearance of HBs may occur while anti-HBc is still being produced. This situation would signal ongoing liver damage.

Edgington and Chisari (1975) propose that cytopathic changes appear in hepatitis B virus infections through five possible mechanisms, antibody-dependent complement-mediated cytolysis, antibody-directed cellular cytotoxicity, T-lymphocyte-mediated cytotoxicity, macrophage-medicated cytolysis, and immune complex injury. Destructive host responses may be directed against viral antigens on the cell surface and to hepatocytic proteins reaching the cell surface. Of these, the cellular immune response is probably the most cytopathic. Eventually, the production of suppressor antibodies in undamaged cells terminates the infection. Failing this, the infection and cytopathic process continues.

The carrier state appears to result from reduced cellular immunity to HBsAg. In otherwise healthy carriers, this reduced immunity does not apply to other viruses. However, chronically immunosuppressed patients, such as those with Down or Sjogren syndrome, chronic renal disease, leukemia, or common variable hypogammaglobulinemia, often become hepatitis B carriers and suffer from chronic hepatitis. Killer lymphocytes, which participate in antibody-dependent cell-mediated cytotoxicity, have been implicated as a mediator of chronic active hepatitis and may also play a part in acute damage as well. They may be the source of anti-HBc, which is a marker of ongoing hepatitis.

Patients with reduced antibody-dependent cell-mediated cytotoxicity generally have less severe liver disease, but are more inclined to form circulating immune complexes and experience extrahepatic manifestations of hepatitis B viral infection. These include periarteritis nodosa, membranous glomerulonephritis, acrodermatitis, Raynaud phenomenon, polyarthritis, and essential mixed cryoglobulinemia. While the exact mechanism of hepatic damage by hepatitis B virus is not clearly worked out, it is apparent that host mechanisms, both cytopathic and suppressive, do indeed play a large part in the clinical picture resulting from the infection.

Epidemiology of Hepatitis B. By testing for HBsAg and anti-HBs in families of antigen-positive blood donors and in controls, Szmuness et al (1975) determined that the incidence of antigenemia was 10 times as high in members of families with B-positive donors than it was among members of families with negative donors. Antibody positivity was 2 to 3 times as high among donor-positive families as controls. About 40 percent of families showed two or more cases, and there was a high prevalance among siblings and parents of index cases. As with hepatitis A infection, clustering appeared to occur to a greater degree among nonwhite, large families, and in families where educational level was low. Occurrence in spouses of positive donors was also low, and this finding suggests that a genetic basis exists for hepatitis B transmissability, supporting the earlier observations of Blumberg (1965). These findings demonstrate the large reservoir of hepatitis B existing in the general population and help to explain the occurrence of cirrhosis of the liver in HBsAg-positive patients who are unaware of ever being infected.

Follow-up study for one to five years of 429 patients with type B hepatitis (Redeker 1975) showed that 90 percent of patients healed completely and became HBsAg negative, 7 percent (30 patients) developed persistent hepatitis, and 3 percent (13 patients) developed chronic active hepatitis. Six of the carriers became negative for HBsAg after periods as long as 14 to 73 months following the acute illness. While no mortality was noted in that study, the rate is about 0.1 percent in patients under 15, 0.9 percent from age 15 to 29, and 2.2 percent for patients over age 29 in other studies (Bryan and Gregg 1975).

Prevention. Immune serum globulin from large donor pools has high mean anti-A titers by passive hemagglutination test (1:1000) and lower titers of anti-HBs (1:500) and anti-HBc (1:800). Since 1972, all preparations have been screened for the absence of HBsAg (Hoofnagle and Waggoner 1980). The small amounts of anti-HBs may make it somewhat protective against small inocula of hepatitis B. It has been shown to be ineffective against larger injections.

Presently, hepatitis B immune globulin with titers of anti-HBs of 1:500,000 is available to confer tempoary passive immunity upon persons with a high likelihood of contracting hepatitis B. Prince (1978) recommends administering B immune globulin acutely to people who have suffered needle sticks with B-antigen-containing blood, to sexual partners of patients with active infections, to people who may have ingested the virus, to newborns with surface and *e* antigenemic mothers, and to workers in dialysis units where hepatitis B is a major problem. If the HBsAg blood can be shown to have anti-e and no DNA polymerase, hepatitis B immune globulin is not necessary. The dosage of this product is 0.06 ml per kg intramuscularly, repeated once in 30 days. This confers effective passive immunity for about four months. If exposure to hepatitis B is continuous, immune globulin should probably be given repeatedly. Hepatitis B immune globulin is well tolerated; the major drawbacks to its use are its expense and the short period of passive immunity engendered by it. Hoofnagle et al (1979) noted a 10.5 percent incidence of subclinical hepatitis B infection in recipients of hepatitis B immune globulin and suggest that the agent may induce passive-active immunity. It should probably not be administered to casual contacts of patients, because the likelihood of infection among them is so slight.

There is great hope that active immunity to hepatitis B may be produced by vaccines containing pure hepatitis BsAg, free of core antigen, *e* antigen, and DNA polymerase. Such vaccines have been shown not to cause hepatitis B in simians and to protect them against later exposure to HB virus (Purcell and Gerin 1975). Another study has also demonstrated this protection and shown that the vaccine causes anti-HBs to appear prior to the challenge with live virus (Buynak et al 1976). In humans, 72 percent of 25 subjects developed anti-HBs levels after receiving one to four monthly injections of a similar HBs vaccine (Tao et al 1978). However, none of six children showed an antibody response. In another trial of vaccine among staff and patients in a hemodialysis unit, Maupas and colleagues (1978) demonstrated a primary antibody response in 93 percent of 162 members of the staff and in 64 percent of 55 patients. An epidemic of hepatitis B was raging in the hemodialysis unit during the two years of this study, and 12 of 24 unimmunized members of the staff developed HBs antigenemia transiently, 8 with hepatitis and jaundice, and 4 without hepatitis. This 50 percent attack rate among unimmunized staff compares with a 5 percent attack rate, demonstrated by transient HBs antigenemia alone, in 8 of the immunized staff members. The benefit conferred by immunization of patients on hemodialysis was equally favorable. Among unimmunized patients, 25 became chronic B virus carriers during the study, and two others had transient HBs antigenemia, an attack rate of 87 percent. Among immunized patients, only 1 developed transient antigenemia and none became chronically infected. In a Korean trial of HBsAg immunization among 115 subjects living in a heavily endemic area, only 1 subject developed clinical hepatitis B and 9 acquired HBs antigenemia in periods of one to almost four years. These attack rates were significantly lower than those in the unimmunized population (Kim et al 1979).

Szmnness et al (1980) have shown in a randomized double-blind trial of HBs immunization among homosexuals that 77 percent of 549 immunized subjects developed high levels of anti-HBs within two months and that this incidence increased to 96 percent after booster doses were administered. During 18 months of follow-up, various hepatitis B "events" ranging from acute hepatitis to surface or core antigenemia, occurred among 1.4 to 3.4 percent of immunized subjects and among 18 to 27 percent of controls who received dummy injections, a highly significant difference.

Barin et al (1979) have characterized the major polypeptide of HBsAg, and found it to have a molecular weight between 5,000 and 10,000. They caution that use of this product for prophylaxis will depend first upon its immunogenicity, and second on the ability to produce it in commercial amounts. These reports collectively afford hope that an effective form of active immunization against hepatitis B is waiting just over the horizon, despite the fact that the entire virion has thus far evaded efforts to culture it.

Virus C (Non-A, Non-B)

Any hope that blood-borne hepatitis would be completely eliminated by screening donors for A and B antigenemia was quickly dashed by the discovery that hepatitis could still be transmitted by blood or blood products containing no evidence of either of these viruses. This result could have been anticipated by acknowledgment of a few scattered reports describing patients who, having recovered from attacks of both hepatitis A and B, later contracted a third form of hepatitis unassociated with any other known virus infection, such as cytomegalic virus or herpes. It was also shown that hepatitis A is rarely if ever associated with transfusional hepatitis, and that carrier states of hepatitis A probably do not exist.

Early on, it was felt that these cases of non-A, non-B hepatitis might represent disease from more than a single additional virus, and such may indeed be the case. However, there is now enough evidence available pointing to the specificity of a third virus that it seems justified to designate it as virus C. It is felt that nearly all of the cases of "nonspecific" hepatitis seen today are due either to virus C, or to its as yet unindicted coconspirators.

The Evidence. It has been shown that when one graphs the incubation periods of all viral hepatitis cases seen in a given period of time, including types A and B, a unimodal distribution curve is formed, stretching from 2 to 26 weeks, with the mode at about 7 weeks. Were the disease due to only two distinct viruses, Mosely (1975) concluded that the curve should have been bimodal, and that the absence of two distinct peaks spoke for the presence of at least a third virus, whose incubation period was intermediate between that of viruses A and B. It was also noted that 50–75 percent of cases of posttransfusion hepatitis showed no evidence of B antigenemia and that the institution of testing for HBs in donor blood, especially that acquired from commercial sources, did not reduce the attack rate of hepatitis following transfusion by more than 25 percent, although it did result in a 50 percent reduction in hepatitis B and in the case fatality rate. The continued appearance of hepatitis B in a small number of recipients of tested blood is attributed to the fact that around 10 percent of B carriers are undetected by present radioimmunoassay techniques. The incidence of posttransfusion hepatitis from blood tested for B antigen ranged from 11 to 45 percent in various studies done between 1975 and 1977, and 63 to 94 percent of their attacks appeared to be unassociated with any of the known viral agents (Alter et al 1978). Furthermore, a number of patients with anti–HBs, a marker of immunity to further infections with that virus, have been found to develop hepatitis after subsequent transfusions. Hepatitis C or other viral agents is probably responsible for almost all of the three to six cases per 1,000 blood transfusions seen in the United States today. One thus presupposes the existence of many asymptomatic carriers of unidentified hepatitis viruses. Dienstag (1981) points out that the elimination of the use of commercial blood donors has doubtless done more than screening for B virus to reduce the incidence of transfusion hepatitis to current levels. Ach et al (1981) indicate that exclusion of all donor blood with alanine aminotransferase levels above 29 IU per liter should reduce the attack rate of non-A, non-B hepatitis among recipients to 6 percent or less.

The disease is frequently anicteric, and often prolonged. Several studies have shown that the incubation period of hepatitis C is around 7 (3 to 14) weeks, averaging 6 to 7 weeks less than the incubation period of hepatitis B. It is a less severe disease acutely than hepatitis B, since only 15 to 30 percent of patients become icteric, compared with the occurrence of jaundice in nearly two-thirds of hepatitis B patients, and aminotransferase levels tend to be less in hepatitis C. Despite this, fulminant hepatitis and fatalities have been reported (Dienstag et al 1977). The disease is more likely to become chronic than is hepatitis B. In one study (Alter et al 1978), serum enzymes remained elevated longer than six months in 46 percent of 26 cases, as compared with similar chronicity among only 6 percent of 19 patients with hepatitis B. The course of the disease may wax and wane, and the prognosis appears to be particularly poor if alanine aminotransferase levels exceed 300 μ per ml. Liver biopsies in 10 such patients with chronic type C hepatitis showed 1 with chronic persistent hepatitis, 8 with chronic active disease, and 1 with cirrhosis. Type C disease may also recur intermittently with acute flares. A study of 6 cases of non-A, non-B hepatitis among dialysis patients (Coursaget et al 1978) confirms the singularity of the disease. All patients had serum antibodies to hepatitis A virus, and all had been actively immunized against BsAg, although only 4 had developed B surface antibodies. All patients developed malaise while aminotransferase levels were elevated, but only 1 patient became icteric. This observation is confirmed by the findings of Haugen (1979) who noted the occurrence of hepatitis among 56 recipients of over 31,000 units of blood, 80 percent of which were given as frozen or washed red cells. Ninety-five percent of the hepatitis was non-A, non-B, and commercially obtained blood was involved in 44 of the cases. By using only blood obtained from voluntary donors, the incidence of hepatitis was reduced from 2.1 to 0.3 per 1,000 transfusions.

The picture that emerges from these seminal observations about type C hepatitis is that of a mild and prolonged disease, which may be commonly associated with resultant chronic active hepatitis, and possibly hepatocellular carcinoma. While the disease is certainly transmitted by blood and by needle sticks, it also appears in sporadic cases unassociated with direct contact with blood or its products (Villarejos et al 1975). The large reservoir of nontransfused carriers also implicates vertical and sexual transmission. Tong et al (1978) have confirmed the transmission of non-A, non-B hepatitis to six of nine infants born to mothers who had acute disease during their last trimester of pregnancy.

The Agent. Trepo et al (1979) have demonstrated a hepatitis C antigen in 12 of 14 patients with non-A, non-B hepatitis, following blood transfusions. Antigenemia preceded elevations in blood aminotransferases, and cleared before enzymes returned to normal in 7 cases. In the remaining 5, antigenemia persisted and was associated in 4 with elevated enzyme levels during a six-month period of observation. The antigen was also detected in the sera of 12 of 30 patients with chronic hepatitis after blood transfusion, and in 6 of 45 patients who had not been transfused. This same group also reports detecting a hepatitis C surface antigen, slightly smaller than hepatitis B virus and immunologically distinct from it, containing DNA and DNA polymerase activity, in the blood of infected patients and chimpanzees (Prince et al 1979). They have also found IgG molecules in the same samples having the characteristics of HBeAg and anti-e and suggest that the hepatitis C virus is related to, but distinct from, hepatitis B virus and may share a similar set of e determinants.

The most striking demonstration of a singular hepatitis C virus was reported by Coursaget and colleagues in 1979, in the urine of two out of three patients with acute non-A, non-B hepatitis and in the blood of one patient. This observation has not been supported however.

ETHYL ALCOHOL

Alcoholism affects an estimated 9 million Americans, and the abuse of alcohol is reported to have cost this country around $31.5 million in 1971, from lost production, health care, vehicular accidents, crime, and social expenditures (Berry 1976). The treatment of alcoholism and related problems in that year was responsible for about 10 percent of all health care costs in the United States, and over 15 percent of hospital charges. A large proportion of the health-related costs of alcoholism are related to the care of patients with liver disease. Cirrhosis of the liver, most of which is related to alcoholism, was responsible for 31,000 deaths among Americans in 1977. Cirrhosis is the seventh highest cause of death among men, the eighth among women. Maximal death rates in both sexes occur during the most productive years of life, from ages 35 to 74. We have indeed a problem of staggering proportions.

Despite much which has been written to the contrary in the past, there is no clear indication that certain racial or ethnic groups are better able to metabolize alcohol than are others. There is some evidence that Orientals may experience more unpleasant early side effects from drinking, such as flushing, tachycardia, and hypotension, but, while this leads to less intake, it is not associated with slower metabolism (Mendelson and Mello 1979). There may be inherited susceptibility to alcoholism. Several studies (Goodwin et al 1974) have indicated that there is an increased trend toward alcoholism in children of alcoholics, even when the children are adopted at birth and raised away from their biological parents by nonalcoholic foster parents.

Tolerance and dependence are two major complications of alcoholism, the former leading to increasing intake because of more rapid catabolism of alcohol, and the latter causing prompt withdrawal symptoms when blood levels decrease. A chronic alcoholic may experience tremors when his blood levels fall modestly, even though such levels would be high enough to cause deep inebriation in a nonalcoholic.

The effects of alcohol are general, causing diseases of the liver, pancreas, and stomach, cerebral degeneration (Wernicke and Korsakoff psychosis), peripheral neuropathies, bone marrow depression, birth defects (the fetal alcohol syndrome), sterility, and cardiomyopathies. The gynecomastia seen in so many alcoholic men appears to result from a decreased production of testosterone by the gonads, which results in increased estradiol receptors in hepatocytes and increased intracellular concentration of estradiol (Eagon et al 1978).

The Metabolism of Alcohol

Almost all ingested ethyl alcohol is metabolized in the liver to acetaldehyde, acetate, acetyl coenzyme A, carbon dioxide, and water. The first step, the conversion of ethyl alcohol to acetaldehyde, is rate limiting and varies considerably among normal individuals. Alcohol metabolism is faster at high blood levels and thus does not follow zero-order kinetics.

The conversion of alcohol to acetaldehyde is accomplished in vitro by three enzymes, alcohol dehydrogenase, catalase, and the cytochrome P450 microsomal ethanol oxidation system (MEOS) in the following manner:

1. Ethanol + Nicotinamide adenine dinucleotide (NAD^+) $\xrightarrow{\text{alcohol dehydrogenase}}$ Acetaldehyde + NADH + H^+

2. Ethanol + hydrogen peroxide $\xrightarrow{\text{catalase}}$ Acetaldehyde + (2) water

3. Ethanol + NADPH + O_2 + H^+ $\xrightarrow{\text{MEOS}}$ Acetaldehyde + (2) water + $NADP^+$

The first reaction is, by far, the most important one, since the rise in the NADH:NAD^+ ratio in vitro is proportional to the rate of ethanol metabolism. Blocking of the catalase system by inhibitors does not appear to alter the in vivo rate of ethanol metabolism (Mezey 1979). The MEO system probably operates at high blood level of ethanol, but this is not certain. Finally, there is some evidence that another form of dehydrogenase, II-alcohol dehydrogenase, operates at higher concentrations of ethanol in humans and may be responsible for the shift away from zero-order kinetics at higher blood levels. It is believed that the metabolism of ethanol is accelerated in chronic alcoholics by more rapid oxidation of NADH, possibly through the induction of sodium, potassium, ATPase activity, with increased production of adenosine diphosphate (ADP) and increased uptake of oxygen.

Acetaldehyde is oxidized mainly in the mitochondria by a dehydrogenase linked to NAD^+. The accumulation of acetaldehyde in the cytosol can inhibit mitochondrial function and may be responsible for pathologic changes (megamitochondria) and enzymic defects noted in heavy users of alcohol. Phenobarbital increases ethanol metabolism, possibly by increasing hepatic blood flow. Fructose, in large doses, may also accelerate the metabolism of ethanol by increasing the oxidation of NADH by glyceraldehyde.

Metabolic Effects of Alcoholic

Mezey (1979) points out that alcohol inhibits gluconeogenesis by increasing NADH:NAD^+. This increases the amount of lactate formed, reducing the amount of pyruvate and phosphoenolpyruvate which participates in gluconeogenesis. This shift in ratio also prevents the entry of amino acids and glycerophosphate into the gluoneogenetic pathway. Hypoglycemia readily results from alcohol overdosage if no exogenous sources of glucose are available. Hyperuricemia may also occur, because the accumulation of lactate decreases distal renal tubular excretion of urates.

Hypertriglyceridemia is commonly seen after alcohol ingestion. This results from increased production and release of lipoproteins. The fat so released may come from the diet or from body stores acutely, and from increased hepatocytic production of fatty acids and decreased degradation in the chronic alcoholic. Fatty acid synthesis is stimulated by increased NADPH, and oxidation of fats is reduced by elevation of the NADH:NAD^+ ratio. These mechanisms are believed to be responsible for the accumulation of hepatocytic fat seen so commonly in alcoholic liver disease.

Changes in the metabolism of drugs by the liver are induced by alcohol. Alcoholism leads to proliferation of hepatocytic smooth endoplasmic reticulum, the site where many drugs, such as diphenylhydantoin, warfarin, and meprobamate, are metabolized. Alcoholics may, accordingly, experience increased tolerance for these agents and, for several weeks after discontinuing alcohol, may require larger doses to produce consistent effects. On the other hands, drugs which, like alcohol, are metabolized in the microsomal system, may be more slowly metabolized than usual, and their effects potentiated thereby. This category includes many tranquilizing and sedative substances, whose administration to alcoholics may produce excessive responses.

Hypermetabolism. Increased oxygen consumption by the liver has been shown to occur in animals fed alcohol over extended periods of time. This is probably linked to excessive production of Na^+, K^+ ATPase, increased oxidation of NADH, and proliferation of smooth endoplasmic reticulum, all of which require energy. Israel and colleagues (1975) have suggested that this increased demand for oxygen may be responsible in part for the centrilobular necrosis which is a hallmark of alcoholic hepatitis, occurring when tissue demands for oxygen exceed the supply delivered to distal hepatic sinusoids. This group has shown that alcohol-fed rats do indeed develop centrilobular hepatic necrosis if placed in a reduced oxygen atmosphere, and that this effect can be averted by pretreatment with an antithyroid drug, propylthiouracil, or by thyroidectomy (Israel et al 1975). These observations in laboratory animals have clear implications for understanding the pathogenesis of alcoholic liver disease in humans.

Pathologic Effects of Alcohol

Ethanol ingestion increases the production and delays the metabolism of fat in hepatocytes. This process occurs regardless of the adequacy of the remainder of the diet in calories and essential nutrients. A spectrum of disease is produced, ranging from simple fatty metamorphosis of the liver, to alcoholic hepatitis, and finally to cirrhosis. Fatty liver is a benign condition and completely reversible with abstinence. Alcoholic hepatitis and cirrhosis lead to marked hepatic dysfunction and permanent changes in the liver.

Early studies on alcohol-fed rats, and on humans, had shown that the ingestion of alcohol caused fatty livers, despite a diet which was otherwise adequate. Rats did not, however, develop alcoholic hepatitis, and efforts to produce the lesion in human volunteers would have been unjustifiable. It was thus a signal breakthrough when Rubin and Lieber (1974) demonstrated that chronic alcohol ingestion in baboons for nine months to four years produced fatty livers in seven animals, alcoholic hepatitis in four, and cirrhosis of the liver in two. Their diet had been isocaloric with controls, contained adequate vitamins, and differed only in that carbohydrate was replaced by alcohol, which accounted for half the total calories ingested.

Control animals in this study had normal liver biopsies throughout, and the liver was abnormal in all of the animals fed alcohol. Fatty metamorphosis was present in all from the earliest biopsies, at one to two months, and increased progressively. Fat accumulated first in centrilobular hepatocytes and then in midzonal areas. As the cytoplasmic inclusions increased in size, cellular walls were broken down and fat cysts were formed between adjacent cells. Hyaline sclerosis, fibrosis of terminal hepatic sinusoids neighboring central veins, occurred in several animals. This perivenular sclerosis has subsequently (Worner and Lieber 1978) been determined to be a good predictor of subsequent cirrhosis in men who continue to drink alcohol following its appearance. The animals with alcoholic hepatitis showed these fatty changes, plus ballooning of hepatocytes (swelling with attenuation of the cytoplasm), inflammation with mononuclear and occasional polymorphonuclear leukocytes, and some hepatocytes containing Mallory hyaline. Hyaline sclerosis was present in many central areas where hepatocytes had disappeared, and proliferation of collagen fibers had occurred widely, often surrounding groups of centrilobular hepatocytes, and occasionally extending from centrilobular to portal areas. Central veins were occasionaly obliterated. In the cirrhotic animals, fibrosis was increased, with formation of micronodules, and progressive loss of normal lobular architecture. Portal areas were infiltrated with lymphocytes and histiocytes. In the cirrhotic baboons, regenerating nodules showed little or no fatty metamorphosis. Laboratory data showed mild elevation of aminotransferase activity in animals with fatty livers, and moderate elevations in animals with alcoholic hepatitis and cirrhosis. At no time (save in one baboon) did levels approach the massive elevations seen in viral hepatitis.

Ultrastructuraly, hepatocytes from fatty livers and from alcoholic hepatitis showed similar changes. Cytoplasmic fat was increased, mitochondria were swollen, and cristae were distorted, smooth endoplasmic reticulum was increased, and rough reticulum was reduced. Hepatocytic membranes, nuclei, and bile canaliculi appeared normal.

These pathologic changes have been described in some detail because they closely parallel changes seen in human alcoholic liver disease and provide a clear basis for distinguishing its various stages from other hepatic disorders seen on liver biopsy. Unfortunately, the discovery on liver biopsy of fatty infiltration, hepatocytic necrosis, Mallory bodies, central and portal fibrosis, cellular infiltration, and bile duct proliferation is not confined solely to alcoholic liver disease. Most of these findings have been seen in a group of 27 nonalcoholic patients, primarily white, middle-aged women, many of whom were obese and diabetic and had coronary artery heart disease (Miller et al 1979). The cause of this condition is not clear, although the occurrence of fatty livers in poorly controlled diabetes is common.

Pathogenesis of Alcoholic Hepatitis and Cirrhosis

It is clear that alcohol is directly responsible for fatty metamorphosis of the liver. It is equally clear that continued use of alcohol can cause progressive hepatic damage, from fatty liver to alcoholic hepatitis and cirrhosis. Furthermore, abstention from further use of alcohol at the fatty liver stage, prior to the onset of alcoholic hepatitis, results in a fairly prompt return of hepatic function and morphology to normal. What is presently lacking is a clear understanding of the one or several changes that convert the relatively benign and wholly reversible condition of fatty metamorphosis to the stage of hepatocellular necrosis, scarring, and at best, only partial reversibility of alcoholic hepatitis. In many clinical instances, alcoholic hepatitis appears to be self-perpetuating, progressing to fulminant hepatic failure or cirrhosis despite adequate dietary replacement and abstinence from further ethanol.

A number of explanations have been given for the phenomena of hepatocellular necrosis and self-perpetuation. First is the attractive theory already mentioned, that increased cellular metabolism results in increased oxygen demand and relative oxygen deficiency in hepatic sinusoidal blood, particularly in blood reaching centrilobular areas. Alcohol has also been shown to damage cytoplasmic microtubules and may thus cause hepatocytic damage by interfering with the secretory activity of the cells. In fact, it is believed that microtubular aggregates result in Mallory bodies (Isselbacher 1977). It has been proposed that this decrease in microtubules in chronic alcoholics may be related to increased amounts of acetaldehyde in hepatocytes (Baronoa et al 1979). Both of these processes may contribute to hepatocytic necrosis.

Autoimmune phenomena may explain the propagation of the necrotic process in alcoholic hepatitis and cirrhosis. Leevy et al (1975) found a decrease in number and reactivity of T-lymphocytes in alcoholics with liver disease; there were a number of lymphocytes that responded to liver extracts with increased transformation and migration inhibition. Lue et al (1979) have also shown that lymphocytes from baboons with alcoholic hepatitis show increased cytotoxicity to host hepatocytes and to nonalcoholic control hepatocytes, when compared with lymphocytes from controls. The hepatocytes from the alcohol-fed animals became necrotic more quickly than control hepatocytes. These results suggest that hepatocellular necrosis in alcoholic hepatitis is probably due in part to increased lymphocytotoxicity and in part to decreased resistance of liver cells.

Fibrosis is, of course, a hallmark of cirrhosis of the liver. There is some evidence that alcoholic cirrhosis can appear both spontaneously and consequent to alcoholic hepatitis, in alcoholic subjects. The fibrosis that follows alcoholic hepatocellular necrosis could be the result of repair following disturbance of the reticular framework of the liver, just as occurs in hepatocytic necrosis from any cause. But direct fibrosis induced by alcohol is another matter. Guzelian and Diegelmann (1979) have shown that type III collagen is produced in excess by regenerating rat hepatocytes when compared to normal hepatocytes, and that the product differs completely from the type I collagen produced by fibroblasts. Alcohol appears to stimulate the production of both type I and type III collagen, and appears to do this by inhibiting the production of lysosomal collagen peptidase in hepatocytes (Henley and Laughrey 1979). This process could clearly operate in the absence of actual necrosis of liver cells, and one would assume that the type of collagen found in patients without necrosis would be primarily type III.

Diagnosis and Management of Alcoholic Liver Disease

Fatty liver and cirrhosis from alcohol ingestion are often diagnosed at routine examinations, the patient frequently being free of symptoms. Fatty liver presents with hepatomegaly, frequently associated with tremulousness, an indication of early alcohol withdrawal. Slight degrees of jaundice may also be present. Cirrhosis may present with gastrointestinal bleeding, ascites, or early hepatic encephalopathy, and occasionally with a fulminant picture.

Alcoholic hepatitis is another matter entirely. The patient is often febrile and shows progressive jaundice. Encephalopathy may be an early symptom and oliguria and the hepatorenal syndrome may be present. At times, tremulousness and hallucinatory activity may make it difficult to distinguish between delirium tremens and alcoholic hepatitis. Jaundice and leukocytosis would, of course, make the latter diagnosis more likely.

The primary element in management is to remove the patient permanently from any further ingestion of alcohol. While simple to say, this is almost invariably difficult to accomplish, and I know of no method which has been uniformly, or even frequently, effective. The use of group discussions, counseling, Alcoholics Anonymous, and intervention therapy have all had some measure of success and should be tried. The more active the role played by the physician in the program of alcohol abstinence, the more effective is the long-term result. Ambulatory patients must be seen frequently so that they learn to recognize the importance of continued abstinence and know that they have access to someone who is willing to listen to their problems. It is helpful to have the confidence of a close relative of the patients, so that renewed use of alcohol becomes known promptly. Recidivism is very high and is better managed with sympathy than with scorn. It is best not to employ disulfiram in patients with alcoholic liver disease, since blockade of acetaldehyde metabolism, should the patient drink again, may aggravate hepatocytic damage. The management of alcoholic patients is very trying, but the rewards can be great and are worth seeking.

Special agents have been employed in management of patients with severe alcoholic hepatitis. Glucocorticoids have not been found to be effective clinically (Depew et al 1980) but have been shown to reduce the inflammatory reaction in successive liver biopsies (Boitnott and Maddrey 1979). Propylthiouracil, given to reduce hepatic metabolism, has been shown to result in a significantly more rapid rate of improvement in hepatic status than did a dummy agent in a double-blind study of 133 patients (Orrego et al 1979). The effect was most striking among patients whose liver function tests were most abnormal and whose serum T_3 levels were lowest. In another randomized trial, 25 of 50 patients were given insulin (24 units) and glucagon (2.4 mg) intravenously, twice daily for three weeks, in an effort to stimulate hepatocytic regeneration (Hatfield et al 1979). While there was a trend toward reduced mortality and more rapid improvement among patients receiving this treatment, the results were short of being statistically significant.

OTHER CHEMICAL AGENTS

Hepatic damage, to paraphrase a statement attributed to Abraham Lincoln, can be caused by almost all drugs some of the time; it can even be caused by some drugs all of the time. If, indeed, one looks extensively through available reports, it is difficult to discover a single chemical agent in use today which has not been implicated as, at the very least, an occasional cause of hepatotoxicity. The situation is compounded further by the fact that people are exposed increasingly today to a variety of potent hepatotoxins dispensed elsewhere than in the pharmacy. They appear naturally in innocent-looking patches of wild mushrooms (phalloidin), in medicinal bush teas (senecio), and on fugus-infected peanuts (aflatoxins). They appear as insecticides and herbicides (chlorinated hydrocarbons), solvents (carbon tetrachloride), and propellants (vinyl chloride). And they may also appear as innocuous food preservatives (nitrites converted to nitrosamines). This sorry state of affairs has prompted an eminent hepatologist, Hyman J. Zimmerman (1978), to observe that "man finds himself in a chemical jungle," surrounded, I might add, by a host of greedy hepatophilic predators.

However, the situation is not all bad. Governmental safeguards are effective enough in many parts of the world to prohibit the release of hepatotoxic drugs for general use, and citizen alertness has been effective in putting reins on the industrial situation. These controls must continue. Self-restraint alone, by even the most enlightened industry, is unlikely to ensure fully against the release in future of markedly hepatotoxic drugs, like carbon tetrachloride and cinophen. Prerelease testing must continue to be mandated and vigorously monitored.

But no amount of policing is going to neutralize humanity's perverse efforts to damage the liver with chemicals. We have already considered the invariable and often devastating effects of ethyl alcohol, that panjandrum of all hepatotoxins. It is a prime example of a chemical that adversely affects all livers in both its original form and also as one of its metabolites (acetaldehyde). Its consumption will doubtless continue well beyond the foreseeable future. And then there is the case of acetaminophen, a benign reliever of headaches and muscular pains and totally harmless if used in modest doses. Individuals have contrived to convert acetaminophen into a deadly hepatotoxin, simply by taking it in large enough amounts to exceed the supply of available conjugants and allow the accumulation of large amounts of deadly electrophilic metabolites that cause hepatic necrosis. Thus, while nature, industry, and the pharamaceutical industry are significant agencies in the propagation of hepatotoxins, people themselves are probably the most significant.

A word must be said in favor of the sapient prescription of known hepatotoxins in the treatment of mortal disease. The hope, of course, is to administer the agents in doses large enough and frequent enough to control the lethal disorder, usually cancer, and yet small enough to prevent serious and irreversible damage to the liver. One attempts to find the therapeutic pharmacokinetic window between the effective dose and the severely hepatotoxic dose, risking the latter while hoping to achieve the former. Regular testing of liver function and occasional biopsies of the liver provide adequate indices of hepatotoxicity. As long as such precautions are regularly taken in oncologic therapy, and as long as patients are aware of their risks, the use of hepatotoxins in this way is fully justifiable.

Why So Many Hepatotoxins?

Being the central collecting station for most constituents absorbed from the gastrointestinal tract, and being the recipient of a major proportion of atmospheric inhalants, the liver is excellently situated to prepare (detoxify) foreign agents for excretion. Since many of these agents are nonpolar and lipid soluble, hepatic enzyme systems must be able to convert them to polar compounds by hydroxylation and conjugation and enable them to be excreted as harmless metabolites into the urine and bile. Low molecular weight conjugates are generally excreted into the urine, while higher molecular weight (over 300) conjugates appear in the bile. Some of the conjugated biliary agents are deconjugated in the intestine, reabsorbed and recirculated, thus prolonging their therapeutic or toxic effects. Hepatic damage may occur as the metabolic capacity of the liver is exceeded by the amount of exogenous agent presented to it (intrinsic, direct, predictable, or invariable hepatotoxins), a dose-dependent type of hepatotoxicity, common to all persons. Or damage to the liver may occur because of some special feature of the host, such as allergy or unusual metabolic processes, causing a type of liver damage (idiosyncratic, indirect, unpredictable, variable) which may be either independent of the dose, or dose related. Frequently, one encounters situations in which both invariable and variable damage occurs, the invariable damage usually being slight, while the specific features of the host lead to more extensive harm. Hepatotoxicity to chlorpromazine, C-17 alkylated steroids, and isoniazid are probably of this type. The percentage of subjects developing liver damage is much greater among invariable than it is among variable hepatotoxins. Most variable hepatotoxins do not cause liver disease in greater than 1 percent of users, unless the disorder is dose related. This complexity of hepatotoxic mechanisms makes classification very difficult and unsatisfactory, since the various permutations of cause and effect defy any rigid nosologic pattern. The best approach, to my way of thinking, is to consider that all hepatotoxins exist along a spectrum, and range from those which are purely invariable, regardless of the host, to those which are purely variable for different reasons. Along the way are many hepatotoxins whose ill-effects are combinations of both invariable and variable susceptibilities. Using selected examples, the accompanying table (Table 10–1) attempts to employ this method of classification.

Pathways of Hepatic Metabolism of Chemical Agents

Some hepatotoxic agents are poorly metabolized and damage hepatocytic membranes or enzyme systems in their unaltered form. The folic acid antagonists, methotrexate, is a potent antineoplastic and hepatotoxic agent for one and the same reason. It inhibits the production of nucleic acids by blocking the enzyme that guides the formation of tetrahydrofolic acid. Prolonged and excessive administration causes fatty infiltration of liver cells, hepatocytic necrosis, and cirrhosis of the liver. On the other hand, we have seen that ethyl alcohol harms liver cells primarily by hastening production and reducing oxidation of lipids, second, by increasing cellular metabolism and producing a trend toward hepatocytic necrosis through relative hypoxia, and third, by leading to a microtubular damage through biotransformation to its metabolite, acetaldehyde.

There are two major hepatocytic enzyme systems responsible for the conversion of fat-soluble drugs to water-soluble compounds. The mixed function oxidase system hydroxylates compounds through a series of enzymic (phase I) reactions. The conjugating system replaces a hydrogen atom on slightly polar groups with a large water-soluble molecule through another (phase II) enzyme system of the smooth endoplasmic reticulum (Branch et al 1975). Both of these systems are subject to induction through the agency of chemicals, such as ethanol, phenobarbital, and diphenylhydantoin, which lead to increased production of metabolites.

The mixed function oxidase system (MFOS) hydroxylates chemical agents by borrowing electrons from NADPH through flavoproteins and converting ferric to ferrous cytochrome P-450. This complex interacts with oxygen and then, having become an agent with high molecular affinity, reacts readily with many other available compounds, becoming oxidized again to the ferric form in the process. The formerly stable compound with which

Table 10–1. Examples of Hepatotoxic Agents, Distinguished by Their Sensitivities, Pathogenetic Mechanisms, and Effects on the Liver

Agent	*Classification*	*Pathogenesis*	*Pathologic Effects*
Carbon tetrachloride	invariable, general, dose dependent	only slight toxicity without biotransformation, which occurs in all but newborns; oxidized to CCl_3 free radicals in cytochrome P-450 mixed function oxidase system (MFOS); causes lipid peroxidation in endoplasmic reticulum, decreased production of lipoproteins, fat retention; Necrosis results from altered membranes.	fatty liver; centrizonal necrosis; cirrhosis; ? mutagenesis
Ethanol	invariable, general, dose dependent	primarily, causes increased synthesis, decreased metochondrial oxidation of fat; increases cellular metabolism, leading to relative hepatocytic hypoxia and necrosis; increases formation of collagen III; converted by alcohol dehydrogenase to acetaldehyde, which is probable cause of microtubular damage and Mallory bodies; autoimmunity to cell constituents and Mallory bodies may contribute to necrosis.	fatty liver; alcoholic hepatitis; micronodular cirrhosis; hepatocellular carcinoma
Acetaminophen	invariable, general, dose dependent	cytotoxicity due to unconjugated metabolite; drug primarily forms nontoxic glucuronides and sulfates; remainder is converted to electrophilic metabolite in MFOS, which immediately conjugates with glutathione and is converted to mercaptapuric acid; excess causes necrosis by binding covalently with nucleophilic cellular macromolecules	centrizonal, hemorrhagic necrosis; chronic active hepatitis (with long-term use)
Aflatoxins	invariable, cytotoxic, dose dependent	inhibits RNA polymerase and impairs synthesis of nucleic acids, either directly, or by hydroxylated metabolites; individual susceptibility varies; increases in association with protein malnutrition.	acute central and midzonal necrosis; microdispersed cytoplasmic fat; bile duct hyperplasia; cirrhosis;

Table 10–1. Examples of Hepatotoxic Agents, Distinguished by Their Sensitivities, Pathogenetic Mechanisms, and Effects on the Liver (Continued)

Agent	*Classification*	*Pathogenesis*	*Pathologic Effects*
C-17 alkylated steroids; Estrogens with phenolic A rings	invariable cholestatic, dose dependent with variable sensitivity (? genetic)	damage to hepatocytic canalicular membranes produces decreased bile flow; variable severity; jaundice is obstructive; process is most marked in patients who also display cholestasis in late pregnancy, which probably has same etiology as drug-induced disorder.	cholestasis; peliosis hepatis; hepatic adenomas; hepatocellular carcinoma; estrogens may also cause Budd-Chiari syndrome
Chlorpromazine	variable, cholestatic hypersensitivity, not related to dose, complicating invariable slight cholestasis	decreased production of bile and increased viscosity of bile due to direct reaction with bile components; increased absorption of water from bile; hypersensitivity manifested by eosinophilia, recurrence with small challenge doses; autoimmunity suggested by nuclear antibodies, possibly increased transformation of lymphocytes.	cholestasis, often prolonged; portal infiltrates, often eosinophilic; slight necrosis; rare cirrhosis
Halothane	variable, general hypersensitivity, not related to dose, complicating invariable slight cytotoxicity	80 percent of patients with liver disease have had prior exposure; drug usually oxidized in MFOS, probably to free radical which binds to cellular macromolecules, causing necrosis; metabolite may also become antigenic, causing autoimmunity; effect aggravated by previous enzyme induction and by hypoxia.	spotty to confluent necrosis, usually centrizonal; cirrhosis with repeated exposure
Phenylbutazone	variable, general hypersensitivity, not related to dose, complicating invariable mild cytotoxicity	possibly induced by a metabolite; half of patients show true hypersensitivity, with onset 1 to 5 weeks after commencing drug, fever, eosinophilia.	spotty to massive necrosis; cholestasis; fatty liver; granulomas, occasional

Table 10–1. Examples of Hepatotoxic Agents, Distinguished by Their Sensitivities, Pathogenetic Mechanisms, and Effects on the Liver (continued)

Agent	*Classification*	*Pathogenesis*	*Pathologic Effects*
Diphenylhydantoin	variable, cytotoxic hypersensitivity, not related to dose, complicating slight invariable cytotoxicity	drug is a potent inducer of microsomal enzymes, possibly leading to initial damage by metabolites; hypersensitivity manifested by fever, eosinophilia, rash, lymphadenopathy, drug antibodies	spotty to massive necrosis; lymphocytic infiltrates
Methyldopa	variable, cytotoxic hypersensitivity, not related to dose, complicating slight invariable cytotoxicity	initial toxicity probably due to arylating (adding aromatic groups to nucleophilic macromolecules) microsomal metabolites produced in MFOS; severe liver disease caused by autoimmune allergy, manifested by fever, hemolysis, nuclear, and smooth muscle antibodies in some patients; inhibits function of suppressor lymphocytes (Kirtland et al 1980)	spotty necrosis; portal infiltrates; bridging necrosis; chronic active hepatitis; granulomas
Isoniazid	variable, general, dose related	variability depends on rate at which patient acetylates drug in liver; toxicity depends on accumulation of electrophilic metabolite in hepatocytes of rapid acetylators; Acetylsoniazid is hydrolyzed to acetylhydrazine, which is converted to activated acylating agent in MFOS; this binds covalently to cellular macromolecules causing necrosis; slow acetylators are protected by producing less acetylhydrazine (45 percent of dose) than do rapid acetylators (94 percent of dose)	spotty necrosis, occasionally confluent or submassive, especially in elderly; chronic active hepatitis

cytochrome P-450 has reacted becomes an avidly electrophilic intermediate and conjugates immediately with glutathione. If adequate amounts of conjugating agent are not available, the intermediate binds covalently to nucleophilic cellular macromolecules, causing necrosis of the cell. Drugs that induce this enzyme system increase the production of the potentially toxic metabolite and may overwhelm the capacity of the next, or conjugative, mechanism to form an innocuous moiety (Mitchell and Lauterburg 1978). This inexpedient aspect of induction is believed to explain why previous ingestion of ethanol worsens the hepatotoxic effects of further amounts, and why phenobarbital pretreatment makes a given dose of acetaminophen more toxic. Table 10-1 lists examples of drug metabolism involving the MFOS.

The conjugating system is largely the same as that responsible for the conjugation of free bilirubin, in which a glucuronide molecule is donated to the fat-soluble free drug from one or two molecules of uridine disphosphate glucuronic acid in the smooth endoplasmic reticulum, under the influence of glucuronyl transferase. It is the major pathway for the excretion of acetaminophen and many other drugs. Conjugation may occur on hydroxide, carboxyl, amine, or sulfhydral groups, with sulfates, acetylates, or mercaptopurates, as well as glucuronic acid and glutathione.

Types of Hepatic Injury

Chemical agents may cause hepatotoxicity either by action of the agent itself or by action of one of its metabolites. The damage to the cell may be generalized or quite specific. Some agents, such as acetaminophen, lead to massive hepatocellular damage, while others, such as chlorpromazine, only reduce bile production and increase its viscosity. Some, such as vinyl chloride, aflatoxins, and estrogens, appear to react with nucleic-acid-replicating mechanisms and may lead to development of mutant cells. Still others form antigens with hepatocytic proteins and lead to continuing autoimmune hepatic destruction in sensitive persons. Almost any imaginable type of hepatic lesion can be caused by at least one chemical agent; so that to know hepatotoxicity thoroughly is to know nearly everything about acute and chronic liver disease.

Acute hepatocellular necrosis is the hallmark of poisoning with carbon tetrachloride and acetaminophen. Both disorders are also typified by centrizonal lesions. Fatty metamorphosis is characteristic of carbon tetrachloride poisoning and is believed to result from decreased production of lipoproteins. Acute necrosis, varying from spotty to bridging and submassive necrosis, is also seen in patients with various types of hypersensitivity hepatitis, such as that resulting from halothane exposure, diphenylhydantoin, and methyldopa.

Cholestasis probably occurs to a limited degree in all patients receiving agents such as chlorpromazine, C-17 alkylated steroids, and estrogens with phenolic A rings. The estrogens appear to reduce sulfotransferase activity, at least in rats, and thus reduce biliary flow. However, actual cholestasis progressing to jaundice is very infrequent with these agents, and the sensitivity to the hormones may be genetic. Jaundice from chlorpromazine, on the other hand, appears quite clearly to be a hypersensitivity type of reaction, since it is usually associated with fever, eosinophilia, and a tendency to recur promptly with reexhibition of the drug.

Chronic active hepatitis has been described as rare consequence of prolonged exposure to a number of agents, including methyldopa, isoniazid, halothane, and nitrofurantoin. Autoimmunity has been invoked as the cause of chronic active drug hepatitis, and the disease often responds to discontinuation of the drug (Zimmerman 1978). The process seen in patients with long continued use of isoniazid, however, appears to result from continued hepatocytic necrosis and repair due to rapid acylation of the drug and formation of toxic amounts of acetylhydrazine from it.

Cirrhosis of the liver is seen in patients subjected to repeated exposure to halothane and carbon tetrachloride and is also seen in patients exposed to aflatoxins. Fortunately, this complication is not encountered often because the causative agent, in most cases, has caused acute injuries which have been followed by interdiction of the offender. Cases that have occurred are primarily among patients receiving long, low-level occupational exposures. Biliary cirrhosis has been described as a rare complication of long-term use of chlorpromazine.

Hepatic neoplasms of many types have been attributed to drugs and environmental agents. Peliosis hepatis, collections of blood-filled cystic structures, while not truly neoplastic, may be associated with tumors. This condition has been described rarely among patients taking anabolic steroids and estrogens for extended periods. Adenomas of the liver are occasionally seen in women taking contraceptive steroids, and may become quite large at times. Hepatocellular carcinomas occur rarely in patients with alcoholic cirrhosis, and may also occur as a consequence of prolonged exposure to aflatoxins. A peculiar type of angiosarcoma has been causally related to exposure to vinyl chloride, a compound used widely in the plastics industry. Similar lesions have been produced in rats exposed to moderate doses of vinyl chloride, so the relationship between the chemical and the hepatic lesion appears to be established. It is believed that hepatic damage results from a toxic metabolite of vinyl chloride, and that it may also be responsible for causing sclerosis of the porta hepatis and portal hypertension in some patients.

Diagnosis of Hepatotoxicity

In most instances, the diagnosis of toxic liver disease depends primarily upon elucidation of the exposure from the patient's history. A careful review of medications, occupational and environmental exposures, and personal habits is accordingly essential to the evaluation of newly diagnosed disease of the liver, especially where the cause is not immediately apparent. Physicians should have ready access to references of known hepatotoxins, for the list of possible offenders is so long that any one person is unlikely to be aware of them all. It is essential also to determine whether any familial or occupational clustering of liver disorders has occurred in the patient's immediate circle, since the product involved may not have been heretofore implicated as a hepatotoxin. This is particularly possible where only small numbers of persons have been exposed to an agent causing a slowly developing asymptomatic disorder, such as occurred in the case of exposure to vinyl chloride, or where a host peculiarity, such as the rapid acetylation of isoniazid, is required before toxicity is fully expressed.

Consultation with Other Sources of Information. In instances of hepatic disease occurring from exposure to an as yet unimplicated hepatotoxin, the importance of consulting current medical references and speaking with one's colleagues cannot be overly stressed. Since liver disease from many agents is due both to the agent and the host's own peculiar sensitivity, the disorder may occur so infrequently that a single physician may not see more than one patient for years. Pooling of personal experiences with those of colleagues increases the denominator in the disease incidence fraction and is likely to reveal some increase in the numerator as well if there is indeed a relationship between the drug and the disease. This type of informational consolidation clearly helped to implicate the regular use of contraceptive steroids in the genesis of hepatic adenomas and the prophylactic use of isoniazid with the infrequent occurrence of hepatitis.

The importance of continuous testing for hepatotoxicity of drugs following their release for general use is illustrated by an experience in the United States during 1979 and 1980. Ticrynafen, a uricosuric antihypertensive agent, had been administered to 4,000 patients in carefully monitored trials for several years prior to its release in 1979. The studies had been conducted in numerous centers, and only one had reported any ensuing abnormalities of hepatic function. These appeared to be mild, infrequent, and readily reversible with discontinuance of the drug. The manufacturer's new drug application mentioned these patients, recalled that only 22 cases of liver injury had been reported among approximately 1 million patients who had received the agent in France during the previous four years, and added that another American study of 500 patients had detected no hepatic damage whatsoever.

Ticrynafen was released with approval of the Food and Drug Administration and prescribed for about 300,000 patients in the ensuing nine months. Information concerning possible hepatotoxicity was prominently included in prescribing literature. By early 1980, approximately 60 patients receiving the drug had developed an illness associated with fever, malaise, elevations of aminotransferases, and abdominal pain. Nearly two-thirds of the patients became icteric. Toxicity occurred within 2 to 12 weeks after exposure to ticrynafen, and five deaths were reported, although the cause of death was not specified in some. A number of patients were rechallenged with the drug after hepatic function tests normalized, and their symptoms promptly recurred (FDA 1980). The 0.02 to 0.03 percent incidence of hepatotoxicity, delayed onset of symptoms, fever, and exacerbation with a single rechallenge dose support the notion that ticrynafen is a variable, hypersensitivity type, cytotoxic agent. It has been removed from sale voluntarily by the manufacturer at the request of the FDA and probably will not return. The fact that the drug may be hepatotoxic and that its therapeutic actions are not unique justifies the recall, despite its convenience and the rarity of the liver problem with which it is associated. The experience with ticrynafen clearly indicates the importance of continued postrelease testing of all new drugs for possible unsuspected toxicity.

The facts of the isoniazid story are curious and underscore another type of problem encountered in relating the use of a drug, an established agent in this case, to infrequent hepatotoxicity. It is known that administration of isoniazid in small daily doses for two to three years is an excellent means for preventing active pulmonary tuberculosis in persons whose tuberculin tests have recently converted from negative to positive, and in young people who have been exposed to a patient with active disease. In most large American communities, detection of tuberculin converters and case contact is the province of public health authorities, who eagerly undertook the responsibility of prescribing isoniazid to appropriate persons at risk. The problem of associating the hepatic disorder with the drug arose because, as patients became ill, they reported to their personal physicians rather than to the agency which had prescribed it. Since individual physicians are quite busy and not generally inclined to write letters or to prepare manuscripts for publication, they discovered that something could go wrong with isoniazid but did not publicize the information widely. What news did return to public health agencies was fragmentary and often inconclusive, to the point where it was commonly ignored. It was only when large prospective studies were done, and the bearing of rapid acetylation on the genesis of the disorder was clarified, that the general medical community became fully aware of the problem (Mitchell et al 1976). While isoniazid is still prescribed today, regular observation and hepatic function testing of patients is employed effectively to limit the incidence and severity of hepatitis.

Prospective diagnosis of hepatotoxicity should be undertaken regularly in patients at high risk. This includes regular hepatic function testing of patients receiving a variety of oncologic drugs, patients on methyldopa and diphenylhydantoin during the early weeks of treatment, and patients with hypersensitivitiy to other drugs. Exposed workers in plastics factories and industries using volatile agents should also be tested regularly, as should women taking contraceptive steroids. Using this approach, disease can be detected early and the drug or exposure terminated before any serious problems occur.

Presenting Symptoms. The presenting symptoms of hepatotoxicity range all the way from simple hepatomegaly to fulminant hepatic failure, cirrhosis, and hepatic neoplasms. In many patients, symptoms do not appear until disease is well advanced. I recall seeing a previously asymptomatic patient who was hospitalized with bleeding esophageal varices and moderate, firm heptomegaly. History of alcohol ingestion, drugs, previous hepatitis, and familial clustering was totally negative, and hepatic function testing was reasonably good. For many years, he had employed carbon tetrachloride as a glue solvent and cleansing agent in his model airplane hobby, working long hours in a small, poorly ventilated room, several times a week. He had noted feelings of giddiness and nausea on occasion, but these symptoms cleared rapidly, and there had never been an acute major episode of illness. Biopsy of the liver showed micronodular cirrhosis, and a portacaval shunt was performed. During the next four years in which the use of carbon tetrachloride was proscribed, he continued to feel well, and had no further bleeding. While this experience does not provide total proof that his exposure to carbon tetrachloride was responsible for the cirrhosis, the circumstantial evidence is fairly persuasive.

Rash, fever, lymphadenopathy, and eosinophilia in association with evidence of acute liver damage strongly suggest an allergic response often seen in patients who develop hypersensitivity hepatitis and is not uncommon in patients with disease resulting from chlorpromazine, diphenylhydantoin, or sulfonamide. Obstructive jaundice, especially if the obstruction is total, may present a considerable problem, since extrahepatic obstruction is a possibility, even though the patient is known to be taking a potentially cholestatic agent. In such patients, it is well to perform hepatic sonograms, looking for dilatation of extrahepatic bile ducts, and to allow a fortnight or so to pass if that study is negative. Generally, drug-induced cholestasis will commence to clear but may not resolve fully within that time, and the diagnosis will become apparent. If improvement does not commence, liver biopsy and percutaneous transhepatic cholangiography will often clarify the question of whether cholestasis was the result of extrahepatic obstruction unrelated to drug ingestion.

Management of Acute Toxic Hepatitis

In most instances, the manifestations of acute toxic hepatitis disappear quite soon after discontinuation of the responsible agent, regardless of whether the liver lesion is primarily hepatocytotoxic or cholestatic. Considerable patience is required at times in awaiting full remission of disease in patients with cholestasis, but gradual improvement occurs almost invariably, once extrahepatic obstruction has been excluded. Patients with hepatocytotoxic lesions respond well unless the disease is fulminating, but some may be left with permanent hepatic scarring, and even a degree of cirrhosis, if preceding necrosis was extensive enough to destroy the hepatic reticular framework in places.

The major therapeutic challenge occurs in patients whose initial lesion results in diffuse hepatic necrosis, or those in whom such a complication is anticipated by calculation of the amount of dose-dependent hepatotoxin ingested. Supportive care is essential in such patients, especially for the maintenance of circulating plasma volume, electrolytic balance, and nutrition. Management of encephalopathy, consumption coagulpathy, and renal complications has already been discussed. If the poison was administered orally, gastric lavage and the use of chelating agents, such as charcoal and cholestyramine, is indicated to reduce the toxic burden on the liver. Hemodialysis may also be slightly beneficial, although this can only be expected to remove the toxin which has not been picked up by the liver on its first passage through that organ. Additional use of glucocorticoids may be helpful where there is reason to suspect that autoimmunity is incriminated in propagation of hepatic injury, and trials of glucagon and insulin as stimulators of hepatic regeneration are worthy of investigation.

In acetaminophen toxicity, a striking breakthrough in therapy has been achieved. Therapy is based on the theory that exhaustion of hepatic stores of glutathione has resulted from excessive production and subsequent conjugation of toxic electrophilic metabolites of the drug in the mixed function oxidase system. The inability of excessive amounts of the metabolite to conjugate with glutathione leads to covalent binding with nucleophilic cytoplasmic macromolecules and cellular necrosis. Patients were given large amounts of a sulfhydryl-containing agent, *n*-acetylcysteine, to form nontoxic conjugates with the excess metabolite, as a substitute for glutathione. The results showed both marked improvement in patients with active acetaminophen toxicity and very mild disease in patients who, by calculation of the dose ingested, would have been expected to have very severe disease (Black 1980). If anyone seeks clear proof of the essential relationship between basic science research and clinical medicine today, here is a shining example.

Management of Chronic Active Hepatitis

Autoimmunity. Chronic active hepatitis (CAH) syndrome may, as has been seen, result from types B and C hepatitis, from certain chemical agents and, in occasional instances, from alcohol. Wilson disease, alpha-1 antitrypsin deficiency, and cytomegalic virus infections may also cause CAH. The picture may finally occur in other patients, usually young women, in the absence of any evidence of toxic agents or viral infections. These patients are frequently found to have circulating antinuclear antibodies, usually without any other signs of lupus erythematosus, and have been designated in the past as having lupoid hepatitis. The flavor of autoimmunity runs through all concepts relating to the pathogenesis of chronic active hepatitis, regardless of cause.

Humoral immunity, manifested by elevated levels of gamma globulin, nuclear, smooth-muscle, and mitochondrial antibodies, and prevelance of mononuclear cells in the liver, appears to be present in most patients with CAH to varying degrees. Antibodies to liver membrane antigens have also been found in many patients (Meyer zum Buschenfelde et al 1979). Humoral immunity is often found, however, to be incomplete. Thus, HBs carriers do not develop anti-HBs, whether they are asymptomatic carriers or have CAH. Healthy carrier of HBs may carry anti-HBe, but patients with CAH do not, and they usually show persistent DNA polymerase activity and circulating Dane particles as well.

Cellular immunity is also reduced in CAH. Lymphocyte stimulation with HBsAg regularly occurs in patients who have recovered from acute infections with B virus. Carriers, and patients with CAH, do not demonstrate this stimulation, and some show a sustained cytotoxicity of lymphocytes to red cells coated with HBsAg. A number of patients have developed often fatal aplastic anemias consequent to viral hepatitis infection (Hagler et al 1975), and some of these have been found to have autoantibodies and cytotoxic lymphocytes. Another demonstration of transient autoimmunity occurred in a patient described by Wilson et al (1980), who developed pure red cell aplasia during an attack of hepatitis. Patient's lymphocytes were transiently cytotoxic to his own and foreign erythrocytes. Many patients with HBsAg-positive CAH also demonstrate prolonged cellular immunity to liver-specific protein and cytotoxicity to hepatocytes grown in culture from several different species.

These, and many other observations, suggest important roles for both T-cell and antibody-dependent cytotoxicity in CAH, regardless of the cause of the syndrome. The disease could result from failure of suppressor T-cells to function normally. This concept is supported somewhat by the observation that CAH, both specific and nonspecific, tends to occur frequently in patients who are immunosuppressed by disease, including patients with collagen disease, cancer, malnutrition, and hereditary hypoimmune disorders, as well as patients being treated with immunosuppressive agents. Most patients appear to have a low-grade immunologic response to the etiologic agent of CAH, be they viruses, immune complexes, or autoantigens, but their reactions are not strong enough to eradicate these agents (Weimar and Schellekens 1979).

Therapy. This sort of thinking has led to therapeutic efforts directed at either suppression of the autoimmune reaction or stimulation of the immunosurveillance mechanism. The first mechanism, primarily through the use of prednisolone, has been widely tested and found to be quite effective in controlling CAH, particularly in HBsAg-negative patients who are also symptomatic (Schalm et al 1976). Eighty-five percent of B-negative patients responded beneficially to this therapy in that study, compared with slightly over half of HBsAg-positive patients. The dose of prednisolone, usually about 20 to 30 mg daily, must often be continued for extended periods of time, and lowered only gradually, with careful monitoring of hepatic function tests and liver biopsies for evidence of recurrent inflammation. A critical review of three glucocorticoid trials (Wright et al 1977) concluded that therapy is of proved efficacy only in patients who are both symptomatic and HBsAg negative, and who have severe histological abnormalities of the liver. Patients who are free of symptoms and have only mild tissue changes should probably be observed regularly without treatment.

A later study (Lam et al 1981) indicates that prednisolone is probably dangerous in patients with chronic viral active hepatitis who are HBsAg positive. Each member of a pair of patients was randomly assigned to drug or placebo, and biochemical remissions appeared to be delayed significantly in the prednisolone group. Mortality was also greater among patients on the glucocorticoid. Among patients with nonviral CAH who respond to glucocorticoid therapy by converting to a histologic picture of persistent hepatitis (portal lymphoid hyperplasia without hepatocellular necrosis) (Zaja et al 1981) have shown that nearly half will relapse to CAH after the drug is withdrawn. Over 80 percent of the relapses responded to treatment, but some developed cirrhosis. This finding indicates that patients with CAH require prolonged surveillance.

Immunostimulation is only in its infancy as a therapeutic tool in CAH, and little can be conclusively said about it. Transfer factor may be both immunologic and antiviral (Pizza et al 1979). In one series of nine patients with chronic active hepatitis associated with HBs antigenemia, transfer factor from patients with acute hepatitis B replicated on lymphoblastoid cells was administered. Seven patients had subjective improvement, five displayed decreased levels of aminotransferases, and liver biopsies in four showed improvement after therapy. Only one patient developed a negative test for HBs antigen. Levamisole (a stimulant of T-cell function), and BCG vaccine (a nonspecific immunostimulant) have also been tried in small studies, and results have been encouraging, particularly in patients with virus B CAH. Much needs to be learned about the possible toxicity of these agents and about their effectiveness over extended periods of time. For the present, glucocorticoid therapy appears to be the most useful and widely available tool in patients who qualify for it, although its value in CAH associated with hepatitis virus B is limited.

REYE-MORGAN-BARAL (RMB) SYNDROME

This curious and often devastating syndrome appears to be the result of altered host responses to viral infections, perhaps genetically determined, with extensive mitochondrial damage occurring acutely throughout the body, but especially in the liver, brain, and kidneys (Haller 1980). Mitochondria in the liver and brain become grossly enlarged, developing an ameboid appearance, and fat accumulates in microvesicular cytoplasmic droplets. Carbohydrate metabolism is deranged by the depletion of urea cycle enzymes, the production of protein by the liver is reduced, and hyperammonemia develops. Progressively severe coma develops associated with cerebral edema, and death results if this complication cannot be controlled. Although no exogenous poisons have been involved in the pathogenesis of this syndrome, Reye et al (1963) noted the similarity of the fatty changes in various organs to those seen also in children with crotalaria intoxication. It is more likely that a toxic metabolite produced in response to a viral insult is responsible for the illness, since patients with RMB syndrome do not excrete the hypoglycin metabolites typical of crotalaria (Tanaka et al 1976).

While RMB syndrome occurs most commonly in children, a few cases have been described in adults as well (Atkins and Haponik 1979). It occurs often during influenza B epidemics, and occasionally after infections with influenza A, varicella, adeno, and Cocksackie viruses. The major criteria for diagnosing this disorder are: (1) a history of recent viral infection; (2) vomiting, often repeatedly, at the onset; (3) progressively severe alterations of the sensorium, ranging from hypomanic behavior to deep coma; (4) absence of a history of drug ingestion; (5) slight hyperbilirubinemia; (6) absence of pleocytosis in spinal fluid. Laboratory data include moderate to marked elevations of serum aminotransferases, prolongation of the prothrombin time, elevated serum ammonia levels, and in children, hypoglycemia. Liver biopsy need not be done when the diagnosis is clearly supported by history and findings but is useful in questionable cases. The biopsy is characteristic in showing enlarged hepatocytes containing tiny cytoplasmic fat droplets, plus minimal hepatocytic necrosis and inflammatory infiltrate.

Treatment of RMB syndrome is primarily supportive, with most attention being given to the monitoring of intracranial pressure, either indirectly by symptoms, or directly, with intracranial sensors in patients with advanced degrees of coma. Patients who die appear to succumb to cerebral edema or herniation of the cerebellar tonsils rather than to hepatic failure, although the hyperammonemia contributes to the encephalopathy. The administration of glucose-, oxygen-, and ammonia-lowering agents is helpful, and mannitol has been found useful in lowering intracranial pressure.

HISTORICAL DIGRESSION

Personages mentioned in this chapter without further reference include: John Langdon Haydon DOWN (1828–1896), British physician, London; Michael Anthony EPSTEIN (1921–), British virologist, London, Bristol, described virus of Burkitt lymphoma, 1964; Ernest William GOODPASTURE

(1886–1960), American pathologist, Nashville, described hemorrhagic pulmonorenal syndrome, 1919; Adolf WEIL (1848–1916), German internist, Dorpat, Wiesbaden; Karl WERNICKE (1848–1905), German neuropsychiatrist, Berlin, Breslau, Halle, described encephalopathy of alcoholics, 1881.

SELECTED REFERENCES

Aach RD, Szmuness W, Mosley JW, et al. Serum alanine aminotransferase of donors in relation to the risk of non-A, non-B hepatitis in recipients. The transfusion-transmitted viruses study. N Engl J Med 304:989–94, 1981.

Almeida JD, Rubenstein D, Stott EJ. New antigen-antibody system in Australia-antigen-positive hepatitis. Lancet 2:1225–27, 1971.

Alter HJ, Purcell RH, Feinstone SM, et al. Non-A, non-B hepatitis: A review and interim report of an ongoing prospective study. In: Vyas G, Cohen SN, Schmid R, eds. Viral hepatitis. Philadelphia: The Franklin Institute Press, 1978:359–69.

Alter HJ, Seeff LB, Kaplan PM, et al. Type B hepatitis: the infectivity of blood positive for *e* antigen and DNA polymerase after accidental needlestick exposure. New Engl J Med 295:909–13, 1976.

Atkins JN, Haponik EF. Reye's syndrome in the adult patient. Am J Med 67: 672–78, 1979.

Barin F, André M, Coursaget P, et al. Vaccin contre l'hépatite B: caractérisation des polypeptides constitutifs de l'enveloppe du virus de l'hépatite B. Ann Microbiol (Paris) 130:505–10, 1979.

Barker LF, Gerety RJ, Tabor E. The immunology of the hepatitis viruses. Adv Int Med 23:327–51, 1978.

Baronoa E, Matsuda Y, Pikkarainen P, et al. Exaggeration of the ethanol-induced decrease in liver microtubules after chronic alcohol consumption: role of acetaldehyde. Gastroenterology 76:1274, 1979.

Berry RE, Jr. Estimating the economic costs of alcohol use. New Engl J Med 295:620–21, 1976.

Black M. Acetaminophen hepatotoxicity. Gastroenterology 78:382–92, 1980.

Blumberg BS, Alter HJ, Visnich S. A "new" antigen in leukemia sera. JAMA 191:541–46, 1965.

Blumberg BS, Friedlaender JS, Woodside A, et al. Hepatitis and Australia antigen: autosomal recessive inheritance of susceptibility to infection in humans. Proc Nat Acad Sci USA 62:1108–15, 1969.

Boitnoit JK, Maddrey WC. Suppression of acute and chronic inflammation by prednisolone in alcoholic hepatitis. Gastroenterology 77:A5, 1979.

Branch RA, Nies AS, Read AE. The liver and drugs. In: Read AE, ed. Modern Trends in Gastroenterology-5. London: Butterworths, 1975:289–317.

Bryan JA, Gregg MB. Viral hepatitis in the United States, 1970-1973: an analysis of morbidity trends and the impact of HBsAg testing on surveillance and epidemiology. Am J Med Sci 270:271–82, 1975.

Buynak EB, Roehm RR, Tytell AA. Vaccine against human hepatitis B. JAMA 235:2832–34, 1976.
Corey LC, Holmes KK. Sexual transmission of hepatitis A in homosexual men. Incidence and mechanisms. New Engl J Med 302:435–38, 1980.
Courouce AM, Trepo C, Jungers P. Progrès recent dans la conaissance des hépatites virales. Nouve Presse Med 8:1731–34, 1979.
Coursaget P, Maupas P, Dubois F, et al. Hépatites non-A, non-B chez six malades hemodialysés. Nouve Presse Med 7:3515–19, 1978.
Coursaget P, Maupas P, Levin P, et al. Virus-like particles associated with non-A, non-B hepatitis. Lancet 2:92, 1979.
Czaja AJ, Ludwig J, Baggenstoss AH, et al. Corticosteroid treated chronic active hepatitis. Uncertain prognosis of chronic persistent hepatitis. N Engl J Med 304:5–9, 1981.
Dane DS, Cameron CH, Briggs M. Virus-like particles in serum of patients with Australia-antigen associated hepatitis. Lancet 1:695–98, 1970.
Denes AE, Smith JL, Maynard JE, et al. Hepatitis B infections in physicians. Results of a nationwide seroepidemiologic survey. JAMA 239:210–12, 1978.
Depew W, Boyer T, Omata M, et al. Double-blind controlled trial of prednisolone therapy in patients with severe acute alcoholic hepatitis and spontaneous encephalopathy. Gastroenterology 78:524–29, 1980.
Dienstag JL. Non-A, non-B hepatitis. Adv. Int Med 26:187–233, 1981.
Dienstag JL, Alaama A, Mosley J, et al. Etiology of sporadic hepatitis B surface antigen-negative hepatitis. Ann Int Med 87:1–12, 1977.
Eagon PK, Imhoff AF, Fisher SE, et al. Mechanism of hyperestrogenization in alcoholics: E_2/T ratio. Gastroenterology 75:961, 1978.
Edgington TS, Chisari FV. Immunological aspects of hepatitis B virus infection. Am J Med Sci 270:213–37, 1975.
FDA: Ticrynafen recalled. FDA Drug Bull 10:3–4 (Feb), 1980.
Feinstone SM, Kapikian AZ, Purcell RH. Hepatitis A: detection by immune electron microscopy of a virus-like antigen associated with acute illness. Science 182:1026–28, 1973.
Flaum A, Malmros H, Persson E. Eine noscomiale ikterus-epidemie. Acta med Scand Suppl 16:544–53, 1926.
Gerber MA, Sarno E, Vernace S. Immune complexes in hepatocytic nuclei of HB Ag-positive chronic hepatitis. New Engl J Med 294:922–25, 1976.
Goodwin DW, Schuksinger F, Moller N, et al. Drinking problems in adopted and non-adopted sons of alcoholics. Arch Gen Psychiatry 31:164–69, 1974.
Guzelian PS, Diegelmann RF. Demonstration of collagen synthesis by the hepatocyte. Gastroenterology 77:A15, 1979.
Hagler L, Pastore RA. Bergin JJ. Aplastic anemia following viral hepatitis: report of two fatal cases and literature review. Medicine 53:139–64, 1975.
Haller J. Intracranial pressure monitoring in Reye's syndrome. Hosp Pract 15:101–8 (Feb), 1980.

Hatfield G, Haines N, Schneider J. et al. A randomized trial of insulin and glucagon for alcoholic hepatitis. Gastroenterology 76:1284, 1979.

Haugen RK. Hepatitis after transfusion of frozen red cells and washed red cells. New Engl J Med 301:393–95, 1979.

Havens WP, Jr. Viral hepatitis. In: Anderson RS, ed. Internal medicine in World War II, vol 3. Infectious diseases and general medicine. Washington DC: Government Printing Office, 1968, pp 331–84.

Henley KS, Laughrey EG. Effect of ethanol on neutral extractable hydroxyproline containing peptides in rat liver. Gastroenterology 76:1284, 1979.

Hoofnagle JH, Seeff LB, Bales ZB, et al. Type B hepatitis after transfusion with blood containing antibody to hepatitis B core antigen. New Engl J Med 298:1379–83, 1978.

Hoofnagle JH, Seeff LB, Bales ZB, et al. Mechanism of action of hepatitis B immune globulin and immune serum globulin. Gastroenterology 76: 1284, 1979.

Hoofnagle JH, Waggoner JG. Hepatitis A and B virus markers in immune serum globulin. Gastroenterology 78:259–63, 1980.

Israel Y, Kalant H, Orrego H, et al. Experimental alcohol-induced hepatic necrosis: suppression by propylthiouracil. Proc Nat Acad Sci USA 72: 1137–41, 1975.

Israel Y, Videla L, Bernstein J. Liver hypermetabolic state after chronic ethanolic consumption: hormonal interrelationships and pathogenic implications. Fed Proc 34:2052–59, 1975.

Isselbacher KJ. Metabolic and hepatic effects of alcohol. New Engl J Med 296:612–16, 1977.

Kim CY, Lim KP, Funakoshi S. Prevention of viral hepatitis, type B, by vaccination with purified hepatitis B surface antigen. Gastroenterology 76:1287, 1979.

Kirtland HH, III, Mohler DN, Horwitz DA. Methyldopa inhibition of suppressor-lymphocyte function. A proposed cause of autoimmune hemolytic anemia. New Engl J Med 302:825–32, 1980.

Koff RS. Viral hepatitis. New York: John Wiley and Sons, 1978.

Krugman S, Overby LR, Mushahwar IK, et al. Viral hepatitis, type B. Studies on natural history and prevention re-examined. New Engl J Med 300: 101–6, 1979.

Lam KC, Lai CL, Trepo C, et al. Deleterious effect of prednisolone in HBsAg-positive chronic active hepatitis. N Engl J Med 304:380–86, 1981.

Leevy CM, Chen T, Zetterman R. Alcoholic hepatitis, cirrhosis, and immunologic reactivity. Ann NY Acad Sci 252:106–15, 1975.

Lue SL, Paronetto F, Lieber CS. Cytotoxicity of lymphocytes in alcoholic fatty liver: responsive role of lymphocytes and target cells. Gastroenterology 76:1290, 1979.

Lurman A. Eine icterusepidemie. Berl Klin Wchnschr 22:20–23, 1885.

Maddrey WC, Boitnott JK. Drug-induced chronic liver disease. Gastroenterology 72:1348–53, 1977.

Magnius LO, Espmark JA. New specificites in Australia-antigen positive sera distinct from LeBouvier determinants. J Immunol 109:1017–21, 1972.

Martin CJ. Concerning the pathology and etiology of the infectious jaundice common at the Dardenelles, 1915. Br Med J 1:445–47, 1917.

Maupas P, Goudeau A, Coursaget P, et al. Immunization against hepatitis B in man: a pilot study of two years' duration. In: Vyas G, Cohen SN, Schmid R, eds. Viral hepatitis. Philadelphia: The Franklin Institute Press, 1978:539–56.

Mendelson JH, Mello NK. Biologic concomitants of alcoholism. New Engl J Med 301:912–21, 1979.

Meyer zum Buschenfelde KH, Hutterrroth TH, Arnold W, et al. Immunologic liver injury: the role of hepatitis B viral antigens and liver membrane antigens as targets. In: Popper H, Schaffner F, eds. Progress in liver disease, vol 6. New York: Grune and Stratton, 1979:407–24.

Mezey E. Ethanol: metabolism and adverse affects. Viewpoints Dig Dis 11: 1–4 (March), 1979.

Miller DJ, Ishimaru H, Klatskin G. Non-alcoholic liver disease mimicking alcoholic hepatitis and cirrhosis. Gastroenterology 77:A27 (Nov), 1978.

Mitchell JR, Lauterburg BH. Drug-induced liver injury. Hosp Pract 13:95–106 (Sept), 1978.

Mitchell JR, Zimmerman JH, Ishak KG, et al. Isoniazid liver injury: clinical spectrum, pathology, and probable pathogenesis. Ann Int Med 84:181–92, 1976.

Mosley JW. The epidemiology of viral hepatitis: an overview. Am J Med Sci 270:253–70, 1975.

Nielsen JO, Dietrichson O, Juhl E. Incidence and meaning of the "e" determinant among hepatitis-B-antigen positive patients with acute and chronic liver diseases: report from the Copenhagen Hepatitis Acute Program. Lancet 2:913–15, 1974.

Okada K, Kamiyama I, Inomata M, et al. E antigen and anti-e in the serum of asymptomatic carrier mothers as indicators of positive and negative transmission of hepatitis B to their infants. New Engl J Med 294:746–49, 1976.

Orrego H, Kalant H, Israel Y, et al. Effect of short-term therapy with propylthiouracil in patients with alcoholic liver disease. Gastroenterology 76: 105–15, 1979.

Paul JR, Gardner HT. Viral hepatitis. In: Coates JB, Jr., ed. Preventive medicine in World War II, vol 5. Communicable diseases transmitted through contact or by unknown means. Washington DC: Government Printing Office, 1960:411–62.

Pizza G, Viza D, Roda A, et al. Transfer factor for the treatment of chronic active hepatitis. New Engl J Med 300:1332, 1979.

Prince AM. An antigen detected in the blood during the incubation period of serum hepatitis. Proc Nat Acad Sci USA 60:814–21, 1968.

Prince AM. Use of hepatitis B immune globulin: reassessment needed. New Engl J Med 299:198–99, 1978.

Prince AM, Trepo C, Vitvitski L, et al. Hepatitis C virus: characterization of virus specific antigens and associated particles. Gastroenterology 77: A33 (Nov), 1979.

Purcell RH, Gerin JL. Hepatitis B subunit vaccine: a preliminary report of safety and efficacy tests in chimpanzees. Am J Med Sci 270:395–404, 1975.

Redeker AG. Viral hepatitis: clinical aspects. Am J Med Sci 270:9–16, 1975.

Reye RDK, Morgan G, Baral J. Encephalopathy and fatty degeneration of the viscera: a disease entity in childhood. Lancet 2:749–52, 1963.

Robinson WS, Lutwick LI. The virus of hepatitis, type B. New Engl J Med 295:1168–75, 1232–36, 1976.

Rubin E, Lieber CS. Fatty liver, alcoholic hepatitis and cirrhosis produced by alcohol in primates. New Engl J Med 290:128–35, 1974.

Schalm SW, Summerskill WHK, Gitnick GL, et al. Contrasting features and responses to treatment of severe chronic active liver disease with and without hepatitis B antigen. Gut 17:781, 1976.

Szmuness W, Dienstag JL, Purcell RH, et al. Distribution of antibody to hepatitis A antigen in urban adult populations. New Engl J Med 295:755–59, 1976.

Szmuness W. Harley EJ, Pribe AM. Intrafamilial spread of asymptomatic hepatitis B. Am J Med Sci 270:293–304, 1975.

Szmuness W, Stevens CE, Harley EJ, et al. Hepatitis B vaccine. Demonstration of efficacy in a controlled trial in a high risk population in the United States. N Engl J Med 303:833–41, 1980.

Takekoshi Y, Tanaka M, Miyakawa Y, et al. Free "small" and IgG-associated "large" hepatitis B e antigen in the serum and glomerular capillary walls of two patients with membranous glomerulonephritis. New Engl J Med 300:814–19, 1979.

Tanaka K, Kean EA, Johnson B. Jamaican vomiting sickness. Biochemical investigation of two cases. New Engl J Med 295:461–67, 1976.

Tao CM, Huang TY, Feng PF, et al. A preliminary study on hepatitis B vaccine. Chinese MJ 4:101–10, 1978.

Tong MJ, Rakela J, McPeak CM, et al. Studies in infants born to mothers with type A hepatitis and acute non-A, non-B hepatitis during pregnancy. Gastroenterology 75:991, 1978.

Trepo C, Hantz O, Vitvitski L, et al. Heterogeneity and significance of HBeAG: characterization of third specificity(e3). Gastroenterology 75: 991, 1978.

Trepo C, Vitvitski L, Prince AM. Demonstration in serum and liver of an antigen specific for long incubation non-A, non-B hepatitis (HCAg). Gastroenterology 77:A44 (Nov), 1979.

Villarejos VM, Visona KA, Eduarte A, et al. Evidence for viral hepatitis other than type A or type B among persons in Costa Rica. N Engl J Med 293: 1350–52, 1975.
Weimar W, Schellekens H. Prophylaxis and therapy of HBsAg positive hepatitis. Biomedicine 30:135–38, 1979.
Wilcox WH. Epidemic jaundice of campaigns. Br Med J 1:297–300, 1916.
Wilson HA, McLaren GD, Dworken HJ, et al. Transient pure red cell aplasia: cell-mediated suppression of erythropoiesis associated with hepatitis. Ann Int Med 92:196–98, 1980.
Woodward JJ. Outline of the chief camp diseases of the United States armies. Philadelphia: JB Lippincott, 1863. Reprinted, New York: Hafner Publishing Company, 1964:193.
Worner T, Lieber CS. Prognostic value of perivenular sclerosis in the progression of alcoholic liver injury. Gastroenterology 75:995, 1978.
Wright EC, Seeff LB, Berk PD, et al. Treatment of chronic active hepatitis. An analysis of three controlled trials. Gastroenterology 73:1422–30, 1977.
Zimmerman HJ. Hepatotoxicity. New York: Appleton-Century-Crofts, 1978.

DISCUSSION QUESTION

A promising new drug has been developed for the treatment of hay fever. How would you investigate its possible hepatotoxicity? Under what circumstances would you approve of its release for general use? Would these circumstances differ if the drug were strikingly effective in the treatment of acute myelogenous leukemia?

CHAPTER 11

Singular Forms of Cirrhosis of the Liver

Numerous types of chronic liver disease can be considered as singular, in that they are both distinctive and uncommon. Knowledge of them has helped to broaden our understanding of hepatic metabolism and of the general disease which is manifested partly in the liver. Each of these disorders has a pattern of genetic inheritance, some more clearly than others, and each may lead to portal hypertension, esophageal varices, and hepatic failure. The forms of cirrhosis to be discussed are those associated with Wilson disease, hemochromatosis, alpha-1-antitrypsin deficiency, cystic fibrosis, and primary biliary cirrhosis.

WILSON DISEASE

The year 1912 was a landmark in neurohepatology. Samuel Alexander Kinnier Wilson (1878-1937) of the National Hospital, Queen Square, London, won both a doctoral degree and a gold medal from the University of Edinburgh for the publication of his lengthy article on "progressive lenticular degeneration associated with cirrohosis of the liver" in that year. And Bruno Fleischer (b1874), of the eye clinic, University of Tubingen, also in 1912, reported on patients with "pseudosclerosis closely related to a formerly unrecognized disease, characterized by tremor, psychic disturbances, brownish pigment in certain tissues, especially the periphery of the cornea, and cirrhosis of the liver." Unknowingly, Wilson and Fleischer had described the same disease almost simultaneously.

Wilson had performed autopsies on two patients with this familial disorder which "occurs always in young people" and "is progressive and invariably fatal." He was impressed with their neurological symptoms, which are now classified as extrapyramidal, consisting of involuntary movements, a rhythmical tremor, aggravated by intention, spasticity of the limbs and face, dysphagia, and dysarthria. He was able to associate these changes with "bilateral symmetrical softening in the lenticular nucleus," involving the putamen primarily and the globus pallidus occasionally. But "the most curious and the most remarkable feature of the familial nervous disease is the constant presence of a profound degree of cirrhosis of the liver. This hepatic cirrhosis does not reveal itself by any symptoms during life, nevertheless it is always found after death" (p.297). Wilson felt that he needed to have autopsy results on a third patient to confirm the invariable presence of cirrhosis as a part of the neurological disease.

Such a patient had indeed been identified on the basis of his neurological presentation, which was exactly the same as the others. There was no evidence of hepatic disease and, to make matters worse, he had decided to spend his declining days in Switzerland's alpine surroundings. Undaunted, Wilson arranged to be notified upon the patient's demise and, when word of that event came, he obtained an autopsy permit, spent 10 gold sovereigns on a ticket to Chexbres, and performed the examination in Switzerland. The autopsy was performed 27 hours after death, and Wilson's notes describe the excellent state of preservation of the body due to the fact that "the sanitorium was at a considerable altitude and the nights very cold." Critchley describes Wilson's own appraisal of his emotional state at that time. His entire thesis depended upon finding an abnormal liver, and wishing to postpone the inevitable, he left the examination of the abdomen until the very last. "Eventually he steeled himself to insert his hand and palpate the liver surface. To his relief he realized that the surface of the shrunken liver was nodular, indicating an advanced degree of cirrhosis. For quite a while he was so overcome by emotion that he could not proceed."*

Wilson acknowledged that six other patients with this disease had been described years before, two having been reported by Sir William Richard Gower (1845–1915) in 1906, one by J.A. Omerod of London in 1890, and three by Ernst Alexander Homén (1851–1926) of Helsingfors (Helsinki), also in 1890. But none before had associated the basal ganglion lesion as clearly as had Wilson with the extrapyramidal symptoms displayed by the patients.

For his part, Fleischer credited Bernhard Kayser (1869–1954), a fellow opthalmologist from Tubingen, with the first description of the corneal pigmentary ring in 1902. One year later, Fleischer saw two more patients and, in 1908, a fourth case was added by R. Salus of the University Eye Clinic in Prague. The specific cerebral lesion was not clear to Fleischer, nor was the familial nature of the disease, but he did recognize that pigmentation was generalized throughout many parts of the body, including skin, blood vessels, liver, and kidneys. Homén and the British physicians were

*Critchley M. The divine banquet of the brain. New York: Raven Press, 1979:190.

unaware of the pigmentary changes in the corneas, and Wilson failed completely to appreciate the significance of the "exceedingly sunburnt" appearance of two of his patients, as well as the true hereditary nature of the illness. Homén felt that the disease was a variety of vascular syphilis, Salus a form of multiple sclerosis. Only Wilson and Fleischer appeared to realize the singularity of this condition.

Speaking in a purely historical sense, hepatolenticular degeneration should properly be known also as Gower-Omerod-Homén-Fleischer-Wilson disease, and the corneal pigmentation as Kayser-Fleischer-Salus rings, but time is saved by our natural tendency to abbreviate. Today, the disorder in all forms, including the premorbid condition, is known as Wilson disease, and the corneal pigmentation, which with good medical care will never be seen again, as Kayser-Fleischer rings. Our debt to medical history is permanently and justly recorded in these eponyms, but it is too bad about Omerod and the others.

Pathophysiology

That abnormally heavy deposition of copper throughout the body was the direct cause of Wilson disease had been suspected for many years preceding Glazebrook's clear demonstration of increased amounts of that element in the liver and brain of a single patient in 1945. Numerous subsequent studies have confirmed and extended this observation, causing Walshe (1967) to estimate that the liver of patients with documented Wilson disease contains 10 to 40 times the normal amount of that element. Copper strongly inhibits tissue enzymes, particularly those with sulfhydryl groups, and pyruvate kinase and membranous ATPase. This poisoning of enzyme systems is believed to be responsible for cytotoxicity in the brain, liver, renal tubules, and bone marrow.

Patients with Wilson disease are almost invariably unable to synthesize the protein ceruloplasmin, which normally carries eight atoms of copper on a single molecule. Isotope studies have shown that the normal liver binds ingested copper to ceruloplasmin which then circulates to the blood or is excreted in the bile. Patients with Wilson disease have low levels of copper excretion into the bile (Strickland 1975). Typically, they have slightly depressed levels of serum copper and markedly increased urinary excretion of copper, in addition to very low levels of ceruloplasmin. Urinary copper levels are believed to rise after the liver becomes saturated with that metal.

Symptoms vary considerably from patient to patient. Many with advanced symptoms of basal ganglion disease show no clinical or laboratory evidence of liver disease, although hepatic copper levels are invariably elevated. Some present with symptoms of subacute or chronic active hepatitis, while other patients show signs of damage to other organ systems, especially the kidneys and the bone marrow. Renal symptoms consist primarily of those related to dysfunction of proximal renal tubules (Fanconi syndrome): aminoaciduria, glucosuria, and phosphaturia, as well as loss of bicarbonate potassium and water. Renal tubular acidosis and osteomalacia may be associated. Marrow dysfunction is manifested as a hemolytic anemia, at times associated with jaundice, and the presence of calcified bilirubinate gallstones. Some patients have nearly normal or only slightly reduced levels of ceruloplasmin but show an inability to incorporate radiocopper into ceruloplasmin (Sternlieb and Scheinberg 1979).

Hepatic changes on biopsy are also quite variable and not diagnostic. Hepatocytes often show some fat and focal regeneration; Mallory hyaline is present at times. Inflammation is uncommon, although occasionally signs of chronic active hepatitis are seen. Fibrotic changes range from periportal accumulations to macronodular cirrhosis. Rubionic staining often shows cytoplasmic accumulations of copper, and hepatic tissue usually shows more than 50 μg copper (normally up to 25 μg) per g of drug weight.

Diagnosis

The objective of diagnosis is to accomplish it before irreversible cerebral and hepatic disease occur. Accordingly, one must have a high index of suspicion, especially among relatives of known patients. One should think of Wilson disease in young patients with chronic hepatitis of unexplained cause, psychoses of recent onset, hemolytic anemias, and renal tubular acidosis (Cartwright 1978). Kayser-Fleischer rings are diagnostic of the disease, are found in all patients with neurological symptoms, and are frequently present prior to the appearance of such complaints. The incidence of Wilson disease is low, somewhat more than 1 in 1 million (Bearn 1957), and the diagnosis is often overlooked. Siblings of patients with the disease should be carefully examined, because they have one chance in four of having the problem. Siblings of parents of patients may also be heterozygotes and should be informed of the problems attached to consanguineous marriages.

A ceruloplasmin level below 20 μg (normally 90 to 130 μg) per dl is not adequate by itself to diagnose Wilson disease, since 10 percent of carriers also have low levels and never develop the illness (Sternlieb 1978). Urinary copper levels over 100 μg (normally 10 to 50 μg) per day are confirmatory, and increased hepatic copper levels are nearly diagnostic. Equivocal urinary copper excretion can be followed by retesting after a dose of penicillamine (500 mg), which chelates excess copper and rapidly appears in the urine. Failure of radiocopper levels to become elevated a day after oral ingestion indicates inability to bind copper to ceruloplasmin and is highly compatible with the diagnosis. Liver biopsy and isotope studies are unnecessary when Kayser-Fleischer rings are present.

Therapy

Penicillamine (dimethyl cysteine), which chelates copper through a single sulfhydryl group per molecule, is the drug of choice in Wilson disease. Through its use, body copper stores can be reduced to normal. Treatment must be lifelong, since there is no easy way to restrict copper intake through diet. Nephrotic complications, fever, rashes, and leukopenia may occur, but often these problems can be controlled by desensitization to the drug. Maintenance dose is around 1.0 g per day, depending on patient's response. The advent of chelation therapy has converted Wilson disease from a uniformly fatal disorder to a curious genetic abormality.

HEMOCHROMATOSIS

Hemochromatosis results when both excessive deposition of iron is present throughout the body, and organ necrosis, fibrosis, and dysfunction have resulted from this abnormality. Symptomatic hemochromatosis does not usually appear until the total body content of iron exceeds 5 to 10 times the normal level (Bothwell and Charlton 1975), although recent studies (Beaumont et al 1979; Cartwright et al 1979) have clearly shown that the metabolic disorder can be identified long before. Lesser states of iron accumulation may appear in generalized or in organ-limited forms, without organ dysfunction, and are called *hemosiderosis*. The causes of hemochromatosis are distinct from the causes of hemosiderosis, the latter being invariably a secondary process, while the former may be either primary (idiopathic) or secondary. Thus. hemosiderosis may occur as a consequence of cirrhosis in alcoholics, but levels of hepatic iron are only 2 to 3 times normal and the deposition of iron does not appear to aggravate the disease. Hemochromatosis, on the other hand, results in much higher concentrations of iron in the liver, and directly causes hepatic necrosis and fibrosis. Confusion frequently results when hepatic damage is found in patients with idiopathic hemochromatosis who happen to be alcoholic as well.

In hemosiderosis, the accumulation of hepatic iron is greatest in Kupffer cells and in portal macrophages; in hemochromatosis, iron accumulates preponderantly in hepatocytes and in bile ductular epithelium. Among patients without cirrhosis, the distribution of iron pigment in liver biopsies provides a helpful index for distinguishing between hemochromatosis and hemosiderosis, but actual measurement of hepatic iron content provides more accurate information.

Normal Metabolism of Iron

In humans, total body iron ranges between 3 and 4 g, two-thirds of which is located in hemoglobin, myoglobin, and cellular-oxidizing enzymes throughout the body. Most of the remainder is stored in the liver, bone marrow, and reticuloendothelial cells, while small amounts are found in many other tissues. Ferrokinetic studies have demonstrated a number of iron pools in the body—the red cell pool, the erythropoietic pool, the storage pool, a small plasma pool, and a labile pool. The plasma and labile pools turn over at rapid rates, the former receiving iron from absorption and from destroyed red cells and enzymes, and the latter acting as an intermediary for plasma pool iron and passing it either to the erythropoietic pool or, when levels are high, to storage. The red cell pool turns over at an intermediate rate; the storage pool is quite stable.

The absorption of iron in the duodenum and jejunum is aided by gastric acidity and by ascorbic acid, and the amount of iron absorbed varies directly with the amount ingested and the degree of deficiency in the body. Absorption in the upper small intestine is probably also aided by the presence of gastric mucoproteins which appear to reduce flocculation of iron. The amount of iron absorbed from food is quite variable, but more is absorbed from meat than from vegetables. The mechanics of epithelial uptake of iron are not known, but the rate of absorption is increased in patients with hemochromatosis, iron deficiency states, anemias resulting from shortened red cell survival, and after portacaval shunts. Patients with malabsorption, iron overloads, erythroid hypoplasia, and achlorhydria absorb iron at a slower rate than normal (Brown 1979).

Upon absorption, iron binds to *transferrin*, a plasma beta globulin (mol wt 75,000), which is synthesized in the liver and has a half-life of 7 to 10 days. Transferrin-bound iron circulates to the labile, hematopoietic, or storage pools, depending on requirements, and excesses beyond current needs are stored in various parts of the body, but particularly in hepatocytes and the reticuloendothelial system of the liver, spleen, and bone marrow, in the form of *ferritin*. This is a large, water-soluble protein (mol wt 460,000), each molecule of which contains 2,000 molecules of ferric oxyhydroxide. Ferritin is made in the liver and elsewhere and has at least two isomeric subunits, the significance of which is not clear. Some ferritin, perhaps that derived from the reticuloendothelial system, circulates in plasma, where its concentration reflects total stores of body iron (Powell et al 1980). The ferritin contained in epithelial cells shed by the intestine is responsible for the small (1 mg) amount of iron lost daily by healthy men and women. Menstruation and increased iron demands during pregnancy account for further losses of body iron and lower levels of circulating ferritin among women. Ferritin and hepatic iron levels vary moderately between healthy men and women, as a reflection of these physiologic differences (Table 11-1). *Hemosiderin* is a large, yellowish brown, water-insoluble, irregular crystalline complex which accumulates intracellularly in various iron overload conditions. It appears to be derived from large accumulations of ferritin molecules.

Table 11-1. Iron Status in Normal Subjects and in Patients Heterozygous and Homozygous for Idiopathic Hemochromatosis (95 percent limits)

	Men			Women		
	Normals	*Heterozygotes*	*Homozygotes*	*Normals*	*Heterozygotes*	*Homozygotes*
Serum iron (μg/dl)	50–162	62–208	173–307	42–160	40–181	145–261
Transferrin saturation%	14–50	19–69	80–100	10–50	10–63	73–90
Serum ferritin (ng/ml)	16–542	15–617	565–11,560	7–330	8–335	106–1,390
Hepatic iron (μg/100 mg wet liver)	0–29	0–282	486–1,417	0–19	0–191	59–1,109

Source: After Cartwright et al 1979.

Idiopathic Hemochromatosis

This disease appears to be inherited as an autosomal recessive characteristic, fully expressed in homozygotes and partially expressed without clinical consequences in many heterozygotes (Cartwright et al 1979). There is an association of HLA antigens A3 and B14 with idiopathic hemochromatosis (Simon et al 1977), and many investigators believe that the genetic tendency can be detected by elevated levels of serum ferritin and suggest that serum ferritin levels may actually be a marker of the hemochromatosis allele (Beaumont et al 1979). While some patients with hepatic iron overloads and normal serum ferritin levels have been found, most investigators believe that there are fewer falsely negative serum ferritin levels in patients with precirrhotic hemochromatosis than there are falsely negative serum iron and transferrin saturation levels in similar cases. Serum ferritin levels are invariably elevated in patients with cirrhotic hemochromatosis, and may be elevated in nonhemochromatotic heterozygotes. Full expression of idiopathic hemochromatosis is probably on the basis of autosomal recessive inheritance (Simon et al 1980).

Pathophysiology. Patients with idiopathic hemochromatosis absorb excessive amounts of ingested iron from the small intestine, also appear to remove iron intrahepatically from transferrin more rapidly than normal (Batey et al 1978), and may show a deficiency in the ability of their reticuloendothelial systems to store iron released from aging red cells (Fillet and Marsaglia 1975). Whatever the cause, massive increases in bodily iron stores appear in untreated patients, and the accumulations are greatest in the liver, pancreas, spleen, heart, pituitary, adrenals, thyroid, and skin. Cutaneous accumulations lead to a dusky grayish brown coloration of the skin, especially in areas exposed to light, and endocrine deficiencies manifested by diabetes, from islet cell dysfunction, hypogonadism from pituitary involvement, and mild degrees of adrenal cortical insufficiency are common. In the pancreas, iron deposition occurs in acinar cells as well, and malabsorption due to exocrine deficiency may be part of the clinical picture. The gland becomes fibrotic, deeply pigmented and atrophic.

Greatest havoc occurs in the liver of patients with untreated hemochromatosis. That the deposition of excessive amounts of iron is responsible for the tissue damage appears to be agreed on generally, but the mechanism of that effect is not clear. Certainly, removal of iron by phlebotomy in patients with hemochromatosis reduces the severity of the hepatic necrosis and fibrosis. Powell et al (1980) quote evidence which suggests that iron increases lysosomal fragility in hepatocytes and may thereby lead to cytoplasmic damage from release of lysosomal enzymes. There is also some evidence that free iron radicals may be formed when hepatocytic storage capacity is exceeded, and that these electrophilic radicals can cause damage to cytoplasmic macromolecules, much as carbon tetrachloride does. Finally, there has been some suggestion that iron stimulates collagen synthesis and may induce hepatic fibrosis without hepatocytic necrosis. The fact that iron deposits primarily into hepatocytes in hemochromatosis, probably because of increased rate of release from transferrin, appears to be of some importance in explaining why liver damage occurs in this disease and not in transfusion hemosiderosis, where iron deposition is primarily into Kupffer cells.

Whatever the reason for hepatic damage, the pathologic changes in the liver can be quite severe and are typified by large accumulations of hemosiderin in parenchymal cells, and in portal and lobular macrophages, and by hepatocytic necrosis and micronodular or macronodular regeneration, plus fibrosis. Proliferation of bile ducts is marked, so that the picture of cirrhosis is complete, and iron deposits are also noted in biliary epithelium. In advanced cases, it may be difficult for the pathologist to tell whether the pigment deposition is a result of primary hemochromatosis or if it is secondary to other forms of cirrhosis. Iron deposits in fibrous strands, a tendency for iron deposition to be in the periphery of the lobule, and the relative lack of inflammation favor primary hemochromatosis, as does a relative paucity of iron in Kupffer cells. In patients without cirrhosis, hemosiderin in the periphery of the lobule favors hemochromatosis, while centrilobular hemosiderin is more likely to be seen in congestive heart failure (Kent and Popper 1968). Actual measurement of tissue iron stores may be necessary in uncertain cases.

Symptoms. The purpose of modern efforts at case finding by testing of family members of patients with known hemochromatosis is, of course, to prevent the patient from ever becoming symptomatic. Where symptoms do appear, they are no different now than they were in an early description by Hanot and Schachmann in 1886, who coined the term bronze diabetes to describe this newly discovered entity. Patients were middle-aged and generally impressive by their deeply pigmented skin, not related to jaundice, and by their large firm livers, abdominal discomfort, and wasting. Diabetes often appeared after the onset of portal hypertension, ascites and generalized asthenia. In fact, Hanot commented in one of his cases about the sudden appearance of a good appetite in a formerly anorectic patient. His and the patient's joy was quickly dispelled when he discovered that the return of appetite was only a symptom of the onset of diabetes. But, since diabetes may precede signs of hepatic insufficiency, liver function testing, serum ferritin measurements and possibly liver biopsy, should be done on all new diabetics in their middle years of life, particularly if there is no family history of that disease. Testicular atrophy and mild degress of adrenal insufficiency may also be found in advanced cases. Congestive heart failure and arthritis, the latter due to chondrocalcinosis, are commonly seen. Hepatocellular carcinomas occur in 15 to 20 percent of patients with associated cirrhosis.

Diagnosis. Diagnosis of idiopathic hemochromatosis may be difficult in the absence of a positive family history. This is particularly true in the alcoholic patient in whom the liver disease precedes the hemochromatosis. The best approach is to measure serum ferritin levels, which are always high in idiopathic hemochromatosis, and to perform direct measures of serum iron and transferrin saturation. Slight to moderately decreased levels of serum iron with heavy saturation of transferrin (approaching 100 percent) are clear evidences of the disease. Following this, a liver biopsy (Figure 11-1) showing massively increased amounts of iron is diagnostic, provided secondary causes of hemochromatosis can be ruled out (see below).

Where doubt remains about the diagnosis, some physicians have been helped by giving the patient deferoxamine, an iron-chelating agent, and measuring the urinary excretion of iron for the following 24 hours. In one study, patients with hemochromatosis excreted an average of 11 mg of iron, while patients with cirrhosis and iron overload excreted only somewhat more than half that amount, and other cirrhotics much less.

Treatment. Treatment of the symptomatic patient consists of conventional management of diabetes and congestive heart failure if present and, most importantly, the removal of excess iron stores. Weekly phlebotomy of 500 ml of blood, continued for up to two to three years, may be necessary to rid the patients of their excessive iron stores. The frequency and amount of blood removal relates, of course, to the patient's tolerance, and serum iron studies

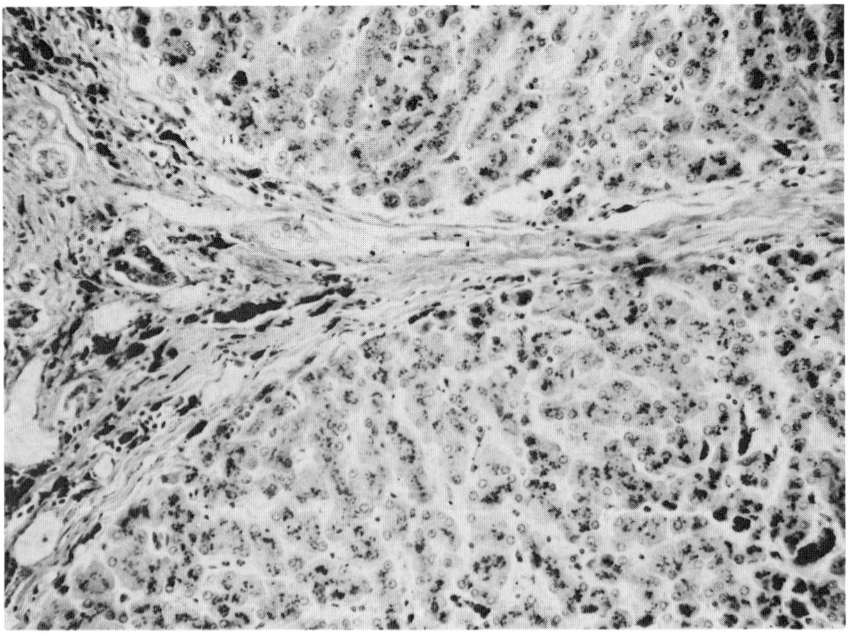

Figure 11-1. Hemochromatosis. Iron pigment is present in hepatocytes, Kupffer cells, and bile ducts. Original magnification x250.

and hemotocrits should be done at monthly intervals during active therapy. Patients generally tolerate the phlebotomies quite well and, when iron stores have been normalized, can usually be maintained well with three or four venesections per year. The effect of phlebotomy in reducing iron stores can be measured by occasional testing with deferoxamine (Baldus et al 1978) and suspending treatment when deferoxamine-chelatable iron falls below 300 μg/kg.

Surveillance. As is also the case with Wilson disease, diagnosis and treatment of the proband with idiopathic hemochromatosis is only a first step in management of the entire problem. While hemochromatosis is almost certainly an autosomal recessive characteristic, the frequency of the responsible gene is high and the incidence of the disease is correspondingly significant. Families of patients should thus be examined for evidence of consanguinity, and first-degree relatives of patients should be tested for evidence of elevated ferritin and serum iron levels. Siblings particularly, who have no evidence of increased iron stores when first seen, should be retested annually, because abnormalities will doubtless eventually occur in those who are actual homozygotes. Routine liver biopsies and HLA typing should probably not be done unless iron status is abnormal, because of the expense and discomfort of these procedures. Evidence indicates that phlebotomy should be undertaken as soon as an asymptomatic homozygote is identified, and continued as often as necessary to maintain iron stores at normal levels.

Secondary Hemochromatosis

Iron may accumulate in the liver as a result of many chronic disorders, especially those which involve defective erythropoiesis or chronic hemolysis (thalassemia major, sickle cell anemia, sideroblastic anemias), portacaval shunting, and excessively high intakes of iron. As has been indicated earlier, these conditions result mainly in siderosis, with iron accumulating primarily in Kupffer cells and hepatic damage being slight, unless the patient also has preexisting liver disease from other causes. A small number of these patients, however, actually develop a secondary form of hemochromatosis, not genetically determined, and may show pancreatic and cardiac dysfunction as well. All patients at risk for siderosis should be regularly observed for signs of secondary hemochromatosis and treated for this disease, should it develop. Since most of these people are already anemic or debilitated by their chronic disease, they should probably be treated with deferoxamine rather than phlebotomy at the start. While the urinary loss of iron with this chelating agent is small compared with the losses obtainable through phlebotomy, the treatment itself is tolerated much better, at least in the early stages.

Secondary hemochromatosis in patients with erythropoietic or hemolytic disorders appears to result from increased absorption of iron. This does not appear to be the case, however, in patients with cirrhosis and portacaval shunts. Since these patients are generally alcoholic as well, it is felt that the combination of ethanol and the large amounts of iron contained in many wines may lead to transient increases in iron absorption. Many male natives of South Africa drink great amounts of beer manufactured in iron pots, and may ingest as much as 50 to 100 mg of iron daily in beer alone. The incidence of siderosis among this population is quite high, especially over age 30, and is 50 to 100 times the incidence in age-matched women. Fifty percent or more of patients with siderosis also have portal fibrosis, and a small number show fully blown hemochromatosis (Bothwell and Isaacson 1962). However, since many South African natives with siderosis do not show evidence of hepatic fibrosis, cirrhosis, or hemochromatosis, it is also possible that genetic conditions are operative, and that the disease state is merely aggravated by the heavy intake of both iron and alcohol. Thus, so-called Bantu hemochromatosis may be a result of both hereditary and environmental circumstances. Each of these mechanisms appear also to be operative in those few cases of hemochromatosis which have been reported among patients ingesting large amounts of inorganic iron for prolonged periods of time.

ALPHA-1-ANTITRYPSIN DEFICIENCY (AatD)

In 1963, Laurell and Eriksson described five adults who were found on immunoelectrophoretic screening to be severely deficient in alpha-1-antitrypsin (Aat), their levels ranging from 2 to 6 percent of normal. Three of these adults also had advanced pulmonary emphysema and chronic bronchitis, and one patient had two first-degree relatives with emphysema and asthma. Following this seminal report, other studies clearly associated the occurrence in adults of chronic pulmonary disease and AatD. Working in a pediatric setting, Sharp et al (1969) described 10 cases of juvenile cirrhosis of the liver associated with AatD in six difference kindreds. This association has also been widely confirmed, and much more has been learned about the inheritance of this genetic defect and the nature of the disorders with which it is related. Hepatic disorders found in children with Aatd include prolonged intrahepatic obstructive jaundice which eventually disappears spontaneously, giant cell hepatitis, hypoplasia of extrahepatic bile ducts, and cirrhosis of the liver. Most adults with AatD show only variably sized hepatocytic inclusions of a diastase-resistant amorphous material which takes up periodic acid Schiff stain, but no other liver disease. Others show cirrhosis of the liver alone, or cirrhosis plus hepatocellular carcinomas. The liver is clearly a major target organ in patients with AatD (Sharp 1976).

Pathogenesis

Alpha-1-antitrypsin is the major component of circulating alpha-1-globulin, and is a potent inhibitor of many proteases, including trypsin, chymotrypsin, elastase, and collagenase. This broad potency has led to the suggestion that its name be changed to alpha-1-protease inhibitor (Jeppson 1978), but the conventional name is preferable for now because of its wide currency. This heterogenous glycoprotein has a molecular weight of 54,000 and consists of a single polypeptide chain with four carbohydrate side chains, mannose, galactose, *n*-acetyl glucosamine, and sialic acid (Morse 1978). Aat is manufactured in hepatocytes, has a half-life of approximately one week, and appears in many bodily secretions, including bile, milk, saliva, semen, cervical fluid, and lymph. Levels increase in the presence of inflammation, malignant neoplasms, and pregnancy. Aat is a major agent in limiting potential bodily injury from inflammatory and destructive agents, and appears to inactivate proteolytic enzymes by combining with them at lysine linkages.

The capacity to produce Aat is genetically determined. Based on their electrophoretic mobility, several different types have been found. They differ primarily in their carbohydrate side chains. The usual type has an intermediate electrophoretic mobility and is designated M, while the slowest type is labeled Z. There is also an S type, intermediate between M and Z, and an F type, which migrates faster than M. Since these glycoproteins are all protease inhibitors (Pi), their hierarchy has been designated as the Pi system. Some patients produce no Aat at all, and are designated Pi-null. The differences between the various forms seems to reside in the number of sialic residues present, type Z probably having none at all (Eriksson and Larson 1975).

The production of Aat is controlled by two codominant autosomal alleles, each of which functions independently of the other. Homozygous patients are labeled ZZ and MM, for example, while others may have more than a single type of Aat present, and are labeled MZ, SZ or Z-null, etc. PiMM occurs in about 90 percent of white people and almost all black Africans. PiMS appears in 7 percent of whites, PiMZ in 3 percent, and the severely deficient types, SZ and ZZ, occur in about 0.12 and 0.02 percent of the population, respectively.

Chronic deficiency of protease inhibitors, by allowing damage from bacterial and leukocytic enzymes to occur, is believed to be responsible for the panlobular emphysema and bronchial fibrosis seen in PiZZ adults. The destructive process in these patients may be protracted by the formation in alveoli of macromolecules consisting of alpha-2-globulin and elastase. Since these macromolecules are only slowly ingested by macrophages, and since the enzyme portion is not inactivated, their formation prolongs the time of alveolar exposure to destructive proteolysis. The cause of the liver disease is far from clear, although both leukocytic and bacterial enzymes have been implicated in the process. Pointing to the low birth weight of many infants with AatD and liver disease, Sveger (1976) has suggested that hepatic damage may actually commence during intrauterine life. PiMZ and PiMS patients do not appear to be at great risk for developing liver disease during childhood, but at least one study has implicated PiMZ in association with hepatic fibrosis, cirrhosis, and hepatocellular carcinoma among adults (Blenkinsopp and Haffenden 1977). Hodges et al (1981) detected the MZ phenotype among 7 of 34 patients with non-B chronic active hepatitis, and in 6 of 28 patients with cryptogenic cirrhosis and suggest Aat phenotyping in all patients with chronic liver disease of unknown cause. Childhood cirrhosis appears to develop in PiZZ patients only, while children with PiSZ develop only mild hapatic function abnormalities. It is not clear why all PiZZ patients do not develop liver disease, and it is not certain why some patients, particularly infants with AatD and liver disease, do not have cytoplasmic inclusions.

The diastase-resistant, PAS-positve hepatocytic inclusions found in patients with AatD are immunologically similar to Aat. Chemically, the molecule is devoid of sialic acid, and this deficiency may account for the inability of hepatocytes to excrete the glycoprotein. The inability of hepatocytes to attach sialic acid to the polypeptide chain may result from slight changes in the amino acid configuration of the protein fraction. On microscopy, inclusion bodies appear to be amorphous and accumulate in the tubules of the rough endoplasmic reticulum. Many patients with these inclusion bodies and AatD do not develop any further hepatic disorder.

Clinical Picture

Aagenaes et al (1974) estimated that 10 to 20 percent of PiZZ infants develop liver disease, and that most of them die from either biliary atresia or hepatocellular dysfunction. Another 10 percent show variable degress of hepatic fibrosis and necrosis as young adults, and 50 percent have cirrhosis or fibrosis in full adulthood. The amount of liver disease is not proportional to the percentage of hepatocytes containing inclusion material. Cottrall et al (1974) have implicated AatD in around 12 percent of all infants with neonatal hepatitis. Among 31 cases of neonatal hepatitis and AatD, Alagille (1978) found that 13 improved partially, 12 developed cirrhosis with portal hypertension, 4 had chronic intrahepatic ductular hypoplasia, and 2 became completely normal. Among 19 PiZZ patients with neonatal obstructive jaundice, Odievre et al (1976) determined that jaundice lasted from two weeks to 10 years, that all had hepatomegaly, 8 had portal hypertension,and only 1 patient had died during a follow-up ranging from six months to 18 years. All but 1 patient had chronic elevations of serum alkaline phosphatase, and slightly under half had modest elevations of aminotransferase levels.

The jaundice was usually obstructive in nature and tends to clear gradually. Most of the patients proceed to develop chronic liver disease. In adults, the disease is usually unsuspected until signs of cirrhosis and hepatic decompensation appear. It has been estimated that from 10 to 50 percent of all adults with hepatocellular carcinoma also have AatD. Chronic liver disease appears only in PiZZ or MZ subjects.

Liver biopsies are typical of AatD only when the eosinophilic inclusions are found (Figure 11–2); their resistance to diastase digestion distinguishes them from collections of glycogen and rules out the possibility of glycogen storage disease. Otherwise the tissue changes in the liver are nonspecific. In infants, giant cell transformation of hepatocytes and hyperplasia of biliary ductules are common in acute stages, and fibrosis followed by micronodular and macronodular cirrhosis gradually supervenes. Patients whose obstructive jaundice improves usually continue to show variable degrees of hepatocellular necrosis in lobular peripheries and mononuclear infiltrates. Among adults, necrosis is usually scanty, but fibrosis and nodular regeneration are prominent. Carcinoma cells, when present, do not contain PAS-positive inclusions.

Treatment. Treatment for the liver disease of AatD is, of course, nonexistent because the proximate cause cannot be altered. Supportive care for complications is similar to that for other hepatic diseases. Hepatic transplantations have been reported in seven patients, three of whom were surviving 13 months to three years after surgery at the time of the report (Hood et al 1980). Pi phenotype changed to MM after surgery and, in successful patients, bilirubin levels and prothrombin times normalized. While this treatment is extremely heroic in its objective, it may be useful in patients with progressive and advanced hepatic dysfunction whose pulmonary reserve remains adequate.

CYSTIC FIBROSIS

A fraction of patients with cystic fibrosis develop a characteristic type of intrahepatic biliary cirrhosis, typified by the fact that it usually involves the liver focally, that liver function generally remains intact, and that a number of lobular bile ducts are plugged with a thick eosinophilic material which is probably analogous to similar matter found as well in the lungs, pancreas, and intestinal tract. Jaundice is rarely seen, and hepatocellular function is good because many parts of the liver are uninvolved by the biliary obstruction. The major complications of this disorder are related to portal hypertension, and include bleeding from esophageal varices and hypersplenism (Stern et al 1976). Encephalopathy rarely occurs, even following a portacaval shunt. The frequency of clinical hepatic disease in cystic fibrosis is quite low, between 2 and 3 percent, but the incidence of periportal fibrosis and bile duct proliferation is considerably higher at

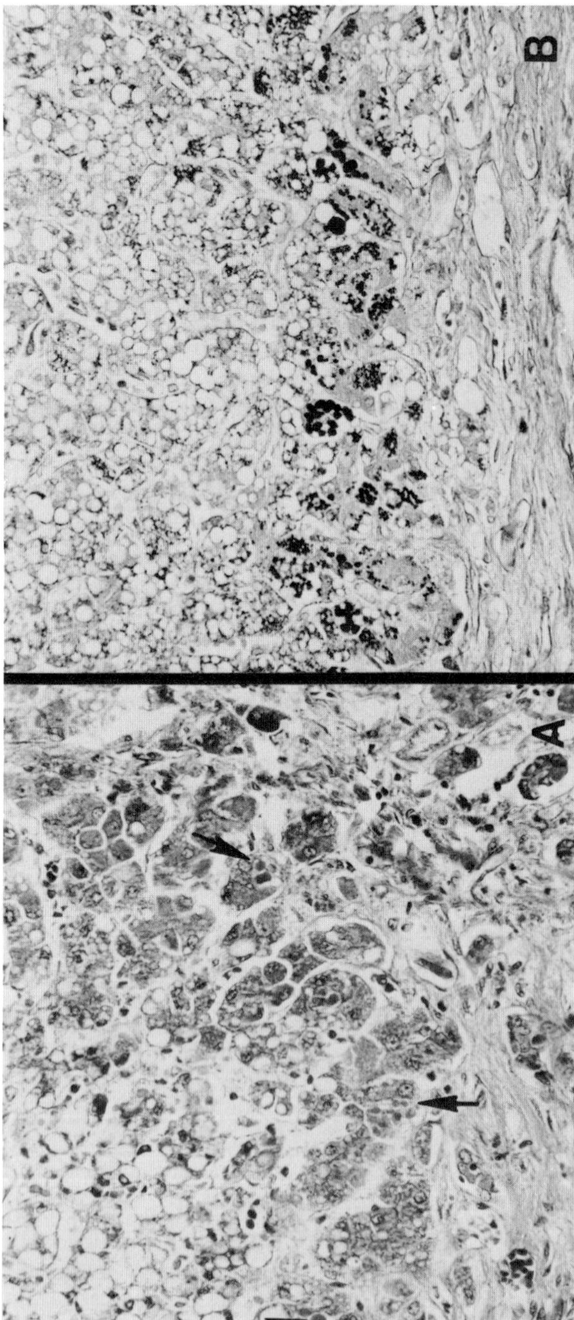

Figure 11–2. Alpha-one-antitrypsin deficiency. *A*, the diagnostic feature is the presence of spherical hyaline eosinophilic bodies in the periportal hepatocytes (arrows). *B*, PAS staining shows that these bodies are diastase-resistant globules. Severe fatty changes are also present. Original magnification x250.

postmortem examination. Either focal or diffuse biliary cirrhosis was found in about 9 percent of autopsies among patients with cystic fibrosis (Craig et al 1957), many of whom died prior to the era of antibiotics and pancreatic enzyme replacement. While there appears to be no way of preventing the development of focal biliary cirrhosis, patients with cystic fibrosis should be followed carefully for indications of variceal bleeding and hypersplenism, and treatment rendered as promptly as possible.

PRIMARY BILIARY CIRRHOSIS (PBC) (CHRONIC DESTRUCTIVE NONSUPPURATIVE CHOLANGITIS)

PBC is a singular disease of unknown etiology. It occurs much more commonly in women (approximately 80 percent) than in men, and is rarely seen before the age of 30 years. It consists of a progressive self-destruction of intrahepatic bile ducts, does not affect extrahepatic ducts, and is closely linked to altered immune mechanisms. Many patients with this disease are asymptomatic despite the evidence on biopsy occasionally of advanced hepatic changes (Fleming et al 1978a), while others suffer progressively from symptoms due initially to cholestasis, and later to hepatic dysfunction and portal hypertension. Pruritus resulting from bile acid retention is the most common presenting complaint, occurring in 46 percent of patients in one large series, and nonspecific symptoms, such as fatigue, abdominal pain, and indigestion (22 percent), are the next most common (Christensen et al 1980). Asymptomatic patients are usually detected when routine blood studies performed for reasons other than hepatic disease reveal evidence of increased serum alkaline phosphatase or hyperlipidemia. There is no way at present of estimating the size of the reservoir of asymptomatic patients, nor is it known how many such patients will ever become symptomatic. At any rate, it is abundantly clear that at least 20 percent of patients with PBC are free of complaints at any one time, that the disease progresses very slightly if at all in some patients, and that it is far from rare.

The lack of diagnostic tests for PBC accounted for its presumed rarity until the 1950s. Clinical attention was drawn primarily to its cutaneous manifestations, occasionally to the pruritus, but more impressively to the collection of flat fatty deposits (xanthelasmata) in the upper and lower eyelids, and to the tuberous fatty nodules (xanthomata) over the elbows and the extensor tendons of the fingers. Pruritus could often be minimized by physicians and treated symptomatically, but the xanthomata could not, primarily because of their cosmetic effects. The association between xanthomata and liver disease was originally reported in 1851 by Addison and Gull, who described three women with obvious PBC, and a fourth patient, a man with diabetes, no jaundice, and flat xanthomata, who probably did not have PBC. Their statement, "In what way the defective action of the liver operates, can, perhaps, be no further explained at present, than by the general theory of disordered circulating fluids,'' could still be truthfully written today, although in more sophisticated language. In the middle of this century, failure to recognize that the fatty cutaneous deposits accompanying cirrhosis were present in only a portion of patients with PBC led, for a short time, to the mistaken use of the term ''xanthomatous biliary cirrhosis,'' to describe the condition, as though xanthomata may also have been blocking the intrahepatic bile ducts. The observation by Christensen et al that less than 25 percent of their 236 patients had xanthomata when first seen gives a clearer percentage of the incidence of this sign in early PBC.

Pathogenesis

As stated in an earlier chapter, the lesion of PBC passes through four pathologically identifiable stages: inflammation of portal areas with granulomas, mononuclear, plasma cell, and histiocytic infiltrates, necrosis of portal bile ducts, and centrilobular cholestasis (stage I); periportal inflammation, proliferation of bile ducts, piecemeal necrosis of hepatic lobules, and more extensive cholestasis (stage II); septal fibrosis, bridging necrosis, or both, with disappearance of bile ducts (stage III); and true cirrhosis with nodular regeneration and variable degrees of inflammation (stage IV) (Figure 11-3). Many patients do not progress from one stage to the next with

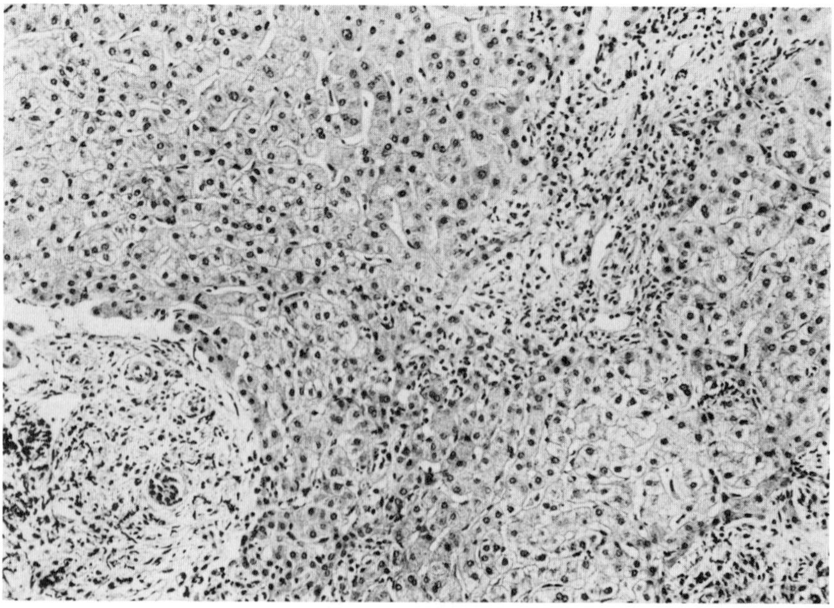

Figure 11-3. Primary biliary cirrhosis. Portal tracts show an irregular expansion with lymphocytic infiltration and fibrosis. The number of bile ducts at this stage is decreased and some are undergoing necrosis. Original magnification x125.

predictable regularity, and some never reach stages III and IV. The course of the disease is often quite prolonged, but from the onset of cholestatic symptoms, death in liver failure occurs with 5 to 10 years among most patients (Sherlock 1978).

Immunological Factors. The not infrequent association of PBC with other collagen diseases, such as scleroderma, rheumatoid arthritis, and Sjogren disease, the hepatic infiltration with lymphocytes and plasma cells, the presence of granulomata, and the absence of any other obvious etiological factors, have led to the investigation of patients for further evidences of possibly altered immune mechanisms. And numerous discoveries have been made which support an autoimmune etiology. Serum gamma globulin levels are commonly elevated, particularly the IgM fraction; mitochondrial antibodies and cryoproteins are found in the serum of 90 percent of patients; T-cell responsiveness is reduced in about 50 percent of patients; and migration inhibition is increased. Mitochondrial antibody is primarily of the IgM category and is specific for the inner membrane lipoprotein of mitochondria. The increased prevalence of hypergammaglobulinemia among asymptomatic relatives of patients with PBC suggests that there might be a genetic pattern to the disorder. Inherited susceptibility to PBC is also supported by the discovery of this disease in four of six sisters and elevated immunoglobulins in six of their children (Jaup and Zettergren 1980). Noting the enhanced toxicity of lymphocytes from patients with PBC for hepatocytes grown in cell culture, and the evidence for destruction of bile ductular epithelium by PBC monocytes, Dienstag et al (1978) investigated the possibility of suppressor T-cell dysfunction in this disease. Nine of 12 patients did indeed show diminished suppressor cell activity, although the suppressor T-cells which were present appeared to function normally in controlling elaboration of IgG by B-cells. They concluded that some B-cells in PBC patients were resistant to the control by suppressor T-cells.

One of the most striking developments in the immunological investigation of patients with PBC was the discovery by Wands et al (1978) of circulating complement-fixing immune complexes in 95 percent of patients. The concentration of immune complexes was quite high, and consumption of complement by both the alternate and classical pathways was also increased. Symptoms of immune complex disease (urticaria, arthritis, nephritis) were lacking, possibly because the complexes were of small size, although large immune complexes have also been found in patients with PBC. The presence of immune complexes could explain the appearance of granulomata, as a reaction to the complexes, in the liver. The immune complexes have been studied further by Gupta et al (1978) and were found to contain IgM, IgG, C_3, mitochondrial antibody, and albumin, thus explaining the previously noted association between the presence of the antibody and immune complexes in PBC. Data to the present thus give a strong immunological flavor to PBC. Autoimmunity may be essential to the fully expressed form of the disease, just as appears to be the case in patients with chronic active hepatitis. The causative or precipitating factor is, however, still not apparent. The sustained high levels of circulating immune complexes in PBC may result from reduced capacity of Kupffer cells to remove them (Lawley et al 1980).

Copper. Accumulation of copper in the liver is markedly increased among patients with PBC (Deering et al 1977), and median levels of hepatic copper may exceed normal levels 10-fold, and be in the same range encountered in patients with untreated Wilson disease. Contrary to the case in Wilson disease, however, ceruloplasmin levels are raised to 50 percent or more above normal in all patients with PBC, rather than being uniformly depressed. Although urinary copper is also increased in patients with PBC, the daily excretion does not approach that seen in patients with Wilson disease. Increased tissue copper has been found in both the spleen and kidneys, and may account for the occasional appearance of renal tubular acidosis due to copper deposition in proximal renal tubules in some patients. Cerebral copper is not increased, but Kasyer-Fleischer rings have been seen in a few patients. There is no evidence for a genetic disorder of copper metabolism in patients with PBC, and current thinking attributes the accumulation of copper solely to decreased bile flow. The accumulation of copper, by forming toxic metabolites, may well enhance liver destruction, just as it does in patients with Wilson disease.

Symptoms and Findings

It has already been indicated that the major symptoms of PBC are similar to those of any other cholestatic disorder, pruritus, and symptoms of conjugated obstructive hyperbilirubinemia being the most common. The typical patient is a middle-aged woman, taking no drugs or alcohol, who is moderately icteric and whose skin is deeply pigmented or excoriated from chronic pruritus. Xanathomata and xanthelasma are found commonly, often without the patient having been aware of them or, because of their gradual development, not relating them to the underlying disease. Some patients have lost weight due to bile deficiency steatorrhea; others may have increased bleeding tendencies due to malabsorption of vitamin K. As the disease advances, more and more evidences of hepatocellular dysfunction occur, including such preterminal events as fetor hepatis, hepatic encephalopathy, gastrointestinal bleeding, and ascites.

The major differential is to rule out extrahepatic biliary obstruction, and this can be readily accomplished by ultrasonography of the upper abdomen, which fails to show evidence of ductal dilatation. Blood chemistries show marked elevations of alkaline phosphatase levels, and these can be confirmed as hepatic by finding similar levels of 5′-nucleotidase or gamma glutamyl transpeptidase elevation. Hyperlipidemia is invariably found, with elevations of both cholesterol and total lipids.

Lipidemias occur in all forms of cholestasis and do not have any value in differential diagnosis. Lipoprotein X, phospholipid 66 percent and cholesterol 25 percent plus small amounts of protein and triglyceride, is characteristic of cholestasis (Sabesin et al 1980). It seems to result from the interaction of bile with serum and migrates between the beta and prebeta bands. The fact that lipoprotein X is also found in lecithin:cholesterol acyltransferase (LCAT) deficiency, has led some investigators to suggest that this enzyme, normally formed in the liver, is deficient in cholestasis. Since LCAT is responsible also for the esterification of cholesterol, its deficiency may account for the decreased percentage of esterified serum cholesterol found in cholestasis. The cause of the hypercholesterolemia of cholestasis is also not clear, but may be due to increased production (no bile salts in small intestine) or lecithin-induced damage to hepatocytic membranes. In PBC, the chronic hyperlipidemia is closely related to the development of xanthomata and xanthelasmata, which may revert somewhat in advanced stages of the disease as hepatic production of lipoproteins and cholesterol diminishes.

The finding of mitochondrial antibodies in patients with obstructive jaundice or elevated serum alkaline phosphatase levels essentially confirms the diagnosis of PBC. Smooth muscle and antinuclear antibodies may also be present, but these are not nearly as diagnostic. Liver biopsies (Figure 10–3) should be performed at least once to diagnose the stage of the disease, and some investigators advise performing annual biopsies in patients with active symptoms and signs.

Treatment

No specific therapy is presently available, but much can be done to comfort the symptomatic patient. Pruritus can be well controlled in most patients by the regular use of the bile acid chelating agent, cholestyramine, starting with 4.0 g qid, and reducing as possible. The only problem with this treatment is that it may aggravate fat malabsorption by reducing micellarization of intestinal fats. Should marked steatorrhea be present, either with or without cholestyramine, medium chain (C_{7-9}) triglycerides can be substituted for usual dietary fats (C_{16-18}). These fats are nutritionally helpful, and are absorbed without hydrolysis and micellarization directly into the portal rather than the lymphatic system.

Fat-soluble vitamin deficiencies can be controlled by the administration of vitamins D and K parenterally and this, along with added dietary calcium, may help to prevent the development of osteoporosis and spontaneous vertebral fractures.

The use of d-penicillamine has recently been advocated for the treatment of patients with PBC, especially for the progressive form, but the results are conflicting. d-Penicillamine can clearly reduce levels of hepatic copper by increasing urinary copper excretion (Deering et al 1977). Epstein et al (1978) suggest that copper depletion may not be the major therapeutic effect of this drug, however, because it also appears to reduce the number of circulating immune complexes and the level of aspartate aminotransferase and immunoglobulins as well and may thus be immunosuppressive. Fleming et al (1978) think that the functional benefits do not parallel the copper losses. Mezey (1978) has also shown that d-penicillamine may reduce the synthesis of collagen by decreasing the activity of hepatic collagen proline hydroxylase, at least in patients with alcoholic hepatitis. Against these optimistic claims, however, is the report of Matloff et al (1979) who showed that a two-year controlled trial of d-penicillamine in 56 fairly well-matched patients with PBC resulted in progression of biopsy changes in about two-thirds of the patients in either group and no significant differences in hepatic functions tests, although cupuresis occurred and hepatic copper levels fell in the treated group. There was a 24 percent death rate in the treated group and a 7 percent rate in patients given the dummy. Furthermore, side effects from the d-penicillamine were found in half of the treated patients, including rash, fever, arthralgia, myalgia, myasthenia, and Goodpasture syndrome. Bone marrow suppression has also been reported from its use. The place of this drug in the therapy of PBC is very unclear at present. Glucocorticoids and azathiaprine have also been tried as immunosuppressive agents, but the former appears to aggravate osteoporosis, and the latter, in controlled studies, was found to be ineffective.

Course

While the lesion of PBC may remain stationary for many years, the course is dismal for patients with progressive disease. Prognosis worsens with the degree of jaundice and the stage of the biopsy, especially at stage IV (Christensen et al 1980). Each of these is a separate aspect of the same problem: a stage IV biopsy shows almost no bile ducts, and it is this feature which is responsible for the hyperbilirubinemia. Similarly, increasing size of the liver is an indication of a poor prognosis and correlates well with the degree of cholestasis. Other poor prognostic signs include the presence of ascites, skin pigmentation, and cholestasis on biopsy involving the periphery of hepatic lobules, rather than only the centrilobular areas. The duration of the disease has no relationship to the mortality risk.

SELECTED REFERENCES

Aegenaes Ø, Fagerhol M, Elgjo, et al. Pathology and pathogenesis in alpha-1-antitrypsin deficient individuals. Postgrad Med J 50:365–75, 1974.

Addison T, Gull W. On a certain affection of the skin. Vitiligoidea-a. plana, tuberosa. Guy's Hosp Rep (2nd ser) 7:265–76, 1851.

Alagille D. Intrahepatic neonatal cholestasis. In: Javitt NB, ed. Neonatal hepatitis and biliary atresia. Washington DC: U.S. Department of Health, Education and Welfare, 1978:177–90.

Baldus WP, Fairbanks VF, Dickson ER, et al: Deferoxamine-chelatable iron in hemochromatosis and other disorders of iron overload. May Clin Proc 53:157–65, 1978.

Batey RG, Petit JE, Nicholas AW, et al. Hepatic iron clearance from serum in treated hemochromatosis. Gastroenterology 75:856–59, 1978.

Bearn AG. Wilson's disease. An inborn error of metabolism with multiple manifestations. Am J Med 22:747–57, 1957.

Beaumont C, Simon M, Fauchet R, et al. Serum ferritin as a possible marker of the hemochromatosis allele. New Engl J Med 301:169–74, 1979.

Blenkinsopp WK, Haffenden GP. Alpha-1-antitrypsin bodies in the liver. J Clin Path 30:132–37, 1977.

Bothwell TH, Isaacson C. Siderosis in the Bantu. A comparison of incidence in males and females. Br Med J 1:522–24, 1962.

Brown EB. Hypochromic anemias. In: Beeson PB, McDermott W, Wyngaarden JB eds. Cecil textbook of medicine, 15th ed. Philadelphia: WB Saunders, 1979:1743–47.

Cartwright GE. Current concepts. Diagnosis of treatable Wilson's disease. New Engl J Med 298:1347–50, 1978.

Cartwright GE, Edwards CQ, Kravitz K, et al. Hereditary hemochromatosis. Phenotypic expression of the disease. New Engl J Med 201:175–79, 1979.

Christensen E, Crowe J, Doniach D, et al. Clinical pattern and course of disease in primary biliary cirrhosis based on an analysis of 236 patients. Gastroenterology 78:236–46, 1980.

Cottrall K, Cook PJL, Mowat AP. Neonatal hepatitis syndrome and alpha-1-antitrypsin deficiency: an epidemiological study in southeast England. Postgrad Med J 376–80, 1974.

Cox TM, Peters, TJ. Uptake of iron by duodenal biopsy specimens from patients with iron deficiency anaemia and primary hemochromatosis. Lancet 1:123–24, 1978

Craig JM, Haddad H, Shwachman H. The pathological changes in the liver in cystic fibrosis of the pancreas. Am J Dis Child 93:357–69, 1957.

Deering TB, Dickson ER, Fleming CR, et al. Effect of *d*–penicillamine on copper retention in patients with primary biliary cirrhosis. Gastroenterology 72:1208–12, 1977.

Dienstag JL, Weake JR, Wands JR. Abnormalities of lymphocyte regulation in primary biliary cirrhosis. Gastroenterology 75:960, 1978.

Epstein O, DeVilliers D, Jain S, et al. The effect of penicillamine on immune complexes and immunoglobulins in primary biliary cirrhosis. Gastroenterology 75:962, 1978.

Eriksson S, Larsson C. Purification and partial characterization of PAS-positive inclusion bodies from the liver in alpha-1-antitrypsin deficiency. New Engl J Med 292:176–80, 1975.

Fillet G, Marsaglia G. Idiopathic hemochromatosis: abnormality in RBC transport of iron by the reticuloendothelial system. Blood 46:1007, 1975.

Fleischer B. Über eine der "Pseudosklerose" nahestande bisher unbekannte Krankheit (gekennzeichnet durch Tremor, psychische Storungen, bräunliche Pigmentierung bestimmter Gewebe, insbesondere auch der Hornhautperipherie, Lebercirrhose). Deutsche Z Nervenheilk 44:179–201, 1912.

Fleming, CR, Ludwig J, Dickson ER. Asymptomatic primary biliary cirrhosis. Presentation, histology, and results with d-penicillamine. Mayo Clin Proc 53:587–93, 1978a.

Fleming CR, Lindor KD, Dickson ER, et al. d-Penicillamine in primary biliary cirrhosis: apparent beneficial effects in spite of a lack of correlation with changes in hepatic copper concentration. Gastroenterology 75: 964, 1978b.

Glazebrook AJ: Wilson's disease. Edinburgh Med J 52:63–87, 1945.

Gower, WR. On tetanoid chorea and its association with cirrhosis of the liver. Rev Neurol Psychiat 4:249–58, 1906.

Gupta RC, McDuffie FC, Dickson ER, et al. The composition of the isolated soluble immune complexes in primary biliary cirrhosis. Gastrotenterology 75:967, 1978.

Hanot V, Schacmann M. Sur la cirrhose pigmentaire dans le diabete sucre. Arch Physiol Norm Path (3rd ser) 7:50–87, 1886.

Hodges JR, Millward-Sadler GH, Barbatis C et al: Heteroozygous MZ alpha$_1$-antitrypsin deficiency in adults with chronic active hepatitis and cryptogenic cirrhosis. N Engl J Med 304: 557–60, 1981.

Homén EA. Eine eigenthumliche Familienkrankenheit, unter der Form einer progressiven Dementia, mit besonderem anatomischen Befund. Neur Centrbl 90:514–18 (17), 1890.

Hood JM, Koep LJ, Peters RL, et al. Liver transplantation for advanced liver disease with alpha-1-antitrypsin deficiency. New Engl J Med 302:272–75, 1980.

Jaup BH, Zettergren LSW. Familial occurrence of primary biliary cirrhosis associated with hypergammaglobulinemia in descendants: a family study. Gastroenterology 78:549–55, 1980.

Jeppson J-O. Alpha-1-antitrypsin: molecular structure, synthesis, metabolism, and physiological role. In: Javitt NB, ed. Neonatal hepatitis and biliary atresia. Washington DC: U.S. Department of Health, Education and Welfare, 1978:135–42.

Kent G, Popper H. Liver biopsy in diagnosis of hemochromatosis. Am J Med 44:837–41, 1968.

Laurell C-B, Eriksson S. The electrophoretic α1-globulin pattern of serum in α1-antitrypsin deficiency. Scand J Clin Lab Invest 15:132–40, 1963.

Lawley TJ, James SP, Jones EA. Circulating immune complexes: their detection and potential significance in some hepatobiliary and intestinal diseases. Gastroenterology 78:626–41, 1980.

Matloff D, Resnick R, Alpert E, et al. *d*-Penicillamine does not alter the course of primary biliary cirrhosis. Gastroenterology 77:A26 (November), 1979.

Mezey E, Potter JJ, Iber FL, et al. Effect of d-penicillamine on hepatic collagen proline hydroxylase activity in alcoholic hepatitis. Gastroenterology 75:976, 1978.

Morse JO. Alpha-1-antitrypsin deficiency. New Engl J Med 299:1045–48, 1099–1105, 1978.

Odiévre M, Martin J-P, Hadochouel M, et al. Alpha-1-antitrypsin deficiency and liver disease in children: phenotypes, manifestations, and prognosis. Pediatrics 57:226–31, 1976.

Omerod JA. Cirrhosis of the liver in a boy, with obscure and fatal nervous symptoms. St. Bart's Hosp Rep 26:57–68, 1890.

Powell LW, Bassett ML, Halliday JW. Hemochromatosis: 1980 update. Gastroenterology 78:374–81, 1980.

Sabesin SM, Bertram PD, Freeman MR. Lipoprotein metabolism in liver disease. Adv Int Med 25:117–46, 1980.

Sharp HL. The current status of α-1-antitrypsin, a protease inhibitor, in gastrointestinal disease. Gastroenterology 70:611–21, 1976.

Sharp, HL, Bridges RA, Krivit W, et al. Cirrhosis associated with alpha-1-antitrypsin deficiency: a previously unrecognized inherited disorder. J Lab Clin Med 73:934–39, 1969.

Sherlock S: Primary biliary cirrhosis. Am J Med 65:217–19, 1978.

Simon M, Bourel M, Genetet B, et al. Idiopathic hemochromatosis. Demonstration of recessive transmission and early detection by family HLA typing. New Engl J Med 297:1017–21, 1977.

Simon M, Fauchet R, Hespel JP, et al. Idiopathic hemochromatosis: a study of biochemical expression in 247 heterozygous members of 63 families: evidence for a single major HLA-linked gene. Gastroenterology 78:703–8, 1980.

Stern RC, Stevens DP, Boat TF, et al. Symptomatic hepatic disease in cystic fibrosis: incidence, course, and outcome of portal systemic shunting. Gastroenterology 70:645–49, 1976.

Sternlieb I. Diagnosis of Wilson's disease. Gastroenterology 74:787–93, 1978.

Sternlieb I, Scheinberg IH. The role of radiocopper in the diagnosis of Wilson's disease. Gastroenterology 77:138–42, 1979.

Strickland GT, Leu M-L. Wilson's disease. Clinical and laboratory manifestations in 40 patients. Medicine 54:113–37, 1975.

Sveger T. Liver disease in alpha-1-antitrypsin deficiency detected by screening of 200,000 infants. New Engl J Med 294:1316–21, 1976.

Walshe JM. The physiology of copper in man and its relation to Wilson's disease. Brain 90:149–76, 1967.

Wands JR, Dienstag JL, Bahn AK, et al. Circulating immune complexes and complement activation in primary biliary cirrhosis. New Engl J Med 298:233–37, 1978.

Wilson SAK. Progressive lenticular degeneration: a familial disease associated with cirrhosis of the liver. Brain 34:295–509, 1912.

DISCUSSION QUESTIONS

1. Seventeen days after attending a conference in Atlantic City, a 33-year-old physician noted the onset of fatigue, slight fever, and dark urine. Examination was normal except for a temperature of 38°C, hyperemia of the pharynx, and tenderness to deep palpation over the right upper quadrant of the abdomen. A distinct hepatic edge could not be felt.

   Laboratory data showed a white blood count of 4,400 per cu mm, with a differential of 50 percent polymorphonuclear leukocytes, 42 percent lymphocytes, 6 percent monocytes, and 2 percent eosinophils. Aspartate aminotransferase was 820 units per ml on the first day, and rose to 2,360 units on the fourth day. HBsAg was negative. Prothrombin content was 65 percent of control values, and serum bilirubin was 5.8 mg per dl total, and 3.6 mg, direct reacting. Alkaline phosphatase was 80 IU per liter.
2. A man of 29 is recovering from infectious hepatitis after two weeks of illness. His bilirubin is 3.0 mg per dl, aspartate aminotransferase 90 units per ml. He feels well and asks permission to return to work as a weight lifter in a carnival. How would you respond to this request? What follow-up would you advise? His mother has just learned of his illness and wants an injection of gamma globulin. How would you respond to this request?
3. What measures should be taken by the director of a blood bank to reduce the spread of blood-borne hepatitis?
4. A 29-year-old woman was hospitalized in the fourth month of her second pregnancy because of jaundice for the preceding two weeks. Earlier in her pregnancy she had been placed on prochlorperazine for severe nausea and occasional vomiting. Her urine became dark in color and her stools turned to a light shade of tan one month later. These symptoms persisted although the drug was

discontinued. Shortly afterward, she noted the gradual onset of itching, and then jaundice. These were associated with progressive anorexia and steady epigastric discomfort, aggravated by meals. Chills, fever, pain in the back, and changes in bowel habits were denied.

On examination, the patient was well developed and showed moderately deep jaundice. Excoriations of the arms and legs were readily apparent. Temperature was 37.8°C. A few spider nevi were visible on the upper anterior chest. The liver was palpable 4 cm below the right costal margin, and the edge was nontender, rounded, and smooth. There was slight tenderness in the upper right quadrant of the abdomen, just below the liver. The spleen was not palpable, and the uterus was appropriately enlarged to just below the umbilical level.

Hematocrit was 36 percent, white blood count 12,100 per cu mm with a slight leftward shift of the differential count. The urine was dark amber in color, but otherwise negative. Stool was very light tan in color, and serum bilirubin was 15 mg per dl, serum cholesterol 445 mg per dl, alkaline phosphatase 238 IU per liter, and aspartate aminotransferase, 210 units per ml. Another urine specimen was positive for bilirubin and negative for urobilinogen.

5. At the time of hospitalization, a 66-year-old woman stated, "I'm yellow. My doctor told me so yesterday." For the previous four months, she had suffered from a persistent feeling of fullness in the epigastrum, and from moderate anorexia, resulting in a weight loss of 10 pounds. Discomfort was often accentuated by eating, after which pain would radiate into the upper lumbar area. Antacids and salicylates failed to relieve the pain, which lasted for several hours after meals. Patient had never suffered from similar symptoms and denied the use of alcohol or any medications other than aspirin.

Her urine became a dark amber color and her stools turned tan simultaneously, about one week prior to admission. The day previous to admission, her physician noted her to be jaundiced for the first time. Mild generalized itching had been present for a few days. The patient denied having nausea, vomiting, melena, dysphagia, chills, fever, or altered bowel habits.

Her previous medical history had been remarkably good, and there had been no major illnesses. A total hysterectomy was performed at age 37 for fibromyomata.

On examination, temperature was 37.2°C, pulse 80, respirations 12, blood pressure 106/85. She appeared to be well developed, slightly obese, alert, and well oriented. There was a slight degree of scleral icterus and a few excoriations on her upper arms. The abdomen was slightly distended and tympanitic, but there was no tenderness, ascites, or evidence of a mass. The liver edge was nontender, smooth and rounded, and palpable 10 cm below the right costal margin. The spleen and gall bladder were not palpable. Rectal examination was normal, but the response to guaiac testing was positive.

6a. An 18-year-old white woman was hospitalized after 10 days of jaundice, which had been preceded nearly two weeks before by chilliness, fever, listlessness, nausea, anorexia, and diarrhea. The chilliness and fever disappeared in four days, but the other symptoms persisted until hospitalization, although with reduced intensity. Two weeks before admission, her urine became tea colored, and one week later she was noted to be jaundiced, and her stools became tan in color. Vomiting, abdominal pain, itching, and rigors were not noted, and there was no history of recent injections, alcohol intake, drug ingestion, or known exposure to persons with hepatitis. Her physician suggested bed rest, but her jaundice had deepened and anorexia intensified during the week prior to admission.

Examination showed a mildly languid but well-oriented woman, who was deeply icteric and slightly tremulous. Asterixis was demonstrable. Temperature was 38.5°C. No spider nevi, palmar erythema, abdominal distention, ascites, edema, or splenomegaly were demonstrable. The liver was palpable 5 cm below the right costal margin, and the edge was smooth, rounded, and tender.

The following laboratory data were obtained initially and on discharge three weeks later:

	Hct %	WBC	Bili mg/dl	Alk phos IU/l	Asp AT U/ml	Pro time pt/control sec	Alb/glob g/dl
Admission	43	4,100	32.0	130	1,005	18/14	3.8/2.8
Discharge	39	5,100	1.2	44	65	15/13	4.2/3.8

The patient had remained icteric listless and with a poor appetite for the first week in the hospital. Spontaneous improvement commenced just as treatment with prednisone was contemplated. At the time of discharge, she was normally alert, free of jaundice and tremor, and her liver edge was just barely palpable.

6b. During the following two years, patient felt entirely well, except for a tendency to tire easily. She then married and, three months later, missed a menstrual period. After another two months, she noted morning nausea, anorexia, and abdominal enlargement. Thinking that she was pregnant, she consulted an obstetrician who noted that the patient was deeply icteric, mildly confused, and had swollen ankles. In retrospect, her husband stated that she had perhaps been jaundiced several weeks and that her urine had been intermittently amber in color for 2 to 3 months. She was hospitalized.

Physical examination showed a deeply icteric patient, who had marked asterixis, and was moderately somnolent. Temperature was 37.4°C. She had palmar erythema, numerous large and small spider nevi, and scattered ecchymoses. The abdomen was distended, shifting dullness was present, and dilated veins were noted in the upper abdomen. The liver was enlarged to 2 cm below the right costal margin, firm, irregular and nontender. The spleen was palpable 5 cm below the left costal margin. There was moderate pitting edema in both legs. Stool was guaiac positive.

Laboratory studies revealed a hematocrit of 32 percent, white blood count of 3,100, total bilirubin of 17.5 mg per dl, alkaline phosphatase of 96 IU per liter, aspartate aminotransferase 280 units per ml, prothrombin time of 22 seconds with a control of 13 seconds, albumin of 1.9 and globulin of 6.4 g per dl.

The patient became progressively more icteric and somnolent and died two weeks after admission following a massive upper gastrointestinal hemorrhage.

7. A 44-year-old woman returned to her physician because of generalized persistent itching for the previous six weeks. Two weeks prior to the onset of this symptom, her physician placed her on sulfasoxazole because of fever, anorexia, myalagia, and slight diarrhea, diagnosed as influenza. Several days after the pruritus began, she discontinued the medication after consulting the physician. She had missed one menstrual period, and denied chills, abdominal pain, alcohol intake or exposure to patients with hepatitis. Recently, she had commenced to bruise easily.

Examination revealed a slightly wasted, deeply icteric woman with excoriations and hyperpigmentation of her shins, forearms, and abdomen. A few spider nevi were present on her shoulders, and a firm, slightly tender and irregular liver edge was palpable 8 cm below the right costal margin. Ascites and edema were absent, but the spleen was palpable 1 cm below the left costal margin.

Hematocrit was 30 percent, white blood count 4,800 per cu mm, with a normal differential count. Urine was dark orange but was otherwise normal. Stools were yellowish brown and showed increased amounts of neutral fat. An upper gastrointestinal series was normal.

Urinary bilirubin was positive, urobilinogen present in small amounts. Total serum bilirubin was 8.4 mg, cholesterol 986 mg, albumin 3.4 g, and globulin 3.9 g per dl. Alkaline phosphatase 178 IU per liter, aspartate aminotransferase 520 units per ml, gamma globulin 38 percent of total globulin, HBsAg negative. Prothrombin content was 24 percent of normal, and rose to 48 percent following parenteral injection of vitamin K.

8. A 58-year-old man was hospitalized because of abdominal swelling of recent onset. He also complained of anorexia and weakness. Ten days prior to admission his urine had darkened and he had begun to experience soreness in the upper abdomen. He had lost 20 pounds in weight during the previous six months, smoked excessively and had a chronic cough.

He appeared cachectic and had moderate scleral icterus. His chest was increased in anteroposterior diameter and hyperresonant to percussion. Scattered rales were audible at the bases of both lungs. The edge of the liver was palpable 10 cm below the right costal margin in the midclavicular line; it was hard and irregular.

Hematocrit was 45 percent, white blood count 12,400. Urine was negative, save for the presence of bilirubin. Serum bilirubin was 2.1 mg, direct reacting 1.5 mg, cholesterol 300 mg, total serum protein 6.8 g per dl. Alkaline phosphatase was 295 IU per liter, aspartase aminotransferase 28 units per ml. A chest X ray showed atelectasis of the right middle lobe and increased bronchopulmonary markings. An upper gastrointestinal series was normal except for leftward displacement of the stomach, presumably by the enlarged liver.

CLINICAL CONFERENCE 5

A 42-year-old woman was hospitalized because of abdominal pain for the previous four days. She had been in good health until two weeks prior to admission, when she developed steady periumbilical pain accompanied by nausea and several episodes of vomiting several hours after she had eaten a very large dinner. Chlorpromazine was prescribed by her physician, and the pain subsided after a period of three hours. Four days before admission she was awakened from sleep by a similar attack, but after two hours the pain radiated into the right upper quadrant of the abdomen and into the back as well. A white blood count at this time was 10,200. Treatment with belladonna was accompanied initially by disappearance of pain, but a stronger attack recurred the day of admission. She noted considerable darkening of her urine and lightening of stools the day before the last attack of pain. On the way to the hospital her husband remarked that her sclerae were slightly yellow in color.

Review of systems revealed that the patient had noted some flatulence during recent weeks. She denied intolerance for fatty food, exposure to drugs or possible hepatotoxins, family history of jaundice, contact with jaundiced persons, or excessive intake of alcohol. She had never previously been jaundiced, but she had been overweight for several years.

She appeared to be acutely ill and in moderate distress from pain in the abdomen. She was well developed and obese. Temperature, 38.5°C; respiration, 24; pulse, 92; blood pressure, 125/75. There was a yellow coloration of her sclerae and skin. The chest was normal, and abdominal examination demonstrated slight hepatomegaly plus tenderness and guarding in the right upper quadrant. Bowel sounds were negative for signs of obstruction. A specimen of stool was light brown and negative for occult blood.

Hematocrit was 53 percent; white blood count, 13,600 with 89 percent polymorphonuclear leukocytes. Analysis of a yellow alkaline urine showed a specific gravity of 1.022, a trace of albumin, three to four white blood cells per high power field, and a positive test for bilirubin. Urobilinogen was present in decreased amounts. Blood glucose was 82 mg; urea nitrogen, 12 mg; serum amylase, 80 Somogyi units; serum protein, 6.2 g (albumin, 4.3 g); total serum bilirubin, 5.2 mg per dl; alkaline phosphatase, 120 IU per liter; and aspartate aminotransferase was 80 units per ml; X rays of the chest and abdomen showed no obvious abnormality.

The patient was treated with intravenous fluids, atropine, and meperidine (Demerol). She was also placed on constant nasogastric suction, and her pain disappeared completely within 10 hours. Abdominal tenderness also diminished considerably. An upper gastrointestinal series was normal. Fever disappeared on the second hospital day, but the liver edge remained palpable, and the jaundice appeared to deepen. Serum bilirubin rose to 9.2 mg, alkaline phosphatase to 200 IU.

On the seventh hospital day she underwent an abdominal operation under halothane anesthesia. Brisk bleeding was encountered at one point during the operation and a transfusion of 2 units of whole blood was given. At surgery a biopsy of the liver was taken (Figure 11-4).

Four days after surgery the total serum bilirubin had fallen to 4 mg and nine days later to 2 mg. Alkaline phosphatase at that time was 60 IU. She was discharged from the hospital three weeks after surgery, at which time the liver was no longer palpable and all tests of hepatic function were normal.

The patient remained well for approximately three months, after which she developed an influenzalike syndrome consisting of chills, fever, and muscular aching. A physician was not called until the reappearance of jaundice was noted. The urine darkened considerably, but the color of her stools remained normal. She was not acutely ill, and she had no complaints other than mild nausea, anorexia, and intermittent chills.

The patient was in no distress on physical examination, but jaundice was quite evident. Vital signs were normal, and no evidence of spider nevi or palmar erythema was noted. The abdomen was slightly protruberant, superficial venous collaterals were not seen, and ascites was not present. The liver was felt 4 cm below the right costal margin; its edge was blunted,

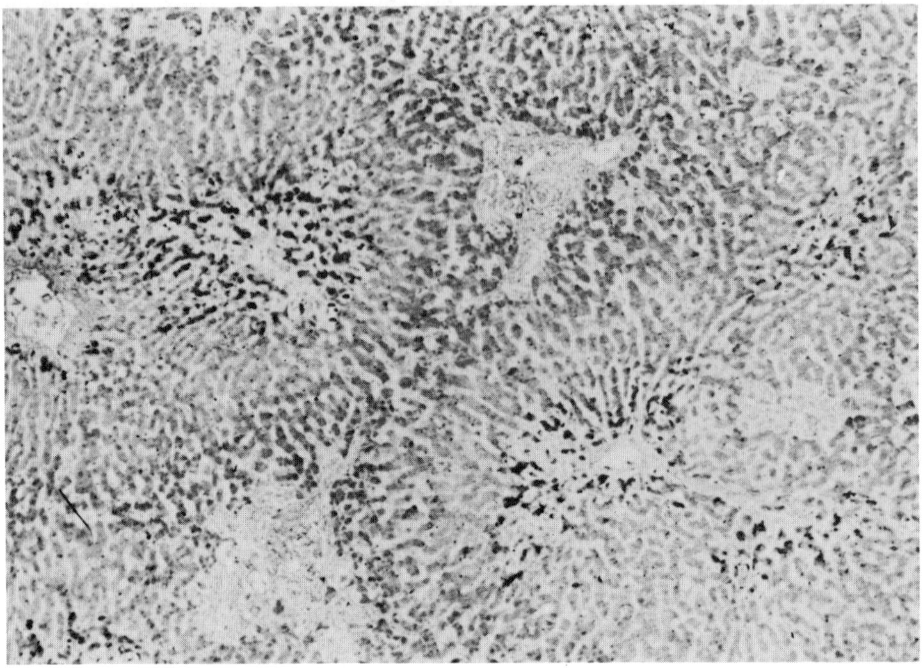

Figure 11-4. Liver biopsy at time of surgery, Clinical Conference 5. Original magnification x30. Courtesy of Dr. Richard J. Stenger.

smooth, and tender. The patient was somewhat lethargic, but she was well oriented, and the balance of the neurologic examination was normal. A stool specimen was brown and negative for occult blood.

Hematocrit was 52 percent; white blood count, 6,400 with 52 percent neutrophils. Analysis of an amber-colored acid urine showed strongly positive tests for bilirubin and urobilinogen, but was otherwise normal. Blood glucose and urea nitrogen were normal. Serum protein was 7.1 g (albumin, 4.0 g); bilirubin, 9.7 mg per dl. Alkaline phosphatase was 50 IU per liter; aspartate aminotransferase 2,600 units and LDH 1,200 units per ml; prothrombin content, 28 percent. The test for HBsAg was negative.

The patient's condition deteriorated rapidly during the second hospital day. She fluctuated between lethargy and hyperactivity and was generally confused and disoriented. A lumbar puncture was normal. X rays of the chest, abdomen and skull gave no additional information. Venous blood ammonia level was 250 μg/dl. Urinary output was only 465 ml on the second day. Early the next day it was noticed that her jaundice had deepened considerably, asterixis was elicited, and deep tendon reflexes were hyperactive. Stupor deepened throughout the day. Serum electrolytes showed CO_2 combining power, 20 mEq; chlorides, 94 mEq; sodium, 132 mEq;

potassium, 5.6 mEq (all per liter). Bilirubin was 27 mg and BUN 43 mg per dl. Prothrombin content had fallen to 12.5 percent.

1. In regard to the jaundice, what is the differential diagnosis for each admission? Support or refute each possibility with appropriate clinical and laboratory data and indicate which type of jaundice you conclude was present at each admission.
2. In regard to the illness, what is the differential diagnosis for each admission? Select the most probable cause(s), and state your reasons for the selection(s).
3. What methods might usefully be applied to manage the patient's latest illness? Why?

CLINICAL CONFERENCE 6

This 48-year-old man states that he was well until four months prior to this hospital admission, at which time he noted the onset of epigastric gnawing pain, which occurred about 90 minutes after meals, did not radiate, and was relieved promptly by the ingestion of antacids. at times the pain would awaken him at night. It became more severe two weeks prior to admission, and antacids began to be less effective in controlling the pain. He drinks four to six glasses of beer every morning and averages another six glasses of beer and "a few shots of whiskey" during the balance of the day. For several months he has also been taking a number of aspirin tablets daily for nervousness. There is no history of nausea, vomiting, loss of weight, or jaundice. There have been no changes in the color or consistency of his stools, and food intolerance, belching, itching, and flatulence are denied.

The vital signs are normal. Patient is well developed and appears to be well nourished. The sclerae are icteric, and the chest is normal. The abdomen is soft and slightly distended. Moderate tenderness is elicited on light pressure in the epigastrium. A fluid wave is absent, but there is shifting dullness in the flanks. Percussion in the midclavicular line reveals hepatic dullness of 16 cm, and the lower edge of the liver is blunt, firm, nontender, and smooth. Rectal examination is normal, and stool is brown and negative for occult blood. Several large ecchymoses are present on both thighs, and a number of small spider nevi are seen on the upper back and chest. Neurologic examination is normal.

Hematocrit was 40 percent; hemoglobulin, 12.8 g per 100 dl; red blood count, 4.1 million; white blood count, 10,200 with a normal differential. Bilirubin was 7.1 mg, direct reacting, 5.0 mg; cholesterol, 666 mg; serum triglycerides, 275 mg; total serum protein, 7.1 g (albumin, 2.2 g) (all per dl). Serum amylase was normal on several occasions, alkaline phosphatase was 160 IU per liter, aspartate aminotransferase 110 units per ml. The urine was amber in color, strongly positive for bilirubin, but otherwise negative. In a

24 hr urine collection sodium content was 6 mEq per liter, and volume was 640 ml.

On the sixth hospital day, the serum bilirubin was 3.5 mg direct and 9.4 mg total. Cholesterol levels fell to 375 mg, but the hematocrit had fallen from 40 percent on admission to 30 percent. Prothrombin content was 35 percent of normal; reticulocytes, 12 percent. An upper gastrointestinal series was normal except for the presence of a deformed duodenal bulb that contained a tiny positive filling defect at the apex. Coarse mucosal folds were seen throughout the stomach. Small intestinal X ray series was normal. After the administration of vitamin K, prothrombin content was 40 percent.

1. In this patient, a considerable amount of data indicate the presence of disease of the liver. To the right of each item in the numbered list place the appropriate letter from the following list:

   A. If the abnormality suggests a hepatocellular disorder
   B. If the abnormality suggests an obstructive disorder
   C. If the abnormality suggests either A or B
   D. If the abnormality suggests neither A nor B

   I. History of alcoholism ____
   II. Spider angiomata ____
   III. Hepatomegaly ____
   IV. Hyperbilirubinemia with bilirubinuria ____
   V. Absence of pruritus with jaundice ____
   VI. Alkaline phosphatase ____
   VII. Aspartate aminotransferase ____
   VIII. Serum cholesterol ____
   IX. Plasma proteins ____
   X. Prothrombin level ____

2. Considering all available data in this case, how do you explain the entire clinical picture?
3. Discuss briefly the significance of the shifting dullness in this patient and the laboratory data which help in its evaluation.
4. Suggest possible mechanisms to account for the abdominal pain.
5. Would it be reasonable and helpful to perform a biopsy of the liver in this patient? Why?
6. What might you expect the biopsy to show?
7. How do you interpret the findings on the upper gastrointestinal series?
8. In what ways and by what mechanisms might this patient's habits influence his gastrointestinal and hepatic disorders?
9. List and briefly give reasons for the types of therapy you would employ in treating these disorders.

CHAPTER 12

The Biliary Tract

We come now to a discussion of diseases of the extrahepatic biliary tract, the most important of which is cholelithiasis and its various complications. Gallstones occur in approximately 10 percent of Americans, the incidence depending on certain variables, such as sex, obesity, diet, pregnancy, associated diseases, and age, each of which will be described where appropriate. Diseases of the gall bladder, almost all of which were related to gallstones or their complications, accounted for 1.7 percent of 24.1 million hospitalizations in the United States during 1972 and 1973, and 2.7 percent of admissions for patients aged 50 or older (Commission on Professional and Hospital Activities 1975). If one assumes that 10 percent of all hospitalized patients have gallstones, it can be estimated roughly that somewhere around 15 percent of patients at risk with cholelithiasis became symptomatic during those years. These calculations may, of course, be somewhat misleading by overestimating the frequency of symptoms, but they do indicate clearly that many patients with cholelithiasis are probably asymptomatic for years at a time, and perhaps permanently. Thus, the mere presence of gallstones in asymptomatic patients does not necessarily indicate that they require treatment.

We have seen earlier that the flow of bile from the liver can be subdivided into two categories, that dependent on the production of bile acids and that which is independent of bile acid production. Bile acid independent bile flow is regulated by the secretion of sodium into the biliary system and by the action of such gastrointestinal hormones as secretin, gastrin, and cholecystokinin. The biliary passages, and particularly the gall bladder, concentrates hepatic bile to as little as one-tenth of its original volume, by the selective reabsorption of water, chloride, and bicarbonate. Thus, gall bladder bile is much more highly concentrated in bile pigments, lipids, bile acids, sodium, potassium, and calcium than is hepatic bile, and almost the entire 3-g bile pool can be accommodated in the resting gall bladder. About 95 percent of the bile acids entering the intestine are reabsorbed passively in the upper small bowel and actively in the ileum, so that only 0.2 to 0.6 g are lost from the pool each day (Figure 12–1).

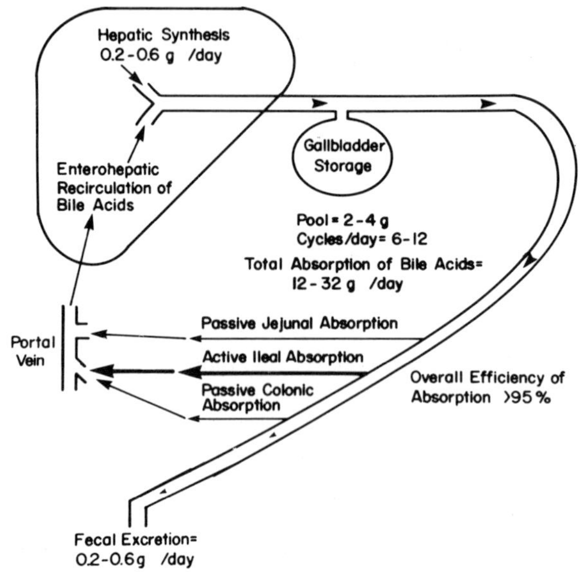

Figure 12-1. Overall economy and enterohepatic circulation of bile acids. After Bennion LJ, Grundy SM. N Engl J Med 299:1164, 1978.

THE BILE ACIDS

Cholic and chenodeoxycholic acids are synthesized in the liver from cholesterol, and are called *primary bile acids* (Figure 12). The former is hydroxylated at C3, 7, and 12; the latter, at C3 and 7. The other major bile acid in bile, deoxycholic acid, is called a *secondary bile acid* because it is formed in the intestine by bacterial dehydroxylation of cholic acid at the C7 position. About two-thirds of the deoxycholic acid is absorbed in the ileum and continues to participate in the enterohepatic circulation of bile acids, although it probably has little value in the micellarization of cholesterol (Thistle et al 1978). This property appears to be reserved primarily to those bile acids which are hydroxylated only at C3 and C7. The secondary bile acid formed in the intestine from dehydroxylation of chenodeoxycholic acid at the C7 position is called lithocholic acid. Upon absorption, lithocholate is rapidly sulfated in the liver and thus becomes less available for reabsorption. The concentration of lithocholic acid in normal bile is, accordingly, very small. The total bile acid pool in humans varies between 2 and 4 g normally, and the mean of its components consist of 40 percent chenodeoxycholic acid, 28 percent cholic acid, and 27 percent deoxycholic acid. The remaining 5 percent is composed largely of lithocholic acid and the 7-beta isomer of chenodeoxycholic acid, ursodeoxycholate. Minute amounts of lithocholate ketone derivatives are also found (percentages derived from data of Northfield and Hoffman 1975).

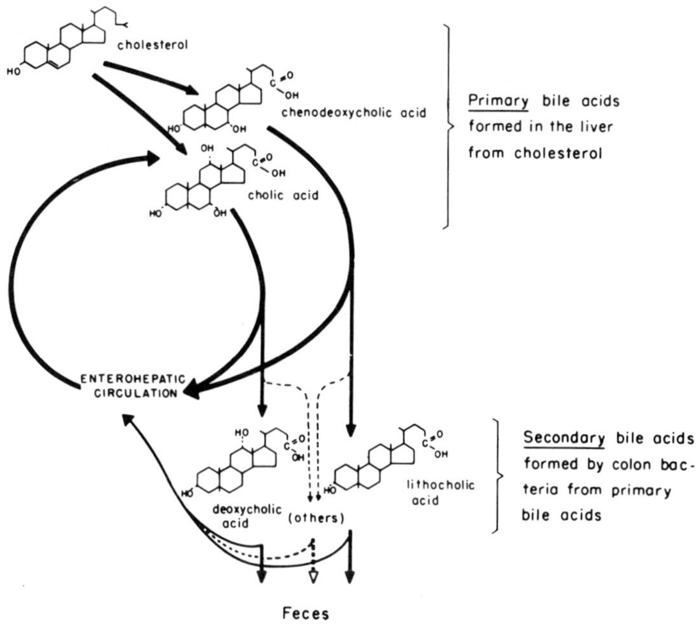

Figure 12–2. Formation of primary and secondary bile acids from cholesterol, and the enterohepatic circulation of bile salts. From Javitt NB. In: Schiff, L, ed. Diseases of the liver, 4th ed. Philadelphia: JB Lippincott, 1945:113. Reprinted by permission.

LECITHIN AND CHOLESTEROL

Cholesterol, which is almost totally insoluble in water, is solubilized in bile by the formation of mixed micelles containing both lecithin and bile acids. Both lecithin and bile acids are amphipathic, in that they contain both hydrophobic and hydrophilic components. Hydrophilic portions of bile acid molecules are both the hydroxy groups and the taurine or glycine conjugate group while the steroid ring is hydrophobic. Lecithin (phosphatidylcholine) contains two long-chain hydrocarbon hydrophobic tails, and a polar phosphoryl choline head, which is hydrophilic. Lecithin-bile micelles, hydrophilic heads ranged outward and hydrophobic tails inward, are soluble in water at a 2 to 1 ratio. The presence of lecithin greatly increases the solubility of cholesterol in the interior of the mixed micelle, at a 1 to 1 ratio. Thus the mixed micelle in solution presents as a spherical particle, cholesterol to the center, dissolved largely in the tails of phosphatidyl choline molecules and to a degree in the sterol components of bile acid molecules. The exterior of the micelle is composed of the hydrophilic hydroxyl and conjugate polar groups of the bile acids, and the phosphoryl choline groups of lecithin (Figure 12-3). The resulting micelle resembles a circle of covered wagons surrounding a community of besieged pioneers in the days of the old West.

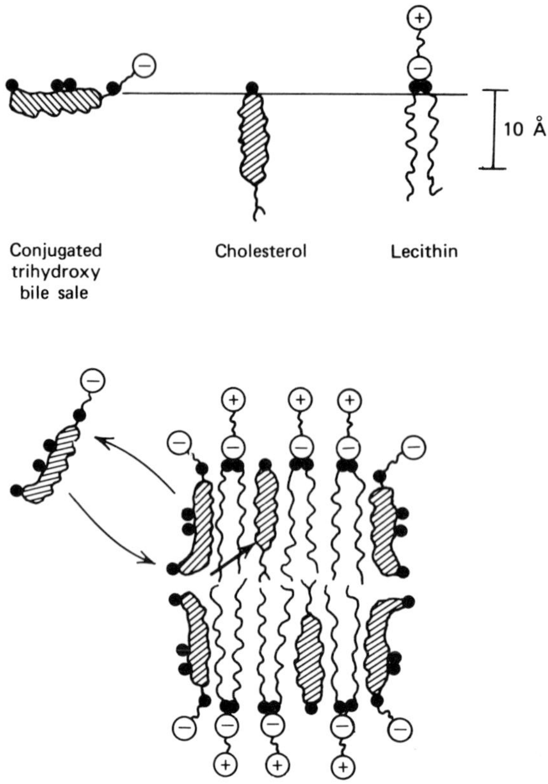

Figure 12–3. Mixed bile acid-lecithin micelle. In the upper part of the diagram, the three lipid molecules are oriented such that their hydrophilic segments are above the line and their hydrophobic segments are below. Bile acids are amphipaths and in aqueous solution form cylindrical aggregates (seen in cross-section in the lower part of the diagram) wherein the hydrophilic groups point outward and the hydrophobic portion is oriented inward. Lecithin is penetrated by water and causes swelling of the micelle. Thus cholesterol (arrow) which is virtually insoluble in water is transported within the hydrophobic center of the mixed micelle in bile, an aqueous solution. Courtesy of Dr. Donald Small. From Schoenfield, LJ. Diseases of the gallbladder and biliary system. New York: John Wiley and Sons, 1977:82. Reprinted by permission.

The solubility of cholesterol in bile is variable, depending as it does on the dilution of the bile, the concentration of total lipids, and the ratio of bile salts to lecithin. Carey and Small (1978) indicate that the relative concentrations of the major bile acids do not seem to affect the degree of cholesterol solubilization, while Thistle et al (1978) believe that deoxycholic acid has very limited effects on solubility. The total lipid content of bile is quite variable from time to time in any one person, and from person to person. Lipid content ranges from 0.2 to 7.9 g per dl in hepatic bile, and from 2.8 to 24.9 g per dl in gall bladdar bile. Accordingly, hepatic bile may often become supersaturated with cholesterol even in normal individuals, especially when the rate of bile flow is low. Supersaturated bile exists in two major states, a *metastable state* in which precipitation is unlikely unless a nidus is present, and a *labile state*, from which spontaneous precipitation is likely to occur. In metastable supersaturation, cholesterol is present in combination with lecithin as liquid crystals. The labile phase contains cholesterol is called *lithogenic*, the degree of lithogenicity being greater in microcrystals of cholesterol precipitate from bile in which labile supersaturation is present. Precipitates which nucleate around a nidus, such as calcium bilirubinate crystals or bacteria, are called heterogeneous calculi; those which precipitate from bile with labile supersaturation are called homogeneous, or pure, calculi (Table 12-1). Bile becomes supersaturated with cholesterol whenever its concentration exceeds the micellar capacity of an existing level of bile acids and lecithin. Because of this tendency for precipitation to occur, bile supersaturated with cholesterol is called *lithogenic*, the degree of lithogenicity being greater in the labile than in the metastable state.

For any given amount of lecithin and bile acids, proportionately less cholesterol is micellarized as the amount of water is increased. Accordingly, supersaturated dilute bile emerging from the liver may be converted to unsaturated bile by absorption of water in the gall bladder. Since the ratio of cholesterol to phospholipids increases at low flow rates of bile, fasting tends to make bile more lithogenic.

THE FORMATION OF GALLSTONES

Gallstones are of three major types, those containing purely cholesterol, those composed only of pigment, and those which contain mixtures of these two major ingredients. Pure stones of either type are quite uncommon, the greatest proportion by far being heterogeneous calculi. For discussion purposes, stones containing less than 25 percent cholesterol by weight are known as *pigment stones*, while those containing larger amounts are called *cholesterol stones*. Approximately one-fourth of all gallstones seen in the United States are pigment stones by these criteria, the remainder

Table 12–1. Steps in the Process of Gallstone Formation

1. Precipitation	cholesterol; calcium bilirubinate; mixed
2. Nucleation	homogeneous: "pure" cholesterol stones in supersaturated bile heterogeneous (stone-forming about a nidus): mucoprotein; calcium bilirubinate; bacteria; ova or worm segments; foreign bodies
3. Accretion	facilitated by stasis in gall bladder or bile ducts; incomplete emptying of gall bladder

being classified as cholesterol stones. Both types of gallstones may contain enough calcium to become radiopaque, this quality being conferred when calcium content exceeds 4 percent of dry weight (Soloway et al 1977). About two-thirds of opaque gallstones are pigment calculi, and about one-fifth of pigment calculi are radiolucent.

Cholesterol Gallstones

The various factors which favor the precipitation of cholesterol in bile are listed in Table 12-2, and the individual headings in that table are treated in detail in Tables 12-3 to 12-7. It appears that patients with cholesterol gallstones exhibit two major abnormalities: a tendency to secrete bile which is supersaturated with cholesterol, and a lower than normal total bile acid pool. There are many variables which contribute to these two abnormalities, and these are summarized in the accompanying tables. Taking as many of these as possible into account, the composite patient at greatest risk for the development of cholesterol gallstones would be an obese Pima Indian woman who has had a previous vagotomy for peptic ulcer disease and an

Table 12–2. Factors that Favor Precipitation of Cholesterol in Bile

1. increased concentration of cholesterol
2. decrement or alterations of bile acid pool
3. decreased phospholipid concentration
4. increased dilution of bile with reduced micellar concentration
5. stasis in gall bladder or bile ducts
6. increased permeability of gall bladder wall to bile acids
7. aging—? decreased bile acids; ? increased stasis

Table 12–3. Factors that Increase Concentrations of Cholesterol in Bile

1. genetic—? increased hydroxy methylglutaryl coenzyme A reductase
2. obesity
3. high caloric diet
4. ? diet high in unsaturated fats
5. hyperglycemia
6. high cholesterol diet
7. decreased conversion of cholesterol to bile acids in liver
8. ? increased mobilization of cholesterol from body stores
9. Estrogens and progestational hormones.
10. reduced chenodeoxycholic:cholic acid ratio
11. reduced rate of total bile acid production and decreased production of phospholipids

Table 12–4. Factors that Cause Decrement or Alterations of Bile Acid Pool

1. decreased conversion of cholesterol to bile acids—genetic (American Indians); progesterone and estrogens; reduced cholesterol 7-alpha-hydroxylase; insulin-treated diabetics; ? use of clofibrate
2. interruption of the enterohepatic circulation—ileal disease, bypass, or resection; untreated pancreatic insufficiency (cystic fibrosis); external biliary fistula
3. decrease in ratio of chenodeoxycholic:cholic acid—pregnancy; estrogens; use of bile acid chelating agents (cholestyramine)
4. reduced synthesis of bile acids by liver in response to decrement in size of pool (defective feedback regulation)—decreased storage time in gall bladder; increased intestinal motility; increased absorption of bile acids in upper intestine

Table 12–5. Factors that Cause Decreased Phospholipid Concentration in Bile

1. decreased production of phospholipids	? low bile output states; low fat diet
2. increased catabolism to lysolecithin	increased phospholipase A in wall of gall bladder, or produced by bacteria

Table 12–6. Factors that Lead to Increased Dilution and Reduced Micellar Concentration in Bile

1. increased bile acid independent bile flow.
2. decreased concentration of bile by gall bladder: chronic cholecystitis, cholesterolosis; Aschoff sinuses

Table 12–7. Factors that Lead to Stasis (Hypotonia, Decreased Emptying, or Both) in Gall Bladder and Bile Ducts

1. low fat diet	5. celiac disease
2. starvation	6. vagotomy
3. diabetes	7. anticholinergics
4. pregnancy	8. vasoactive intestinal polypeptide, gastric inhibitory polypeptide, ? glucagon

ileal bypass procedure for obesity, is a hyperlipidemic diabetic taking insulin, a low fat diet, and clofibrate, and is in the third trimester of pregnancy.

This absurd formulation stresses much that is currently known about the etiology of cholesterol stones. There does indeed appear to be a hereditary predisposition toward stone formation, and this may involve either an increase in the enzyme which monitors the rate-limiting step in the synthesis of cholesterol, a decrease in the enzyme which converts cholesterol to bile acids, or both. Levels of 3-hydroxy, 3-methylglutaryl coenzyme A (HMGCoA) reductase, the enzyme controlling the conversion of HMGCoA to mevalonic acid in the cholesterol pathway, have been found to be increased in liver biopsies from patients with cholesterol gallstones. There is also evidence that cholesterol 7-alpha hydroxylase, the controlling enzyme in the conversion of cholesterol to bile acids, is reduced (Bennion and Grundy 1978). It is not clear, however, that these abnormalities are truly genetic. In support of a genetic factor in the etiology of cholesterol gallstones is the finding of Bennion et al (1979) that the bile of both male and female Pimas tends to be in a metastable state of supersaturation even at puberty. Progression to a labile state during puberty and beyond occurs more rapidly in women, and is associated with a failure to increase the size of their bile acid pools. One might suspect that decreased levels of cholesterol hydroxylase, perhaps due to estrogenic activity, would explain this sexual difference.

Obesity has been found to be clearly associated with increased concentrations of cholesterol in bile, as has a high calorie diet, even among patients who are not obese. These changes are also associated with decreased synthesis of bile acids and phospholipids, which accelerates the trend toward supersaturation of bile with cholesterol.

Reduction of the bile acid pool may be caused by decreased production of bile acids, interruption of the enterohepatic circulation by ileal resection or bypass, and defective feedback regulation of pool size. Reduction in the size of the bile acid pool usually leads to increased synthesis by the liver, but decreased storage time in the gall bladder, increased intestinal motility, and increased absorption of bile acids in the upper intestine might lead to more rapid cycling of bile acids. The regulator of bile acid sythesis may perceive this state of affairs as indicating a normal-sized pool, and synthesis would not be increased. Furthermore, the bile acid profile might be changed by action of substances, such as estrogens, which appear to increase the synthesis of cholic acid at the expense of chenodeoxycholate. This leads to elevations in bile of the secondary bile acid derived from cholic acid, deoxycholic, and this is not believed to be an effective solubilizer of cholesterol (Thistle et al 1978). The use of clofibrate and the employment of insulin in diabetics also appear to decrease the production of bile acids.

Stasis, or incomplete emptying of the gall bladder occurs in many patients following vagotomy, and is an occasional complication of diabetic neuroenteropathy. While this element alone does not predispose to the formation of gallstones and may indeed allow more time for water absorption with an associated reduction in the lithogenicity of bile, stasis of lithogenic bile also provides more time for heterogeneous nucleation and accretion of gallstones to occur (LaMorte et al 1979). Furthermore, there is considerable evidence that decreased tone of gall bladder musculature, with resultant increased size and decreased emptying, may be partly responsible for the common association of cholelithiasis with pregnancy (Braverman et al 1980). Return of tone after pregnancy may account for some of the few cases of spontaneously disappearing gallstones which have been noted in the past (Dworken 1960;Wolpers 1968).

Pigmentary Gallstones

Pigment stones affect a different population than that at risk for cholesterol stones. Sex ratios are equal, aging leads to considerable increases in incidence, and the incidence is high among patients with hemolytic anemias, alcoholic cirrhosis of the liver, and chronic infections of the bililary tract (Table 12–8). Biliary stasis appears to play a large role in their development. Especially in the Orient, pigment stones are found fairly frequently in large bile ducts rather than in the gall bladder. Concentrations of bile acids, phospholipids, and cholesterol are not abnormal in patients with pigment stones, and many of them do have increased amounts of unconjugated bilirubin in their bile (Soloway et al 1977). Where infection is present, this increased degree of deconjugation has been ascribed to bacterial glucuronidases. The cause of deconjugation in uninfected bile may be due to naturally occurring mucosal glucuronidases or to the possibility that patients excrete a greater proportion of unconjugated hepatic bilirubin than usual.

Hypotonia of the gall bladder may favor the precipitation of calcium bilirubinate by allowing more concentration of bile to occur, the opposite of the effect of concentration on cholesterol solubility. Decrease in pH with concentration may also favor this precipitation. Once calcium bilirubinate and other calcium salts precipitate, it is believed that stone formation occurs along a glycoprotein matrix contained in mucus, since these substances avidly bind calcium salts.

Table 12–8. Factors that Favor the Development of Pigment (less than 25 percent cholesterol) Gallstones

1. any hemolytic disorder: associated with increased glucuronidase activity
2. alcoholic cirrhosis of the liver
3. chronic biliary tract infections
4. ? low fat diet
5. aging

INFLAMMATORY DISEASES OF THE GALL BLADDER

Acute and Chronic Cholecystitis

Inflammatory diseases of the gall bladder are almost invariably the result of previous cholelithiasis. In less than 10 percent of all cases, acute inflammation may occur without gallstones, either as a result of stasis due to prolonged fasting or inactivity or rarely from ischemia secondary to vascular diseases, such as periarteritis. Bacterial infection does not appear to be present at the onset of cholecystitis, but it is a common complication after two or three days of acute inflammation. The mechanism by which stasis induces damage to the wall of the gall bladder is not known, but it is believed that at least a portion of the damage may be due to the action of lysolecithin. This compound is produced from lecithin by the action of phospholipase A, an enzyme which has been shown to be present in small amounts in the mucosa of the gall bladder (Sjodahl and Wetterfors 1974). An association has recently been noted between the use of thiazide diuretics and acute cholecystitis (Rosenberg et al 1980). The reason for this relationship is not clear.

Pathology. The acutely inflamed gall bladder shows both edema and erythema of the wall grossly, and infiltration with round cells and polymorphonuclear leukocytes and vascular dilitation on microscopy. Occasional microerosions of the epithelium may be seen, at times associated with necrosis or gangrene of the gall bladder wall. Chronic inflammation is associated with thickening of the wall, reduced or normal size of the gall bladder, and fibrosis. At times, where a calculus has lodged in the neck of the gall bladder, blocking movement of bile in either direction, the organ may become markedly distended to several times its normal size, a condition known as hydrops of the gall bladder. Should the contents of a hydropic gall bladder become infected, a true abscess, or empyema, may appear.

The visceral peritoneum of the gall bladder is commonly involved in acute and chronic inflammatory processes, so it is not unusual to find such organs adherent to adjacent structures, especially the duodenum. Pressure from a large gallstone in an adherent gall bladder may lead to necrosis of the wall of that organ, with creation of a cholecystoduodenal fistula. A large calculus may thus proceed directly from the gall bladder into the intestine and lodge at the next normally narrowed area downstream in the intestine, the ileocecal valve. Failure of the stone to proceed beyond this site results in intestinal obstruction, a condition known as *gallstone ileus*. The cholecystoduodenal fistula is permanent and is readily diagnosed on plain radiographs of the right upper quadrant by the presence of air outlining the biliary tract.

Smaller gallstones commonly leave the gall bladder through the biliary ductal system, either with or without symptoms. They may lodge in the ampulla of Vater, a state known as choledocholithiasis, or they may pass readily into the intestine. Small gallstones have been identified in the stool of many patients with cholecystitis. Patients with transient choledocholithiasis frequently develop mild, transitory episodes of obstructive jaundice, while patients with stones lodged in the common bile duct have more prolonged obstruction, often followed by infections of the biliary tree, or *cholangitis.* Failure to relieve these obstructions promptly may lead to severe ascending cholangitis and even to abscesses in the liver. Localized hepatic abscesses may also result from direct perforation of an infected gall bladder into the substance of the liver. Repeated attacks of cholangitis, or recurrent infections of the extrahepatic biliary tree due to old inflammatory strictures, may, in the absence of corrective surgery, result in chronic obstructive jaundice, hepatocellular damage, and secondary biliary cirrhosis.

Free perforation of an infected gall bladder into the peritoneal cavity is fortunately quite rare. The resulting bile peritonitis is usually walled off quickly by the omentum, but not until considerable damage is done, probably by the action of lysolecithin, to surrounding viscera. Bile peritonitis may also be the result of blunt trauma to the abdomen with rupture of the liver or the extrahepatic biliary tree, and of penetrating wounds in the upper right quadrant. The possibility of secondary bile peritonitis is a persuasive reason against performing a percutaneous biopsy of the liver on a patient with possible total obstruction of the biliary tree.

Symptoms and signs of gallstones, even those associated with chronic cholecystitis, are often totally absent. In fact, it has been estimated that as many as half of all patients with gallstones experience neither symptoms nor complications from them. Certain vague symptoms, such as belching, flatulence, fatty food intolerance, and bloating, are probably no more common in patients with cholelithiasis than they are in an age- and sex-matched population without gallstones (Price 1963). The occurence of gallstones in patients with these symptoms is merely coincidental.

Steady, severe abdominal pain, usually located in the upper right quadrant of the abdomen and commonly referred directly through to the back and, at times, to the tip of the right scapula, is the hallmark of biliary ductal spasm. Symptoms seem to appear when a strong contraction of the gall bladder forces calculi into its ampulla or into the cystic duct, where they may impact and wholly or partially obstruct the flow of bile. Although this pain has commonly been designated "biliary colic," it is rarely intermittent or crampy and the term "colic" should not be used, since it is inaccurate. "Biliary spasm" is a more apposite description. Fever and leukocytosis are uncommon in patients with uncomplicated biliary spasm, and abdominal findings are usually limited to variable degrees of tenderness and perhaps muscular spasm in the upper right quadrant. Numerous observers have indicated that the pain of biliary spasm may appear in other parts of the abdomen, especially the epigastrium and the upper left quadrant, but its character is generally steady, boring, and severe (Schoenfield 1977).

Attacks of biliary spasm resulting from cholelithiasis usually occur some hours following a large meal, during a period of maximal contraction of the gall bladder. Patients are commonly awakened from sleep by the pain during the early hours of the morning. The extreme discomfort usually lasts for several hours and then subsides gradually. Spasmolytic analgesic agents, such as meperidine, are useful in relieving the pain, while morphine and codeine should be avoided since they may aggravate biliary spasm. Over 80 percent of patients with acute biliary spasm experience spontaneous relief of their symptoms.

Patients with *acute cholecystitis* experience the same sort of pain as do patients with biliary spasm alone. However, in the former situation, pain is more prolonged, abdominal tenderness and rigidity more marked, and fever and leukocytosis are usually associated. True rigors associated with the fever indicate biliary sepsis and require prompt blood cultures and administration of antibiotics prior to obtaining definitive bacterial reports. In these cases, it is wise to provide antibiotic coverage against both aerobic and anaerobic organisms, since either type may be involved. Approximately one-third of patients with acute cholecystitis are found to have bacterbilia (Csendes et al 1975), and in nearly 40 percent of these anaerobic organisms predominate (Nielsen and Justesen 1976). Sepsis is more common in patients with choledocholithiasis than it is in patients with acute obstructive cholelithiasis. The bacteria found are invariably enteric organisms, but there is no certainty regarding the route of infection. They are probably blood borne, since there are no data supporting the possibility that bacteria may be secreted by the liver, or that they may pass upward into the gall bladder from the unobstructred ductal system. Stasis of bile flow appears to be a major determinant for the development of sepsis. The effectiveness of an antibiotic depends more on achieving adequate blood and tissue levels than it does on obtaining high concentrations in the bile (Keighley et al 1976).

Ascending cholangitis is suspected when rigors and fever are associated with progressive obstructive jaundice. It is important to remember that cholangitis from choledocholithiasis may occur without any associated pain, especially in older patients. In fact, choledocholithiasis is a common cause of fevers of unknown etiology, regardless of a patient's age. The fever may remit after a period of several hours, only to recur some 10 or 12 hours later (Charcot intermittent fever) and may, occasionally, be associated with indications of gram-negative sepsis.

Hydrops of the gall bladder is diagnosed on examination by palpation of a globular, distended organ below the right costal margin, moving with respiration. The organ may not be tender and, unless empyema is present, the patient may not be febrile. Pressure on the abdomen should be exerted very gingerly in examining a palpable gall bladder, since overly enthusiastic, or repeated, examinations have been known to rupture that organ, especially when gangrene is also present. Should an infected gall bladder perforate spontaneously, a subhepatic abscess is a common complication.

Diagnosis

The diagnosis of cholelithiasis in a patient who has had a single or several attacks or probable biliary spasm is best confirmed by performing a single-dose oral cholecystogram, and repeating it the second day if the first series does not show concentration of the iodinated dye in the gall bladder. Repeat examination may further aggravate renal function in patients with kidney disease. The absence of opacification on the second day among patients who have indeed taken the cholecystographic agent and who do not have liver disease can be taken as a near-certain assurance of gall bladder disease, usually chronic cholecystitis with cholelithiasis. It is wise to conform this probability with ultrasonography, if this technique is readily available. This study can usually determine both the size and contents of the gall bladder and, if calculi are present, reveal the telltale echoes with anechoic areas behind them (Figure 8–18). Of course, the finding of radiopaque stones in a nonfilling gall bladder, or radiolucent stones in a functioning gall bladder on cholecystography, requires no further confirmatory studies. The day may soon come when ultrasonography will take precedence over, or even replace, oral cholecystography, since it is quite accurate and has the advantage of requiring no X-ray exposure and no ingested agents. Furthermore, sonography can be performed accurately even in patients who are icteric or who have chronic liver disease. For the present, however, since expertise in this study is still limited and costs of the procedure are significantly higher, oral cholecystography remains the preferable initial procedure. In the icteric or septic patient, since oral cholecystography is likely to be unsuccessful, sonography should be the primary diagnostic procedure.

Radionuclide scanning of the biliary tract (cholescintigraphy) shows great promise as a diagnostic tool in biliary tract disorders, even in the presence of mild degrees of jaundice. ^{99m}Tc–pyridoxylidene glutamate (PG) and ^{99m} Tc–dimethyl iminodiacetic acid (HIDA) are taken up avidly by hepatocytes following intravenous injection, and are secreted rapidly into the biliary tract in sufficient isotopic concentrations to allow identification of the extrahepatic biliary tree, gall bladder, and duodenum by gamma camera scintigraphy within one hour after administration.

Jaundice does not interfere with biliary excretion of the tagged compounds unless bilirubin levels exceed 5.0 mg per dl. In patients with hepatocellular jaundice, the bile duct system may not be visualized after administration of HIDA, but visualization of the duodenum speaks against biliary obstruction, and occasionally enough isotopic concentration appears in the gall bladder among patients with hepatitis to allow identification of that organ. Some patients with hepatocellular disease show gall bladder visualization at 24 hours without demonstrating intestinal activity of the isotope. If neither gall bladdor nor intcstinal activity appears in a full day, complete biliary tract obstruction is likely to be the cause (Rosenthall et al 1978).

In patients with acute cholecystitis and in patients with other causes of cystic obstruction, administration of these cholephilic isotopes leads to prompt appearance within one hour of ductal and intestinal radioactivity without visualization of the gall bladder. Thus, Down et al (1979) demonstrated that scintigraphy with PG documented the presence of acute cholecystitis in 65 of 66 patients with acute abdominal pain. PG scanning had a 99 percent sensitivity compared with sensitivities of 75 and 54 percent respectively for oral cholecystography and ultrasonography in the same group of patients. The specificity of PG scanning, its negativity in the absence of acute cholecystitis, was 86 percent. Some authors suggest that the specificity of cholescintigraphic diagnosis of cystic duct obstruction is improved by administering cholecystokinin and a second dose of isotope to patients whose gall bladder does not visualize in two hours. This reasoning is based on the suspicion that the isotope may not enter a full gall bladder despite patency of the cystic duct.

Weissman et al (1980) divide the distribution of HIDA into four nonbiliary phases, the blood pool phase (1–5 minutes after injection), the hepatocytic phase (5–20 minutes), the renal excretion phase (5–15 minutes), and the intestinal phase (30–60 minutes). They have shown that scintigraphy may also be useful in demonstrating certain cardiovascular (cardiac chamber enlargement, aneurysms), hepatic (metastases, abscesses), urinary tract (renal masses, urteral obstruction), and intestinal (displacements, malrotations) abnormalities if frequent and appropriate scintiphotos are taken in the minutes following the administration of the isotope.

Treatment

Surgical Therapy. The patient who has had biliary spasm or acute cholecystitis should be treated promptly by cholecystectomy, usually within several days of the disappearance of symptoms. The likelihood that further attacks will occur and the possibility of more severe complications are so great that advising delay, especially in patients who show no contraindications to surgery, is foolhardy. Wenckert and Robertson (1966) showed that at least one-third of patients who had weathered an attack of cholecystitis had serious recurrent problems within 11 years of the original diagnosis. Of course, one must be selective in advising surgery, since some patients with renal or cardiac disease may be such poor risks that careful follow-up is preferable. Roughly 10 percent of patients operated on for cholecystitis will also have common duct stones. Because of this, cholangiograms should probably be performed routinely at the time of surgery.

For the patient who has had no symptoms and is found to have gallstones incidentally on routine examination or while having other abdominal X-rays taken, the disposition is not so clear. Perhaps as many as 80 to 90 percent of these patients will have no symptoms from gallstones during the next decade, and there is no way of predicting which are most likely to have trouble. It was formerly felt that patients with multiple small stones were more likely to have subsequent difficulty than were those with single stones, but this distinction is no longer certain. In the present state of knowledge, it is probably best to inform the patient of the existence of gallstones, advise follow-up and suggest surgery at the onset of symptoms. The only exception to this suggestion may be among insulin-dependent diabetics, who might best be operated upon, even though free of symptoms, when the diagnosis is made. In such patients the increased risk of biliary sepsis and the increased likelihood of complications after emergency surgery appear to support prophylactic cholecystectomy.

Any of the complications of cholelithiasis, of course, require urgent surgery, as soon as the condition of the patient is stabilized. But the best way to treat the complications is to prevent them. Most patients with biliary sepsis have had previous intimations of cholelithiasis, and alertness of the patient and physician to these symptoms, plus early surgery, will avoid future problems.

Dissolution of Gallstones. As soon as the various factors responsible for the solubilization of cholesterol in bile were clarified, it was inevitable that efforts would be made to reduce the lithogenicity of bile, and thus to dissolve cholesterol gallstones, without surgery. It seemed apparent that reduction in the synthesis of cholesterol itself would probably be self-defeating, because this would at the same time reduce the production of bile acids as well. Feeding of choline, the precursor of lecithin, soon proved to be ineffectual in reducing bile saturation.

The administration of bile acids by mouth was approached with some hesitancy because their laxative effects had been known and used therapeutically for many years, and might have proved to be a significant deterrent to long-term therapy. When trials were made, however, it was found that stool frequency responses to oral bile acids varied considerably from patient to patient, and that the diarrhea tended to subside with regular use (Thistle el al 1978). The administration of cholic acid raised the concentration of this normal bile constituent and its secondary derivative, 7-deoxycholic acid, to 75 to 90 percent of total bile acids but did not appreciably change the lithogenicity (cholesterol saturation) of the bile. The administration of chenodeoxycholate, on the other hand, increased its concentration to 75 to 95 percent of total bile acids, and in many cases decreased bile saturation as well. Lithocholate, the secondary 7-deoxy form of chenodeoxycholic acid, was increased only slightly in the bile, presumably because it is sulfated in its first pass through the liver after absorption in the intestine and then no longer participates in the enterohepatic circulation. Thus, chenodeoxycholate was employed in several small clinical trials and in a single national study.

Early results indicate that feeding chenodeoxycholic acid in divided doses of less than 15 mg per kg per day, leads to total dissolution of cholesterol gallstones in just under 25 percent of patients after two years and to a partial response in another 15 percent. With doses exceeding 15 mg per kg, complete dissolution occurs in 50 percent of patients and partial dissolution in 33 percent. Large solitary stones, calcified stones, and stones in gall bladders unable to concentrate cholecystographic contrast substances do not appear to respond, or respond poorly, to this therapy (Hoffman et al 1978). Side effects, other than diarrhea, are minimal, and there is little evidence of significant hepatotoxicity or alterations in serum lipids.

Ursodeoxycholic acid, the 7 beta epimer of chenodeoxycholate, also appears to be effective in reducing bile saturation with cholesterol, and at doses which may be less than half as great. Administration of urso leads to smaller biliary concentrations of lithocholic acid as well and, since this secondary bile acid probably has mild hepatotoxic effects in small doses, urso may actually be preferable to chenodeoxycholate. Added benefits of urso over cheno include an apparent decrease in the synthesis of cholesterol and a reduced tendency to cause diarrhea (Stiehl et al 1978). The only bile acids found to be effective in the dissolution of gallstones thus far are those which are hydroxylated only at the 3 and 7 positions. Cholic acid, a trihydroxy form, may have been effective if its concentration in bile could have been increased without simultaneous elevations of its less effective 3,12 hydroxy secondary derivative, deoxycholate.

The major drawbacks to the regular use of chenodeoxycholate in gallstone dissolution are the length of time required (approximately one year), and the fact that bile lithogenicity reappears promptly after therapy is discontinued. Reappearances of gallstones may take several years, however, and many patients might wish to risk this eventuality if surgery could possibly be avoided. Although the permanent place of dissolution therapy in the management of cholesterol gallstones is not clear at present and will depend on such factors as cost and compliance, its success in many patients is a grand example of the prompt and useful application of laboratory discoveries to patient care.

THE CHOLECYSTOSES

There are a number of noninflammatory, benign hyperplastic disorders of the gall bladder which occur with enough frequency to be mentioned briefly. These include adenomyomatosis, cholesterosis, and procelain gall bladder. These disorders do not produce any distinctive symptoms yet may produce singular pictures on radiography. Procelain gall bladders are agreed to be premalignant conditions and should be immediately removed.

Adenomyomatosis is primarily a hypertrophy of the gall bladder mucosa, with mucosal folds often penetrating into and through the muscularis, producing deep sinuses (Aschoff-Rokitansky) which are clearly apparent as spicules on the margin of the gall bladder shadow on cholecystography. The disorder may be generalized throughout the gall bladder or localized. In the absence of gallstones, this condition is of no special clinical significance.

Cholesterosis of the gall bladder is caused by diffuse infiltration of the mucosa with lipid-filled macrophages. The major lipid is esterified cholesterol which appears to have been absorbed from bile by an unknown process (Feldman and Feldman 1954). Its appearance has no relationship whatsoever to levels of cholesterol in the serum or bile. Grossly, the mucosa of the gall bladder is diffusely red, save for numerous yellowish white nodules disseminated over the surface, the entire picture resembling the surface of a strawberry. The disorder itself is often readily diagnosed on radiography, and probably has no particular clinical significance.

Procelain gall bladder refers to the deposition of a radiopaque layer of calcuim salts evenly throughout the submucosa. The disease is probably a cholecystosis because, in many cases, there is no evidence of chronic inflammation or scarring. It is commonly associated with dysplastic changes of the overlying mucosa, and coexisting carcinomas of the gall bladder are present in approximately one-fourth of patients (Polk 1966) The radiologic picture of a delicate ringlike structure in the upper right quadrant of the abdomen is distinctive and is often found fortuitously on X rays taken for other reasons.

PRIMARY SCLEROSING CHOLANGITIS

This is a rare disorder in which progressive fibrosis occurs in all or in segments of the extrahepatic biliary tree, leading to progressive obstruction of the flow of bile. At times, the process may involve larger intrahepatic ducts as well. The cause is unknown, but up to 25 percent of patients have associated chronic ulcerative colitis, and a few have retroperitoneal fibrosis. The course of primary sclerosing cholangitis is very long, the severity of symptoms being proportional to the degree of biliary obstruction. Patients tend to have pruritus and signs of hyperlipidemia, including xanthomatoses. Rigors and fever are commonly noted in connection with episodes of bacterial cholangitis. In time, biliary cirrhosis, portal hypertension, and variceal hemorrhage may develop. Should surgery be nesessary, patients usually tolerate it well because hepatocullar function is rather well preserved.

The clinical picture at onset is much like that seen in primary biliary cirrhosis, with which this disorder may be confused. However, the prevalence of sclerosing cholangitis in men and the absence of mitochondrial antibodies help clarify the picture. Precise diagnosis can best be made at surgery but, at times, delineation of the extrahepatic biliary tree by endoscopic or percutaneous cholangiography reveals the characteristic beading and narrowing of the lumen. Laboratory data reveal obstructive findings with marked elevations of alkaline phosphatase and cholesterol, moderate aminotransferase elevations, and variable degrees of hyperbilirubinemia. Fat malabsorption due to inadequate amounts of bile salts entering the intestine is a common complication, although weight and appetite are usually quite normal during most of the course of the disease.

The response of primary sclerosing cholangitis to the administration of glucocorticoids for extended periods of time, can, in my experience, be quite gratifying. In many patients it is possible to maintain benefits on alternate-day therapy, with consequent reduction of side effects. Therapy results in reduction of jaundice and malaise, without improvement of elevated phosphatase levels. The mechanism of this response is not clear, because often no active ductal inflammation is found. Pruritus is usually responsive to the administration of cholestyramine, and episodes of cholangitis usually improve with administration of ampicillin, cephalosporins, or animoglycoside antibiotics.

CARCINOMA OF THE EXTRAHEPATIC BILIARY TRACT

Carcinoma of the gall bladder is an uncommon disorder, occurs two-thirds of the time in women over the age of 60, and is associated with gallstones in 90 percent or more of patients. The possibility of its occurrence, however, is not a very strong reason for the removal of asymptomatic gallstones, since the incidence of adenocarcinomas of the gall bladder in such patients is 1 percent or less. Most people believe, however, that chronic cholecystitis is in some way responsible for the subsequent development of cancer (Bismuth and Malt 1979).

When the disease becomes symptomatic, it may cause pain similar to that of biliary spasm, often associated with obstructive jaundice. At this stage, the condition is usually inoperable because of local spread to liver and metastases to regional lymph nodes. Decompression of the gall bladder and internal biliary deviation procedures are usually advisable. Efforts are being made to devise beneficial chemothereapeutic protocols for this disease, but there is as yet no reliable therapy. Radiation may be useful at times.

Carcinoma of the extrahepatic bile ducts is more prevalent in men, and usually presents as gradually progressive obstructive jaundice, often without pain. When pain does appear, it is usually late in the disease and suggests perineural involvement. According to data collected by Schoenfield (1977) biliary ductal carcinomas occur with about one-fifth the frequency of carcinomas of the gall bladder, and one-eighth the frequency of pancreatic carcinomas. The major sites of predilection are the bifurcation of the common hepatic duct, the middle of the common bile duct, and the ampulla of Vater. Vaterian carcinomas tend to be exophytic and often protrude into the lumen of the duodenum; they may accordingly bleed slowly and lead to detectable levels of occult blood in the stool.

When ductal carcinomas occur in the ampulla or in the common bile duct, the resulting obstruction usually causes painless distention of the gall bladder. The presence, then, of an enlarged, nontender gall bladder is a characteristic sign in patients with obstructive jaundice of a distal malignant obstruction. This finding is called the *Courvoisier sign* and serves to distinguish obstructive jaundice caused by gallstones, intrahepatic cholestasis, or tumors proximal to the common bile duct from tumors of the common duct, head of the pancreas, or ampulla of Vater. Ductal obstruction by gallstones usually does not lead to Courvoisier sign because distention is unlikely to occur in a gall bladder fibrosed by previous inflammation.

Bile duct carcinomas are fairly frequently found in societies where infections with the liver fluke, *Clonorchis sinensis,* is common. It is believed that the chronic obstruction by these agents leads to inflammation which, in turn, leads to dysplastic effects of possibly carcinogenic bile sterols. Though very rare, there is also an increased incidence of bile duct carcinoma among patients with chronic ulcerative colitis.

The diagnosis of bile duct carcinomas is not difficult if the gall bladder is distended. In higher lesions, however, one has to entertain the gamut of intrahepatic and extrahepatic possibilities. Utrasonography, with its ability to demonstrate dilated intrahepatic and extrahepatic ducts, has been very helpful in recent years, while additional invasive studies such as percutaneous and retrograde cholangiography are usually diagnostic.

Therapy is limited to surgery, and the results are usually dismal. Bypass procedures are often possible so that jaundice can be relieved, the most useful being implantation of the common bile duct above the obstruction end to end to a loop of jejunum brought into the field after transection of the small intestine below the ligament of Treitz (Roux loop). To date, chemotherapy has not been rewarding.

HISTORICAL DIGRESSION

Proper names referred to in this chapter include: Ludwig ASCHOFF (1866–1924), German pathologist, Freiburg; Jean Martin CHARCOT (1825–1893), French neurologist, Paris; Ludwig Georg COURVOISIER (1843–1918), Swiss surgeon, Basel; Karl Freiherr von ROKITANSKY (1804–1878), Austrian pathologist, Vienna; César ROUX (1857–1934), Swiss surgeon, Lausanne.

SELECTED REFERENCES

Bennion LJ, Grundy SM. Risk factors for the development of cholelithiasis in man. New Engl J Med 299:1161–67, 1221–27, 1978.

Bennion LJ, Knowler WC, Mott DM et al. Development of lithogenic bile during puberty in Pima Indians. New Engl J Med 300:873–76, 1979.

Bismuth H, Malt RA. Current concepts in cancer. Carcinoma of the biliary tract. New Engl J Med 301:704–60, 1979.

Braverman DZ, Johnson ML, Kern F, Jr. Effects of pregnancy and contraceptive steroids on gall bladder function. New Engl J Med 302:362–64, 1980.

Carey MC, Small DM. The physical chemistry of cholesterol solubility in bile. Relationship to gallstone formation and dissolution in man. J Clin Invest 61:998–1026, 1978.

Commission on Professional and Hospital Activities. Hospital mortality, PAS Hospitals, 1972–1973. Ann Arbor, Mich., 1975.

Csendes A, Fernandez M, Uribe P. Bacteriology of the gallbladder in normal subjects. Am J Surg 129:629–31, 1975.

Down RHL, Arnold J, Goldin A, et.al. Comparison of accuracy of $_{99}{}^{m}$Tc-pyridoxylidene glutamate scanning with oral cholecystography and ultrasonography in diagnosis of acute cholecystitis. Lancet 2:1094–97, 1979.

Dworken HJ. Recent experiences with spontaneously disappearing gallstones. Gastroenterology 38:76–86, 1960.

Feldman M, Feldman M, Jr. Cholesterosis of the gall bladder. An autopsy study of 165 cases. Gastroenterology 27:641–48, 1954.

Hoffman AF, Thistle JL, Klein PD, et al. Chemotherapy for gallstone dissolution. II. Induced changes in bile composition and gallstone response. JAMA 239:1138–44, 1978.

Keighley MRB, Drysdale RB, Quoraishi AH. Antibiotics in biliary disease: the relative importance of antibiotic concentrations in the bile and serum. Gut 17:495–500, 1976.

LaMorte WW, Schoetz Jr DJ, Birkett DH, et al. The role of the gall bladder in the pathogenesis of cholesterol gallstones. Gastroenterology 77:580–92, 1979.

Nielson ML, Justesen T. Anaerobic and aerobic bacteriological studies in biliary tract disease. Scand J Gastroent 11:437–46, 1976.

Northfield TC, Hofmann AF. Biliary lipid output during three meals and an overnight fast. I. Relationship to bile acid pool size and cholesterol saturation of bile in gallstone and control subjects. Gut 16:1–17, 1975.

Polk HC, Jr. Carcinoma and the calcified gall bladder. Gastroenterology 50: 582–85, 1966.

Price WH. Gallbladder dyspepsia. Br Med J 2:138–41, 1963.

Rosenberg L, Shapiro S, Slone D, et al. Thiazides and acute cholecystitis. N Engl J Med 303:546–48, 1980.

Rosenthall L, Shaffer EA, Lisbona R, et al. Diagnosis of hepatobiliary disease by $_{99}$mTc-HIDA cholescintigraphy. Radiology 126:467–74, 1978.
Schoenfield LJ. Diseases of the gall bladder and biliary system. New York: John Wiley and Sons, 1977.
Sjodahl R, Wetterfors J. Lysolecithin and lecithin in the gall bladder wall and bile: their possible roles in the pathogenesis of acute cholecystitis. Scand J Gastroent 9:519–25, 1974.
Soloway RD, Trotman BW, Ostrow JD. Pigment gallstones. Gastroenterology 72:167–82, 1977.
Stiehl A, Czygan P, Lommerell B, et al. Ursodeoxycholic acid versus chenodeoxycholic acid. Comparison of their effects on bile acid and bile lipid composition in patients with cholesterol gallstones. Gastroenterology 75:1016–20, 1978.
Thistle JL, Hofmann AF, Ott BJ, et al. Chemotherapy for gallstone dissolution. I. Efficacy and safety. JAMA 239:1041–46, 1978.
Weissman HS, Sugarman LA, Frank MS, et al. Serendipity in technetium-$_{99}$m dimethyl iminodiacetic acid cholescintigraphy. Radiology 135: 449–54, 1980.
Wenckert A, Robertson B. The natural course of gallstone disease: 11-year review of 781 nonoperated cases. Gastroenterology 50:376–81, 1966.
Wolpers C: Spontanauflösung von Gallenblasensteinen. Dtsch Med Wochenschr 90(2):2525–32, 1968.

DISCUSSION QUESTION

A 52-year-old male executive given only to social drinking and asymptomatic save for occasional flatulence is told following a complete physical examination with X rays that his gall bladder "does not function" and should be removed. Comment on all appropriate aspects of this problem.

CLINICAL CONFERENCE 7

A 19-year-old black man is hospitalized for the eighth time, complaining of having had attacks of severe pain in the right upper quadrant of the abdomen radiating into the back during the previous 12 days. Each attack lasts several hours and is associated with nausea and upper abdominal bloating. When the pain is more severe, he feels it also in his right shoulder. It is not aggravated by bending over or breathing deeply. Following the disappearance of the pain, he is weak for several hours.

This type of abdominal pain is completely new to the patient, although since childhood he has experienced episodes of pain in the midabdomen lasting several days at a time. He also has frequent pains in the wrists, hands, and back that are unassociated with swelling or tenderness in his joints.

There is no clear relationship between any of his abdominal pains and his diet. For the past five years recurrent skin ulcerations have appeared around both lateral malleoli. These ulcerations tend to heal slowly and leave large scars. Early in life he was noted to be jaundiced, and this has continued until the present time. With some episodes of abdominal pain, the jaundice seems to become more marked. The patient has also been told that he is anemic and has been transfused with eight units of blood over the years.

On examination he is well developed, weighs 137 pounds, and stands 73 inches tall. He is acutely ill because of abdominal pain. Scleral icterus is marked. Examination of the chest is negative except for a grade 1 systolic apical murmur. The heart is not enlarged, and the lungs are clear. Examination of the abdomen reveals marked tenderness and muscle spasm in the right upper quadrant, without a palpable mass. Bowel sounds are normal, and there is no distention of the abdomen. His spleen is enlarged and descends 8 cm below the left costal margin on inspiration. Superficial ulcerations are present on the lateral aspect of both ankles.

Initial laboratory data show a hemoglobin of 7.0 g per 100 dl; hematocrit, 23 (usually 21 to 25) percent; reticulocytes, 9 (usually 6 to 8) percent; and a white cell count of 20,000. The smear shows anisocytosis, hypochromia, stippled forms, sickled cells, and target cells. A two-hour urine shows a positive test for bilirubin and contains 6 Ehrlich units of urobilinogen. Serum iron is 120 μg; total iron-binding capacity, 270. In the next few days the following laboratory data are obtained (expressed as mg per dl unless otherwise stated): bilirubin, 10.8 total, 5.3 direct; urea nitrogen, 11; fasting glucose, 90; serum electrolytes, normal; alkaline phosphatase, 95 IU per liter. Total serum proteins are 8.6 g per dl, albumin, 4.7; aspartate aminotransferase, 45 (15 to 40) units; serum amylase 45 (4–25) μ per ml. A stool specimen is guaiac negative. Three months earlier the total bilirubin had been 7.7, the direct 0.8. A plain film of the abdomen was taken (Figure 12–4).

Briefly discuss the mechanisms of this patient's illness, touching on the significance of his history, the meaning of the laboratory data, the importance of the X ray, and the probable cause of his new symptoms. Explain particularly the significance of the changes in serum bilirubin values and indicate what the principal features of his treatment should be.

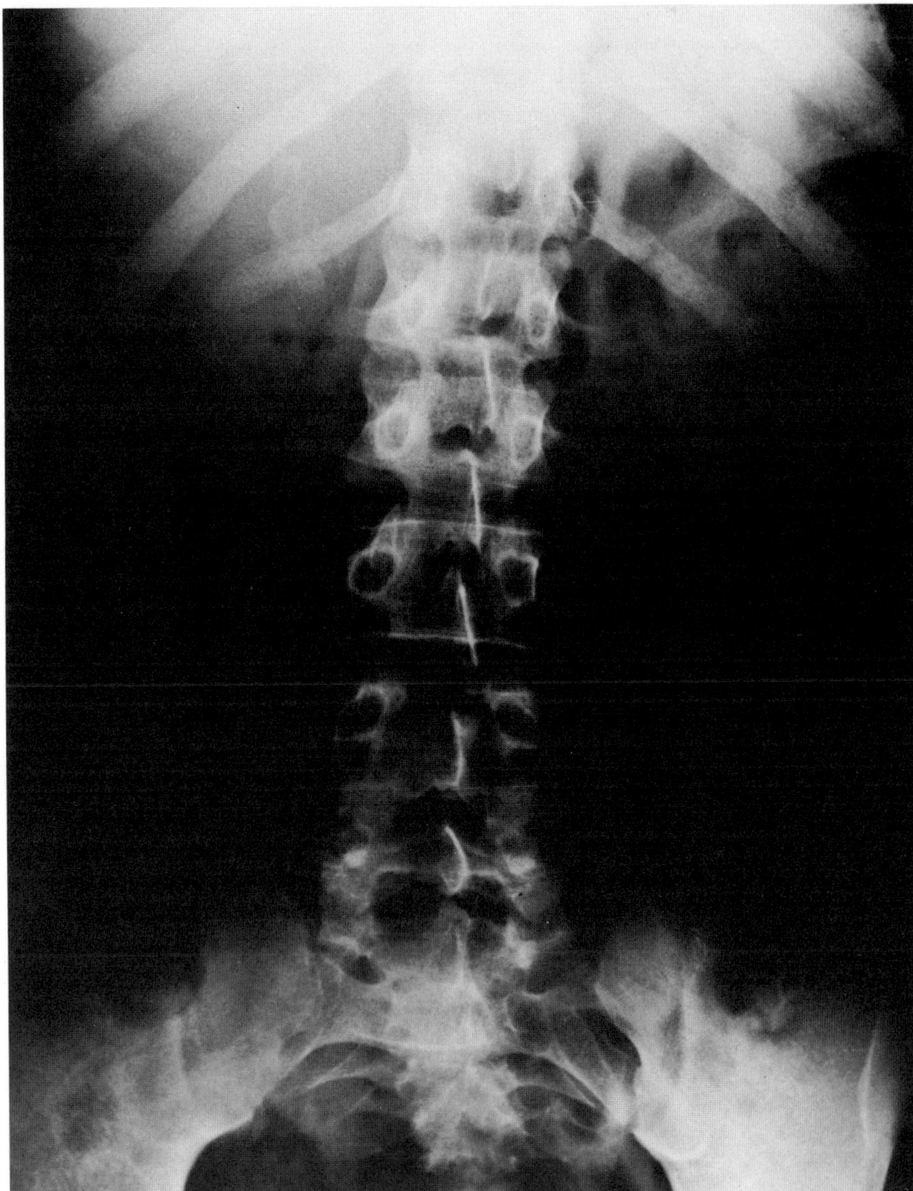

Figure 12-4. Plain film of abdomen, Clinical Conference 7.

CHAPTER 13

The Pancreas: Physiology, Inflammations, and Neoplasms

Like a nuclear power plant, the pancreas operates effectively and quietly when all its synthetic and conveyance systems are in order but is capable of rampant self-destruction and regional catastrophe whenever these normal mechanisms go awry. The damaged pancreas can be literally destroyed by its own synthetic products, digestive enzymes of great potency. This chapter reviews the synthetic capabilities of the pancreas, then highlights agents and mechanisms which are believed to suborn them.

ANATOMY AND DEVELOPMENT

The pancreas is a long, narrow gland which lies transversely across the upper abdomen in the retroperitoneal space. Its head nestles against the inner curve of the C-shaped loop formed by the curve of the upper duodenum. The body and tail of the gland rise upward and to the left from the head and lie behind the stomach. Embryologically, the pancreas arises from a dorsal and a ventral epithelial duodenal bud, each of which develops both ductular and acinar tissue. By the second month of fetal life, these buds fuse into a single organ, the ventral bud forming the head of the adult pancreas, the dorsal bud developing into the body and tail. In humans, the proximal portion of the dorsal bud duct (Santorini) usually atrophies completely, while the body and tail portion remain as the distal section of the adult pancreatic duct (Wirsung). The proximal portion of the adult duct of Wirsung is formed from the duct of the original ventral bud. Rarely, the proximal end of the dorsal bud duct persists into adulthood as an accessory pancreatic duct entering the upper duodenum.

Acinar (exocrine glandular) and ductular tissue arises from multiple sites along the primordial epithelial buds, and islet cell tissue (Langerhans) arises from other sites on the buds. During early fetal life, these two separate tissues mix with one another, but each retains its own distinctive character, acinar tissue being linked to the ductular system, and islet tissue having no ductal connections, thus qualifying as endocrine glands. Distinct islet and acinar tissue are detectable by the 19th week of fetal life (Patten 1953). Occasionally, anomalous pancreatic rests may persist into adult life as functioning acinar tissue located in the wall of greater curve of the distal stomach or the inner curve of the duodenum. These rests usually have their own secretory ducts, respond to normal pancreatic stimuli, and cause no functional problems. Their identification may lead to diagnostic problems, however, when they are found as negative filling defects in the stomach or intestinal wall on X ray study of the upper gastrointestinal tract, and they must be distinguished from neoplastic tissue.

Pancreatic acinar cells have the shape of a truncated pyramid and are arranged around a central lumen in a circular fashion. There is only one type of acinar cell. The central lumina empty into progressively larger intercalated and collecting ducts which eventually join the duct of Wirsung. This main pancreatic duct enters the ampulla of Vater where, in 80 percent of individuals, it is joined with the common bile duct. Occasionally, the junction with the common bile duct is proximal to the ampulla, and in a few cases the pancreatic duct and the common bile duct join the duodenum separately.

Pancreatic islet cells are of at least three different types, designated alpha, beta, and delta. A recent short investigation revealed no clue relating to the absence of gamma cells from this system of nomenclature, so their absence must remain an enigma to those students of medicine who are devoted to a sense of Greek orderliness, and they should trouble themselves no further. Bothersome enough is the fact that some investigators now classify delta as A_1 cells and alpha as A_2! We will keep the matter as simple as possible, using the somewhat recondite alpha, beta, delta system.

All islet cells contain granules, those in delta cells being less dense and smaller than those in alpha and beta cells. Islets are richly supplied with blood, and their tissue mass is about two percent of pancreatic weight (Cardell 1978). Islet cell mass consists of 20 to 35 percent alpha cells, 60 to 75 percent beta cells, and 5 percent delta cells. Alpha cell granules contain only glucagon, and they are soluble in water and insoluble in alcohol. Beta cells contain insulin in alcohol-soluble granules. The granules of delta cells have been shown, at least in tumors, to contain a variety of polypeptide hormones, usually one to the exclusion of the others in any single case. Thus gastrin has been found to be the sole consituent of delta cell adenomas in patients with the Zollinger-Ellison syndrome; vasoactive intestinal polypeptide, the sole constituent in patients with the Verner-Morrison (watery diarrhea, achlorhydria, hypokalemia) syndrome (1974), and somatostatin has been identified in another case (Krejs et al 1979).

EXOCRINE PHYSIOLOGY

Acinar cells comprise 95 percent of the cellular population of the exocrine pancreas. Their cell membranes contain specific receptors for cholinergic (parasympathetic) and various polypeptide (secretin, cholecystokinin) agonists. Acetylcholine and cholecystokinin (CCK), after membrane depolarization, activate the 3′5′-guanosine monophosphate pathway and, in the presence of calcium, cause marked enzymic secretion by acinar cells. Binding of vasoactive intestinal polypeptide and secretin to acinar receptors activates the 3′5′-adenosine monophosphate shunt and causes increased production of bicarbonate, sodium, and water and increased secretion of enzymes by acinar and proximal ductular cells. Bicarbonate is secreted in exchange for chloride, and sodium for hydrogen, resulting in decreased pH of blood leaving the actively secreting pancreas.

Intracellular transport in acinar cells has been worked out in some detail (Webster et al 1977)(Figure 13–1). Almost all enzymic proteins are produced from amino acids brought to the acinar cells, and not from the preexisting cytoplasmic proteins. Enzymes are synthesized on ribosomes of the endoplasmic reticulum, and are then sulfated, glycosylated or combined with metallic ions in the Golgi apparatus. They emerge from Golgi structures as condensing vacuoles, which are then concentrated into membrane-wrapped zymogen granules. Upon stimulation with CCK or acetylcholine, zymogen granules migrate to the apex of the acinar cell, combine their membranes with that of the cell, and extrude their protein (enzymic) contents into the acinar lumen. CCK and acetylcholine also increase the synthesis of enzymes. Drugs, such as colchicine and vinblastine, which inhibit cellular microtubules, reduce the transport and release of protein and the production of zymogen.

The functional state of pancreatic acinar tissue is dependent on the existing milieu. Fasting and total parenteral nutrition lead to reduction in the synthesis of protein, decrease in the amount of nucleic acids, and diminished cellular volume and enzymic production. The response of acinar tissue to feeding following a period of fasting is markedly less than the secretory response produced when an unfasted animal is fed. This hypotrophic response is probably mediated by the absence of both CCK and acetylcholine and not by protein deprivation since, as has been noted, it occurs in well-fed individuals who have been nourished parenterally. Pancreatic atrophy has also been noted after hypophysectomy and is believed to be the result of the absence of growth hormone. Acetylcholine and gastrin cause hypertrophy of acinar cells, but both hypertrophy and hyperplasia are caused by CCK.

Pancreatic Enzymes

Acinar cells produce at least six proteolytic enzymes, plus amylase, lipase, colipase, trypsin inhibitor, and ribonuclease (Wormsley 1977; Figarella 1973; Creutzfeldt and Schmidt 1970). The proteolytic enzymes include trypsinogen (two varieties), chymotrypsinogen (three varieties), proelastase, procarboxypeptidases A and B, and prekallikrein (Table 13–1). Each of the proteolytic enzymes is secreted as an inactive precursor. Trypsi-

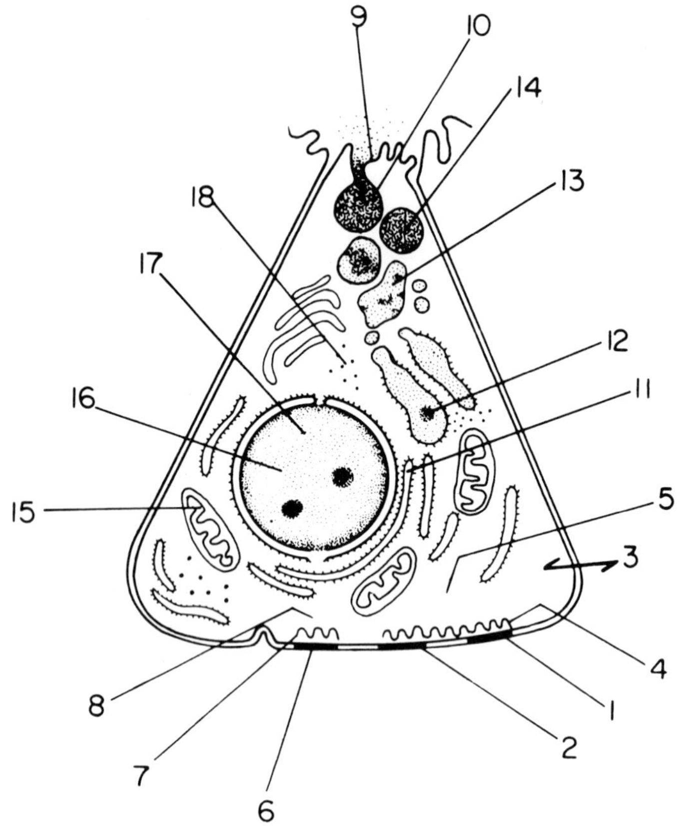

Figure 13–1. This represents diagrammatically pancreatic function at the cellular level. Presumably, changes that occur after feeding also occur after administration of polypeptide and cholinergic agonists. The initial step in agonist action involves binding of polypeptide hormones or neurotransmitters to postulated receptors. (1) binding of acetylcholine to receptor; (2) binding of cholecystokinin-pancreozymin (CCK-PZ) or gastrin to receptor; (3) change in intracellular calcium; (4) activation of guanyl cyclase; (5) synthesis of 3′,5′-cyclic GMP; (6) binding of secretin or vasoactive intestinal peptide (VIP); (7) activation of adenyl cyclase; (8) synthesis of 3′,5′-cyclic AMP; (9) activation of secretion. It is postulated that 3′5′-cyclic AMP and 3′5′-cyclic GMP interact in some way to initiate mechanism of secretion; (10) turnover of membranes; (11) digestive proteins are synthesized on attached ribosomes and then transported through the endoplasmic reticulum into the intracisternal space; (12) synthesized proteins are transported through intracisternal spaces to the Golgi complex; (13) glycosylation, condensation, and encapsulation occur in the Golgi complex; (14) maturation and storage of zymogen granules; (15) increased energy production; (16) initiation of transcriptional events involving synthesis of messenger RNA, ribosomal RNA, and transfer RNA; (17) activation of events at the nuclear level which lead to pancreatic regeneration, hypertrophy, and growth; (18) synthesis of structural proteins on unattached ribosomes. (From Webster PD, III, Black O, Jr, Mainz DL, et al. Gastroenterology 73:1434–49, 1977. Reprinted by permission.)

Table 13–1. Protein Constituents of Pancreatic Acinar Secretions

Lipases	
Prophospholipase A_2[a]	hydrolyzes lecithin and cephalin to lysolecithin, in presence of bile salts and calcium; releases histamine from mast cells
Esterase	hydrolyzes carboxylic esters (cholesterol), and short chain fatty acids in triglycerides (tributyrate) in presence of bile salts
Lipase	hydrolyzes triglycerides with long chain (C16-18) fatty acids to monoglycerides, in presence of bile
Colipase	binds to lipase, prevents surface denaturation by bile salts.
Amylases	
Alpha-amylase (up to 6 varieties, probably all derived from single precursor)	splits carbohydrates to di- and tri-saccharides and dextrins
Proteases	
Endopeptidases	
Trypsinogen (2 varieties)[a]	hydrolyzes lysine, arginine linkages in polypeptides; active form activates other proenzymes
Chymotrypsinogen (3 varieties)[a]	splits aromatic amino acid bonds (tryptophan, phenylalanine, tyrosine) in polypeptides
Proelastase[a]	hydrolyzes neutral aliphatic peptide linkages
Exopeptidases	
Procarboxylase (carboxypeptidase) A	cleaves C-terminal aliphatic or aromatic residues from polypeptides
Procarboxylase (carboxypeptidase) B[a]	cleaves C-terminal arginine or lysine residues from polypeptides
Kallikreinogen (prekallikrein)[a]	liberates kallidin II (lysylbradykinin) from alpha-2 globulin; kallidin II converted to kallidin I (bradykinin) by plasma aminopeptidase
Trypsin Inhibitor	binds tightly to trypsin, cannot be hydrolyzed
Ribonuclease	splits nucleoproteins in bacteria and food
Serum Proteins	
Albumin	
Immunoglobulins A, G and M	

a. Enzymes secreted as inactive precursors. Trypsinogen is activated by enterokinase, and the others are activated by trypsin.

nogen is converted to trypsin rapidly by cleavage of its six terminal amino acids in the presence of the duodenal enzyme, *enterokinase*. Trypsin then rapidly activates the other proteolytic precursors, and also is weakly able to convert additional trypsinogen by a process called autocatalytic activation, which is facilitated by the presence of calcium (Hadorn 1974).

Enterokinase (mol wt 200,000) is the key to the proteolytic cascade of pancreatic enzymes. It is a glycoprotein produced in the brush border of duodenal epithelium and released by interaction with bile acids and by CCK. It contains both a light and a heavy carbohydrate chain and, unlike other brush border enzymes, appears to be partly synthesized in the cytosol of the epithelial cell. Congenital enterokinase deficiency causes severe protein malabsorption, even though pancreatic production of protease precursors is adequate. Fortunately, disorders that reduce other brush border enzyme production, such as celiac sprue, do not lead to deficiencies of enterokinase because of its intracellular production.

Trypsin hydrolyzes basic amino acid bonds, chymotrypsin splits aromatic amino acid bonds, and elastase cleaves the peptide bonds joining aliphatic amino acids, as well as digesting the elastin of meat. The carboxypeptidases remove the terminal amino acids from polypeptides, the A variety following previous digestion by chymotrypsin and elastase, the B variety after digestion by trypsin. Amino acids and dipeptides are the final products of these digestive activities. The presence of trypsin in the intestine also seems to mediate feedback inhibition of the pancreas by reducing the production of CCK.

Amylase and lipase are secreted from acinar cells in their active forms. Amylase splits most ingested carbohydrates to disaccharides and trisaccharides, and to dextrins. Lipase cleaves two fatty acid molecules from triglycerides by hydrolysis, leaving residues of fatty acids and monoglycerides. This process functions only with triglycerides containing fatty acids with chains of 16 to 18 carbon atoms. Colipase overcomes the inhibitory effects of bile acids on lipase, and trypsin inhibitor limits the activity of trypsin, especially in the ductal system of the pancreas.

Zymogen granules consist of all of these enzymes. The proportions of the various enzymes may not be fixed, since while most investigators have found that pancreatic enzymes are secreted in fixed proportions, a few have not (Rinderknecht et al 1978). Concentrations of trypsinogen and proelastase usually do parallel one another, but the relative concentrations of amylase, chymotrypsinogen, and trypsin inhibitor may be variable.

The concentration of bicarbonate in pancreatic secretions is up to sixfold greater than in extracellular fluid. Centroacinar and intercalated ductal cells have active bicarbonate and sodium pumps, and the secretion of water is passive in parallel with ionic concentrations. The most heavy secretion of bicarbonate appears to be in the ducts just distal to the acini. All pancreatic enzymes are denatured by acid and require an alkaline medium for their digestive activities.

The Control of Pancreatic Secretion

While there is a small basal secretion of pancreatic juice, flow rates are mainly mediated by stimulants. Agents responsible for this stimulation have already been noted. Secretin produces a secretion rich in bicarbonate, low in chloride, and transiently high in enzymic content. VIP produces a response qualitatively similar to that of secretin, but much less in quantity. CCK and acetylcholine act on different receptors and potentiate the effect of secretin by increasing enzymic extrusion. While cholinergic and CCK effects are similar, they appear to be mediated differently (Korman 1979). Other hormonal effects include the mildly stimulatory effect of gastrin on both bicarbonate and enzymic secretion, the inhibitory effects of pancreatic polypeptide on CCK, the inhibitory effect of motilin on secretin, and the inhibition of secretin by glucagon. There is also the curious effect of chymodenin, which appears only to stimulate the flow of chymotrypsinogen. Enkephalin has been shown to inhibit pancreatic secretion, at least partly by suppressing the release of secretin (Konturek et al, 1979).

Since so many different stimulatory and inhibitory influences may be operating at any one time, it is not clear how the final secretory picture is orchestrated. As in the stomach, there is a cephalic phase of pancreatic secretion as well. This can be demonstrated by sham feeding and is abolished by vagotomy, but it is not known whether vagal stimulation affects the pancreas directly or operates by way of gastrin, secretin, or CCK. The effect of CCK itself may be partially mediated by cholinergic innervation, since atropine reduces its efficacy, though vagotomy does not. Most agree, however, that CCK and secretin are the major mediators of pancreatic secretion. Secretin is released by the presence of acid in the duodenum, while CCK is released by amino and fatty acids, as well as HCl. The flow produced by secretin is high in volume, bicarbonate, and water, and also contains moderate amounts of enzymes. The flow induced by CCK is thick, low in bicarbonate, and highly concentrated in enzymic activity. Secretin has also been shown to have a trophic effect on the pancreas in rats (Morisset et al 1979).

The Measurement of Pancreatic Exocrine Function

The secretory function of the pancreas can be measured clinically and specimens obtained for cytological study by aspirating duodenal contents following the administration of a pancreatic stimulant. A small-bore polyvinyl tube, weighted at the end with a metal bucket or mercury-filled balloon, is passed through the nose and the end is maneuvered fluoroscopically until it lies in the descending duodenum, beyond the ampulla of Vater. One can then stimulate the pancreas with either a test meal (Lundh 1962) or intravenously administered secretin. The test meal described by Lundh contains dried milk, vegetable oil and dextrin, six percent fat, five percent protein and 15 percent carbohydrate. If secretin is employed, the dose is one unit per kg, which is increased to as much as four units per kg if the results are equivocal and the test is repeated.

Lundh measured only the proteolytic content of aspirated duodenal juice, collected during a two-hour period. Tryptic activity ranged from 180 to over 600 μg per ml in normal patients, and was well below these levels in patients with chronic pancreatitis and pancreatic carcinoma. The secretin test normally produces 2.0 ml or more of volume per kg, maximal bicarbonate concentration of 90 mEq per liter or more, and 6.0 or more Somogyi units of amylase per kg in the 80-minute period following the administration of the stimulant (Dreiling and Wolfson 1979). Both tests are about 90 percent accurate in demonstrating pancreatic insufficiency, and there is little evidence that one is any better than the other. Using CCK in addition to secretin, measuring other enzymes, or giving secretin subcutaneously instead of by vein does not appear to sharpen the sensitivity of the test. Dreiling claims that the secretin test is superior to the Lundh test in being able frequently to distinguish the secretory pattern of pancreatic cancer from that of pancreatitis. He indicates that the pattern of secretion in chronic pancreatitis leads to good flow with abnormally low levels of bicarbonate concentration, while in cancer the flow is reduced and bicarbonate concentration remains normal.

Although physiologically interesting, neither of these tests is used extensively today. For diagnostic purposes, they have generally been replaced by other tests that can often detect pancreatic lesions at an earlier stage and that do not involve the discomfort of a nasal tube.

Other Methods of Detecting Pancreatic Abnormalities

Stool Fat Content. Fat malabsorption occurs when pancreatic production of lipase is reduced to extremely low levels, approaching 10 percent of normal. Stools then appear to be bulky and oily, odor becomes noisome, and the color often changes to a pale yellow tint. The addition of Sudan III, a lipid stain, reveals large globules of fat in a small specimen of stool examined microscopically. Further examination may also show striated muscle fibers, as an indication of inadequate tryptic and elastase activity. Quantitative measurements of stool fat in a patient with a significant lipolytic deficiency reveals that more than 10 percent of ingested fat is excreted in the stool. Luk (1979) has shown that the Sudan III-microscopy test is both sensitive and specific. Since quantitative measurements of stool fat are more difficult and more expensive, qualitative screening is preferable.

The discovery of increased amounts of neutral fat in the stool is not, in itself, proof of pancreatic insufficiency, since it may also be a result of inadequate micellarization of fat by bile salts. However, when other suggestive evidence of pancreatic insufficiency is present, and nothing indicates that bile metabolism is abnormal, increased stool neutral fat (steatorrhea) is strongly supportive of that diagnosis. As will be discussed in a later chapter, there are many other causes of steatorrhea, but in these cases most of the fat is in the form of partially hydrolyzed residues, so that lipid droplets are not found in the untreated specimen.

Serum Amylase and Lipase Levels. These tend to rise in cases of acute inflammation of the pancreas and in pancreatic ductal obstruction. They are normal in most patients with chronic pancreatic insufficiency and in pancreatic carcinoma. Reabsorption of amylase in the renal tubules is reduced in patients with acute pancreatitis, and urinary levels are thus proportionately increased over serum levels (Johnson et al 1976). When serum levels are only moderately elevated, and the diagnosis of pancreatitis is in doubt, it is often helpful to measure the ratio of urinary amylase clearance to that of creatinine (C_{am}/C_{cr}). Normally, this ratio is less than 5 percent. In patients with hyperamylasemia due to pancreatitis, the average C_{am}/C_{cr} is 9.8 percent and, in nearly every case, is over 5.3 percent (Warshaw and Fuller 1975). In patients with hyperamylasemia due to causes other than panceatitis, such as intestinal ischemia, cholecystitis, peptic ulcer, parotitis, and peritonitis, the ratio remains normal because the renal tubular lesion does not develop. The nature of the renal lesion itself is not clear, but it appears to be fully reversible in most cases after recovery from pancreatitis. All but 5 percent of the amylase filtered at the glomerulus is reabsorbed in the renal tubules. The C_{am}/C_{cr} ratio should be used with caution in patients with hyperamylasemia who also have preexisting advanced renal tubular damage, since a high ratio in such cases may be falsely indicative of pancreatitis (Levitt and Johnson 1978).

Serum Lipase. These levels also tend to rise in patients with pancreatitis. Lipase levels rise simultaneously with amylase, but stay elevated for longer periods of time. While useful, this test is not employed as widely as the amylase test, and is rarely necessary for diagnosis if serum and urinary amylase levels are measured.

Isoamylases. It is important to remember that not all of the amylolytic activity measured in the blood is of pancreatic origin. Some may arise from an isoamylase produced in salivary glands, but it is usually a simple task to detect the presence of salivary disease by symptoms and examination. Other carbohydrate-splitting activity may occasionally arise from large amylase-globulin complexes (macroamylases) (Berk et al 1967). These enzymes are of no particular clinical significance of themselves, although they may be elevated in patients with acute liver disease. Macroamylases are too large to be filtered at the glomerulus. Thus, the C_{am}/C_{cr} in macroamylasemia is very low, ranging from 0.2 to 0.45 percent (Levitt et al 1969).

Plain Abdominal Radiographs. Are often useful in supporting a clinical impression of acute pancreatitis. Opaque pancreatic calcifications are commonly seen in patients with chronic pancreatitis and suggest an acute relapse when associated with recurrent abdominal pain. Fine pancreatic calcifications suggest alcoholic pancreatitis, and large chunky concretions in the major pancreatic ducts are most commonly seen in patients with familial pancreatitis. Areas of bowel adjacent to an inflamed pancreas may develop limited segments of visceral peritonitis by direct spread and thus become dilated and partially filled with air. This localized ileus may lead to the presence of dilated sentinal loops of small intestine in proximity of the pancreas, usually in the upper left quadrant of the abdomen (Figure 13-2), or dilatation of the distal portion of the transverse colon without gas in the descending colon, the colon cut-off sign. Patients with pancreatitis also develop inflammatory ascites at times, which may be detectable on plain films.

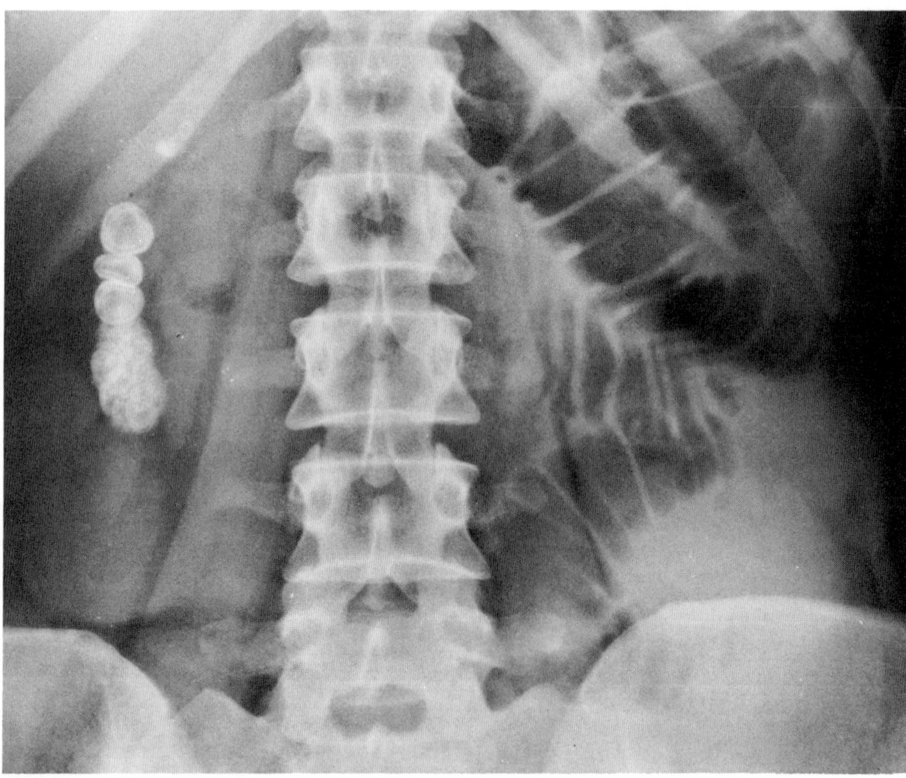

Figure 13–2. Plain abdominal film of patient with acute pancreatitis. Note the numerous radiopaque gallstones on patient's right, and dilated "sentinal loops" of small intestine on the left side.

Ultrasonography and Computed Tomography. These have provided clinicians with their first opportunity to outline the borders and evaluate the texture of the pancreas in unoperated patients. These techniques have revolutionized pancreatic diagnosis and, where available, have proved to be of incalculable benefit. The size, borders, and consistency of the pancreas can be clearly delineated. A diffusely enlarged gland with blurred borders is suggestive of pancreatitis. Cancer often presents as localized solid areas of enlargement (Figure 13-3) and pseudocysts as fluid-filled masses (Figure 13-4). At times, the distinction between benign and malignant enlargements is not clear and the techniques can be used as a guide for obtaining thin-needle biopsies of the pancreas. The cost of tomographic scanning makes sonography the first-level diagnostic study; the former procedure should be used only if sonographic diagnosis is inconclusive. Both procedures may be inconclusive in patients with dilated loops of intestine, ascites, or marked obesity.

Retrograde Pancreatography. This technique allows the clinician to visualize clearly the main pancreatic duct, detecting abnormalities in the wall suggestive of pancreatitis, areas of stenosis, and obstructions suggesting pancreatic carcinoma. Pseudocysts of the pancreas can also be filled by this technique. However, the place of this middle-aged technique in pancreatic diagnosis is unclear since the advent of sonography and computed tomography. This endoscopic procedure is expensive and in centers where it is not employed frequently, often prolonged and uncomfortable to the patient. I would classify it as a third-level diagnostic procedure at this time, and suspect that its use will decrease in the future. Tests of pancreatic function and disease have been critically reviewed by Arvanitakis and Cooke (1978).

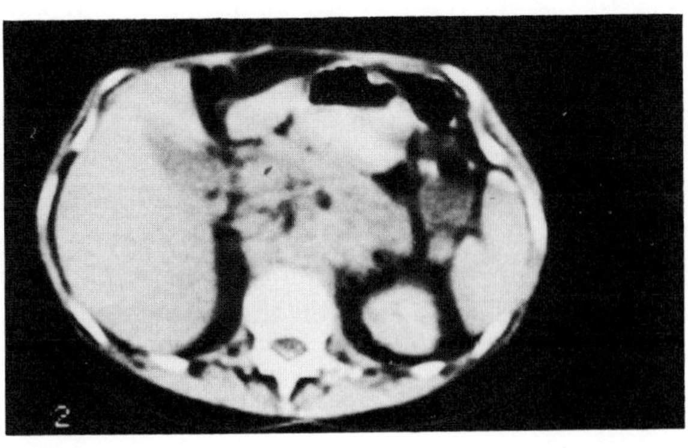

Figure 13-3. Computed axial tomogram in a patient with pancreatic enlargement due to cancer of that organ. The pancreas is the solid central organ overlying the opaque vertebra. The lucent areas in the center of the pancreas are due to ductal dilatation. Courtesy of Dr. Ralph Alfidi.

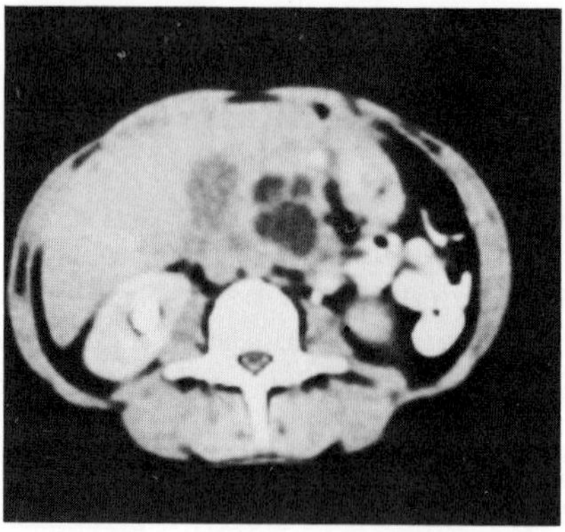

Figure 13–4. Computed axial tomogram in a patient with a pancreatic pseudocyst. The cyst itself is represented by the large lucent area in the center of the swollen pancreas. Courtesy of Dr. Ralph Alfidi.

INFLAMMATORY DISEASES OF THE PANCREAS

Pancreatic inflammatory disease may be characterized by acute attacks alone, by chronic disease with acute relapses and gradual autodestruction of the gland, or by progressive chronic pancreatic destruction without any acute flares. The end stage of the chronic disorder is marked exocrine deficiency, after more than 90 percent of acinar tissue has been destroyed, and occasionally endocrine deficiency (pancreatogenous diabetes) as well. A large number of agents, both extrinsic and intrinsic, have been implicated as causes of acute and chronic pancreatitis, but alcoholism and biliary tract disease are far and away the most common. Other agents that have been identified are hyperlipidemia, hypercalcemia, drugs, hereditary disorders, pancreatic neoplasms, chronic renal failure, viral infections, trauma, duodenal diverticula, malnutrition, and vascular disorders. In 16 series of cases of acute pancreatitis reported between 1959 and 1975, over 5,000 patients were identified. Biliary tract disease was implicated as the cause of pancreatitis in 37 percent, alcoholism in 42 percent, and all other causes were included in the remaining 21 percent (Schmidt and Creutzfeldt 1976, with additions). The incidence of alcoholic pancreatitis tended to be higher among patients studied in the United States and South Africa and depended closely upon the characteristics of the population served.

Pathogenesis

The lesions of pancreatitis depend on destruction of acinar and ductular tissue by activated pancreatic enzymes, particularly phospholipase A, chymotrypsin, kallikrein, and elastase. Trypsin probably functions more as enzyme activator in pancreatitis than as a destroyer of tissue, while lipase participates mainly in extrapancreatic fat necrosis. By releasing lysolecithin from phosphatidylcholine, phospholipase A can cause marked tissue destruction and release of histamine. Chymotrypsin causes both edema and hemorrhage, while kallikrein and elastase lead to vascular destruction, hemorrhage, vasodilatation through histamine release, and migration of polymorphonuclear leukocytes to the area of tissue destruction. The ability of trypsin to cause coagulation necrosis of acinar tissue is probably limited by the presence of trypsin inhibitor.

How do proenzymes, particularly trypsinogen, become activated while still in the pancreas? While the answer to this question still remains elusive, it is clear that activation does indeed occur. A number of plausible explanations have been advanced, and it is apparent that different causative agents operate through different mechanisms.

Reflux of duodenal contents or bile into the pancreatic duct appears to be the most likely cause of pancreatitis associated with diseases of the biliary tract, duodenal obstruction, and duodenal diverticula located adjacent to the ampulla of Vater. Refluxed constituents include lysolecithin, trypsin, and bile acids as well as enterokinase, agents which, in combination, have been shown to cause pancreatitis experimentally. Kelly (1976) identified one or more gallstones in the stool of 38 of 45 patients following an attack of gallstone pancreatitis. He suggests that these stones had become impacted temporarily in the ampulla and facilitated the reflux of bile into the pancreatic duct under increased pressure. Increased pressure could have damaged acinar cell membranes and permitted activation of intracellular zymogens. Another possible explanation is that a calculus, temporarily lodged in the sphincter of Oddi, may splint that structure enough to allow reflux of duodenal secretions to occur. Increased pressure against the sphincter with eventual weakening and reflux has been suggested to be the major mechanism of the pancreatitis that occurs in patients with partially obstructed afferent duodenal loops following a Billroth II gastrojejunostomy and in patients with large duodenal diverticula adjacent to the ampulla of Vater. When duodenal obstruction of a similar degree is established in dogs, pancreatitis occurs almost invariably, unless the pancreatic duct has also been ligated.

Spontaneous activation of proteolytic enzymes intraductally has been found in two patients with pancreatitis by Renner et al (1978). In each case, pancreatic secretions were obtained by deep catheterization of the pancreatic duct transduodenally so that secretions were obtained from the body of the pancreas. Both patients showed free proteolytic activity, higher than normal levels of enzyme production, and increased sensitivity to stimulation by secretin. It is not clear how the proteases had been activated, but there was no evidence that reflux was responsible. Similarly, White and Allan (1974) described a patient with a cancer of the head of the pancreas totally obstructing the pancreatic duct and preventing biliary or duodenal reflux. The proximal pancreatic duct was drained surgically to reduce pain, and the initial secretions obtained showed no proteolytic activity. A week later, secretions showed chymotryptic activity and, shortly after, the patient developed an attack of pancreatitis. Subsidence of pain was later associated with disappearance of chymotrypsin and increase of trypsin inhibitor levels. While not indicating how the chymotrypsinogen was activated, this case does suggest that pancreatic trypsin inhibitor is a potent protective agent against pancreatitis in vivo. It is possible that the neoplasm itself produced a trypsin activator.

Sustained pancreatic hypersecretion has been implicated as the cause of the pancreatitis that occurs so commonly among chronic alcoholics and among patients with hypercalcemia. A single dose of alcohol is not a particularly potent stimulus of pancreatic secretion, but Sarles et al (1977) showed a significant increase of bicarbonate and water secretion in dogs after 24 months of alcohol feeding and attribute this to pancreatic ductal hyperplasia. After three months, the protein secretory response to CCK also appears to be heightened. This pancreatic secretion contains increased calcium and mucoprotein and often contains calcium carbonate and protein precipitates. It is believed that these precipitates may cause plugging of smaller pancreatic ducts, leading to localized areas of pancreatic necrosis. Lactoferrin, a protein not normally found in pancreatic juice, has been identified regularly in secretions of patients with alcoholic chronic calcifying pancreatitis and may indicate a genetic predisposition to that disorder.

Calcium excess may also lead to pancreatic hypersecretion. Ionic calcium is essential to both acinar and ductal secretion, and both rise considerably in the presence of calcium excess (Petersen and Iwatsuki 1978). It is likely that this response, possibly associated with decreased amounts of trypsin inhibitor, may lead to acinar damage, especially if ductal plugs of calcium carbonate are also present. Clinically, pancreatitis has been found to complicate about 10 percent of hypercalcemic states, such as hyperparathyroidism.

Hyperlipidemic states, especially types I and V which are associated with chylomicronemia, are commonly associated with recurrent pancreatitis. Patients with type IV hyperlipidemia are also at risk when their serum lipids rise, especially after ingestion of alcohol or while taking estrogenic therapy, and chylomicronemia transiently appears. The form of pancreatitis may be the result of substrate excess and possibly of lipase induction. Local release of free fatty acids is believed to be responsible for initiating the tissue damage, followed by enzymic activation and further tissue destruction.

Viral damage to acinar cell membranes is felt to be the cause of pancreatitis accompanying mumps, and certain cocksackie and ECHO-virus infections. Usually attacks of viral pancreatitis are short-lived, mild, and nonrecurrent.

Drug-induced pancreatitis is a recognized entity, but the mechanisms involved are not clear at present (Mallory and Kern 1980). Drugs which have been definitely associated with acute pancreatitis include: azathioprine, estrogens, tetracycline, sulfonamides, and sulfonamide derivatives like furosemide and the chlorthiazides. Probably associated drugs include L-asparaginase, chlorthalidone, corticosteroids, ethacrynic acid, phenformin, and procainamide. Hypercalcemia caused by overbalanced parenteral alimentation or by vitamin D overdosage may also cause pancreatitis. The pancreatitis seen occasionally among kidney recipients is believed to be a result of azathioprine toxicity. Acute pancreatitis from drugs may, at times, be very severe and even fatal.

Protein malnutrition has been implicated as a cause of chronic calcifying pancreatitis (Sarles 1974). The pancreatic lesion is identical to that seen in patients with chronic alcoholism and is distinguished by the fact that it occurs in much younger individuals. In Kerala state, India, chronic calcific pancreatitis is the cause of death in 5.5 percent of the general autopsy population and is believed to result from malnutrition. The mechanism of action of protein malnutrition is not clear, but apparently involves the precipitation of abnormal proteins in smaller pancreatic ducts.

Pathology

Acute pancreatitis is of variable severity. In mild cases, the gland is focally or diffusely edematous and shows only slight round-cell infiltrates on microscopy (interstitial pancreatitis). Severe cases are characterized by marked acinar destruction with hemorrhage, extensive leukocytic infiltrates, and necrosis of peripancreatic fat (hemorrhagic pancreatitis) (Figure 13–5). The severity appears to rest directly on the amount of enzymes released locally, especially those like kallikrein, elastase, and phosapholipase that appear to cause the most tissue and vascular damage.

Foulis (1980) has described two histologic patterns of acute necrotizing pancreatitis which may relate to the etiologies of the disease. The first pattern, seen primarily in pancreatitis associated with cholelithiasis or alcholism, consists primarily of ductal inflammation and periductular acinar necrosis. There is a marked acute inflammatory infiltrate in these cases, and ducts are often blocked with proteinaceous material. Perilobular necrosis, the second pattern, seems to be related to ischemia and occurs mainly among patients who have been in shock. Pancreatic acini farthest from lobular arteries are at greatest risk, and ductal inflammation is absent in the pure form.

Pseudocysts are often found in or around the pancreas, varying from less than 1 cm to 20 cm or more in diameter. These are due to rupture of pancreatic ducts with penetration of active enzymes beyond the boundary of the pancreas. Penetrations are walled off in the retroperitoneal space and may

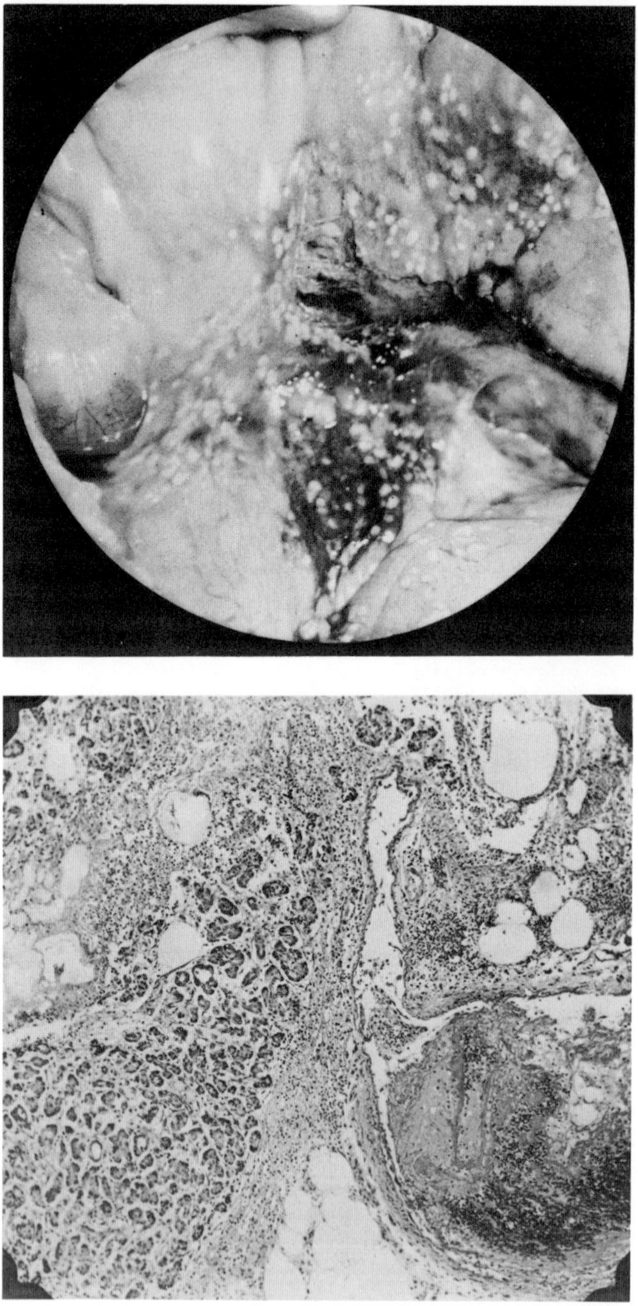

Figure 13–5. Acute hemorrhagic pancreatitis and fat necrosis. Upper picture shows gross hemorrhage and necrosis of mesenteric fat. Lower picture is a low-power photomicrograph showing the extravasation of blood and a heavy inflammatory infiltrate around the pancreatic tissue in the lower left portion of the picture. Courtesy of Dr. Jerry Wolkoff.

eventually drain spontaneously when they communicate with the ductal system. Occasionally pseudocysts become infected and develop into abscesses. Their contents invariably contain enzymic activity and hemoglobin metabolites. They are called pseudo rather than true cysts because they are not lined by epithelial tissue.

Chronic pancreatitis is characterized by scarring, atrophy, and calcification in the gland (Figure 13–6). Total acinar tissue mass is markedly reduced, and islet cell tissue is also diminished in severe cases. The calcifications are intraductular and appear to result from precipitation of calcium carbonate in mucus plugs. The acinar tissue drained by obstructed ducts is usually atrophic. Chronic, thick-walled pseudocysts may also be present, and the cellular infiltrate usually consists of lymphocytes and plasma cells.

Symptoms and Signs: Acute Pancreatitis

Upper abdominal pain is the cardinal symptom of pancreatitis, and occurs in over 95 percent of cases. The pain is usually steady and agonizing and, as an indication of its retroperitoneal origin, commonly penetrates through to the midback. Patients are usually uncomfortable lying in one position, and frequently find some relief by flexing their back and drawing their knees toward the abdomen. Nausea, vomiting and fever appear in more severe cases. The upper abdomen is tender, and varying degrees of reflex muscle spasm may be noted if localized parietal peritonitis is present. In extreme cases, the entire anterior abdominal wall may become rigid, resembling the clinical picture of a perforated peptic ulcer. Rarely, proteolytic enzymes escape into the subcutaneous layers of the abdomen and cause localized ecchymoses in the flanks (Gray-Turner sign) or in the periumbilical area (Cullen sign). Localized areas of subcutaneous fat necrosis may also be seen as a consequence of lipolytic activity. The abdomen is frequently distended due to reflex ileus from peritonitis, and auscultation reveals diminished or absent bowel sounds. Small to moderate amounts of ascitic fluid may also be detectable as a response to exudation caused by peritonitis.

Signs of hypovolemia, ranging from tachycardia to shock and anuria, are common in patients with severe (hemorrhagic) pancreatitis. Hypovolemia results from capillary damage secondary to elastase and kallikrein release, and from ileus which allows for the accumulation of fluid in the intestinal "third space." Circulating blood volume may decrease to as little as 50 to 60 percent of normal, and the hematocrit tends to increase, though not in direct proportion to the volume loss, since bleeding into tissues and the peritoneal cavity also occurs.

Pulmonary dysfunction is encountered frequently in patients with acute pancreatitis, as many as 50 percent showing reductions in P_{aO_2} (Carey 1979). Severe respiratory distress and cyanosis may accompany massive

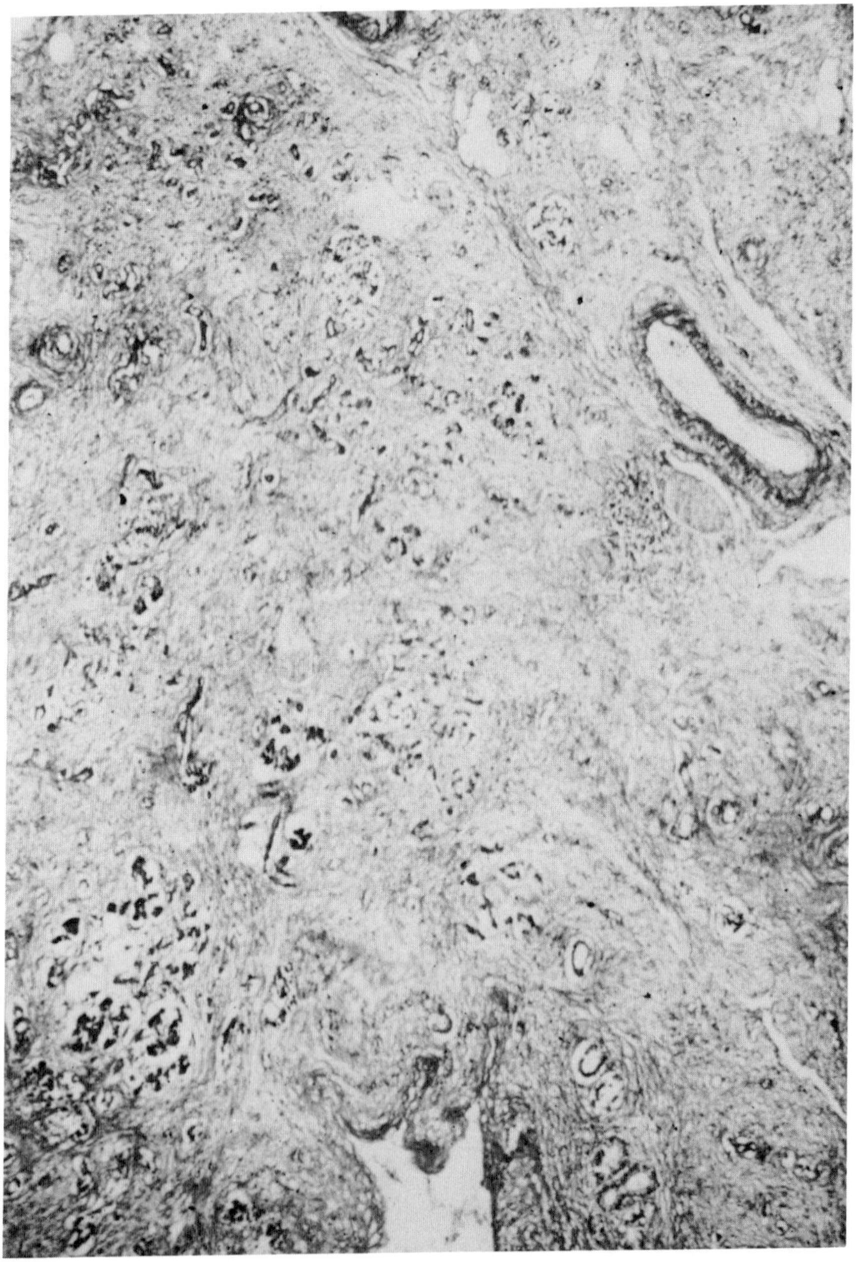

Figure 13–6. Chronic pancreatitis. Pancreatic acinar tissue has been replaced almost completely by fibrosis; ductal remnants remain. Original magnification x60.

acute pancreatitis. Lee et al (1979) indicate that hypoxemia results from alveolar-capillary block due to interstitial pulmonary edema secondary to increased pulmonary vascular permeability. Reduced cardiac output resulting from hypovolemia and cardiomyopathy and pleural effusions also contribute to hypoxemia. Jacob et al (1980) suggst that the hypoxemia may result from complement activation and aggregation of granulocytes in pulmonary capillaries.

The renal tubular damage which is responsible for the transitory increase in C_{am}/C_{Cr} in acute pancreatitis, may lead to more extreme renal dysfunction with a fall in renal blood flow and glomerular filtration rate in severe cases. While the resultant azotemia is worsened by hypotension, progressive renal failure may occur without a fall in blood pressure.

Disseminated intravascular coagulation is an occasional critical complication of massive pancreatitis. This appears to be the result of activation of the coagulation cascade by the intravascular release of kallikrein.

Hypocalcemia with reduction of free and albumin-bound calcium levels is frequently found in patients with severe acute pancreatitis. It appears to be the result of transient resistance to parathormone and possibly from hypomagnesemia rather than to the formation of calcium soaps by released fatty acids. Hypocalcemic tetany is uncommon in these patients, because there is usually an associated parallel decrease in serum albumin levels.

The poor prognostic signs for survival in acute pancreatitis have been listed by Hermon-Taylor (1977). These include age over 55 years, associated diabetes mellitus, sustained fever, respiratory distress, pulse rate greater than 120 per minute, systolic blood pressure less than 100 mm Hg, albumin less than 3.0 g per dl, white blood count over 20,000 per cu mm, hematocrit less than 30 percent, a rising blood urea nitrogen level, serum calcium less than 7.5 mg per dl, and a P_{aO_2} less than 60 mm Hg.

Symptoms and Signs: Chronic Pancreatitis

Abdominal pain and variable degrees of intestinal malabsorption are the characteristic findings in patients with chronic pancreatitis. Pain is by far the more common symptom, and its chronicity leads frequently to narcotic addiction. The addition of addiction to a chronic pain state makes therapy in these cases uncommonly difficult, because physicians are often at a loss to know whether a patient's pain is the result of pancreatitis or of narcotic dependence. Patients with chronic pancreatitis may develop exacerbations of acute pancreatitis, but these attacks are rarely of great severity. The pain of chronic pancreatitis has been attributed to perineural inflammation of retroperitoneal sensory nerves.

Intestinal malabsorption is the direct result of advanced pancreatic insufficiency and is commonly associated with loss of weight, often with a good appetite, and stool findings, already described, suggesting steatorrhea.

Fat-soluble vitamin deficiencies are common, vitamin K depletion being demonstrated by prolonged prothrombin times, and vitamin D deficiency by hypocalcemia and, eventually, osteomalacia. Occasionally, patients may also be depleted in vitamin B_{12} and demonstrate an associated macrocytic anemia. Malabsorption of B_{12} may be the result of deficient enzyme production by the pancreas, and failure to release the vitamin from its "r" factor binding salivary protein. This could block the ability of intrinsic factor to bind B_{12}, and thus reduce the uptake of the vitamin in the terminal ileum, although this possible mechanism has been disputed (Steinberg et al 1979).

Diabetes mellitus is not uncommonly associated with chronic pancreatitis, and can only be treated with insulin replacement. Vascular, neurological, and other complications of pancreatogenous diabetes appear to be no different than those associated with the familial adult-onset form of the disease.

Hereditary Pancreatic Disorders

Familial pancreatitis is an uncommon disorder which has been described in a number of kindreds (Comfort and Steinberg 1952). There are at least two types, one of which is associated with aminoaciduria. The disorder is transmitted as an autosomal dominant, is associated with recurrent attacks of pancreatitis commencing in childhood or early adulthood, and commonly eventuates in advanced ductal calcification and pancreatic acinar insufficiency. Its signs and symptoms do not differ from those of other types of pancreatitis. It should be suspected whenever a first-degree relative also has the disease. Hyperlipidemic pancreatitis is also genetic in origin, and so possibly is the susceptibility to alcoholic pancreatitis.

Cystic fibrosis of the pancreas is far more common and occurs only in homozygotes as a recessive characteristic. While not usually associated with attacks of pancreatitis, cystic fibrosis is a common cause of pancreatic exocrine deficiency. The disease is apparently the result of chronic ductal obstruction by thick mucus, with resultant dilatation of proximal ducts and acinar degeneration. Pancreatic insufficiency may be present at birth and is occasionally associated with meconium ileus, a state of intestinal obstruction by ascitic fluid proteins undigested by pancreatic proteases. Diagnosis is confirmed by finding more than 60 mEq per liter of sodium and chlorides in sweat.

Diagnosis of Pancreatitis

Acute pancreatitis is diagnosed most commonly by detecting elevations of serum, urinary, and ascitic amylase levels in patients with abdominal pain. Abdominal sonography and plain abdominal radiographs are often confirmatory. An upper gastrointestinal series will commonly detect expansion of the duodenal C-loop with flattening of mucosal folds resulting from enlargement of the head of the pancreas. There may also be anterior displacement of the stomach or duodenum, especially if a pseudocyst is present (Figure 13-7). The detection of calcifications in the pancreas suggests

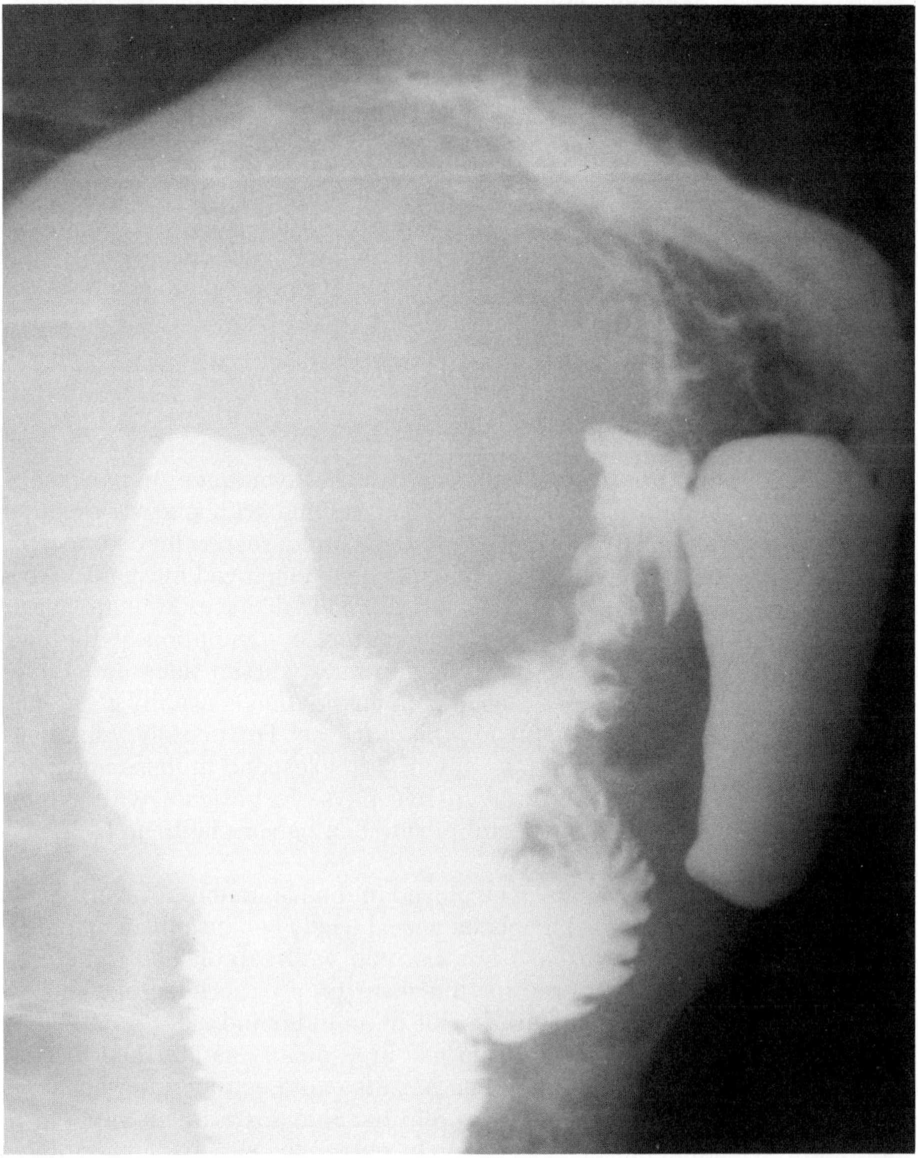

Figure 13-7. Lateral film of barium-filled upper gastrointestinal tract showing marked anterior displacement of the stomach and descending duodenum by a retroperitoneal pancreatic pseudocyst. Courtesy of Dr. Jerry Wolkoff.

that the acute attack is superimposed upon chronic disease. More complex diagnostic studies are rarely indicated.

Chronic pancreatitis is diagnosed most readily by the detection of calcifications in the pancreas, associated with evidence of exocrine or endocrine deficiency. Examination of stool for fat and meat fibers and secretin-stimulated pancreatic drainage studies are invaluable ancillary procedures, which often indicate the type and amount of treatment required. In patients with sustained pain or chronic hyperamylasemia, retrograde pancreatography may demonstrate areas of ductal narrowing or small pseudocysts.

Care must be taken in all patients with pancreatitis to detect which of the known causes of the disease are most likely to be responsible. Thus, every patient should be questioned about drug or alcohol ingestion, and studies should be undertaken to demonstrate the presence of hypercalcemia, hyperlipidemia, peptic ulcer, and biliary tract disease. Evidence is strong that adequate treatment of the proximate cause of pancreatitis will often prevent further attacks.

Treatment of Pancreatitis

Acute pancreatitis is treated primarily by avoidance of pancreatic stimulation, replacement of deficient blood volume with plasma or other expanders, correction of electrolytic deficits, and respiratory support if needed. Continuous nasogastric suction has been employed for many years, but there are no data that support its value, in mild disease. Anticholinergic drugs have been used to reduce parasympathetic stimulation of the pancreas, but the side effects of these agents may worsen ileus and tachycardia. The need for frequent doses of pain medication is usually great, and meperidine appears to be useful for this purpose. Fortunately, almost 90 percent of patients with edematous pancreatitis respond to these nonspecific measures usually within three to five days. In patients with diffuse hemorrhagic pancreatitis, the mortality rate can be very high, up to 80 percent.

A trypsin inhibitor has been employed in the treatment of severe acute pancreatitis, but the results have been poor, largely because the medication must be given after the disease has become well established. Similarly, glucagon has been found to reduce the severity of experimental pancreatitis, especially if it is administered prior to an ethionine diet (Manabe and Steer 1979), but appears to be of no use in clinically established disease (Olazabel and Fuller 1978). Cimetidine has also not been found to be useful in shortening the course of acute pancreatitis. Somatostatin, an inhibitor of pancreatic secretion, has been shown to be extremely effective in improving survival among dogs with experimental pancreatitis (Usadel et al 1980). Therapy with this polypeptide hormone has also shown some benefit in early studies of human pancreatitis.

In desperately ill patients who are not responding well to conservative measures, some success has been reported from the use of peritoneal lavage with large volumes of electrolytically balanced solutions (Cooperman 1978). This procedure can remove large amounts of vasoactive pancreatic enzymes, can be undertaken in intensive care units, and has been reported to be very beneficial at times for short periods, although controlled studies have not been reported. Similarly, exploratory laparotomy may be used as a third-stage procedure. The objective is to drain retroperitoneal and lesser omental collections of fluid, remove necrotic portions of pancreas, and to provide better organ drainage by catheterizing the common bile duct or the pancreatic duct. Laparotomy in acute necrotizing pancreatitis is a desperation procedure: mortality is high; postoperative healing is often poor. This procedure should be reserved only for those patients showing steady clinical deterioration.

Local complications of acute pancreatitis are pseudocysts, pancreatic abscesses, and pancreatic ascites. Any pseudocyst that does not regress spontaneously in size to less than 4 cm in diameter should probably be drained. They may be associated with chronic pain or sustained hyperamylasemia, and they may become infected or rupture spontaneously into the peritoneal cavity (Figure 13-8). Thus, failure to regress adequately in several weeks calls for intervention, which usually involves forming a surgical cystogastrostomy. Cysts have also been drained successfully without laparotomy by percutaneous needle aspiration after localization by sonography or computed tomographic scanning (Smith et al 1979). Pancreatic abscesses are heralded by elevations in fever and white blood count and must be surgically drained without delay to prevent generalized sepsis. Pancreatic ascites is also an indication for laparotomy, since its appearance is a nearly certain indication of pancreatic ductal rupture.

Chronic pancreatitis is best treated expectantly. If recurrent pain is a problem and ductal strictures can be demonstrated on retrograde pancreatography, surgical relief of the obstructions may be beneficial. For fibrous obstructions at the distal end of the pancreatic duct, a plastic procedure on the sphincter of Oddi may be sufficient to promote adequate flow and relieve pain. Where strictures are multiple along the course of the duct, it becomes necessary to open the duct longitudinally and to anastomose the entire cut surface to a Roux loop of jejunum (Puestow and Gillesby 1958). Prinz et al (1978) reported substantial relief in 81 percent of 77 patients operated on for the pain of chronic alcoholic pancreatitis, and followed for 2 to 21 years. Whatever surgical procedure is employed must be carefully tailored to the specific needs of the patient.

Chronic pancreatic exocrine deficiency requires adequate replacement with oral pancreatic enzymes before and during meals. The preparation used should have adequate enzymic activity and be presented in an adequately digestable form (Graham 1977). Measures should be taken to ensure that gastric pH is kept above 4.0 to avoid enzymic inactivation in the stomach. This is best accomplished by simultaneous administration of ant-

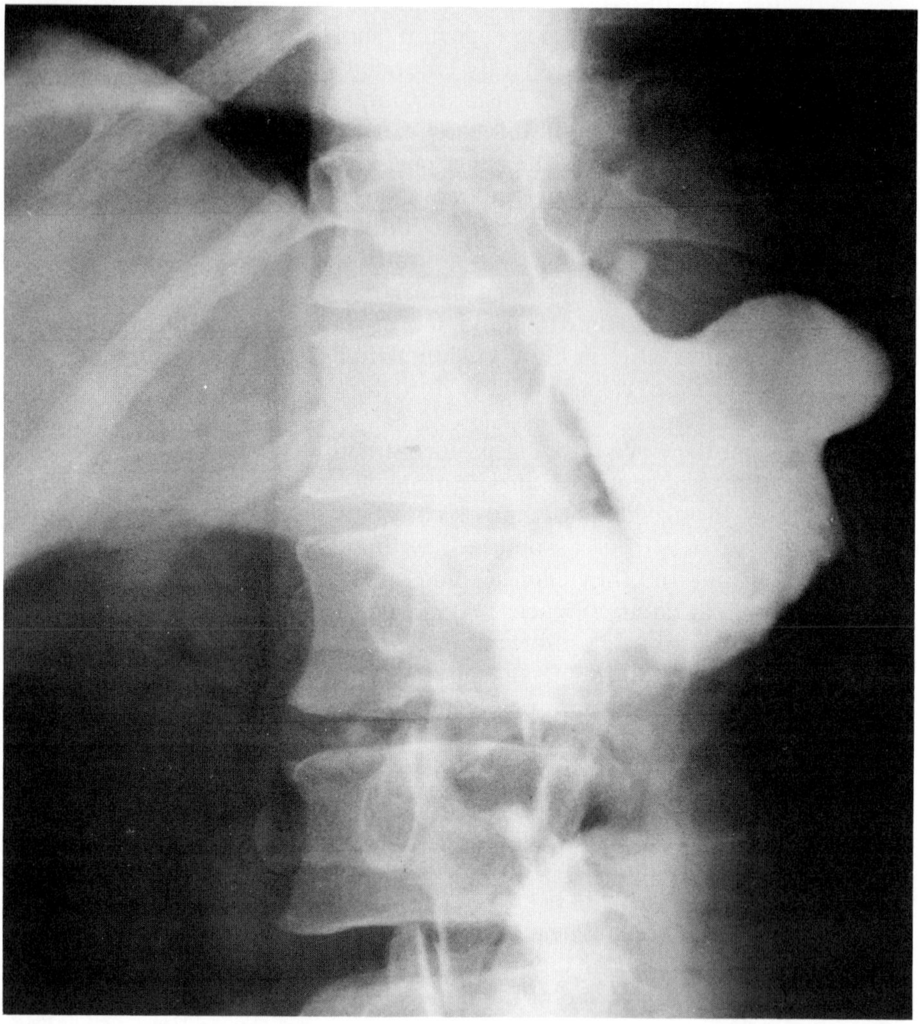

Figure 13-8. Oblique film of upper abdomen after injection of radiopaque dye into a pancreatic pseudocyst at surgery. Courtesy of Dr. Jerry Wolkoff.

acids or cimetidine. Fat-soluble vitamin supplements should also be given, for there is evidence that tissue levels of vitamins A, D, and K may be low even though steatorrhea has been fairly well controlled (Dutta et al 1979).

Prevention of Further Attacks of Pancreatitis

There is clear evidence that removal of gallstones will prevent further attacks in patients with gallstone pancreatitis. It is similarly proved that correction of hypercalcemia by parathyroidectomy in patients with hyperparathyroidism will also prevent further attacks of pancreatitis, and that correcting hypertriglyceridemia with a low fat diet is useful in lipidemic patients. There is also evidence that abstinence from alcohol is very beneficial to patients with alcoholic pancreatitis. But, as is the case in patients with alcoholic liver disease, encouraging the patient to become abstinent is very difficult. Counseling, group therapy, disulfiram, and prolonged follow-up have had modest successs.

CARCINOMA OF THE PANCREAS

Aside from aging itself, there are few known or suspected risk factors for adenocarcinoma of the pancreas. In an interview study of 369 patients with proven cancer of the pancreas and 644 control patients, MacMahon et al (1981) have shown an unanticipated correlation between cancer of the pancreas and the ingestion of three or more cups of coffee per day. This association applies to both men and women, but its real significance must await confirmation in other studies. The disease has shown a gradually increasing incidence in the United States during the last quarter century, having risen about 25 percent among both sexes. It is the fourth highest cause of cancer deaths among men over age 54, and among women over age 75. For 1980, the American Cancer Society estimates an incidence of 24,000 new cases, and nearly 21,000 deaths from carcinoma of the pancreas, about 5 percent of all deaths from cancer during the year. The five-year survival rate is less than 1 percent.

Maruchi et al (1979) have published demographic data on 113 patients with carcinoma of the exocrine pancreas seen in a single county during a 35-year period. Sixty-two percent of patients were men, 75 percent were over 59 years of age at the time of diagnosis, 20 percent had primary carcinoma at another site earlier or concurrently, and the incidence of pancreatic carcinoma in male metal workers was over five times the frequency of those occupations in the general male population. The head of the pancreas was involved in over two-thirds of the cases. There was a suggestion that diabetes was more common among women with cancer of the pancreas.

The tumor is usually solid, but occasionally presents as a large polycystic structure. Carcinomas of the pancreas are usually well-differentiated ductular tissue and may at times contain mucin-secreting cells. Bockman et al (1979) present evidence that indicates that the ductular tissue, at least in experimental pancreatic tumors, is derived from dedifferentiating acinar cells. Zymogen granules disappear, and acinar cells form into adenomatous tubular structures.

Cancers of the pancreas may start in any portion of the organ, but appear to be somewhat more common in the head. Spread is both by local invasion of surrounding organs, and by metastases to lymph nodes, lung, and liver.

Symptoms and Signs

Cancer of the pancreas usually has a most insidious onset. In many cases, patients are not aware of illness until obstructive jaundice develops from blockage of the common bile duct by the neoplastic mass in the head of the pancreas. Pain is the classical symptoms of tumors of the body and tail of the pancreas and usually represents perineural involvement by neoplastic tissue. The pain tends to be most prominent in the midback and quickly becomes steady and agonizing. As in chronic pancreatitis, patients tend to bend forward at the waist and draw up their knees in an effort to relieve the discomfort. Loss of weight may be the result of anorexia consequent to the pain, or it may also result from malabsorption secondary to blockage of the pancreatic duct, or from diabetes due to loss of islet cells. A few patients may develop peripheral thrombophlebitis in one or several veins. This condition was clearly described by Trousseau (1865), who considered this "phlegmatia alba dolens" to be an epiphenomenon caused by cancer at several different primary sites. Mental depression has also been considered to be symptomatic of pancreatic cancer. It does not appear to be a reaction to the diagnosis itself, since many patients are otherwise free of symptoms.

Clinical signs of pancreatic carcinoma are often very scarce. Physicians must have a high index of suspicion regarding the disease and carefully study all patients with suggestive symptoms, especially if they are in their middle years. A new pain in the back without antecedent injury, new onset diabetes in a patient without familial history for the disease, an unexplained episode of depression or thrombophlebitis, and an attack of pancreatitis in a patient with no known cause for the disease—all should make one suspicious of pancreatic carcinoma. An abdominal mass is usually not felt until very late in the course. Obstructive jaundice is also a very late sign and is usually accompanied by a palpably enlarged gall bladder (Courvoisier sign). An audible bruit in the upper abdomen suggests compression of a large abdominal artery (aorta, celiac axis, splenic) by a mass. In most early cases, the physical examination is quite normal, and one must rely on diagnostic studies.

Diagnosis

DiMagno et al (1977) performed an evaluative study of diagnostic techniques in patients with cancer of the pancreas. Ultrasonography alone was positive in 85 percent of patients with pancreatic disease, and in 10 of 14 patients with pancreatic cancer. Pancreatic function testing was positive in 12 of these patients. These tests also detected patients with pancreatitis, and false negative results were infrequent. To improve the specificity of preoperative testing, the authors recommend following a positive ultrasound or pancreatic function test with retrograde pancreatography or arteriography, the specificity of the former test being about 90 percent.

Unfortunately, this study did not lean heavily on signs and symptoms in supporting a diagnosis of pancreatic cancer, pancreatitis, or other disease in their patients. Personal experience convinces me that a high index of suspicion in a patient with suggestive symptoms and a positive sonogram is indication enough for surgical exploration. In such patients, it would be difficult to postpone surgery on the basis of a negative pancreatogram, unless serious counterindications to laparotomy are present. What this study does clearly demonstrate, however, is that our available diagnostic procedures are finally able to give us useful information about a previously inaccessible organ. Much of the inaccessibility of the pancreas has been dispelled by computed tomographic scanning of the abdomen. Early experience with this procedure and with scan-directed flexible needle biopsies indicates that diagnosis of pancreatic cancer need no longer be as delayed as it was in the past.

Treatment

Extirpation is the only treatment for pancreatic cancer, and all too often this is impossible to accomplish. On most occasions, the surgeon can do no more than perform a cholecystoenterostomy to prevent or relieve jaundice, and a gastrojejunostomy to relieve potential gastric or duodenal obstruction by the neoplasm. Where the tumor has not invaded locally, a total pancreatectomy is performed, and among such patients, a small percentage of long-term survivals may result. They develop permanent diabetes and pancreatic exocrine insufficiency, but these can be treated with proper supplements.

For inoperable patients, chemotherapy has a little to offer. In a few patients, there has been a beneficial response to courses of adriamycin and 5-fluorouracil, but most often in patients with a large tumor mass these drugs are ineffective. Focused high-voltage X ray therapy may also offer benefits for palliation.

HISTORICAL DIGRESSION

Proper names employed without reference in this chapter include: Thomas Stephen CULLEN (1868–1953), American gynecologist, Baltimore; George Grey TURNER (1877–1951), British surgeon, London; Paul LANGERHANS (1847–1888), German pathologist, Berlin, described pancreatic islets in 1869; Giovanni Domenico SANTORINI (1681–1737), Italian anatomist, Pisa and Venice; Johann Georg WIRSUNG (1600–1643), German anatomist, Padua and Augsburg, described pancreatic duct in 1642.

SELECTED REFERENCES

Arvanitakis C, Cooke AR. Diagnostic tests of exocrine pancreatic function and disease. Gastroenterology 74:932–48, 1978.

Berk JE, Kizu H, Wilding P, et al. Macroamylasemia: a newly recognized cause for elevated serum amylase activity. New Engl J Med 277:941–46, 1967.

Cardell BS. The pancreas. In: Symers WS, ed. Systemic pathology, 2nd ed, vol 3. Edinburgh: Churchill Livingstone, 1978: 1332–73.

Carey LC. Extra-abdominal manifestations of acute pancreatitis. Surgery 86:377-42, 1979.

Comfort MW, Steinberg AG. Pedigree of a family with hereditary chronic relapsing pancreatitis. Gastroenterology 21:54–63, 1952.

Cooperman AM, Hoerr SO. Surgery of the pancreas: a text and atlas. St. Louis: CV Mosby, 1978:90–91.

Creutzfeldt W, Schmidt H. Aetiology and pathogenesis of pancreatitis. (Current concepts.) Scand J Gastroenterol 5 (Suppl 6):47–62, 1970.

DiMagno EP, Malagelada J-R, Taylor WF, et al. A prospective comparison of current diagnostic tests for pancreatic cancer. New Engl J Med 297: 737–42, 1977.

Dreiling DA, Wolfson P. New insights into pancreatic disease revealed by the secretin test. Dev Dig Dis 2:155–70, 1979.

Dutta SK, Costa BS, Russell RM, et al. Fat soluble vitamin deficiency in treated patients with pancreatic insufficiency. Gastroenterology 76:1126, 1979.

Figarella C. Les protéines du suc pancréatique humain. Arch Fr Mal App Dig 62:337–53, 1973.

Foulis AK. Histological evidence of initiating factors in acute necrotising pancreatitis in man. J Clin Pathol 33:1125–31, 1980.

Graham DY. Enzyme replacement therapy of exocrine pancreatic insufficiency in man. Relation between *in vitro* enzyme activities and *in vivo* potency in commercial pancreatic extracts. New Engl J Med 296:1314–17, 1977.

Hadorn B. Pancreatic proteinases. Their activation and the disturbances of this mechanism in man. Med Clin North Am 58:1319–31, 1974.

Hermon-Taylor J. An aetiological and therapeutic review of acute pancreatitis. Br J Hosp Med 18:546–52, 1977.

Jacob HS, Craddock PR, Hammerschmidt DE, et al. Complement induced granulocyte aggregation. An unsuspected mechanism of disease. N Engl J Med 302:789–94, 1980.

Johnson SG, Ellis CJ, Levitt MD. Mechanism of increased renal clearance of amylase/creatinine in acute pancreatitis. New Engl J Med 295:1214–17, 1976.

Kelly TR. Gallstone pancreatitis: pathophysiology. Surgery 80:488–92, 1976.

Konturek SJ, Tasler J, Schally AV, et al. Enkephalin inhibits the release and action of secretin on pancreatic secretion. Gastroenterology 76:1174, 1979.

Korman LY, Gardner JD. Functionally distinct modes of action of CCK and cholinergic agents on pancreatic acinar cells. Gastroenterology 76: 1175, 1979.

Krejs GJ, Orici L, Conlon JM, et al. Somatostatinoma syndrome. Biochemical, morphologic and clinical features. New Engl J Med 301:285–92, 1979.

Lee BC, van der Zee H, Malik AB. Pathogenesis of pulmonary edema in acute experimental pancreatitis. Surg Forum 30:420–22, 1979.

Levitt MD, Johnson SG. Is the C_{am}/C_{cr} ratio of value for the diagnosis of pancreatitis? Gastroenterology 75:118–19, 1978.

Levitt MD, Rapapport M, Cooperband SR. The renal clearance of amylase in renal insufficiency, acute pancreatitis and macroamylasemia. Ann Intern Med 71:919–25, 1969.

Luk GD. Qualitative fecal fat by light microscopy: a sensitive and specific screening test for steatorrhea and pancreatic insufficiency. Gastroenterology 76:1189, 1979.

Lundh G. Pancreatic exocrine function in neoplastic and inflammatory disease: a simple and reliable new test. Gastroenterology 42:275–80, 1962.

MacMahon B, Yen S, Trichopoulos D et al: Coffee and cancer of the pancreas. N. Engl J Med 304:630–33, 1981.

Mallory A, Kern F. Jr. Drug-induced pancreatitis: a critical review. Gastroenterology 78:813–20, 1980.

Manabe T, Steer MJ. Experimental acute pancreatitis in mice. Protective effects of glucagon. Gastroenterology 76:529–34, 1979.

Maruchi N, Brian D, Ludwig J, et al. Cancer of the pancreas in Olmsted County, Minnesota, 1935–1974. Mayo Clin Proc 54:245–49, 1979.

Morisett J. Solomon TE, Grossman MI. Effect of secretin and caerulein on pancreatic weight, DNA synthesis and DNA content. Gastroenterology 76:1206, 1979.

Olazebel A, Fuller R. Failure of glucagon in the treatment of alcoholic pancreatitis. Gastroenterology 74:489–91, 1978.

Patten BM. Human embryology, 2nd ed. New York: Blakiston Company, 1953.

Petersen OH, Iwatsuki N. The role of calcium in pancreatic acinar cell stimulus-secretion coupling: an electrophysiological approach. Ann NY Acad Sci 307:599–617, 1978.

Prinz RA, Kaufman BH, Folk FA, et al. Pancreaticojejunostomy for chronic pancreatitis: 2- to 21-year follow-up. Arch Surg 113:520-25, 1978.

Puestow CB, Gillesby WJ. Retrograde surgical drainage of the pancreas for chronic relapsing pancreatitis. Arch Surg 76:898–907, 1958.

Renner IG, Rinderknecht H, Douglas AP. Profiles of pure pancreatic secretions in patients with acute pancreatitis: the possible role of proteolytic enzymes in pathogenesis. Gastroenterology 75:1090–98, 1978.

Rinderknecht H, Renner IG, Douglas AP, et al. Profiles of pure pancreatic secretions obtained by direct pancreatic duct cannulation in normal healthy human subjects. Gastroenterology 75:1083–89, 1978.

Sarles H. Chronic calcifying pancreatitis—chronic alcoholic pancreatitis. Gastroenterology 66:604–16, 1974.

Sarles H., Tiscornia O, Palasciano G. Chronic alcoholism and canine exocrine pancreas secretion. A long-term follow-up study. Gastroenterology 72:238–43, 1977.

Schmidt H, Creutzfeldt W. Etiology and pathogenesis of pancreatitis. In: Bockus HL, ed. Gastroenterology, 3rd ed, vol. 3. Philadelphia: WB Saunders, 1976:1005–19.

Singh M, Webster PD, III. Neurohormonal control of pancreatic secretion. A review. Gastroenterology 74:294–309, 1978.

Smith FR, Barkin JS, Pererias R, et al. Therapeutic percutaneous aspiration of pancreatic pseudocysts. Gastroenterology 76:1250, 1979.

Steinberg WM, Curington CW, Toskes PP. Evidence that failure to degrade r-binder is unimportant in the pathogenesis of cobalamin malabsorption in patients with chronic pancreatitis. Gastroenterology 76:1255, 1979.

Toskes PP, Dawson W, Curington C, et al. Non-diabetic retinal abnormalities in chronic pancreatitis. New Engl J Med 300:942–46, 1979.

Trousseau A: Clinique medicale de l'hotel-dieu de Paris, 2nd ed, vol. 3. Paris: J-B Balliere et Fils, 1865:660–63.

Usadel KH, Schwedes U, Leuschner U, et al. Treatment of acute-Pancreatitis with somatostatin. Natl Pancreatic Cancer Proj Newsl 5:19, 1980.

Verner JV, Morrison AB. Endocrine pancreatitis islet disease with diarrhea. Report of a case due to diffuse hyperplasia of nonbeta islet tissue with a review of 54 additional cases. Arch Intern Med 133:492–500, 1974.

Warshaw AL, Fuller AF, Jr. Specificity of increased renal clearance of amylase in the diagnosis of acute pancreatitis. New Engl J Med 292:325–28, 1975.

Webster PD, III, Black O, Jr, Mainz DL, et al. Pancreatic acinar cell metabolism and function. Gastroenterology 73:1434–49, 1977.

White TT, Allan BJ. Intrapancreatic activation of proteases in the etiology of pancreatitis and cancer of the pancreas. Med Clin North Am 58:1305–10, 1974.

Wormsley KG. Pancreatic exocrine physiology. Br J Hosp Med 18:518–27, 1977.

DISCUSSION PROBLEM

A 53-year-old white man with a long history of moderate ingestion of alcohol, consisting of three to four shots a day, develops steady and deep nonradiating epigastric pain, followed shortly by the onset of clay-colored stools, amber-colored urine, and slight generalized pruritus. He denies taking any drugs or medication, has noted no change in appetite, and has lost no weight in the six weeks of illness.

On examination, patient is icteric with normal vital signs. Examination of the abdomen is completely normal. No masses are found, and the liver and gall bladder are not palpable. An abdominal computed tomographic scan reveals diffuse enlargement of the pancreas, moderate enlargement of the gall bladder which contains several opaque shadows, and dilatation of the extrahepatic and intrahepatic bile ducts.

Comment on the differential diagnosis in this case. Indicate what further diagnostic procedures are necessary, and how the results of each would affect your management.

CHAPTER 14

The Small Intestine and Colon: Structure and Function

We come now to consider a section of the alimentary tract which is second in importance only to the liver in the essential nature of the functions which it serves. The intestine must be able to digest a variety of nutrients after their initial exposure to pancreatic enzymes and bile, and then be able to transport them, all the while conserving bodily electrolytes and water and protecting itself against infectious agents ingested with the diet. It is essential to our independent life. We can live on alimentary feedings, albeit with difficulty, lacking an esophagus, stomach, or colon; we cannot do so without a small bowel.

ANATOMY

The small intestine in autopsy specimens measures about 600 to 700 cm in length and is divided into three segments. The upper segment, the duodenum, is distinguishable from the remainder grossly by its retroperitoneal location, and microscopically by the presence of submucosal Brunner glands. The two lower segments, the jejunum and ileum, are not grossly distinguishable from one another, are convoluted, and are suspended from a common mesentery. Morson and Dawson (1979) calculate that the jejunum occupies about 40 percent of the mesenteric small intestine, the ileum the remainder. Ancient descriptions of length of the duodenum (12 fingers = 25–30 cm) and of the ileum (21 hands = 200 cm) are at some variance from contemporary estimates. The upper three-fourths of the duodenum are supplied by the gastroduodenal artery, while the remainder of the duodenum and the balance of the small intestine are supplied by branching arcades of the superior mesenteric artery. All venous return empties into the portal system, and lymphatic drainage is into the thoracic duct by way of regional ducts and nodes.

When viewed grossly, the inner surface of the small intestine is seen to be thrown up into numerous, rather closely packed traverse folds (plicae circularis, folds of Kerckring) which serve to increase the mucosal surface area. The surface area is increased still further by the fact that the mucosa itself is thrown up into myriads of projections, called *villi*. The villous pattern of the small intestine is most impressive when viewed through a hand lens. One sees numerous, tightly packed fingerlike projections of the mucosa. Occasionally these are convoluted and leaf or spade shaped. On microscopy, villi occupy up to 75 percent of mucosal thickness, measure from 320 to 570 μm in height, and are quite slender (Fig. 14-1). The villous surface is covered with narrow columnar epithelium (absorptive cells) and occasional goblet cells. Absorptive cells predominate over the entire villus, but a greater proportion of goblet cells is present at the base. At 430 magnifications, the luminal edges of the absorptive cells are seen to be tipped with a thin, somewhat densely staining brush border. Villous epithelium rests on a lamina propria containing small lymphatic channels, a few lymphocytes, plasma cells, and stroma. Villi arise from mucosal crypts, and one sees lymphocytes, plasma cells, Paneth cells, and occasional granular endocrine cells in the basal epithelial populations. Mononuclear cells in the lamina propria increase progressively in the jejunum and ileum and coalesce in

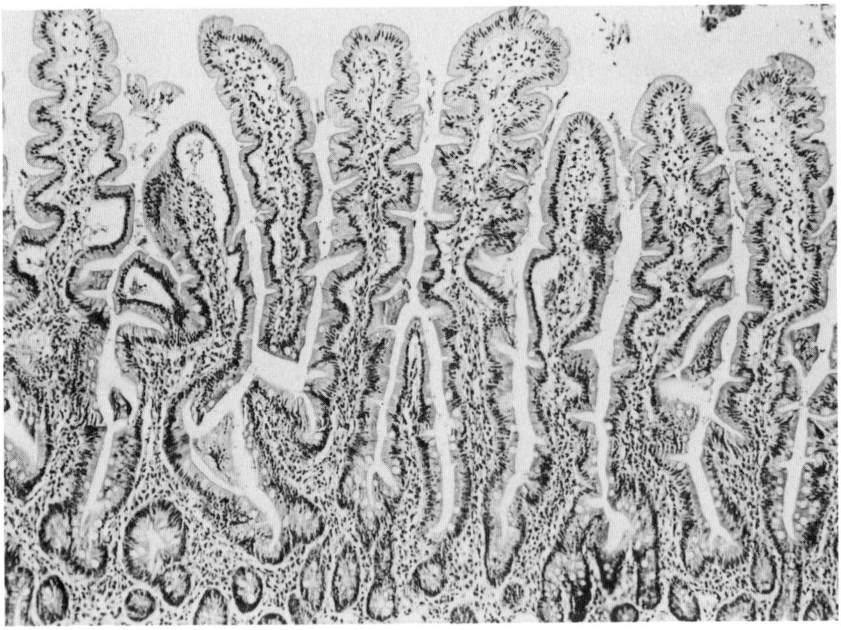

Figure 14-1. Biopsy of normal jejunal mucosa. Note elongated, closely packed villi, whose total height occupies at least 75 percent of the entire mucosal thickness. Epithelial cells are columnar, and nuclei are located at the bases of the cells. A distinct, darker gray brush (microvillous) border can be distinguished, especially at villous tips. The lamina propria contains a moderate number of mononuclear cells (lymphocytes and plasma cells). Original magnification x80.

areas as follicles with germinal centers, called Peyer patches. The epithelium over Peyer patches is frequently nonvillous and probably nonabsorptive. Morson and Dawson indicate that villi in the duodenum have broader bases than do those in the lower small intestine, and that villi from the upper small intestine are more likely to have saw-toothed margins than do villi in the ileum. Ileal villi also tend to be longer and less straight and contain more goblet cells. Underlying the lamina propria and radiating strands into the villi is a thin layer of longitudinal muscle, called the *muscularis mucosae*, and below this a moderately thin layer of submucosa, consisting of lymphoid cells, loose connective tissue, vessels, lymphatics, and nerve (Meissner) plexi. The small intestine is completely invested by two layers of smooth muscle deep to the submucosa, an inner circular layer and an outer longitudinal layer. Nerve plexi (Auerbach) are present throughout this layer. Where present, the outer serosal layer is composed of a single layer of cuboidal cells.

I have indicated that the absorptive surface of the small intestine is increased considerably by the presence of circular folds and villi. Further massive increases of surface area are appreciated when the brush borders of absorptive cells are viewed under the electron microscope (Figure 14–2). This area consists of myriads of short, straight microvilli which have both absorptive and synthetic (enzyme-producing) functions. Each microvillus has a trilayered surface membrane from which tiny projections emerge, forming the fuzzy coat of the epithelium. Adjacent epithelial cells are bound to one another at their luminal ends by filamentous areas, called *tight junctions*, which limit absorption between cells.

The colon measures about 150 cm in length and is considerably larger than the small intestine in diameter. It is joined to the small intestine at the ileocecal valve, which rests in the lower right quadrant of the abdomen. The blind portion of the colon lying below the ileocecal valve is called the cecum, and the appendix protrudes from the medial wall of the cecum as a long, narrow diverticulum. Proceeding distally, the cecum is contiguous with the ascending colon which rises to the level of the underside of the liver, and turns obtusely in a medial direction at the hepatic flexure, continuing upward and to the left as the transverse colon. At the left lateral margin of the peritoneal cavity, the colon makes an acute downward bend, at the splenic flexure, and is designated as the descending colon. The descending colon progresses distally to the level of the true pelvis, where another obtuse angulation occurs, directed medially, at the sigmoid flexure. The sigmoid colon is shaped rather like a question mark, and is about 35 cm in length. This connects, in turn, with the rectum, whose terminal portion (the rectal ampulla) is considerably larger in diameter than the sigmoid. The rectum is approximately 20 cm long and is divided into segments by three successive semilunar valves. The transverse colon and sigmoid are completely invested with peritoneum, the ascending and descending colon are covered with peritoneum, anteriorly alone and the rectum has no peritoneal covering.

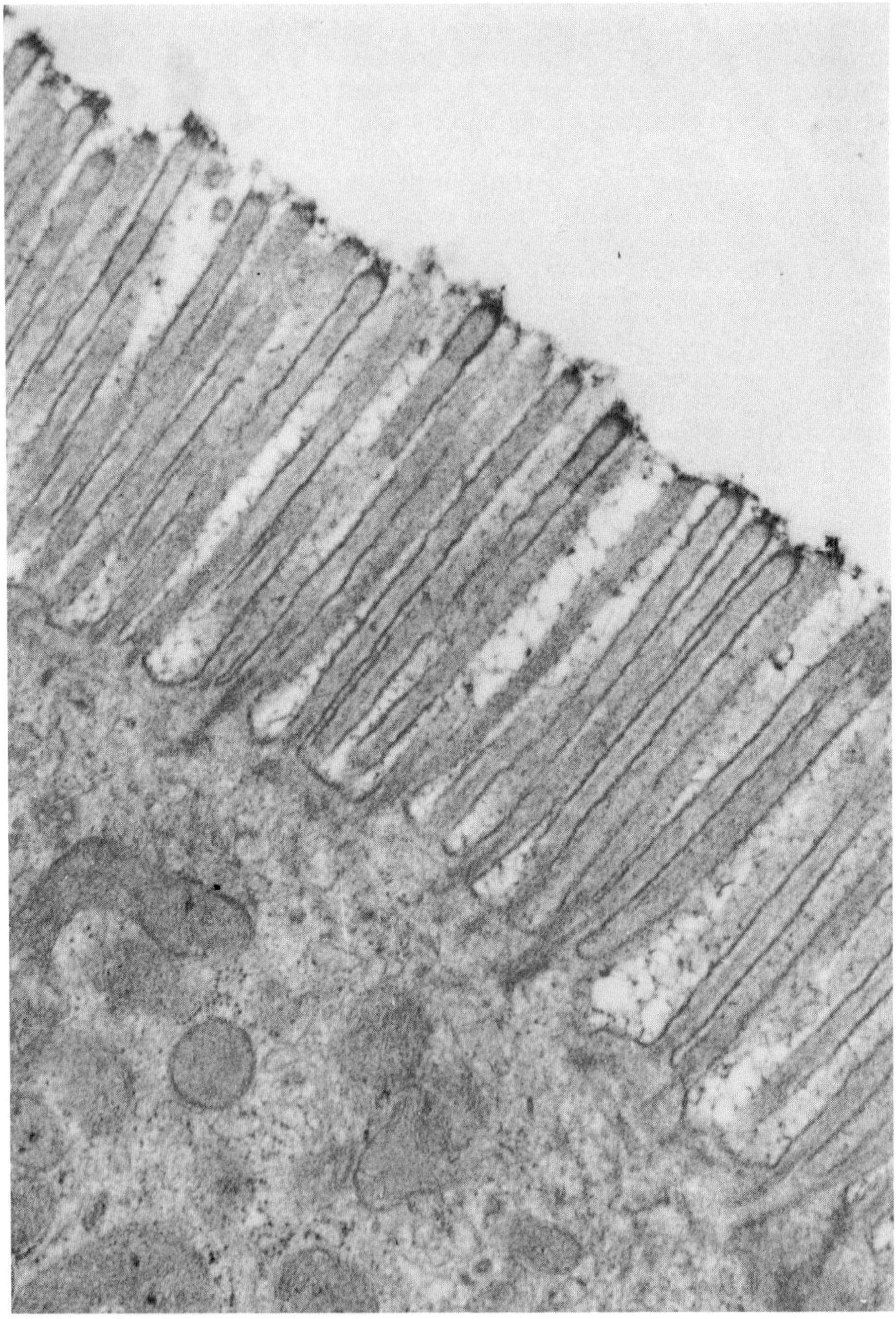

Figure 14-2. Microvilli on the luminal margin of a single jejunal epithelial villous tip cell. Disaccharidases and petidases are elaborated at this border membrane. Original magnification x343,000. Courtesy Dr. William Morningstar.

Grossly, the colon is distinguished from the small intestine not only by its greater diameter, but also by the fact that it is thrown into regular sacculations, or haustra, from cecum through sigmoid. These sacculations are caused by three longitudinal muscular bands which run the length of the colon, the taenia coli, and are shorter than that organ. The taeniae are analogous to the outer longitudinal muscle of the small intestine but do not form a complete coat. The circular muscular layer of the colon is complete. Both muscular coats are complete in the rectum. Colonic blood supply from the cecum to splenic flexure arises from three major branches of the superior mesenteric artery. The inferior mesenteric artery supplies the descending colon and the upper rectum, while the middle hemorrhoidal artery comes from the internal iliac artery, and the inferior hemorrhoidal artery arises from the pudendal vessels.

The colonic epithelium consists of tightly packed straight glands, or crypts. The tubular portions of these glands consist primarily of goblet cells, while the surface epithelium is primarily composed of columnar cells plus a few goblet cells. The lamina propria is quite cellular and contains fibroblasts, lymphocytes, plasma cells, macrophages, and some lymphoid follicles. Lymphatic channels are scarce. Epithelial cells do have microvilli, but they are shorter and more scanty than in the jejunum. There is also a continuous muscularis mucosae.

EMBRYOLOGY

The temporal differentiation of the small intestine is outlined in Table 14–1. The complexity of this process indicates pathways for a number of teratological and genetic defects. Failure of rotation of the intestine between the 6th and 10th weeks of embryonic developments can lead to a variety of malrotations which may be either asymptomatic or may lead to obstructions of the intestine during postnatal life. Localized duplications of the intestine, some in communication with the main lumen and others completely separate, may occur. They usually lie in the mesentery, occasionally contain functioning oxyntic mucosa, and thus may ulcerate or cause obstructive kinks in the intestine. The vitelline duct, connecting the primitive gut to the yolk sac, may persist in toto and lead to an umbilico-intestinal fistula, or incompletely regress to a fibrous strand, which may in life form the axis for later obstructive volvulus. Persistence of the enteric end of the vitelline duct causes formation of an ileal (Meckel) diverticulum. Meckel diverticula may twist, causing volvulus, or may lead to ileal ulcerations and hemorrhage resulting from acid-peptic secretion by areas of gastric epithelium contained in their mucosa. They may also become obstructed by intestinal contents and acutely inflamed, much like the pathophysiology of appendicitis. The intestine, finally, may not return to the abdominal cavity after the 10th week and present, at birth, as a small or large umbilical hernia.

Table 14-1. Structural and Functional Differentiation of the Developing Small Intestine

Age of Embryo (weeks)	*Length (mm) Crown to rump*	*Stage of Intestinal Development*
2.5	1.5	gut contiguous with yolk sac
4	5	simple tube lined by layer of epithelium, 4 cells thick
5	8	lengthens into a single loop
6	12	loop begins to rotate around superior mesenteric artery
7	17	intestine elongates rapidly, and all but duodenum and distal colon herniate into umbilical cord; alkaline phosphatase, leucine aminopeptidase, and ATPase present in epithelial cells
8	19–23	epithelium becomes columnar, one cell thick; villous proliferation begins in duodenum, jejunum, occluding duodenum
9	30	duodenum patent; Auerbach plexi present; beta-adrenergic receptors demonstrable; alpha receptors appear later
8–10	23–40	microvilli appear on epithelial cells; goblet cells appear
10	40	intestine reenters abdomen, jejunum to the left, ileum to the right, cecum fixed in lower right quadrant; crypts of Lieberkühn present; active transport of glucose and ability to absorb lipids demonstrable; dipeptidase and adenylate cyclase activity present
		mitochondrial enzymes, nonspecific esterases present
11	56	intestinal musculature present; disaccharidases, active transport of amino acids demonstrable
13	65	Meissner plexi, peristalsis present; pinocytotic vesicles, inclusions in epithelial cells (? able to absorb macromolecules)
	78	Kerckring folds, Brunner glands present; villi now present throughout small intestine

Table 14-1. Structural and Functional Differentiation of the Developing Small Intestine (continued)

Age of Embryo (weeks)	*Length (mm) Crown to rump*	*Stage of Intestinal Development*
15	110	mast cells in lamina propria; lymphopoiesis begins in submucosa
16	112	Proliferation of intestinal glands
	120	increased jejunal transport of glucose
17		increased dipeptidase, disaccharidase activity
20	160	Peyer patches well developed in submucosa, muscularis — will increase in amount until age 10; muscularis mucosae identified
24	203	ascending colon, hepatic flexure identifiable, Paneth cells appear, increased lactase activity in jejunum, with decreasing gradient to ileum
32		Kerckring folds throughout small intestine
38	350	intestine has elongated 1,000-fold since fifth week; at birth, small intestine is over 1 m long, colon approximately 17 cm
Postnatal period		lipid absorption increases due to increased production of bile salts; glucose absorption increases; secretory IgA appears gradually; epithelial cells have ability at birth to form chylomicrons; lactase activity gradually decreases

Source: Adapted from Grand RJ, Watkins JB, Torti FM. Development of the human gastrointestinal tract. A review. Gastroenterology 70:790–810, 1976.

A number of genetic disorders can also lead to congenital abnormalities. Limited ability to absorb specific amino acids may lead to Hartnup disease (inability to absorb neutral amino acids) or cystinuria. Deficiencies of brush border enzymes may cause intolerance for certain disaccharides, especially lactose. Inability to produce secretory IgA (hypogammaglobulinemia) may lead to increased intestinal bacterial flora and malabsorption. Failure of development of mesenteric lymphatics may lead to lymphangiectasia and fat malabsorption, and inadequate myenteric plexus function may cause inadequate peristalsis, bacterial overgrowth, and malabsorption (intestinal pseudo-obstruction). Chloridorrhea is a rare condition associated with the inability to exchange chloride for bicarbonate in the lower small intestine while exchange of tissue hydrogen ion for luminal sodium continues normally. It results in chronic diarrhea and metabolic alkalosis and is believed to be due to a genetic developmental defect.

EPITHELIAL RENEWAL

Mitotic replacement of epithelial cells occurs in villous crypts and in the lower portions of villi. Columnar absorptive cells (enterocytes), mucous cells, enteroendocrine cells, and Paneth cells appear to emerge from a common stem cell. Enterocytes and mucous cells migrate from crypt to villous tip in five to six days before being extruded, enteroendocrine cells migrate somewhat more rapidly, and Paneth cells remain in the crypts for several weeks (Eastwood 1977). There is a gradient from high to low of disaccharidase, DNA, and protein content and mucosal thickness from jejunum to ileum. The S, or DNA synthetic, phase of mitotic activity is increased, and cell renewal is prolonged in patients with peptic ulcer and uremia. Methotrexate and starvation, parenteral hyperalimentation, and beta-adrenergic stimulation inhibit cell renewal and S-phase activity. Radiation inhibits all phases of the mitotic cycle. Cell renewal is hastened by bacterial and viral infections, celiac sprue, lactation, administration of growth hormone and thyroxine, alpha-adrenergic stimulation, and intestinal resections, especially of the upper portion. The effect of intestinal resection is at least in part humorally mediated, since it appears in the unoperated member of parabiotic-paired rats. The mucosa is thinner in germ-free than in normal rats, and the population of mucosal lymphocytes and plasma cells is reduced. The rate of epithelial growth may be dependent to a degree on subepithelial factors, since projections of epithelium into underlying mesenchyme have been noted during organogenesis, and continuing immaturity of fibroblasts, as in adenomatous polyps, is associated with increased epithelial proliferation. The rate of proliferation of crypt cells is inversely proportional to the population of epithelial villous cells.

Mucosal Production of Antibodies

In addition to epithelial renewal, mucosal protection is also provided by the production of immunoglobulins (antibodies). Mucosal antibodies protect the host from proliferation of bacteria and viruses, and prevent penetration of the mucosa by enterotoxins and by luminal antigens (Walker and Isselbacher 1977). Intestinal secretions contain all antibody classes, but contrary to other body fluids, secretory IgA is present in the greatest quantity. IgA concentrations average 0.2–0.3 mg per ml, IgM about 5 percent of this, IgG somewhat less than IgM, and IgE is present only in minute amounts (Brown 1978).

Intestinal IgA, M, and E are produced largely in mucosal plasma cells. These, in turn, have arisen in mesenteric lymph nodes and in Peyer patches as lymphoblasts. The conversion of lymphoblasts to plasma cells is facilitated by the action of helper, thymus-derived, lymphocytes. Thymus-deficient "nude" mice are unable to synthesize effective levels of IgA and are highly susceptible to enteric infections. Unlike circulating IgA, enteric IgA is dimeric rather than monomeric. It is attracted to epithelial cells in the gut mucosa, especially to those in glandular crypts, where it is coupled to secretory component, a glycoprotein. Secretory IgA, IgA linked to secretory component, is released by epithelial cells and proceeds to coat the entire microvillar margin. It is believed that secretory component prevents destruction of IgA by intercellular lysosomes and by luminal enzymes. The secretion of polymeric IgM is similar to that of IgA. The monomeric immunoglobulins, G and D, are released with other serum proteins at villous tip cells without secretory component and are probably not produced in the intestinal mucosa. Monomeric IgE is produced by mucosal plasma cells but is not linked to secretory component; it is degraded extensively in epithelial cells and in the lumen of the intestine.

Mucosal antibody responses are mediated by specialized epithelial M cells, which are located in the ileum overlying Peyer patches. These M cells are capable of absorbing macromolecules and transmitting them to underlying lymphoblasts, which then produce antibodies. This is not the sole mechanism, however, for initiating the production of intestinal antibodies. It has been shown in mice (Owen et al 1979, 1980), for example, that Giardia muris organisms penetrate between epithelial cells and are apparently ingested by epithelial macrophages which prepare the antigens for presentation to lymphocytes. They do not adhere to M cells. In immunocompetent mice, this incursion is followed by the extrusion of lymphocytes into the intestinal lumen, and attachment of these to the Giardia organisms.

Being polymeric in structure, IgA is well adapted for blocking bacterial- and toxin-binding sites and forming immune complexes with these agents on the surfaces of epithelial cells. This complexing process prevents the entrance of bacteria and toxins into epithelial cells and also facilitates the destruction of the foreign agents by prolonging their exposure to intestinal digestants. IgM operates in a similar fashion and provides supplementary protection against mucosal absorption of bacteria and toxins, especially in patients with IgA deficiency syndromes. Patients with deficiencies of both IgA and IgM (common variable immunodeficiency) and patients without helper T-cell activity (ataxia telangiectasia) do indeed suffer from increased intestinal infections and, possibly due to reduced defense against oncogenic viruses and other antigens, from an increased incidence of cancer.

INTESTINAL MOTILITY

It has been recognized for centuries that phasic intestinal peristalsis occurs, especially in the upper small intestine, even without stimulation by feeding. Early anatomists, in fact, were impressed enough by the "emptiness" of the upper small bowel at autopsy, especially when compared with the "fullness" of the colon and lowermost small intestine, to memorialize that observation in the name, jejunum, by which that portion of the intestine has since been known. It is only in recent years, however, that the importance of this interdigestive motility has come to be recognized (Vantrappen et al 1977). Present thinking ascribes the low bacterial content of the upper small intestine to two essential factors: (1) interdigestive motility, and (2) the production of mucosal antibodies. In the absence of either, there is pronounced tendency for intestinal bacterial overgrowth to occur.

The empty small intestine has been found to undergo cycles of peristaltic activity (interdigestive motor complexes) each lasting about 85 minutes. The first phase of each cycle is one of essentially absent propulsive motility; this is followed by a second phase of irregular myoelectric spikes and contractions. The third phase consists of a burst of rhythmic propulsive contractions (11–12 per minute) lasting for 5 or 6 minutes and progressing distally over a 32- to 36-cm segment of intestine. This phase has been shown to start in the stomach, duodenum, or jejunum, and is followed by the final phase, in which activity slows. The interdigestive motor cycle is interrupted by eating, when it is replaced by irregular propulsive complexes for a period of three to four hours. Interdigestive motility is reduced in many patients with bacterial overgrowth in the small intestine and is interrupted by vagotomy. Insulin, motilin, somatostatin, and possibly gastrin appear to stimulate the interdigestive motor complex. The effect of somatostatin is blocked by atropine (Lux et al 1980). Motor complexes in the duodenum are preceded by an increase in gastric acidity and followed by a rise in the production of bicarbonate and amylase by the pancreas, suggesting that this electrical activity has both motor and secretory implications (Vantrappen et al 1979). Using intracerebral endorphin and enkephalin, Burks and Galligan (1980) found significantly increased intestinal transit times in rats, an effect which was abolished by vagotomy, a finding which supports the notion that central factors also control intestinal motility. Martin et al (1980) have shown that invasive bacteria, non-invasive bacteria producing enterotoxins, and ethanol also tend to increase intestinal motility in rabbits and may in part contribute to the diarrhea caused by these agents.

Colonic motility is also phasic, and consists primarily of two wave types, segmenting and propulsive. During extended periods, the colon may show little or no electrical activitity. Segmenting waves occur every few minutes, while propulsive waves may occur no more often than several times per day. Peristalsis is initiated frequently by eating, which causes emptying of the ileum (gastroileal reflex), and peristalsis in the colon (gastrocolic reflex). These reflexes are mediated by the autonomic nervous system and are inhibited by atropine. Cholecystokinin also stimulates the distal colon, and its effect is not blocked by atropine (London et al 1980).

The ileocecal valve is a true sphincter, whose resting pressure is higher than that in the ileum and cecum. It relaxes when ileal pressures rise and tightens when cecal pressure is increased, thus serving to prevent cecoileal reflux. In the anal area, there are two sphincters, the upper receiving autonomic innervation, the lower, somatic. Proximal peristalsis relaxes the upper sphincter and tightens the lower portion, causing the urge to defecate. Colonic pressure is decreased if contents are soft and bulky, and transit time is also reduced. Low-residue diets lead to increased luminal pressure and to constipation.

INTESTINAL MICROFLORA

Approximate numbers and types of microorganisms vary greatly from site to site in the normal gastrointestinal tract (Table 14–2). In general, the

Table 14–2. Normal Gastrointestinal Microflora

Site	*Concentration of Organisms*	*Types of Organisms*
Stomach	less than 10^3 per ml	primarily gram-positive *Staphylococci, Streptococci, Lactobacilli;* occasional *Candida.* Few aerobic coliforms
Duodenum-jejunum	less than 10^5 per ml	similar to stomach; no anaerobes
Distal ileum	10^7 –10^8 per ml	obligate and facultative anaerobes (gram-positive-*Lactobacilli;* gram negative-*Bacteroides*)
Colon	10^{10} – 10^{11} anaerobes and 10^8 facultative anaerobes per g	*Bacteroides* outnumber gram positive anaerobics; facultative anaerobes consist of coliforms, *Streptococci, Lactobacilli* (5% of total); small numbers *Clostridia, Staphylococci,* spore-forming organisms, *Proteus, Candida, Torula, Aspergillus*

bacterial population increases markedly from stomach to colon. Anaerobic organisms are not found above the lower ileum and make up over 95 percent of fecal flora, and gram-negative anaerobes (*Bacteroides* group) tend to predominate over gram-positive anaerobes. Diet appears to play very little part in overall gut ecology, except in the breast-fed infant whose stool contains primarily bifido bacteria, few or no putrefactive (*Bacteroides*) organisms, and is acidic rather than alkaline in pH.

Relative sterility of the upper alimentary tract contents appears to be maintained by gastric acidity, bile acid secretion, mucus production, gastrointestinal motility, and antibody production (King and Toskes 1979). Aberrations in any one of these cleansing factors leads to bacterial overgrowth, with resultant malabsorption. Malabsorption from bacterial overgrowth will be discussed later in several different contexts, but has, in general, been found to be the result of two major factors: (1) intraluminal deconjugation of bile salts with reduction of total conjugated forms to below the amount required to form micellar solutions of lipids (critical micellar concentration), and (2) damage to intestinal mucosa, producing partial villous atrophy, decreased production of brush border enzymes, and loss of blood and plasma proteins. Nutrient malabsorption occurs whenever bacterial concentrations exceed 10^7 per ml, especially when anaerobic forms predominate.

MECHANISMS OF INTESTINAL ABSORPTION

The Transport of Electrolytes and Water

One never ceases to wonder at the immense work of which the intestine is capable, involving the bidirectional transport of ions and water in immense quantities each day and the processing of a nearly infinite variety of foodstuffs, all performed while avoiding any material changes in bodily homeostasis. To summarize this activity, we begin with a short tabular and narrative survey of ionic transport and the movements of water, and proceed thence to consideration of nutrient absorption.

Transport of water and electrolytes is bidirectional at many points, and one speaks of net absorption or net secretion based on the arithmetical total of fluxes in both directions. It is generally believed that most intestinal secretion occurs at the bases of villous crypts, while absorption occurs at epithelial cells along the villi. Absorption and secretion often occur simultaneously. Two types of transport are identified: passive transport, which is a flux of a constituent along an electro-chemical or osmotic gradient, or movement in company with another constituent which is being actively transported (solvent drag); and active transport, which is energy dependent and carrier mediated. The energy source is usually through the activity of cyclic adenosine 5′-monophosphate (cAMP). In the case of solvent drag, transport can progress against a gradient and still be a passive process. Thus, passive transport is not limited solely to movement along a concentration gradient (Krejs and Fordtran 1978).

The transport of water in the intestine appears to be purely passive and depends upon osmotic gradients between fluids in the lumen of the bowel and in extracellular spaces, on hydrostatic gradients developed in spaces between epithelial cells when ions (especially Na^+ and Cl^-) are pumped into these spaces by active transport from intracellular cytoplasm, and on hormonal activity. Water is transported through "pores" located near the tight junctions between epithelial cells; it is not absorbed at brush borders. Tight junctions bind the luminal end of one columnar cell to its neighbors, and the sizes of the pores appear to be larger in the jejunum (leaky tight junctions) than in the ileum and colon. Because of this, the secretion of water is less in the ileum than it is in the jejunum, and the tighter junctions in the lower small intestine favor the overall absorption of water. Prostaglandins, vasoactive intestinal peptide and gastric inhibitory peptide cause net secretion of water, while increased release of cAMP is associated with inhibition of the absorption of water (Field 1974).

The movement of electrolytes is summarized here and in Table 14-3:

- Sodium is actively absorbed in the jejunum, ileum, and colon. In the jejunum it is ionically transported with glucose or animo acids, or absorbed in exchange for H^+. In both cases, it is promptly pumped into intercellular spaces at the basolateral membrane of the epithelial cell, in company with HCO_3^-. Active absorption of NA^+ does not occur in the absence of HCO_3^-. From the intercellular spaces, NA^+ can be absorbed into the vascular space if pressure gradients favor that movement, or secreted into the gut in ionic form. HCO_3^- is only absorbed, because its negative charge prohibits transport through positively charged junctional pores. Sodium is actively absorbed in the ileum and colon, paired to Cl^-, the latter being actively exchanged for HCO_3^-. Na^+ may also be absorbed independently of Cl^- in the ileum (Frankel and Hopfer 1980). It is actively pumped into intercellular spaces, along with Cl^-, and absorbed into vascular spaces as neutral NaCl. Sodium is also passively transported (solvent drag) through jejunal tight junctions in both directions and to a lesser extent in the ileum, but not in the colon.
- Potassium movement is entirely passive throughout the intestine.
- Chloride is passively transported by solvent drag in the jejunum, but not in the ileum or colon, where it is actively absorbed in exchange for bicarbonate. It is actively secreted in the jejunum (Davis et al 1980) and may also be actively secreted in the ileum as well.
- Bicarbonate is actively absorbed in the jejunum and actively secreted in the ileum in exchange for chloride.

Table 14-3. Intestinal Transport of Electrolytes and Water

Jejunum	*Ileum*	*Colon*
Sodium Active absorption per brush borders (1) coupled to glucose or amino acids and (2) in exchange for H^+; actively pumped at basolateral membrane to intercellular space; active absorption occurs only in presence of HCO_3^-	mechanisms (1) and (2) apply, but little glucose available; (3) neutral NaCl absorption in exchange for H^+ and HCO_3^-; NaCl to vascular space, since no electrical gradient develops; (4) independent Na^+ absorption.	mainly, active ionic absorption, not coupled to glucose, controlled by aldosterone; plus mechanism (3) coupling possibly to short chain fatty acids (acetate, butyrate, propionate)
	Active secretion (?cAMP)	same as ileum
passive absorption per solvent drag at tight junctions	process less than in jejunum because of smaller (less leaky) pores at tight junctions	
passive secretion proportional to potential difference developed by unpaired anion absorption with glucose	process less than in jejunum because of reduced luminal glucose	minimal (75 mEq Na^+ enter from ileum daily, 4 mEq excreted)
Chloride active absorption	per neutral NaCl carrier	same as ileum
none	*active secretion* (?cAMP)	same as ileum
passive absorption per solvent drag with Na^+, K^+, etc.	none	none (36 mEq Cl^- enter from ileum daily, 2 mEq excreted)
Bicarbonate actively absorbed	same as jejunum	
	active secretion in exchange for chloride. Also secreted with cAMP stimulation	same as ileum *absorbed* after displacement by organic anions (lactate, etc.) (74 mEq HCO_3^- enter from ileum daily, 30 mEq excreted)
Potassium passively absorbed and secreted throughout intestinal tract		(44 mEq K^+ enter from ileum daily, 3 mEq excreted)

Table 14–3. Intestinal Transport of Electrolytes and Water (continued)

Jejunum	*Ileum*	*Colon*
Water passively absorbed and secreted throughout intestinal tract, largely based on osmotic gradients, hydrostatic pressure in intercellular spaces, and hormonal effects (VIP, GIP, etc.); transported exclusively through tight junctions		(600 ml H_2O enter from ileum daily, 100 ml excreted.) Major anions in stool water are short chain fatty acids produced by bacterial fermentation of carbohydrates

The transport of water and electrolytes depends on many variables, including the composition and the tonicity of intestinal contents and the segment of intestine being considered. Hormonal effects on secretion must also be reckoned with in determining the net movement of ions and water at any one time. Glucocorticoid deficiency, for example, decreases the absorption of Na^+ and Cl^-, while excesses increase the secretion of HCO_3^- (Sellin and Field 1980). A great variety of theoretical situations can be postulated, encompassing all these changeable factors. The sum total of the processes shaping the movements of ions and water remains "a riddle wrapped in a mystery inside an enigma."* While a great deal is indeed known, a unified concept of ionic transport is lacking. Its development remains for the future.

Digestion and Absorption of Carbohydrates (Table 14–4)

Approximately one-half of ingested calories is in the form of carbohydrate, and of this, 60 percent is in the form of starch, 30 percent as sucrose, and the balance as lactose (Gray 1975). Some dietary carbohydrates (raffinose, stachyose) are indigestible in the upper small intestine, are converted by bacterial digestion to short chain fatty acids, hydrogen, and carbon dioxide, and account for the intestinal gas caused by certain foods, such as beans. Starches and glycogen (alpha 1,4 polysaccharides) are acted on by salivary and pancreatic amylases and converted to dextrins (octosaccharides-average), maltose and maltotriose. Further digestion of these and ingested disaccharides (sucrose, lactose) is carried

*Winston S. Churchill, radio broadcast, 1 October 1939.

Table 14-4. Digestion and Absorption of Dietary Carbohydrates

Effectors	*Functions*
salivary, pancreatic amylases[a]	starch → dextrins, maltose, maltotriose
brush border oligosaccharidases	hydrolyze sucrose, maltose, maltotriose, lactose
transport with Na	glucose, galactose, xylose absorption ($C_6 > C_5$)
transport without Na	fructose absorption

a. Cellulose, stachyose not affected.

out by brush border carbohydrases (oligosaccharidases, disaccharidases). Cellulose, a beta 1,4 polysaccharide, is not digested by human amylases.

Disaccharidases are specific glycoproteins that hydrolyze sucrose, maltose, and lactose. They are present, especially in the jejunum, only on mature villous epithelium, but less in the brush border of the oldest villous tip cells. In general, the hydrolytic process is very rapid and is rate limiting only for the absorption of lactose.

Eighty percent of ingested dietary carbohydrate is digested to glucose, and the absorption of glucose requires a specific active membrane transport mechanism. The transport carrier requires a five-carbon ring on the sugar, hydroxylated at C_2. The process is facilitated by a sixth carbon atom. Thus, hexoses are absorbed more readily than pentoses. As implied in the previous section, the absorption of glucose (and galactose) requires Na^+ at another brush border site and results in intracellular glucose concentrations many times greater than luminal levels. Intracellulary, the glucose is released from its membrane carrier and diffuses into the vascular space, while the Na^+ is actively pumped out of the cell to the intercellular epithelial space. The absorption of fructose is independent of the glucose-galactose pathway and does not require contemporaneous absorption of Na^+.

Hydrolysis at brush borders is, of course, inhibited by deficient production of disaccharidases and also by a buildup of unabsorbed glucose in the brush border (produce inhibition). Thus, transfer of glucose across the villous membrane appears to be the rate-limiting step in the digestion-absorption process. In addition to Na^+ insufficiency, hypomotility also seems to slow absorption.

Digestion and Absorption of Proteins (Table 14-5)

Protein provides from 11 to 14 percent of total calories in the average diet, and approximately 45 g of nutritionally balanced protein are required by a 70-kg man. In addition to dietary protein, the body must also reabsorb

Table 14-5. Digestion and Absorption of Dietary Protein

Effectors	*Functions*
gastric proteases	large polypeptides, free amino acids (AA) from protein
pancreatic proteases	small (2-6 AA) polypeptides, free AA, from large polypeptides
brush border aminopeptidases	Tetra, Tri, dipeptides, from larger peptides
active transport	
dipeptide carrier	rapid absorption dipeptides
Na-dependent AA carrier (2 or more systems)	slow absorption: branch > straight chain AA
cytoplasmic peptidases	AA (intracellular)

endogenous proteins which reach the intestine in the form of digestive gland secretions, mucus, desquamated cells, and plasma proteins. Daily stool losses of protein average 1 to 2 g (Freeman and Kim 1978).

Gastric peptic activity produces mainly polypeptides with N-terminal phenylalanine and leucine, plus a few free amino acids. Pancreatic proteolysis results in free amino acids and small (2 to 6 amino acids) polypeptides. There are at least two major brush border absorption systems for the active transport of protein digestion products, one for amino acids and one for dipeptides and tripeptides. There is a decreasing gradient for amino acid and dipeptide absorption from jejunum to ileum. Matthews and Adibi (1976) indicate that the dipeptide transport carrier system is more efficient than the amino acid carrier, and is probably of more importance in human nutrition. Luminal dipeptides disappear with equal speed from the jejunum and the ileum, but the ileal disappearance is due to increased hydrolysis rather than to increased absorption. For the first 48 hours of neonatal life, infants are capable of absorbing whole proteins and large macromolecular fragments, such as antibodies. Adults can also absorb some macromolecules, but these are probably not nutritionally useful. They may function as antigens.

Brush border enzymes (aminopeptidases) convert polypeptides to tripeptides and tetrapeptides. Triglycine appears to be absorbed intact by the peptide carrier, but trileucine must be further hydrolyzed to leucine and dileucine prior to absorption. Tetraglycine is converted to triglycine and glycine at the brush border and, because the peptide absorption system is faster than the amino acid carrier mechanism, a tetraglycine solution is absorbed more rapidly than an equimolar solution of glycine alone.

The absorption of luminal amino acids is also an active carrier-mediated process, coupled to the absorption of Na^+. Sodium need not be present in the diet, because it may be concentrated at the brush borders from vascular stores. Amino acid absorption occurs over a wide range of pH but is reduced at levels below 2.5. There are at least two, and perhaps more, active carrier systems for amino acids, one for neutral (leucine, phenylalanine, etc.), and the other for basic (lysine, arginine, cystine) varieties. Others have been suggested for dicarboxylic acids and for glycine. Patients with Hartnup disease cannot absorb neutral amino acids, like tryptophan and phenylalanine, but can absorb dipeptides. Consequently, they may develop a pellagralike picture due to nicotinic acid deficiency but do not show protein malnutrition. Patients with cystinuria cannot transport dibasic amino acids and also have a similar defect in renal tubular reabsorption.

Among the various amino acids, branched chain forms (methionine, leucine, valine) show the highest rate of absorption, while glutamic and aspartic acids show the lowest (Adibi 1978). The presence of side chains and the absence of electrical charges appear to enhance the affinity for epithelial absorption sites. The presence of high affinity types in a mixed solution of amino acids further competitively inhibits the absorption of lower affinity types.

Protein fractions absorbed by the peptide carrier are hydrolyzed to amino acids by cytoplasmic peptidases. Transport of these to blood is probably by simple membrane diffusion, similar to the glucose-galactose pathway.

Digestion and Absorption of Fats (Table 14-6)

Fat differs from other nutrients and from electrolytes by being insoluble in water. Davenport (1978) points out that it is this very property of lipids that makes them essential constituents in cellular membranes. The lack of solubility in water also requires a distinctive mechanism for intestinal

Table 14-6. Digestion and Absorption of Dietary Fat

Effectors	*Function*
lingual lipase	limited hydrolysis of triglycerides
duodenal phospholipids/bile acids	emulsification of lipids
pancreatic phospholipase A_2	phospholipid hydrolysis
pancreatic colipase	binds to surface fatty acids on phospholipids
pancreatic lipase	C_1, C_3 hydrolysis of triglycerides
bile acids	Form micelles → diffusion through unstirred layer
epithelial brush borders	absorb fatty acids and C_2 monogylcerides
cytoplasmic activity	triglycerides reconstituted in enterocyte
cytoplasmic B apoproteins	chylomicrons formed in enterocyte
basolateral membrane transport	conveys chylomicrons to lymphatics

digestion and absorption of fats. Borgström (1980) indicates that a small percentage of free fatty acid is necessary on the surface of fat droplets for binding colipase to its surface, and that enough lipase is usually present in-pharyngeal secretions (lingual lipase) to accomplish this limited hydrolysis. The absence of colipase in the duodenum causes malabsorption of fat, even when lipase concentrations are adequate (Gaskin et al 1980). Long-chain triglycerides, even when emulsified by phospholipids and bile acids in the presence of colipase, are not immediately available for hydrolysis by pancreatic lipase, unless limited hydrolysis of the phospholipid (phosphatidyl choline) component has occured through the action of pancreatic phospholipase A_2. This latter action releases free fatty acids at the surface of the droplet for colipase binding. The sequence of events in the intestinal digestion of triglycerides is then as follows: emulsification of fat by biliary phospholipids and bile acids, partial hydrolysis of surface phospholipids by pancreatic phospholipase, with release of surface fatty acids, binding of pancreatic colipase (previously bound to lipase) to droplet surface by fatty acids, action of lipase on triglycerides.

Following hydrolysis, chyme contains free fatty acids and monoglycerides, which are esterified at the C_2 position. Reesterification with free fatty acids at C_1 and C_3 does not occur in the jejunum. Since hydrolysis proceeds rapidly and is not the rate-limiting step in the digestion and absorption of lipids, the concentrations of free fatty-acids and monoglycerides in the upper intestine increase rapidly after a fatty meal. These products of fat hydrolysis form micelles with conjugated bile acids in the intestinal lumen, provided that the concentration of the bile acids is at or above the critical micellar level. If this level is not reached, or if bile acids have been deconjugated by intestinal bacteria, micelles do not form and the absorption of lipids is markedly delayed. So long as lipase activity is present, however, lipid absorption does occur in the absence of bile salts, albeit more slowly, less efficiently, and at lower levels of the small intestine. In addition to free fatty acids, monoglycerides, and bile salts, cholesterol- and fat-soluble vitamins are also found in intestinal micelles.

Since micelles remain in solution in the unstirred aqueous layer bathing epithelial brush borders, they bring lipids into proximity with the cellular absorbing surface. Fatty acids and monoglycerides diffuse rapidly from these micelles and are absorbed by gradient in the duodenum and jejunum. Whole micelles are not absorbed, and the major reabsorption of bile acids occurs in the lower ileum (Hofmann 1977).

Monoglycerides are converted to triglycerides in the supranuclear cytoplasm of intestinal epithelial cells, and some free fatty acids are joined to glyceryl-phosphate to form phospholipids. Medium-chain (C_8-C_{12}) fatty acids are transmitted to portal capillaries, while longer chain fatty acids, triglycerides, and cholesterol are formed into chylomicrons, by surface coating with a cytoplasmic apoprotein, beta lipoprotein. Rachmilowitz et al (1978) have shown that human intestinal mucosa synthesizes apoproteins from dietary amino acids. Rubin et al (1980) have shown in elegant cytological studies that apoprotein B is probably synthesized in supranuclear rough endoplasmic reticulum, is transmitted to smooth endoplasmic reticulum on absorption of fat, coats the surface of chylomicrons intracellularly, and remains on these surfaces while and after the chylomicrons are extruded into the lamina propria via basolateral epithelial cell membranes. Chylomicrons cannot be formed in the absence of beta lipoprotein. A recessive genetic disorder, a-betalipoproteinemia, is characterized by steatorrhea, deficiency of essential fatty acids and fat-soluble vitamins, and neurological damage. The intestinal biopsy in these patients is characterized by the presence of numerous, untransportable cytoplasmic fat droplets in the jejunal epithelium.

Chylomicrons are transported from epithelial cells to intracellular spaces, whence they are transferred to mesenteric lymphatics. Here again, congential or acquired blockade to mesenteric lymphatics can result in an obstructive disorder known as lymphangiectasia. Absorption of long-chain fatty acids is diminished and steatorrhea appears, proportional to the percentage of long-chain fatty acids in the diet. Patients with lymphangiectasia also develop hypoproteinemia due to loss of circulating proteins into the gut lumen secondary to lymphatic blockade. They also develop lymphocytopenia because of inability of mesenteric lymphocytes to gain access to circulating blood, and show decreased resistance to infections.

Normal stool losses of fat (generally fatty acids and soaps) are less than 5 g per day and are not dependent upon dietary intake. Nutrient fat is essentially fully absorbed by healthy subjects, and the small amounts of lipid in the stool are largely of bacterial origin.

Absorption of Water-Soluble Vitamins

Choline, thiamin, folic acid, nicotinic acid, and riboflavin are each absorbed from the upper intestine by carrier-mediated, active transport processes. Ascorbic acid is actively absorbed in the ileum. Sodium is required for the absorption of ascorbic acid, folic acid, nicotinic acid, and thiamin, but not for the absorption of riboflavin or choline (Rose 1980). Thiamin absorption probably also requires oxygen, and the carrier appears to be a pyrophosphokinase, since the vitamin is phosphorylated in the transport process. Folic acid is derived from dietary pteroylheptaglutamate, which is hydrolyzed in cellular lysosomes by folate conjugase. The absorption of riboflavin is membrane limited but enhanced by bile acids. The vitamin is probably phosphorylated in the absorptive process. Since the absorption of all water-soluble vitamins requires intact brush borders, it is clear that disorders that interfere with this membrane will be associated with vitamin deficiencies. Because of its applicability to the testing of malabsorption, the absorption of vitamin B_{12} is discussed in Chapter 15.

HISTORICAL DIGRESSION

Proper names used in this chapter without reference include: Leopold AUERBACH (1828-1897), German physiologist, Breslau; Johann Conrad BRUNNER (1653–1727), German anatomist, Mannheim, Heidelberg; Hans Christian Joachim GRAM (1853–1958), Danish pharmacologist, pathologist and internist, Copenhagen; HARTNUP is derived from the surname of the affected family, also called H disease. Disorder is fully described in Baron DN, Dent CE, Harris H, et al. Hereditary pellegra-like skin rash with temporary cerebellar ataxia, constant renal amino-acidura, and other bizarre biochemical features. Lancet 2:421–28, 1956; Theodorus KERCKRING (1640–1727), German anatomist, Amsterdam, Hamburg; Johann Nathanel LIEBERKUHN (1711–1756), German anatomist, Berlin; Johann Friedrich MECKEL, Jr. (1781–1833), German anatomist and surgeon, Halle; Georg MEISSNER (1829–1905), Swiss anatomist and physician, Basel, Gottingen; Joseph PANETH (1857–1905), Swiss anatomist and physician, Basel, Gottingen; Joseph PANETH (1857–1890), Austrian physiologist, Vienna; Johann Konrad PEYER (1653–1712), German physician and anatomist, Schaffhausen.

SELECTED REFERENCES

Adibi SA. Intestinal absorption of amino acids and peptides. Viewpoints Dig Dis 10:1–4, 1978.

Borgström B. Importance of phospholipids, pancreatic phospholipase A_2, and fatty acid for the digestion of dietary fat. *In vitro* experiments with the porcine enzymes. Gastroenterology 78:954–62, 1980.

Brown WR. Relationships between immunoglobulins and the intestinal epithelium. Gastroenterology 75:129–38, 1978.

Burks TF, Galligan JJ. Centrally mediated inhibition of intestinal transit: role of endogenous opioid peptides. Gastroenterology 78:1146, 1980.

Davenport HW. A digest of digestion, 2nd ed. Chicago: Year Book Medical Publishers, 1978: 123–37.

Davis GR, Morawski SG, Santa Ana CA, et al. Active chloride secretion in the normal human jejunum: a property that may regulate normal absorption rate. Gastroenterology 78:1153, 1980.

Eastwood GL. Gastrointestinal epithelial renewal. Gastroenterology 72:962–75, 1977.

Field M. Intestinal secretion. Gastroenterology 66: 1063–84, 1974

Frankel MH, Hopfer U. Independence of sodium transport from chloride in rabbit ileum brush border membranes. Gastroenterology 78:1167, 1980.

Freeman HJ, Kim YS. Digestion and absorption of protein. Ann Rev Med 29:99-116, 1978.

Gardner JD, Brown MS, Laster, L. The columnar epithelial cell of the small intestine: digestion and transport. New Engl J Med 283:1196–1202, 1264–71, 1317–24, 1970.

Gaskin KJ, Durie PR, Hill RE, et al. Colipase in pancreatic insufficiency. Gastroenterology 78:1170, 1980.

Gray GM. Carbohydrate digestion and absorption. Role of the small intestine. New Engl J Med 292:1225–30, 1975.

Hoffmann AF. Fat absorption and malabsorption: physiology, diagnosis and treatment. Viewpoints Dig Dis 9:1–4, 1977.

King CE, Toskes PP. Small intestinal bacterial overgrowth. Gastroenterology 76:1035–55, 1979.

Krejs, Fordtran JS. Physiology and pathophysiology of ion and water movement in the human small intestine. In: Sleisinger MH, Fordtran JS, eds. Gastrointestinal disease, 2nd ed. Philadelphia: WB Saunders, 1978: 297–335.

London R, Cohen S, Snape W, Jr. The action and role of cholecystokinin on distal colonic function. Gastroenterology 78:1210, 1980.

Lux G, Femppel J, Lederer P, et al. Somatostatin induces interdigestive intestinal motor and secretory complex-like activity in man. Gastroenterology 78:1212, 1980.

Martin JL, Justus PG, Mathias JR. Altered motility of the small intestine in response to ethanol: an explanation for the diarrhea associated with the consumption of alcohol. Gastroenterology 78:1218, 1980.

Matthews DM, Adibi SA. Peptide absorption. Gastroenterology 71:151–61, 1976.

Morson BC, Dawson IMP. Gastrointestinal pathology, 2nd ed. Oxford: Blackwell Scientific Publications, 1979: 211–33.

Owen RL, Allen L, Stevens DP. Intraepithelial trapping of *Giardia* by macrophages in Peyer's patches of normal and nude mice—an intestinal defense and antigen processing mechanism. Gastroenterology 78:1232, 1980.

Owen RL, Nemanic PC, Stevens DP. Ultrastructural observations on Giardiasis in a murine model. I. Intestinal distribution, attachment, and relationship to the immune system of *Giardia muris*. Gastroenterology 76:757–69, 1979.

Rachmilewitz D, Albers JJ, Saunders DR, et al. Apoprotein synthesis by human duodeno-jejunal mucosa. Gastroenterology 75:677–82, 1978.

Rose RC. Water-soluble vitamin absorption in intestine. Ann Rev Physiol 42:157–71, 1980.

Rubin CE, Perkins WD, Surawicz CM, et al. Ultrastructural apoprotein B localization within human jejunal absorptive cells during fat absorption. Gastroenterology 78:1248, 1980.

Sellin J, Field M. Glucocorticoids and ileal ion transport. Gasteroenterology 78:1257, 1980.

Vantrappen G, Janssens J, Hellemans J, et al. The interdigestive motor complex of normal subjects and patients with bacterial overgrowth of the small intestine. J Clin Invest 59:1158–66, 1977.

Vantrappen G, Peeters TL, Janssens J. The interdigestive complexes of man have both secretory and motor components. Gastroenterology 76:1264, 1979.

Walker WA, Isselbacher, KJ. Intestinal antibodies. New Engl J Med 297: 767–73, 1977.

DISCUSSION QUESTION

A healthy woman of 26 years developed severe viral gastroenteritis during the 10th week of her first pregnancy and remained quite ill for six days. There was no evidence of impending abortion, and the remainder of her pregnancy was uneventful except for the fact that labor occurred in the 37th week and the infant weighed only 2 kg at birth. Based on your knowledge of embryology and intestinal physiology what abnormalities might you anticipate in this infant?

CHAPTER 15

Disorders of Intestinal Absorption

Review of the preceding chapter suggests many ways in which the multiple functions of the small intestine may be subverted and lead to absorptive disorders. And the chances are great that any mechanism that can be devised by the reader does indeed have its counterpart in nature! There is a great variety of intestinal absorptive diseases, and it is the aim of this chapter to categorize them, give specific mechanisms in each category, and suggest modes of diagnosis and treatment.

There are two major groups of absorptive disorders, those due to *maldigestion* of nutrients in the intestinal lumen or at the mucosal brush border, and those due to *malabsorption* of properly digested nutrients as a result of abnormalities in the intestinal mucosa. Maldigestion and malabsorption often coexist, the one process being secondary to the other, or both processes being caused by a single agent. Bacterial overgrowth syndromes are examples of the latter category; maldigestion occurs because of luminal deconjugation of bile acids, malabsorption because of patchy inflammatory atrophy of the villous epithelium.

CAUSES OF MALDIGESTION

Pancreatic Insufficiency

The causes and treatment of this disorder have already been discussed. Pancreatic insufficiency is a common feature of chronic calcific pancreatitis and carcinoma of the pancreas; it is almost invariably encountered in patients with cystic fibrosis. In the absence of pancreatic enzymes, all categories of food are poorly digested, and stools are loaded with fat (steatorrhea) and nitrogenous nutrients (creatorrhea).

Deficiency of Conjugated Bile Acids Due to Cholestasis, Bacterial Overgrowth, or Hypomotility

Deficiency of conjugated bile acids leads to defective micelle formation of fats in the intestine and results in a reduction of the lipid surface area exposed to the action of colipase and lipase. Absorption of fatty acids and monoglycerides is also reduced because of the relative inability of fats to penetrate the unstirred aqueous layer surrounding intestinal villi. Conjugated bile acid levels may be low because of decreased entry into the intestine, increased deconjugation, or poor mixing of chyme.

Intrahepatic cholestasis and obstructive disorders of the biliary tree are major causes of maldigestion. Inadequate mixing of chyme with bile in the upper intestine, as in certain patients with gastrojejunostomies, may also lead to maldigestion. Inadequate mixing also occurs in patients with diabetic enteropathy, scleroderma (progressive systemic sclerosis), intestinal pseudo-obstruction, and other disorders which interfere with intestinal motility. Most motility disorders are also associated with bacterial overgrowth in the intestinal contents, and since bacteria are capable of deconjugating bile acids, this condition reduces conjugated bile acid levels below critical micellarizing levels and results in steatorrhea. The fact that the malabsorption of diabetic enteropathy and of intestinal pseudo-obstruction usually do not respond well to antibiotics, however, suggests that intestinal motility itself is important to the digestive process.

Bacterial overgrowth appears also in patients with partially obstructed blind loops of the intestine and occurs occasionally in the afferent loop following gastroenterostomies, and in patients with multiple jejunal diverticulosis. Bacterial overgrowth leads to malabsorption through at least two different mechanisms, the deconjugation of intraluminal bile salts and damage to intestinal mucosa, causing villous atrophy. Patchy villous atrophy and invasion of the lamina propria by mononuclear cells has been found in patients with obstructed blind loops. It has been found also that certain coliform organisms produce enterotoxins which are capable of causing this damage, and it has been suggested that these bacterial products might be the cause of the diffuse mucosal lesion seen in patients with tropical sprue (Klipstein and Schenk 1975). The malabsorption and the mucosal lesion of tropical sprue respond very well to the administration of broad-spectrum antibiotics and often to poorly absorbed sulfonamides.

We have previously noted that patients with IgA deficiency commonly develop bacterial overgrowth in the small intestine. This condition too is often associated with malabsorption, diarrhea, and villous atrophy on small intestinal biopsy, similar to the picture seen in tropical sprue. The response to antibiotics is frequently very gratifying.

Low Intraduodenal pH

Perhaps the most classical example of this form of malabsorption occurs in patients with gastrin-secreting delta cell adenomas of the pancreas (Zollinger-Ellison syndrome). Extremely large volumes of acid gastric secretion continually pour into the duodenum and overwhelm the effect that pancreatic and biliary bicarbonate usually have in raising intraduodenal and jejunal pH. Pancreatic enzymes are produced normally in these patients, but are inactivated in the acidic duodenal environment. This state of affairs results in a malabsorptive picture similar to that seen in patients with pancreatic insufficiency. Watery diarrhea in these patients is probably caused by hydroxylation of unabsorbed unsaturated fatty acids due to bacterial action in the lower small bowel and colon. These hydroxy fatty acids have been shown to damage the colonic mucosa, much as castor oil does, and to provoke marked increases in watery secretion. Oleic acid (C_{18}) is an example of a dietary monounsaturated fatty acid that is common in the diet and which, if not absorbed in the small intestine, becomes saturated by hydroxylation and leads to this sort of watery diarrhea (Phillips 1975). The diarrhea of gastrinomas frequently responds very well to the administration of cimetidine, occasionally in twice the usual dosage, and occasionally supplemented with anticholinergics.

Primary and Secondary Disaccharidase Deficiencies

Primary disaccharidase deficiencies are congenital disorders, and usually consist of the lack of a single brush border enzyme. While histological changes are not present, the absence of enzyme activity can be definitively diagnosed by measuring glucose production from an intestinal biopsy incubated with the suspect disaccharide. Patients complain of cramps, bloating, and often diarrhea whenever the offending disaccharide is ingested. Bloating and gas are produced by fermentation of the disaccharide in the lower bowel and colon as a result of bacterial action. Unabsorbed disaccharides increase the osmolarity of intestinal contents and lead to increased secretion of water by the intestinal mucosa, with resultant osomotic diarrhea. Lactase deficiency is the most common of these syndromes. Patients can digest all but milk sugar. Sucrase-isomaltase deficiency is less common. Each of these diseases is genetically determined.

Lactase deficiency is extremely common in black and Semitic peoples. Since deficiency does not usually appear until adulthood, most patients have had no trouble digesting milk in childhood. Their deficiency is merely an aggravation of a condition, decreased lactase production, common to all adults. Frequently mild lactase deficiency is subclinical until patients develop increased rapidity of gastric emptying, as is the case following subtotal gastric resection for peptic ulcer.

Sucrase-isomaltase deficiency is an uncommon recessive disorder that always appears to involve deficiency of both enzymes. Trehalase deficiency is extremely rare and involves difficulty in digesting trehalose, a carbohydrate found in mushrooms and other plants. Any disaccharidase or oligosaccharidase deficiency is treated most effectively by avoiding the incriminated carbohydrate. Lactose-poor diets are not difficult to follow, but the avoidance of sucrose and maltose can be very trying. Such patients can usually digest lactose well and can substitute pure glucose for sucrose.

Secondary disaccharidase deficiencies are usually multiple, and result from damage to brush borders secondary to other forms of absorptive disorder, especially sprue, lymphoma, bacterial overgrowth, and extensive Crohn disease. Treatment varies, depending on the cause of the underlying disorder.

CAUSES OF MALABSORPTION (TABLE 15-1)

Primary absorptive disorders are caused by destruction of small intestinal epithelium, delayed renewal of epithelium, and defective transport of absorbed nutrients in the epithelial cells or in mucosal lymphatics. The absorptive defect may encompass all nutrients, including electrolytes and water, or it may be monospecific, as in the case of pernicious anemia (malabsorption of vitamin B_{12}), Hartnup disease (inability to transport neutral amino acids), cystinuria (inability to transport dibasic amino acids), and chloridorrhea (inability to exchange Cl^- for HCO_3^-). When the absorptive disease also reduces brush border enzymes, it leads to secondary maldigestion of carbohydrates and proteins. And often, as we have seen in the case of bacterial overgrowth syndromes, malabsorption and mucosal damage result from or occur simultaneously with a disease which is also maldigestive. Thus, the distinction between malabsorption and maldigestion is somewhat artificial; it can, however, be useful to physicians in developing orderly thought processes for the diagnosis and treatment of individual patients with absorptive disorders.

Destruction of epithelial cells is classically associated with the lesion of celiac sprue. Villi become atrophic, microvilli disappear from individual cells, epithelial mitoses increase, and the lamina propria is infiltrated with lymphocytes and plasma cells. But this lesion is not distinctive, for it is also associated with acute gastroenteritis of viral or bacterial origin, various protein allergies, kwashiorkor, eosinophilic gastroenteritis, bacterial overgrowth syndromes, and tropical sprue. The same basic lesion also occurs in patients with immunodeficiency syndromes and with giardiasis (Hoskins et al 1967). The lesion of immunodeficiency, however, is distinguished by the absence of plasma cells (Trier 1977), and in giardiasis the invasive protozoan can frequently be seen. Because of their reduced immunity, giardiasis is a common problem among patients with hypogammaglobulinemia.

Delayed renewal of epithelial cells results most commonly from exposure to radiation and to drugs which interfere with the mitotic cycle. Radiation leads to decreased mitotic activity in mucosal crypts and reduction in the size of villi or even to their disappearance. Focal necrosis may also occur. Folic acid antagonists, such as methotrexate, also reduce mitotic

Table 15–1. Components of Digestion and Absorption, and Pathophysiology of Absorptive Disease

Region	*Digestive or Absorptive Function*	*Requirements for Function*	*Interrupted by*
Mouth and pharynx	chewing	proper dentition	dental defects, edentia
	polysaccharide hydrolysis	salivary glands	glandular atrophy (Sjogren syndrome)
	swallowing	neuromuscular integrity	disorders of the brainstem (bulbar poliomyelitis, basilar artery thrombosis), neuromuscular disorders (amyotrophic lateral sclerosis) myopathies
Esophagus	conveyance	neuromuscular integrity	achalsia, diffuse spasm, scleroderma, intestinal pseudo-obstruction
		patency	Zenker diverticulum, strictures, neoplasms
Stomach	early proteolysis	chief cells (pepsinogens), oxyntic cells	atrophic gastritis, gastric resection, vagotomy
	mixing and regulated emptying	neuromuscular integrity	vagotomy, diabetic enteropathy, scleroderma, amyloidosis, intestinal pseudo-obstruction
		patency	
Pancreas	digestion of fats, proteins, bicarbonate	acinar capacity	chronic pancreatitis, cystic fibrosis, cancer
		responsiveness to CCK and secretin	gastrojejunostomy, celiac sprue
			? celiac sprue
		duodenal pH above 6	hyperacidity, Zollinger-Ellison syndrome
		brush border enterokinase	absent in patients with enterokinase deficiency, reduced in patients with mucosal atrophy
	alkaline pH	capacity to secrete bicarbonate	chronic pancreatitis, carcinoma, cystic fibrosis
	conveyance of enzymes to duodenum	patency of ductal system	pseudocysts, carcinoma
		access of secretions to chyme	hypomotility, obstructed afferent loop, gastrojejunostomy

Table 15–1. Components of Digestion and Absorption, and Pathophysiology of Absorptive Disease (continued)

Region	*Digestive or Absorptive Function*	*Requirements for Function*	*Interrupted by*
Liver and biliary tract	disperse fat in micellar solutions	synthesis of bile salts, adequate bile pool	advanced hepatocellular disease illeal resection; ingestion of chelating agents
	conveyance of bile	patent biliary tree	cholestasis, neoplasms, biliary fistulas
	storage and release of bile	responsive gall bladder	vagotomy, celiac sprue, excessive VIP, ? obstruction of cystic duct
Duodenum and jejunum	disaccharide hydrolysis	normal brush border enzymes	primary disaccharidase deficiency (lactase, sucrase-isomaltase); deficiency secondary to celiac sprue, bacterial overgrowth, enterotoxins (tropical sprue).
	peptide hydrolysis	normal brush border enzymes	celiac sprue, tropical sprue, overgrowth, etc.
	monosaccharide absorption	normal brush border enzymes	glucose-galactose malabsorption
		adequate absorbing surface	sprue syndromes, giardiasis, etc.; short small intestine
	amino acid and peptide absorption	adequate absorbing surface	Hartnup disease, cystinuria; sprue syndromes
	fatty acid and monoglyceride absorption	conjugated bile acids and sterility of intestinal contents	hepatic disease, biliary obstruction, decreased bile acid pool; bacterial overgrowth, hypomotility (anaerobes deconjugate and dehydroxylate bile acids)
		adequate absorbing surface	sprues, Whipple disease, short small bowel, etc.
	ability to form chylomicrons	epithelial betalipoproteins	abetalipoproteinemia

Table 15-1. Components of Digestion and Absorption, and Pathophysiology of Absorptive Disease (continued)

Region	*Digestive or Absorptive Function*	*Requirements for Function*	*Interrupted by*
	lymphatic transport	intestinal lymphatics	lymphangiectasia, Whipple disease, lymphosarcoma, ? congestive heart failure
	mixing of chyme	neuromuscular integrity	scleroderma, diabetic enteropathy, intestinal pseudo-obstruction
	absorption of iron	HCl; intact epithelium	epithelial destruction; gastric achlorhydria
Lower ileum	absorption of vitamin B_{12}	gastric intrinsic factor	pernicious anemia; advanced atrophic gastritis
		salivary factor	?
		splitting of r factor-B_{12} complex	? pancreatic insufficiency
		intestinal sterility	bacterial overgrowth consumes luminal B_{12}
		normal ileum	ileal resection or bypass; ? Crohn disease
	absorption of vitamin C	intestinal sterility	bacterial overgrowth
		normal ileum	see above
	absorption of bile salts	normal ileum	see above
Colon	Cl^- exchange for HCO_3^-	?	chloridorrhea
	absorption Na^+ and water	isosmolar chyme	disaccharidase deficiency, lactulose, Mg^{++}
		absence of dihydroxy fatty and bile acids	ileal disease or resection; steatorrhea
		normal bacterial ecology	certain antibiotics lead to overgrowth of *Clostridium difficile*, causing pseudomembranous colitis.
		normal mucosa	ulcerative and invasive colitides; radiation
		patency	carcinomas, strictures, diverticulitis
		? short chain fatty acids	

activity and lead to steatorrhea. Neomycin administration is occasionally associated with decreased mitoses, villous edema, increased macrophages in the lamina propria, and reduced content of plasma cells. Chronic ischemia may also lead to malabsorption by causing spotty necrosis of crypts and shortening of villi.

Defective transport in epithelial cells has already been discussed in connection with abetalipoproteinemia, in which cellular ability to form chylomicrons is defective. Fat accumulates in epithelial cytoplasm, but mucosal architecture is otherwise unaffected.

Defective transport in mucosal lymphatics is the characteristic lesion of lymphangiectasia, which was described in Chapter 14, and in *Whipple disease.* This curious disorder is the result of infection with an as yet unclassified microorganism. The intestinal mucosal biopsy is diagnostic in showing that the lamina propria is filled with large macrophages containing Schiff stain positive material in their cytoplasm. Lymphatic obstruction apparently results from these accumulations, and the absorption of fat is markedly retarded. Although villi are enlarged by the lymphatic obstruction, the epithelium is commonly normal. The affecting microorganisms can be seen in the lamina propria on electron microscopy. Whipple disease occurs primarily in middle-aged white men and is associated with generalized lymphadenopathy, polyarthritis, and marked wasting.The condition usually responds well to long-term administration of antibiotics (Bayless 1970).

Celiac Sprue

This fascinating and fairly common disorder has been variously known during the last 50 years as Gee-Heubner-Herter disease, celiac disease, idiopathic steatorrhea, nontropical sprue, and gluten-sensitive enteropathy. Its present name was advocated by Rubin et al (1970) to indicate the identity of the celiac disease of children with the nontropical sprue of adults. Celiac sprue is a type of panmalabsorption associated with (1) diffuse villous atrophy, particularly in the upper small intestine, and (2) complete remission in response to the removal of all dietary sources of wheat protein (gluten). There is not only a clear familial predisposition to the disease (MacDonald et al 1965), but there is evidence that susceptibility is genetically determined (Trier et al 1978). The term *sprue* itself is of obscure Dutch or Flemish origin, and means "to sprinkle."

The microscopic lesion is characterized on jejunal biopsy by atrophy of intestinal villi, distortion of columnar epithelium into a more cuboidal shape with loss of microvilli and brush border, loss of nuclear polarity, and infiltration of round cells and plasmocytes into the lamina propria. Villous atrophy is often detectable by examination of a biopsy with a hand lens and is clearly demonstrated on light microscopy (Figure 15-1). The decrease of surface area resulting from atrophy of both macrovilli and microvilli (Figure

15–2), and the loss of brush border enzymes leads to extensive malabsorption. Since the process is most severe in the upper small bowel and does not usually involve the ileum, the absorption of bile acids, vitamin B_{12}, and ascorbic acid is normal.

Celiac sprue results from mucosal sensitivity to wheat, rye, oat, or barley glutens, which reside in the alcohol-soluble protein fractions of these grains. This discovery was made in the Netherlands in 1950 by W.K. Dicke, who reported his findings in a doctoral thesis submitted to the University of Utrecht. He noted that patients with celiac disease, who had improved spontaneously during the years of the German occupation of the Lowlands in World War II, tended to relapse unexpectedly following the Allied victory. Feeling that diet must be the key to this puzzle, he deduced that the major change with the coming of peace, other than for total calories, was the return of wheat flour, a commodity that had been unavailable during the last years of the Occupation. He observed that his patients again went into remission when they returned to a diet free of wheat, and that the remission persisted even though they consumed wheat starch (Dicke et al 1953). These observations were confirmed by other groups (Anderson et al 1952), and it is now universally agreed that peptides derived from wheat are responsible for the lesion of celiac sprue.

It has been shown that intestinal mucosal cells from patients with active celiac sprue will develop microvilli and brush border enzymes when cultured in a medium free of gluten (Falchuk et al 1974). However, the addition of gluten to cultures of apparently normal epithelial cells from patients in remission from celiac sprue does not adversely affect these cells. This suggests that the toxicity of gluten is mediated by an endogenous cofactor which must be contained in cells populating the lamina propria. A current theory (Trier et al 1978) holds that this cofactor is generated by interepithelial and lamina proprial lymphocytes in response to binding of gluten to genetically determined receptors on epithelial membranes. Gluten becomes immunogenic, and specific antibodies, sensitized lymphocytes, and destructive lymphokines are generated that destroy epithelial cells and produce an inflammatory reaction. The fact that at least three genetic markers have been identified in many patients with celiac sprue, HLA-B8 (88 percent), HLA-DW3 (88 percent), and a separate gene on B-lymphocytes (90 percent), makes this autoimmune hypothesis an attractive one. Since 20 percent of normal people also have HLA-B8 histocompatibility antigens, it is apparent that no single gene controls the sensitivity to celiac sprue. Pena et al (1978) suggest that the sensitivity to celiac sprue is controlled by two nonlinked genetic loci, homozygosity for the B-cell gene, and either antigen DW3 or an antigen usually associated with it. It is supposed that these genes code for surface proteins which form receptors for gliadin and thus initiate the process.

Dermatitis herpetiformis, an autoimmune cutaneous disorder producing multiform grouped papular, vesicular, and bullous lesions on many parts

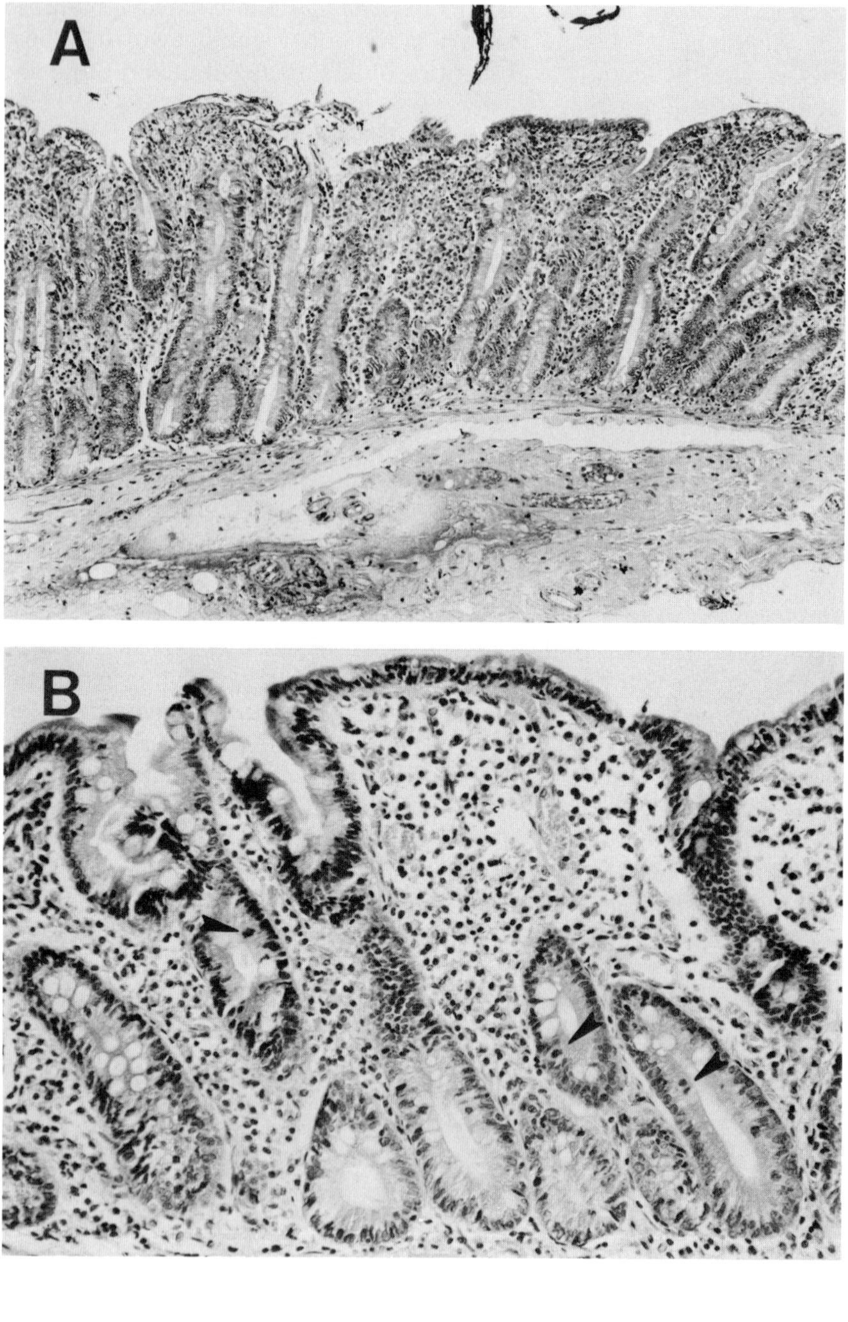
A
B

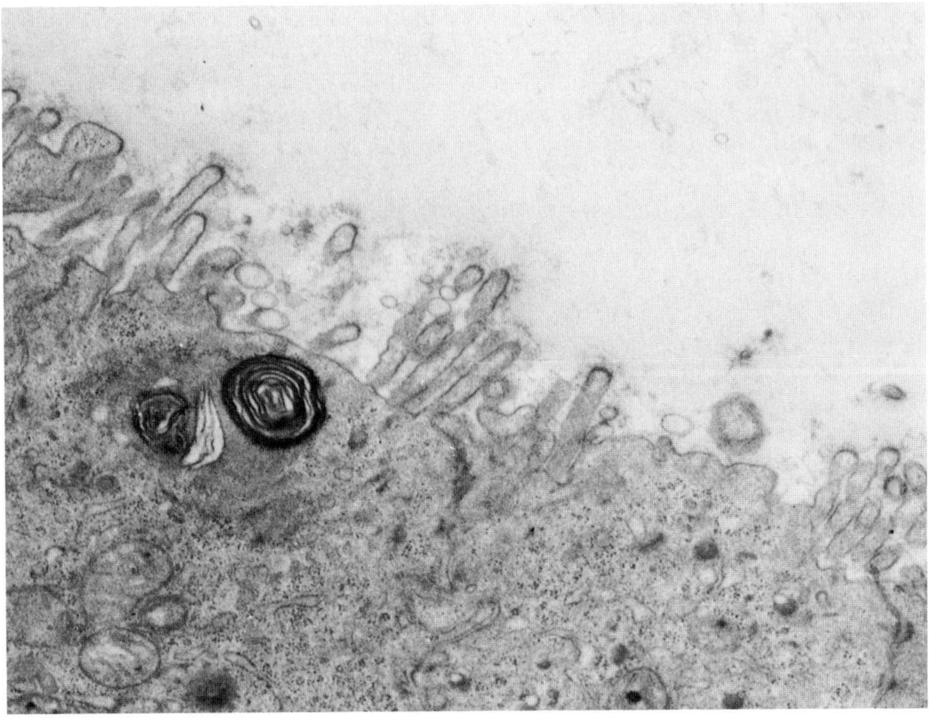

Figure 15-2. Electron photomicrograph of jejunal microvillous border in a patient with untreated celiac sprue. Note the marked destruction of the microvillous border and the disappearance of enzymic particles from microvillar tips. Compare with normal cell border, Figure 14-2. Original magnification x17,000. Courtesy of Dr. William Morningstar.

Figure 15-1. Jejunal biopsy from a patient with untreated celiac sprue. *A*, the loss of villi is almost total, and those that remain are very short and blunt. Surface epithelium is less columnar, and lamina propria is also more cellular than normal; compare with Figure 14-1, normal mucosa. Original magnification x100. *B*, Higher power view of same specimen showing thin mucosa, loss of epithelial brush border, and loss of basal nuclear polarity in epithelial cells. Lining cells show active regeneration manifested by abundant mitotic figures (arrowheads). The lamina propria is edematous, hyperemic, and infiltrated by plasma cells and lymphocytes. Original magnification x 200.

of the body, has been associated with the duodenojejunal lesion of celiac sprue in about two-thirds of cases (Roberts-Thomson et al 1977). Around 64 percent of patients with dermatitis herpetiformis are also of HLA type B8. However, there is an equal frequency of the celiac sprue lesion in dermatitis patients with and without type B8, and there are certainly many patients with celiac sprue who do not develop dermatitis. These findings indicate that while the susceptibilities to celiac sprue and to dermatitis herpetiformis have some features in common, they also have certain genetic features that are not always, but may at times be, shared. The skin lesion of dermatitis herpetiformis responds well to the administration of sulfones, but a gluten-free diet is usually necessary to control the alimentary lesion. There is some evidence to suggest that the skin lesion may be responsive to gluten withdrawal in patients who also have celiac sprue.

The physiologic effects of celiac sprue are widespread. Not only are the hydrolysis and absorption of oligosaccharides and oligopeptides reduced, but there is evidence that the release of enterokinase is also impaired and leads to reduced activation of trypsinogen with, as a result, reduced activation of other pancreatic proteases. Furthermore, celiac sprue apparently leads to decreased responsiveness of the gall bladder to cholecystokinin, (CCK), resulting in reduced luminal concentrations of bile salts after meals. There may be reduced responsiveness of the pancreas to secretin as well. Water-soluble vitamins and iron are also malabsorbed. Finally, it appears that the diseased intestinal mucosa of sprue patients leads to active secretion of water, sodium, and potassium, causing losses of these substances and reduced absorption of glucose and vitamins, which are dependent on active absorptive fluxes of sodium.

Refractory Sprues

This is the generic term applied to those diseases which resemble celiac sprue in all other ways, including the jejunal biopsy, but are not responsive to the removal of dietary gluten. In most instances, refractoriness is due to failure of adherence to an adequate dietary regimen by patients with true celiac sprue, and is thus more apparent than real. Therefore, all patients with suspected, yet unresponsive, celiac sprue should be hospitalized and placed on a carefully monitored gluten-free diet before searching for other diagnoses.

Intestinal Lymphomas. These may present with malabsorption and villous atrophy. Their symptoms do not respond to gluten withdrawal, and as a group, patients appear to experience more abdominal pain and fever. Rebiopsy and gastrointestinal X rays may demonstrate infiltrative lesions. Splenomegaly and lymphadenopathy support the diagnosis of lymphoma. Isaacson and Wright (1978) have described this spruelike picture in patients with malignant histiocytosis of the intestine.

True Refractory Sprue. This is clinically identical to responsive sprue and may have presented originally as the responsive disease. Continuation of a gluten-free diet does not seem to help, though frequently patients benefit from the administration of glucocorticoids. The prognosis is poor, unless nutrition is supported by parenteral hyperalimentation. Many patients with responsive sprue that later exaggerates despite continuing dietary precautions are found to have developed lymphomas or other malignancies. Cooper et al (1980) describe 55 such patients, 23 of whom developed histiocytic lymphomas, 4 Hodgkin disease, and 28 various cancers, particularly of the digestive tract.

Collagenous Sprue. This is typified by failure of response to gluten withdrawal and, in time, by the laying down of collagen in the lamina propria. It is fortunately an extremely rare condition and can be treated only by parenteral hyperalimentation.

Tropical Sprue

Attention has already been drawn to the fact that this disorder usually responds well to the administration of broad-spectrum antibiotics. It also regresses when folic acid is administered, but the response to antibiotics is usually better and more permanent. Intestinal flora are markedly increased in patients with tropical sprue, but no single causative agent has been identified. The place of malnutrition in its etiology is not certain, but it is clearly not the result of folic acid exclusion alone, else it would be common among North American alcoholics, which is decidedly not the case.

The disease differs clinically from celiac sprue in that patients with tropical sprue show more glossitis and more evidence of megaloblastosis. They also show some evidence of increased intestinal permeability, by virtue of the fact that they tend to absorb a considerable proportion of sucrose in the unhydrolyzed state. The mucosal atrophy appears to be somewhat more spotty than in celiac sprue, and most significantly the occurrence of tropical sprue is confined to certain geographic areas, notably India, the Far East, and the Carribean. But even within geographic areas, the incidence of tropical sprue is variable from place to place. Stefanini (1948) performed a singular study on tropical sprue, observing nearly 1,100 cases among 12,500 Italian prisoners of war confined to a single camp in the Himalayan foothills during a period of three years. The disease was seasonal and, most notably, did not occur among prisoners at other camps, living in similar quarters and eating a similar diet. In 1944, the incidence rate reached nearly 60 cases per 1,000 prisoners. An infectious agent is certainly the most likely cause.

APPRAISAL OF PATIENTS WITH ABSORPTIVE DISORDERS

History and Examination

There is a certain deductive logic which can be applied to the evaluation of a patient with an absorptive disorder. The history of loss of weight that is out of proportion to the intake of food is the foremost consideration, even though it may not be the patient's primary complaint. At times, patients may be more impressed with a change in stool quality from normal to a bulky, pale yellow, and foul-smelling character. Flatulence and abdominal bloating, largely from the fermentation of unabsorbed sugars in the colon, may be prominent. Watery diarrhea may appear as a result of the effect of dihydroxy bile acids or fatty acids on the colonic mucosa.

The effects of specific deficiencies may also be present. Deficiency of vitamin K may lead to an increased tendency to bruise and bleed, while decreased protein absorption, together with loss of plasma proteins into the gut lumen, may result in hypoalbuminemia and edema. Failure to absorb vitamin D and the increased concentration of labile fatty acids in the intestinal lumen may lead, in the first instance, to decreased absorption of calcium, and in the second to increased formation of nonabsorbable calcium soaps in the intestine. The net result of these processes is hypocalcemia, which may result in tetany if albumin losses have not been parallel to calcium losses and the plasma content of ionized calcium falls. Bone pain and spontaneous fractures may appear as a result of osteomalacia secondary to hypocalcemia and hypoproteinemia, and secondary hyperparathyroidism consequent to calcium malabsorption. Deficiencies of water-soluble vitamins are suggested by the presence of glossitis (folate, niacin, or thiamin deficiencies), or pains and paresthesias in the extremities (thiamin deficiency). Signs of deficiencies of vitamins C and B_{12} are uncommon in patients with celiac sprue, probably because these vitamins are absorbed in the lower ileum, which is usually unaffected by the sprue lesion. More localized symptoms, such as obstructive jaundice, attacks of upper abdominal pain, or recent-onset diabetes bring obstructive disorders of the biliary tract or diseases of the pancreas into consideration.

Certain historical data help in the evaluation of absorptive disorders. In patients whose presumptive tests indicate maldigestion, a history of attacks of recurrent abdominal pain since childhood and a family history of similar problems suggest familial pancreatitis. A history of alcoholism and abdominal pain indicate chronic calcific pancreatitis, while the sudden onset of maldigestion in midlife suggest cancer of the pancreas, especially if steady abdominal or back pain or diabetes of recent onset are present. Maldigestion in a child or youth with chronic respiratory infections suggests cystic fibrosis.

In patients with suspected malabsorption, a recent camping trip or visit to an endemic area suggests giardiasis, while a sojourn in the tropics leads one to suspect the existence of tropical sprue. Bacterial overgrowth should be suspected in patients with malabsorption and a history of previous gastric surgery, while radiation enteritis should be surmised in a patient previously exposed to X ray therapy. Onset of malabsorption in a middle-aged man with a previous history of arthritis or spondylitis suggests the possibility of Whipple disease, while a preceding history of Raynaud phenomenon or dysphagia is indicative of scleroderma.

But whatever impressions are gained from history taking must be confirmed by the use of various diagnostic studies. A progressive sequence of diagnostic testing in patients with suspected malabsorption is given in Figure 15-3.

Serum Carotenoids

Vegetable carotenoids and retinol synthesized from beta-carotene in the intestinal mucosa are fat soluble and poorly absorbed from the intestine in patients with fat malabsorption. Since carotenoids are easily measured in the blood, and since levels remain detectable for some hours after ingestion, their determination is a very simple and useful screening test in patients with suspected fat malabsorption. Provided that one can be certain that the patient has been consuming a diet containing moderate amounts of vegetables or liver, a fasting serum carotenoid level below 80 μg per dl is strongly suggestive of fat malabsorption. Where some doubt exists about the dietary intake of carotenoids, one may measure the serum levels before and two or three hours after the ingestion of vitamin A (50,000 units)—the vitamin A tolerance test. Failure of serum levels to rise more than 20 μg over fasting is suggestive of fat malabsorption. However, since results are not highly specific, they should always be checked by determining stool fat levels.

Examination of the Stools for Fat

Since steatorrhea is the common denominator for all types of panabsorptive disorders, the first, most simple, and most important test to be performed is the microscopic examination of a stool specimen with Sudan III, both before and after treatment of the specimen with heat and 36 percent acetic acid. Sudan III stains neutral fat droplets and melted fatty acid crystals reddish pink, and the acetic acid converts unstainable calcium and potassium soaps to stainable free fatty acids. If the stool contains a large number of Sudan-III-staining droplets prior to its exposure to acetic acid and heat, the increased amount of triglyceride in the stool suggests that the causative disorder is primarily maldigestive rather than malabsorptive, since dietary neutral fats are apparently not being hydrolyzed. Such stools

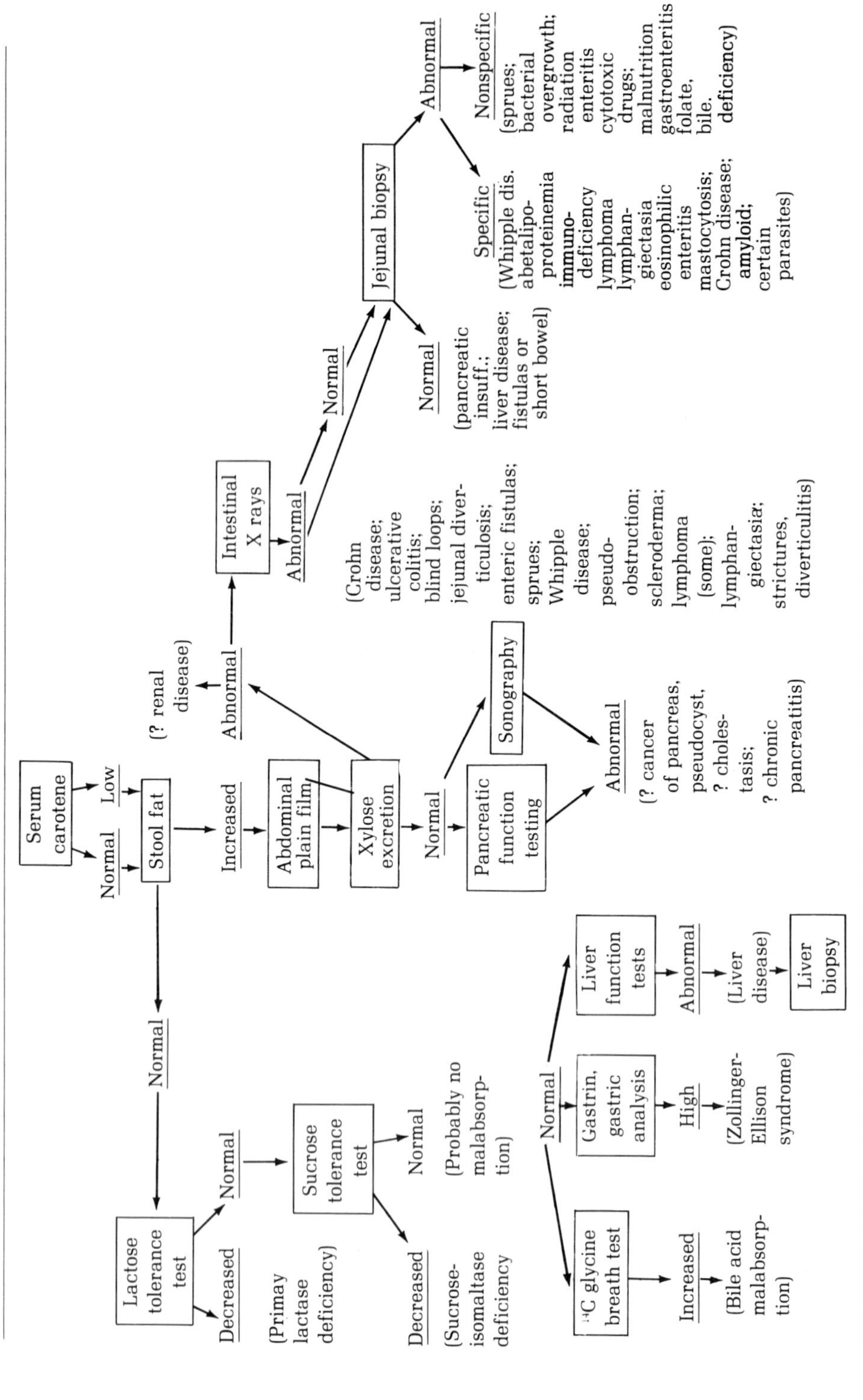

Figure 15–3. Pathways of diagnostic testing in patients with chronic diarrhea and suspected malabsorption

would appear in patients with pancreatic insufficiency (chronic pancreatitis, cancer of the pancreas, cystic fibrosis) or decreased micellarization of fat resulting from inadequate enteric bile acids, or from increased deconjugation of bile acids in the intestine. An increased number of striated and often nucleated meat fibers may also be seen, particularly in patients with pancreatic insufficiency. A preponderance of Sudan-positive droplets only after the application of acetic acid and heat suggests that digestion is apparently normal but absorption is deficient.

Despite being disarmingly simple and inexpensive, the Sudan III test is a remarkably exact method for determining the presence of steatorrhea and for indicating the cause. Luk (1979) reports comparing the results of this simple procedure with the results of quantitative stool fat examinations in 320 patients, 192 of whom did not prove to have steatorrhea. Thirty-five of the 128 patients, with steatorrhea had pancreatic insufficiency; the remainder, other types of malabsorption. All of the patients with pancreatic insufficiency showed neutral stool fat on Sudan testing, and all of the patients with other forms of malabsorption showed split fats (after acetic acid and heat). There were no false negative tests (sensitivity 100 percent). Seven patients with nonpancreatitic steatorrhea showed neutral fat in their stools, as did 2 of the controls (specificity 94 percent). Only 8 of the controls showed increased split fats (specificity 96 percent). When performing the Sudan test it is important to remember that barium combines with stool fat and makes it unstainable, thus leading to false negative results, while the administration of mineral oil or the use of glove lubricants for obtaining rectal stool samples will cause falsely positive results.

The Sudan test is almost invariably adequate for the diagnosis of steatorrhea, especially if it is repeated on two or three specimens of stool. Quantitative determinations are complicated by the necessity of collecting stools for 72 to 96 hours before analyzing them. Such a measurement is rarely necessary in clinical practice, being more useful as a research tool, when balance studies are being performed, or if data regarding the precise degree of response to a new therapeutic regimen are required. A normal subject ingesting 70 to 100 g of fat daily should excrete no more than 6 to 7 g, or a total that is no greater than 10 percent of the amount ingested. In health, essentially all dietary fat is absorbed, regardless of the amount ingested. The fat which appears in the stool of healthy subjects is largely of bacterial origin.

As can be seen from Figure 15–3, the finding of normal amounts of stool fat in patients with chronic diarrhea does not exclude primary disaccharidase deficiency. Where these disorders are suspected, lactose and sucrose tolerance tests may be indicated.

Plain Abdominal Films

An X ray of the abdomen often detects calcifications of the pancreas and may also reveal localized areas of ileus in patients with different types of fat malabsorption, especially those with intestinal pseudo-obstruction and Crohn disease. At times the air mucosal interface in bowel loops reveals distinct mucosal abnormalities. While rarely diagnostic, plain abdominal films may, if abnormal, provide distinctive evidence of intestinal or colonic disease.

The Xylose Tolerance Test

This test is widely used to distinguish between those cases of steatorrhea that are due to maldigestion and those that are purely the result of intestinal epithelial dysfunction. Xylose is a pentose sugar that is fairly well absorbed and unchanged by enterocytes and is quickly excreted into the urine because it is not metabolized in the liver. Thus, the appearance of normal amounts of xylose in the urine after oral ingestion suggests that epithelial absorptive function is also normal.

The appearance of xylose in the urine depends also on normal renal function. A healthy subject will excrete 20 percent or more of an oral dose (either 5 or 25 g) into the urine within five hours after ingestion, provided that adequate amounts of water (about 500 ml) have also been consumed. In a patient with steatorrhea who excretes normal amounts of xylose, it can be reasonably concluded that the fat malabsorption is the result of maldigestion rather than mucosal disease. Such results suggest pancreatic insufficiency, decreased levels of conjugated bile acids in the upper small intestine, or excessive HCl production in the stomach (Zollinger-Ellison syndrome). Further tests should be done to rule out these disorders, as indicated in Figure 15–3.

When xylose excretion is below normal levels, one may tentatively conclude that steatorrhea results, at least in part, from mucosal dysfunction. Prior to accepting the validity of this conclusion, however, clinicians must assure themselves that nonintestinal disorders, such as gastric retention, inadequate urine flow, and renal disease, are not interfering with the reliability of the test, and that no anatomical intestinal bypasses capable of carrying xylose around the upper small intestine exist. While patients with bacterial overgrowth syndromes (blind loops, jejunal diverticulosis, scleroderma) frequently develop patchy atrophy of the small intestinal mucosa, their reduced excretion of xylose is most likely to be the result of bacterial metabolism of the pentose. Elderly persons and patients with hypothyroidism or cirrhosis of the liver and ascites may also show reduced excretion of xylose in the absence of significant small intestinal mucosal disease. In patients with renal insufficiency, the determination of serum levels of xylose has been found to be an acceptable alternate measure of intestinal absorption. A concentration of 8 to 28 mg per dl is normally reached within an hour after the oral ingestion of a 5-g dose.

Lactose and Sucrose Tolerance Tests

These tests are very helpful in the diagnosis of specific primary disaccharidase deficiencies. The lactose tolerance test is usually performed first, because lactase deficiency is much more common than isomaltase-sucrase deficiency. In searching for patients with primary disaccharidase deficiencies, a normal xylose test result should be obtained prior to performing the lactose test, since patients with xylose malabsorption will not be able to absorb glucose derived from lactose and may, in addition, have a disaccharidase deficiency secondary to the primary epithelial disorder.

Both tests depend on the presence of brush border disaccharidases capable of hydrolyzing disaccharides to monosaccharides, and upon normal epithelial cells capable of absorbing glucose. Two hours after the ingestion of 100 g of either lactose or sucrose, serum glucose levels normally rise 25 percent or more over fasting. The failure of glucose levels to increase to that extent suggests a specific disaccharidase deficiency. One may test the validity of this impression by placing the patient on a diet excluding the suspect disaccharide or, if the test is available, by direct measurement of the disaccharidase activity from a jejunal biopsy obtained by peroral suction.

Qualitative information may also be obtained during disaccharide tolerance testing by recording the patient's symptomatic reactions to the test sugar. Commonly, disaccharidase-deficient patients will experience abdominal cramps, intestinal hurry, bloating, and occasionally, diarrhea within an hour or so after the ingestion of the specific sugar. To make this phase of the test more valid, it is important that the patient not be informed of the exact nature of the test substance.

Radioactive Breath Testing

^{14}Carbon labeling has been useful in measuring certain aspects of malabsorption and may prove to be the avenue for simplifying testing procedures. The end point of these tests is the measurement of radioactivity of expired air following the administration of a labeled test substance. ^{14}C-glycine conjugates with bile acids, and is excreted into the intestine, reabsorbed and becomes a member of the bile acid pool. Early appearance of the label in breath carbon dioxide after ingestion indicates rapid intestinal deconjugation of bile acids and suggests either small intestinal bacterial overgrowth or ileal dysfunction. In the latter situation, conjugated bile salts are not reabsorbed at normal rates, flow into the colon, and are deconjugated by normal colonic flora.

When ^{14}C is used as a label on triolein, one normally notes a prompt rise in breath $^{14}CO_2$, indicating that hydrolysis of the triglyceride has occurred and the resulting fatty acids and monoglycerides have been absorbed.

Failure of this elevation to occur suggests malabsorption of fat. Patients with mucosal disease and with deficient micellar concentrations of intestinal bile salts also show delayed absorption of ^{14}C-labeled fatty acids, while patients with pancreatic insufficiency could be expected to show delayed production of $^{14}CO_2$ with the triglyceride (triolein) but not with the fatty acid. Because of the instability of ^{14}C and its long half-life, there has been reluctance to use this isotope widely, especially in children. But preliminary experience with ^{13}C-labeled triglycerides and fatty acids in children (Watkins et al 1980) has shown that breath testing is of considerable diagnostic use and is safe because of the stability of the isotope.

Folic Acid Determination

Macrocytic anemias are encountered with considerable frequency in patients with malabsorption states, and in many of these the serum folate levels are below the normal minimum of 3.0 ng per ml. Serum folic (pteroylglutamic) acid is derived from a variety of foods containing polyglutamates which must be hydrolyzed by brush border enzymes prior to absorption. Since folic acid is essential for the production of nucleic acids, its deficiency is fairly quickly reflected in tissues with short turnover times, such as the blood and intestinal mucosa. The characteristic hematological change is a maturation arrest, manifested by a megaloblastic marrow, macrocytic anemia, and granulocytopenia. Macrocytosis may also be seen in the intestinal epithelium.

Since folate hydrolysis and absorption occurs maximally in the jejunum, the process is most inhibited by diseases that lead to extensive reductions in jejunal mucosal brush border enzymes and surface area, such as the sprue syndromes, and is usually unaffected by diseases that lead to reductions of lower small intestinal surface area, such as Crohn disease and short small intestinal syndromes. Folic acid levels may be considerably elevated in malabsorptive states associated with bacterial overgrowth and normal jejunal function, such as blind loops and jejunal diverticulosis. In these conditions, excess folate is produced by bacterial flora, absorption of the vitamin is normal, and fat malabsorption results from bacterial deconjugation of luminal bile acids. Thus, determination of folic acid levels, whether low or elevated, give considerable pathophysiologic guidance in the diagnosis of patients with fat malabsorption.

Vitamin B_{12} Absorption

A number of patients with fat malabsorption show serum levels of vitamin B_{12} (cobalamin) below the normal minimum of 90 pg per ml. Since this vitamin is linked to the release of folic acid from folate pools, its deficiency also results in macrocytic anemia. However, the half-life of vitamin B_{12} is very long, averaging nearly four years, due in large part to the fact that it participates in the enterohepatic circulation. Thus, macrocytosis due to B_{12} deficiency takes a long while to develop, even though malabsorption is present. Because of this, it is well to perform isotope absorption tests of cobalamin in patients with suspected malabsorption, even if serum levels are within the normal range.

The absorption of vitamin B_{12} can be briefly summarized: (1) the average American diet provides about 5 to 15 μg per day; (2) it is promptly bound to salivary "r" protein in the mouth and esophagus; (3) unbinding takes place in the upper small intestine, possibly through the mediation of pancreatic proteases; (4) two molecules of B_{12} then complex with two molecules of the glycoprotein, intrinsic factor, and pass unabsorbed through the upper intestine; (5) unbinding of this complex takes place at specific ileal receptors, and free cobalamin is transferred to plasma transcobalamin II. A small amount of free B_{12} is absorbed by diffusion in the upper intestine but quantities are not large enough to fulfill normal requirements. Cobalamin is also produced by colonic bacteria, but this is not absorbable in the colon.

Keeping this fairly complex absorptive process in mind, physicians must decide in specific cases of B_{12} malabsorption exactly where the defect lies. Following administration of a flushing dose of parenteral B_{12} (100 to 1,000 μg), a tracer dose of ^{60}cobalt-vitamin B_{12} is given by mouth (Schilling test). Normal subjects excrete no less than 5 percent of a 2-μg dose of labeled B_{12} or 10 percent of a 0.5-μg dose in the urine during the ensuing 48 hours. If these limits are not reached, vitamin B_{12} malabsorption exists. If this malabsorption is corrected by a second tracer dose of ^{60}Co-B_{12}, plus active intrinsic factor, it may be concluded that the patient has true pernicious anemia. When malabsorption of the tracer is corrected by pretreatment of the patient with broad-spectrum antibiotics for several days, it can be assumed that the abnormality resulted from binding of B_{12} by intestinal bacteria, and that significant bacterial overgrowth exists. This degree of bacterial overgrowth is often seen in patients with partially obstructed blind loops, jejunal diverticulosis, and peristaltic disorders, such as intestinal pseudo-obstruction, scleroderma, and diabetic enteropathy.

If the addition of intrinsic factor and antibiotics does not correct malabsorption of ^{60}Co-B_{12}, one must think of dysfunction of the lower ileum as the culprit. This problem does arise in many patients with Crohn disease, those who have had previous ileal resections, and patients in whom the ileum has been previously bypassed for the control of obesity. The lesion of tropical sprue may also involve the lower ileum and interfere with B_{12} absorption, but the lesion of celiac sprue does not extend that far distally into the small intestine.

Other Plasma Abnormalities in Malabsorption

Prolongation of the one-stage prothrombin time and its correction by the parenteral administration of vitamin K in a patient not receiving oral antibiotics indicates that liver function is normal and that enteric vitamin K, being lipid soluble, is being lost in the stool, along with fat.

Hypophosphatemia and hypocalcemia may result from the loss of vitamin D, another fat-soluble dietary constituent. This disturbance may result in osteomalacia and spontaneous periosteal fractures in adults, and in rickets among children. Hypocalcemia may also result from the combination of luminal calcium with free fatty acids, and the formation of poorly absorbed calcium soaps. Such a situation, hypocalcemia without hypophosphatemia, suggests that steatorrhea is not a result of lipase deficiency, since calcium saponifies only with free fatty acids and not with the triglycerides.

Decreased serum levels of free calcium are often associated with clinical tetany, a common symptom of absorptive disorders. Since a large fraction of serum calcium is normally bound to serum albumin and is not available to modulate muscular contractility, tetany may be encountered at relatively higher total calcium levels when albumin content is normal, and at lower total calcium levels when albumin levels are also depressed. Thus, a patient with malabsorption is often protected from having tetany by the fact that a proportionate degree of hypoalbuminemia is also present.

Hypocalcemia often leads to hypertrophy and occasionally adenomas of the parathyroid glands, a condition known as secondary hyperparathyroidism. Such patients may mobilize large amounts of calcium from their bones, and thus have normal or even slightly elevated levels of serum calcium and low serum phosphorus levels. Osteomalacia and spontaneous fractures may also occur. Serum parathormone levels are elevated. If the malabsorption in these patients responds to therapy, parathyroid function usually returns to normal. However, in some instances parathyroid hyperfunction continues autonomously after the malabsorption is corrected (tertiary hyperparathyroidism), and surgical removal of parathyroid tissue is required to control it.

Hypoalbuminemia is a common consequence of malabsorption. In patients with small intestinal diseases, such as Crohn disease or the sprues, large amounts of albumin are lost through the inflamed intestinal mucosa (protein-losing enteropathy), and losses are beyond the hepatic capacity to synthesize protein. Malabsorption of dipeptides and amino acids also contributes to the hypoproteinemia. Patients with pancreatic insufficiency may also become hypoalbuminemic because of decreased luminal proteolysis. Dependent edema of the extremities is usually the earliest symptom of hypoalbuminemia.

Barium Contrast Radiologic Studies

Many absorptive disorders are associated with radiological abnormalities of the small intestine, particularly alterations of the normally delicate mucosal pattern of the jejunum (Figure 15–4). They may also cause changes in the motility of the intestine, leading to disruption of the normally

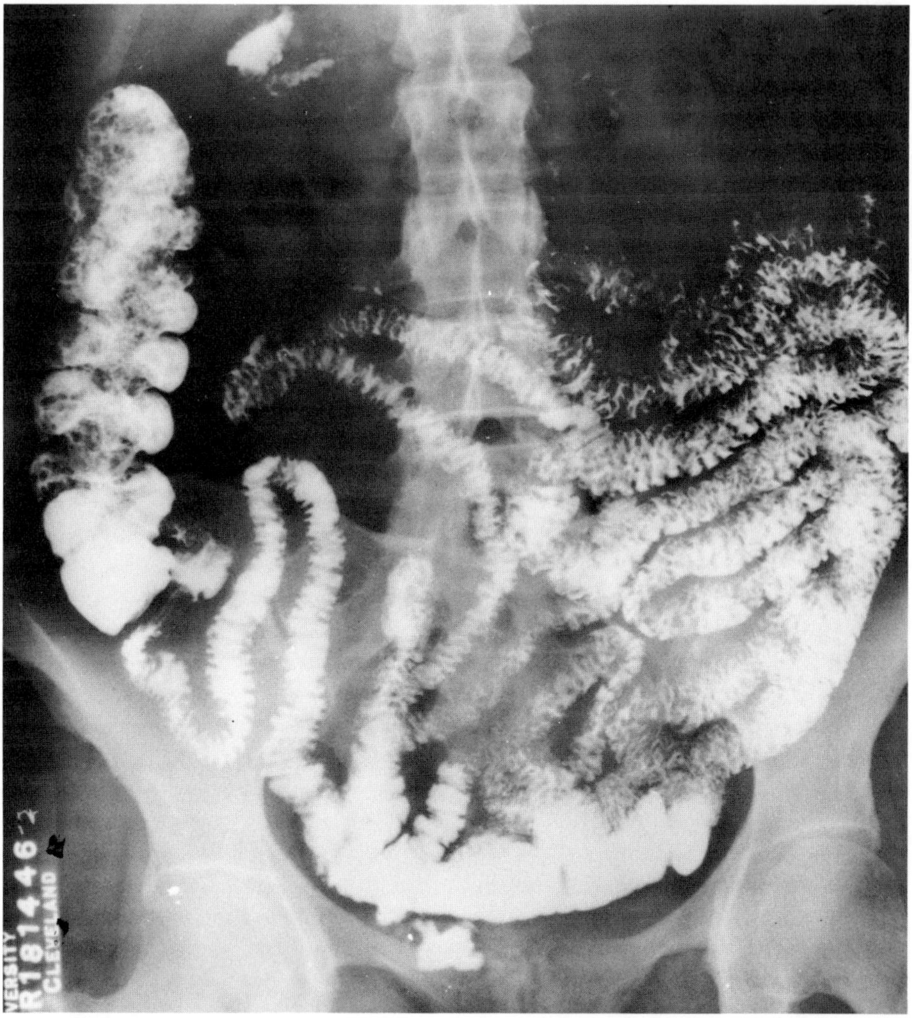

Figure 15-4. Normal radiographic appearance of jejunum, ileum, and ascending colon. The delicate tracery of mucosal folds is quite apparent throughout the small intestine. This pattern is clearly different from the haustral configuration of the right side of the colon. A small amount of barium remains in the stomach (upper center) overlying the vertebral column, and in the duodenal bulb (beneath the right 12th rib).

continuous barium column. The changes caused by various diseases are rarely specific, but may be highly suggestive to the trained observer. The Zollinger-Ellison syndrome, for example, is often accompanied by gastric rugal hypertrophy, edematous mucosal folds in the upper small intestine, and unusually located or multiple peptic ulcers. Patients with carcinomas of the pancreas or pancreatic pseudocysts may demonstrate rightward displacement of the descending limb of the duodenum, compression of the lumen of the second or third parts of the duodenum, or anterior displacement of the stomach. Crohn disease is typified by segments of narrowed small intestine with effaced valvulae conniventes (circular folds), often interspersed between normal-appearing bowel segments. A similar picture may be caused by intestinal lymphomas. Whipple disease and intestinal lymphagiectasia cause areas of mucosal edema (Figure 15–5). Blind loops and diverticula of the small intestine, the functional status of an existing gastroenterostomy, the existence of enteric fistulas, and the presence of radiation enteritis are all demonstrable by barium studies. Disordered motility, delayed transit, flocculation of barium, and disruption of the barium column are commonly found in the sprue syndromes, intestinal pseudo-obstruction, scleroderma, and diabetic enteropathy. (Figure 15–6).

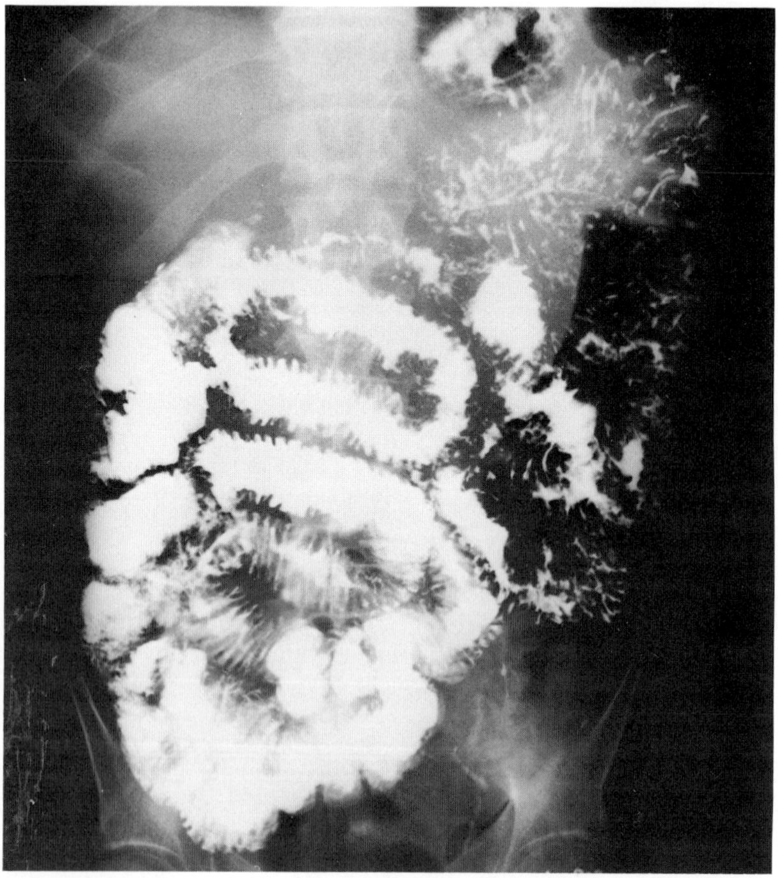

Figure 15–5. Small intestinal radiograph in a patient with Whipple disease. The mucosal folds are thickened by edema from lymphatic obstruction and by the mucosal infiltrate. Compare with normal pattern, Figure 15–4.

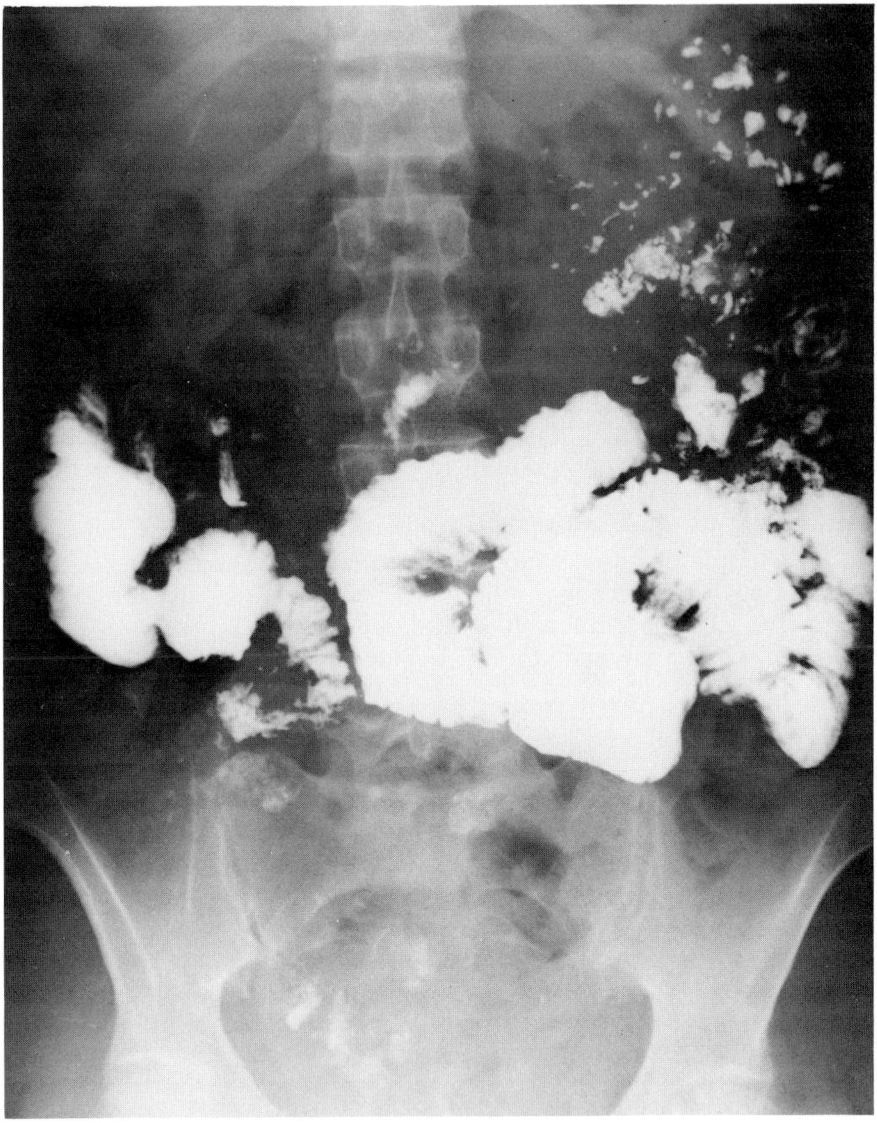

Figure 15–6. Lower small intestinal radiograph in a patient with celiac sprue. The intestinal loops appear to be dilated, and the fine mucosal pattern has become very coarse. The barium column is fragmented. This is a nonspecific pattern suggesting malabsorption.

Peroral Biopsy of Jejunal Mucosa

Any patient with steatorrhea associated with an abnormal xylose test should be subjected to a peroral small intestinal biopsy. A number of satisfactory instruments are available to perform this procedure, which can be done relatively easily and with minimal discomfort to the patient. The biopsy capsule is placed with fluoroscopic guidance, and a small piece of mucosa is sucked into a port in the capsule, and cut either by releasing a spring-cocked capsular knife or by traction on a pull-wire connected to a knife blade in the capsule. The biopsy, upon removal of the capsule, should be lain flat, mucosal side upward, on a small piece of filter paper and fixed immediately in Bouin solution. Regular and special stains can then be performed.

Small intestinal biopsies will be normal, abnormal specific, or abnormal nonspecific. The normal biopsy (Figure 14–2) shows multiple regular villi whose height is about four times the depth of villous crypts. Epithelial cells are columnar, nuclei are arranged in an orderly fashion at the base of the cell, and a definite brush border is visible at villous tips. The lamina propria contains a few mononuclear and plasma cells, as described in the previous chapter, and lymphatics are small and often not clearly visible. Jejunal biopsies are normal in pancreatic insufficiency and liver disease. Abnormal specific lesions are either diffuse or patchy. Whipple disease (Figure 15–7), abetalipoproteinemia, and immunodeficiency are the only abnormal diffuse mucosal diseases specifically recognizable on biopsy. Jejunal mucosa in Whipple disease is characterized by the presence in the lamina propria of huge macrophages, filled with Schiff positive glycoprotein. Lymphatics may also be dilated. In abetalipoproteinemia, one sees large fat droplets in the luminal end of epithelial columnar cells, especially in those close to villous tips. The biopsy of patients with immunodeficiency is typified by the absence of plasma cells from an otherwise normal, or somewhat atrophic musoca. Diagnostic, but spotty, lesions may be found in patients with specific infections, particularly giardiasis, lymphagiectasia, lymphomas, Crohn disease, and eosinophilic enteritis (Figure 15–3).

While striking, the atrophic changes of the jejunal mucosa in the sprue syndromes is not specific. Biopsies thus have to be interpreted in light of the patient's history, other findings, and response to therapy. Villous atrophy can often be detected by examination of the biopsy with a hand lens before fixation. Villi may be either very short, or completely absent, the crypt-to-villus height ratio often being below unity. On microscopy, epithelial cells often appear to be more cuboidal than columnar, brush borders are absent, and mitoses in villous crypts are increased (Figure 15–1). Electron microscopy also shows marked disruption of microvilli. What villi remain are blunted as well as shortened. The lamina propria, as previously described, shows an increased mononuclear population, both lymphocytes and plasma cells. This picture is seen in celiac sprue, unclassified sprue, bacterial over-

Figure 15–7. Whipple disease. *A*, there are many macrophages with foamy cytoplasm in the lamina propria of the jejunal mucosa. *B*, the use of periodic acid Schiff (PAS) stain and diastase shows that the cytoplasmic inclusions take up the stain and are resistant to the enzyme, and are thus not glycogen. This finding is diagnostic of Whipple disease. Villous crypt cells appear pale because they do not take up the stain. Original magnification x200.

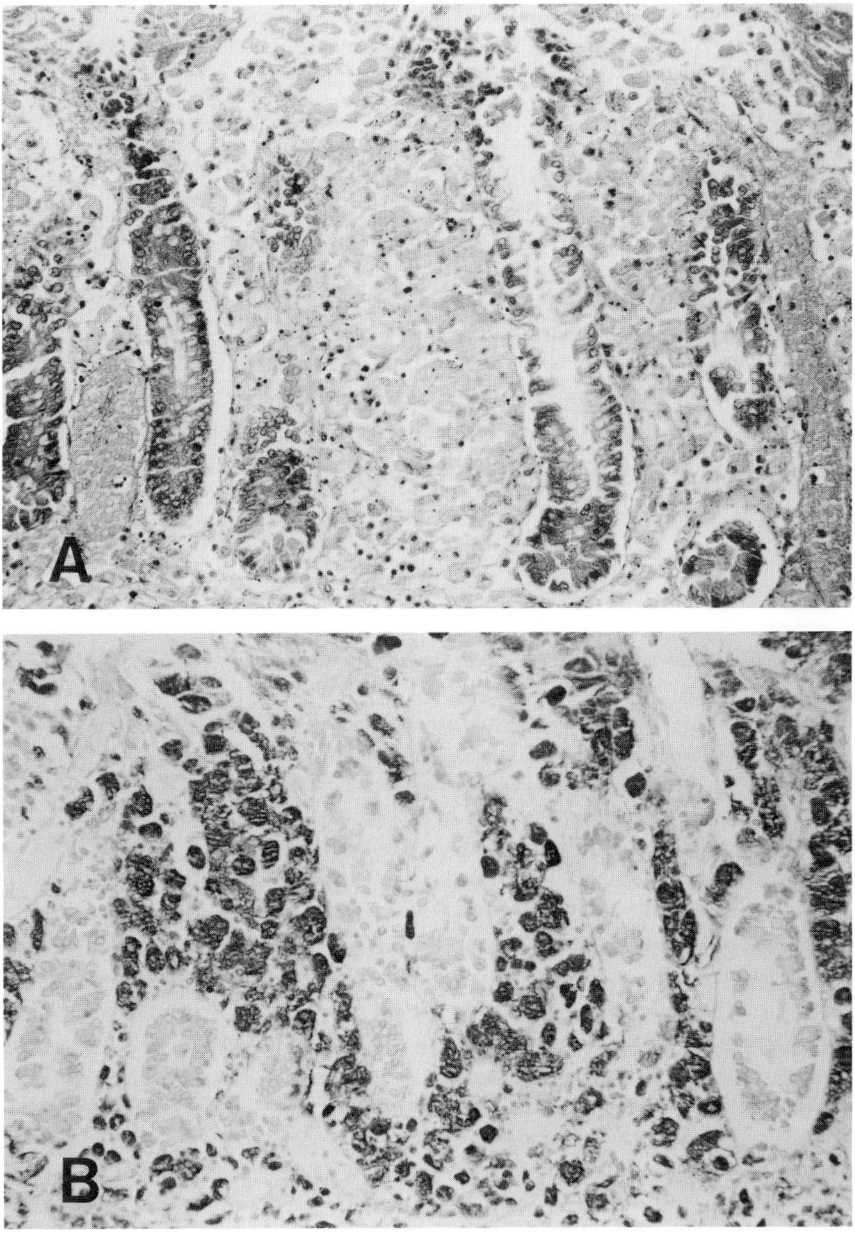
A
B

growth syndromes, bacterial dysentery, viral gastroenteritis, and tropical sprue. Although the lesion is usually most severe in the sprue syndromes, a specific diagnosis cannot be made from the biopsy alone.

THERAPY OF MALABSORPTION SYNDROMES

A variety of therapeutic agents and programs is available for the treatment of the causes and effects of malabsorption (Table 15–2). These can be classified as specific therapy, where the cause is known and can be effectively treated; exclusion therapy, where the mechanism of the illness is rather well recognized and can be controlled only by avoiding precipitating agents; ameliorative therapy, where either the cause of the disease is unknown or is not directly treatable; and replacement therapy, where malabsorption is the result of specific deficiencies which can be replaced, or produces certain deficiencies which can be corrected.

Specific Therapy

Specific therapy of malabsorption is related particularly to infections, such as giardiasis and Whipple disease, where chemotherapy can effectively obliterate the causative microorganism. Giardiasis is quite responsive to atabrine or metronidazole, and recurrences are few unless the patient has an underlying immunodeficiency state. In Whipple disease, while the causative microorganism has not been identified, the infection responds well to the long-term administration of antibiotics. Surgery is specific treatment in those patients with intestinal blind loops, strictures, and fistulas that are capable of being corrected, or in those few patients with gastrinomas (Zollinger-Ellison syndrome) which can be extirpated completely.

Exclusion Therapy

This is best illustrated by the extremely beneficial responses of patients with celiac sprue to gluten-free diets. Gluten sensitivity remains throughout life but, aside from an increased risk of lymphosarcoma and other malignant neoplasms, patients with celiac sprue can remain totally asymptomatic on a diet free of wheat, barley, and oat protein. Similarly, patients with primary disaccharidase deficiencies can remain well by avoiding lactose, sucrose, or maltose as the case may be, and patients with Hartnup disease and cystinuria respond well if neutral amino acids, in the former case, and dibasic amino acids, in the latter, are avoided. Certain patients with secondary deficiencies of disaccharides due, for example, to mucosal damage from radiation or Crohn disease, may respond partially to disaccharide exclusion.

Table 15–2. Representative Therapeutic Agents in a Variety of Absorptive Disorders

	Anti-biotics	*Ca/Mg*	*Chol-esty-ramine*	*Cimet-idine*	*Folic acid*	*Gluco-corti-coids*	*Gluten-free diet*	*Lactose-free diet*	*Medium-chain trigly-ceride*	*Meto-clopra-mide*	*Metro-nida-zole*	*Pan-creatic supp.*	*Paren-teral hyperali-mentation*	*Sur-gery*
Abetalipoproteinemia									X					
Blind loop syndrome	X													occ
Celiac sprue							X							
Crohn disease		occ	occ		occ	X		occ	occ				occ	occ
Eosinophilic gastroenteritis						X								occ
Giardiasis											X			
Ileal dysfunction		X	X											
Immunodeficiency states	X							occ	occ					
Intestinal pseudo-obstruction	X	occ								X			X	
Jejunal diverticulosis	X													
Lactase deficiency								X						
Lymphangiectasia									X					
Pancreatic insufficiency				X								X		
Radiation enteritis	occ	occ	occ		occ	occ							occ	occ
Scleroderma	X									X				
Short small bowel		X	occ										occ	
Tropical sprue	X				X									
Whipple disease	X													
Zollinger-Ellison syndrome				X										occ

occ = occasionally

Ameliorative Therapy

This consists of attempts to bypass the malabsorptive lesion, or to improve it with nonspecific management. Medium-chain triglycerides are often beneficial in patients with abetalipoproteinemia because they undergo epithelial transport without conversion to chylomicrons; they are also handled well by patients with lymphangiectasia, because they are transported into portal venous rather than lymphatic channels. Since medium-chain triglycerides do not require micellarization or hydrolysis for absorption, they may also be useful in the treatment of patients with reduced bile acid pools and with pancreatic exocrine deficiency.

Cholestyramine is often helpful in reducing the diarrhea of patients with ileal dysfunction. By chelating bile acids in the small intestine, this agent makes them less susceptible to bacterial deconjugation in the colon, and thus less likely to produce damage to colonic musoca. It must be remembered, however, that cholestyramine may well reduce the bile acid pool and thus contribute to decreased micellarization of fats in the upper small intestine.

Glucocorticoids are employed commonly in patients with Crohn disease as anti-inflammatory agents and may be extremely beneficial, at least for short periods of time. These agents also benefit patients with eosinophilic gastroenteritis and radiation enteritis at times. Both eosinophilic gastroenteritis and Crohn disease are of unknown etiology, and the responses to glucocorticoids are frequently unpredictable and impermanent. Continued use of this therapy may be associated with complications of its own, especially growth failure in children and osteoporosis in adults.

Broad-spectrum antibiotics are extremely helpful in reducing bacterial overgrowth in patients with basically incurable diseases, such as scleroderma, amyloidosis of the intestine, and intestinal pseudo-obstruction. Reduction of bacterial flora leads to the correction of mucosal damage and to reduced deconjugation of intestinal bile acids, with resultant improvement in fat absorption. Sustained benefit can often be achieved by using antibiotics on a permanent, intermittent schedule.

The use of cimetidine in the Zollinger-Ellison syndrome can also be considered ameliorative therapy. Reduction in gastric secretion of HCl improves the efficiency of small intestinal pancreatic enzymes and improves absorption, as well as facilitating the healing of gastric and intestinal ulcers. At times, this therapy can initiate prolonged remissions in the disease, without actually changing the heavy autonomous secretion of gastrin.

Agents such as metoclopramide and urecholine, which stimulate intestinal motility, may benefit patients with the enteropathy of diabetes, scleroderma and pseudo-obstruction. Increasing motility appears to stimulate mixing of intestinal chyme and movement of bacteria into the lower intestine. The effects are usually not sustained, and prolonged use of these agents has not been completely satisfactory.

The reduction of nutrients to their simplest forms in so-called elemental diets may be beneficial to patients with otherwise untreatable and extensive small intestinal deficiency, including advanced Crohn disease, radiation enteritis, short small intestine, and pseudo-obstruction. Proteins carbohydrates, and fats are ingested respectively as dipeptides and amino acids, monosaccharides, and medium-chain triglycerides. Vitamins and minerals are added to the oral feedings in amounts large enough to meet normal requirements. Such diets have been shown to reduce malabsorption and to diminish diarrhea, but they have the major disadvantages of great expense, poor taste, and monotony. Futhermore, some patients cannot tolerate the diarrhea that occasionally occurs, and that may be poorly responsive to psyllium hydrophylic mucilloid, loperamide, or diphenoxylate. In my experience, most patients will consume oral elemental diets for only short periods of time, although they may benefit considerably from these exposures.

Parenteral hyperalimetation is a form of intravenous elemental diet, wherein total balanced nutrition is provided by continuous or intermittent intravenous solutions. While soybean emulsions, 5 percent dextrose, and 5 percent amino acid solutions can be dripped slowly into a large brachial vein, patients are most comfortable when an indwelling catheter is placed into a large central vein, usually the superior vena cava via the external jugular. Catheters may be left in place for extended periods of time, and with careful dressing changes, infection is a minimal problem. A fully balanced diet can be administered, including 3,000 or more kcal per day. Severely undernourished patients may thus regain lost weight and experience great relief from their symptoms by virtue of the fact that they are not using their intestinal tracts. In some cases of Crohn disease, parenteral hyperalimentation is associated with improvement of the inflammatory process. The immunodeficiency of malnutrition is also frequently corrected. By the use of a silastic catheter tunneled under the skin of the chest wall, and then into a large cervical vein, permanent parenteral hyperalimentation is now possible. Patients are able to administer their own daily nutritional requirements over a period of 10 to 12 hours with specially designed pumps and in a number of instances have been able to return to work. In certain cases, this treatment may be lifesaving, and because of this its expense is worthwhile.

Replacement therapy

The use of pancreatic supplements in patients with pancreatic insufficiency has been discussed in Chapter 13 and is a prime example of replacement therapy in malabsorption. Ionic replacement with calcium, magnesium, and potassium is also often indicated in patients with chronic malabsorption. One must additionally be mindful of vitamin needs in planning a program for patients with chronic malabsorption. Careful attention to these minutiae can produce satisfactory results even in patients with the most resistant forms of absorptive disorders.

HISTORICAL DIGRESSION

Proper names mentioned without reference in this chapter include: Paul BOUIN (1870–1962), French histologist, Algiers, Nancy, Strasbourg; Burrill Bernard CROHN (1884–), American gastroenterologist, New York, described terminal ileitis in 1932; Samuel Jones GEE (1839–1911), British physician, London; Alfred GIARD (1846–1908), French zoologist, Paris; Christian Archibald HERTER (1843–1910), American physician, New York; Otto Johann Leonhard HEUBNER (1843–1926), German pediatrician, Leipzig, Berlin; Wilhelm Dusan LAMBL (1824–1895), Polish pathologist, Cracow; Robert Frederick SCHILLING (1919–), American physician, Boston, Madison; Tage SJOGREN (1859–1939), Swedish physician, Jönköping, described sicca syndrome in 1933; George Hoyt WHIPPLE (1878–1976), American pathologist, Baltimore, Rochester (New York), Nobel laureate 1934 with Minot and Murphy.

SELECTED REFERENCES

Anderson CM, Frazer AC, French JM. Coeliac disease: gastrointestinal studies and the effect of dietary wheat flour: Lancet 1:836–42, 1952.

Bayless TM. Whipple's disease: new concepts of therapy. Adv Intern Med 16: 171–89, 1970.

Cooper BT, Holmes GKT, Ferguson R, et al. Celiac disease and malignancy. Medicine 59:249–61, 1980.

Dicke WK, Weijers HA, van de Kamer JH. Coeliac disease. II. The presence in wheat of a factor having a deleterious effect in cases of coeliac disease.

Donaldson RM, Jr. Small bowel bacterial overgrowth. Adv Intern Med 16:191–212, 1970.

Falchuk ZM, Gebhard RL, Sessoms CS, et al. An *in vitro* model of gluten sensitive enteropathy. The effect of gliadin on intestinal epithelial cells in organ culture. J Clin Invest 53:487–500, 1974.

Hoskins LC, Winawer SJ, Broitman SA, et al. Clinical giardiasis and intestinal malabsorption. Gastroenterology 53:265–79, 1967.

Isaacson P, Wright DH. Intestinal lymphoma associated with malabsorption. Lancet 1:67–70, 1978.

Klipstein FA, Schenk EA. Enterotoxigenic intestinal bacteria in tropical sprue. II. Effect of the bacteria and their enterotoxins on intestinal structure. Gastroenterology 68:642–55, 1975.

Luk GD. Qualitative fecal fat by light microscopy: a sensitive and specific screening test for steatorrhea and pancreatic insufficiency. Gastroenterology 76:1169, 1979.

MacDonald WC, Dobbins WO, Rubin CE. Studies on the familial nature of celiac sprue using biopsy of the small intestine. New Engl J Med 272:448–56, 1965.

Pena AS, Mann DL, Hague NE, et al. Genetic basis of gluten-sensitive enteropathy. Gastroenterology 75:230–35, 1978.

Phillips SF: Diarrhea-a broad perspective. Viewpoints Dig Dis 7: 1-4 (November) 1975.

Roberts-Thomson IC, Stevens DP, Michel B, et al. Factors influencing small bowel changes in dermatitis herpetiformis. Aust NZ J Med 7:356–62, 1977.

Rubin CE, Eidelman S, Weinstein WM. Sprue by any other name. Gastroenterology 58:409–13, 1970.

Stefanini M. Clinical features and pathogenesis of tropical sprue. Observations on a series of cases among Italian prisoners of war in India. Medicine 27:379–427, 1948.

Trier JS. Diagnostic usefulness of small intestinal biopsy. Viewpoints Dig Dis 7:1–4, 1977.

Trier JS, Falchuk ZM, Carey MC, et al. Sprue and refractory sprue. Gastroenterology 75:307–16, 1978.

Watkins JB, Park R. Perman J. Detection and identification of fat malabsorption with non-radioactive $^{13}CO_2$ breath tests. Gastroenterology 78:1288, 1980.

DISCUSSION QUESTIONS

1. A 40-year-old man commenced having recurrent episodes of abdominal distention terminated by the passage of bulky malodorous stools at age 30. Over the the years episodes became more frequent and lasted for longer periods of time, up to several weeks. Each was accompanied by a loss of 10 to 12 pounds, most of which was regained when symptoms abated. For the last five months, symptoms have been more severe and prolonged than ever. He passes up to six frothy loose stools daily and has noted increasing weakness, tingling in his extremities and a tendency to bruise more readily than usual.

Examination reveals a poorly nourished man whose skin is pale and shows several truncal ecchymoses. Vital signs are normal. The tongue is red and fairly well papillated. The abdomen is distended, and loud infrequent borborygmi are audible. No masses are felt. Gentle tapping over the zygomatic arch provokes spasm of facial muscles (Chvostek sign). There is slight ankle edema, but sensory examination and tendon reflexes are normal.

Stool is strongly positive for Sudan-III-staining droplets after treatment with acetic acid and heat, and muscle fibers are not seen. Hematocrit is 25 percent, white blood count, 2,900 per cu ml. Ninety percent of the polymorphonuclear leukoctyes show more than two lobes, and red blood corpuscles are macrocytic. Serum calcium is 6.4 (9 to 11)* mg, and albumin is 1.9 (3.5 to 5.5) g per dl. Prothrombin level is 24 (90 to 100) percent of normal. After ingestion of 25 g of d-xylose, 1.5 g appeared in the urine during the ensuing five hours. Schilling test without intrinsic factor was normal.

1. What is the most likely mechanism of this illness?
2. How do you establish the diagnosis?
3. What is the explanation for each abnormal laboratory result?
4. What treatment would you suggest?

2. A 68-year-old man complains that he has lost 60 pounds and has become progressively weaker since the death of his wife two years ago. Appetite has been poor, and he has had much flatulence, although this symptom antedates the others by several years. For six months, he has noted progressively severe weakness and numbness in his lower extremities.

He shows evidence of wasting and pallor. Mucous membranes are pale. Vital signs are normal, save for a regular pulse rate of 110. The abdomen shows slight distention but no palpable organs or masses, and neurologic examination reveals absent Achilles reflexes as well as diminished vibratory and position senses in the ankles and feet.

Stool is moderately positive for fat and negative for muscle fibers. Hematocrit is 25 percent. White blood count is 3,100, and red cells are macrocytic on smear. Serum calcium, albumin, and prothrombin content are normal; 6.0 g of xylose are excreted after an oral dose of 25 g. Shilling test shows 1 (10 or more) percent excretion of the label in 24 hours, and the result is not corrected with addition of active intrinsic factor. Gastric aspirate shows a pH of 1.7.

1. What is the nature of this absorptive disorder?
2. What changes would you expect to see in a random biopsy of the jejunum?
3. How do you explain the abnormal laboratory data?
4. What study is most likely to reveal a definitive diagnosis?

3. A 21-year-old man complains of having had a persistent daily cough productive of thick yellow sputum for two years. He has also been short of breath, and for seven years he has had frequent chest colds and sinusitis attacks. Since the age of four he has had a ravenous appetite, and he passes several oily stools each day. Weight and development are normal, and he denies any bleeding tendency or abdominal pain.

*Normal laboratory values are shown in parentheses.

Examination shows a temperature of 37.8°C and a respiratory rate of 26. There are multiple nasal polyps, and his chest is increased considerably in anteroposterior diameter. There is diffuse hyperresonance over the lungs, as well as scattered wheezes and rhonchi. The abdomen is normal.

A randomly obtained sample of stool is strongly positive for fat without heating, and also shows many muscle fibers. D-Xylose excretion is 1.2 g following a dose of 5 g. Hematocrit is 46 percent, and white blood count is 11,800 with 80 percent polymorphonuclear forms. A chest X ray shows evidence of emphysema and increased bronchial markings bilaterally.

1. Explain the nature of this patient's malabsorption.
2. How would you localize the site of the absorptive disorder?
3. What diseases could be responsible? Which is most likely? Why? How would you prove it?
4. According to your answers to the previous question, how would you treat his malabsorption?

CLINICAL CONFERENCE 8

A 58-year-old male boxmaker complains of having had anorexia, bulky stools, and up to three bowel movements per day for two years. He has lost 50 pounds during this time, and four weeks ago he experienced the onset of progressively increasing abdominal and ankle swelling. Eight years ago a subtotal gastric resection was performed for a gastric ulcer. He tolerated this operation well, except for occasional fullness in the upper abdomen after meals. This sensation was usually relieved by belching, although at times he vomited bile-stained material.

Physical examination shows a wasted man with normal vital signs and a transverse upper abdominal scar. There is marked pitting edema of groins, scrotum, penis, and legs, and there is a soft mass to the right of the umbilicus. Peristaltic activity is visible in this mass.

Laboratory data reveal an anemia whose smear shows many macrocytes and hypochromic cells. Stool smear contains many yellow globules of fat, 10 to 75 μ in diameter, both directly and after hydrolysis. Plasma albumin is 2.8 g per dl; serum carotene is 83 (normal 80 to 300) μg per dl. Upper gastrointestinal X rays show a gastric pouch with normal mucosal folds. The gastroenterostomy empties promptly without marginal ulcer, and the efferent loop fills readily, showing a feathery mucosal pattern. The afferent loop fills only with difficulty and retains barium for 72 hours. A 5-g dose of xylose produces a urinary excretion of 0.8 g. Serum B_{12} on two occasions is 60 to 65 (160 to 900) pg, and serum folate levels are 22 and 25 (4 to 18) ng per ml. A Schilling test without intrinsic factor reveals 2.9 percent excretion in 24 hours.

1. What is the most likely cause of pain in this patient?
2. How do you explain his loss of weight and edema?

3. What are the possible causes of his steatorrhea and anemia?
4. What further information would you like to have?
5. How would you treat this patient? Is it premature to begin treatment?

A bone marrow aspirate shows megaloblastosis. The lowest pH of gastric juice after stimulation is 2.8. A second Schilling test made after ingestion of 20 ml of normal human gastric juice shows 3.2 percent excretion in 24 hours. A 72-hour stool collection contains 39 g of fat per day on a 100-g fat diet. Innumerable colonies of *Escherichia coli* are grown from a culture of duodenal fluid, and a jejunal biopsy shows fingerlike villi. His hematocrit rises slightly, and he is given monthly injections of vitamin B_{12}. Three months later the hematocrit has fallen to the initial level.

6. How do you explain the anemia and steatorrhea now?
7. What single agent might treat both his steatorrhea and his anemia?

He is given a course of ampicillin for 21 days. His hematocrit rises again to 38 percent. D-xylose excretion is now 1.1 g in five hours after a 5-g dose. Stool fat is 20 g per day on a diet containing 100 g fat. Schilling test reveals 15 percent excretion; serum B_{12} is 300 pg/ml, and serum folate is 8 ng/ml. The patient feels somewhat improved, and the edema has disappeared. His weight has fallen to 60 kg, and serum albumin has increased to 3.5 g per dl.

8. How do you explain the partial hematologic response? What additional information would you need to treat his anemia?
9. How do you explain the decrease in steatorrhea? What could you do now to stop the steatorrhea completely? Describe the medical and the surgical therapy that might accomplish this end.
10. The patient's weight at 18 was 83 kg. How do you explain his loss of weight?

Serum iron is 6 μg per dl, and iron-binding capacity is 344 μg per 100 dl. Treatment with pancreatin and iron is started. He gains weight steadily to 69 kg. His hematocrit is 45 percent, and his albumin is 4.5 g per dl.

11. What multiple causes for steatorrhea exist in this patient?
12. What multiple causes for anemia does he have?

CLINICAL CONFERENCE 9

A 33-year-old woman with seven children has had attacks of abdominal pain for the past 25 years. These attacks occur two to three times per year and continue for 7 to 10 days. The pain is a deep aching sensation in the left upper abdomen and left lower chest. At times cramps associated with nausea and vomiting occur in the middle and left upper abdomen and last for 2 to 5 minutes. The cramps recur at 30- to 90-minute intervals and are associated with nausea and vomiting. Her pain is frequently aggravated by food and is unaffected by antacids, but assuming a fetal position affords some relief from pain. Earlier attacks of pain were accompanied by bouts of diarrhea consisting of five loose bowel movements per day and, occasionally, bulky stools.

Her growth and development were unremarkable up to age 17, when she weighed 51 kg and stood 152 cm tall. Menarche occurred at age 13 and menses were regular. Pregnancies were all carried to term. Her education was interrupted by the frequent attacks of abdominal pain.

She was first hospitalized at age 14 for abdominal pain and leukocytosis. An appendectomy was performed, but the appendix was normal. She was next admitted at age 17 with epigastric pain, nausea, and vomiting. Vital signs were normal, and the liver was palpable and slightly tender. Liver function tests were normal. Blood glucose was 50 mg per dl. Her symptoms disappeared spontaneously.

At age 33, she weighed 36.8 kg and complained initially of vague, postprandial, left upper quadrant discomfort. There was no polyphagia, polyuria, or polydipsia, nor was there a family history of diabetes mellitus. A glucose tolerance curve showed a fasting level of 83 mg per dl, rising in a half hour to 160, at one hour to 158, at two hours to 151, and at three hours to 111. Her hematocrit was 41 percent with a hemoglobin of 14.3 g and a normal blood smear. Serum amylase ranged between 40 and 70 (80 to 180) Somogyi units on several determinations.

1. What are the likely causes of this sort of pain? Why?
2. What is probably causing her diarrhea? Is it related to her loss of weight?
3. How do her continuing fertility and lack of anemia provide clues to her disease?
4. What is the significance of the glucose tolerance curve?

She was hospitalized for investigation of weight loss. Examination reveals a well-developed, poorly nourished, 34.1 kg woman whose vital signs are normal. There are no signs of vitamin deficiency. Tenderness is present in the left upper quadrant of the abdomen and in the left costovertebral area. Serum iron is 100 μg per dl. A stool specimen is pale yellow, greasy, and bulky. Sudan III stain without heating shows many large globules of fat and muscle fibers per high-powered field.

5. What is the probable cause of the fat in this stool? How does this test distinguish between normal and increased quantities of fat?

Should a Sudan-III-stained preparation from a normal stool show fat globlules? Why?

6. What further tests would confirm the suspicion of steatorrhea and the general type?

A 72-hour stool collection while the patient was ingesting 100 g of fat daily contained 105 g of total lipid. In the urine in the five-hour period following the oral ingestion of 5 g of xylose, 1.2 g was excreted. Serum carotene was 50 μg per dl, and the prothrombin time was 28 seconds with a control of 14 seconds. A plain film of the abdomen revealed extensive calcification of the pancreas.

7. What physiologic process is comprised in this patient: digestion or absorption?
8. What further information about possible gastric or ileal surgery do you need to exclude a sequel to surgery as the cause of her steatorrhea?
9. Does the presence of pancreatic calcification exclude extrapancreatic causes of steatorrhea?
10. What test might now be employed to prove precisely that pancreatic insufficiency is the cause of the steatorrhea in this patient?

Medical history did not reveal any evidence of gastric surgery with duodenal bypass. Her appendectomy had not been complicated by perforation or abscess. No small intestine was removed. Duodenal intubation was performed and the pancreas was stimulated by the intravenous administration of 75 units of purified secretin. Maximal bicarbonate concentration of 33 mEq per liter was revealed in one 20-minute collection. Total volume collected in 80 minutes was 90 ml. Cytology was negative.

The patient was begun on pancreatin, USP 0.6 g every waking hour. Within one week, the 24-hour stool fat had fallen to 8 g per day on a 100-g fat diet, and she gained 1.75 kg.

11. What are the most likely causes of this patient's pancreatitis?
12. What additional information do you need to identify the exact cause of the pancreatitis? Why is it important to know?

A gall bladder X ray did not reveal stones. Biliary drainage was carried out using first 75 ml of 33 percent vol/vol magnesium sulfate and then 75 ml of olive oil as stimulants. No crystals were seen in the sediment.

13. How may gallstones be associated with pancreatitis? Is it a common association?

14. Why was duodenal drainage for calcium bilirubinate and cholesterol crystals performed notwithstanding a well-visualized gallbladder?

Further history revealed that the patient drank beer nightly as a sedative. She denied taking wine, whiskey, or any other alcoholic drinks, although her liver was palpable and slightly tender on admission. This cleared when she gained weight following pancreatin therapy. Liver function studies were normal. Serum cholesterol was 141 mg per dl, and serum triglycerides were 105 (30 to 130) mg after an 8-hour fast. Multiple serum calciums were below 9.4 mg per dl; 24-hour urinary calcium excretion was normal. The alkaline phosphatase was 85 IU per liter. A 24-hour urine amino acid chromatogram revealed excessive lysine and leucine.

15. How commonly is alcoholism associated with pancreatitis? Is it likely that his patient has alcoholic pancreatitis?
16. What further studies might define the etiology of this patient's pancreatitis?
17. What is the mechanism for calcium malabsorption in steatorrhea?
18. Why isn't this patient anemic?
19. What is the significance of the aminoaciduria?

Further history was obtained by an inquisitive medical student: the patient's father died during a severe bout of abdominal pain. Information from a pathologist confirmed that the patient's father had died with calcific pancreatitis. Investigations of her sisters and child over several years have confirmed the presence of pancreatitis in several of them as well.

The patient has survived 12 years since the original diagnosis, has had two more children, and has cared for her large family without difficulty. Her weight has stabilized at 45 kg. She has rare attacks of pain and only one bowel movement per day. Her most recent two-hour postprandial blood sugar was 95 mg per dl.

CHAPTER 16

Diarrhea and Constipation: Mechanisms, Classification, and Illustrations

DIARRHEAL DISORDERS

While everyone knows what diarrhea is, many find it difficult to define its minimal clinical limits. Just as a single swallow does not make a summer, so also does one loose stool not usually constitute pathological diarrhea. For our purposes, clinical diarrhea will refer to the passage of successive loose or watery stools over a period of more than a few hours. Diarrhea can also be physiologically defined as a net accumulation of fluids and electrolytes in the intestinal lumen, resulting from increased secretion, decreased absorption, or both (Binder 1980), bearing in mind the fact that the small intestine both secretes and absorbs simultaneously, but that net absorption normally exceeds net secretion.

The distinction between *diarrhea* and *dysentery* should also be made clear. The former term refers to the character of the stools alone, while the latter refers both to symptoms of intestinal dysfunction, such as abdominal cramps and tenesmus, and to abnormalities in stool characteristics, chiefly the presence of blood and mucus. Thus, a patient with a diarrheal disorder may have dysenteric symptoms without dysenteric stools, while patients with dysenteric stools almost invariably have dysenteric symptoms as well. Dysenteric symptoms result from intestinal hypermotility and distention, while the presence of dysenteric stools suggests that ulcerative lesions have appeared in the intestinal mucosa. In the following discussion, the term *dysentery* will be confined to those diseases in which mucosal damage is a prominent feature.

Classification of Diarrheas

Diarrheal disorders may be acute or chronic, and of one or more of four general types: osmotic, secretory, exudative, or limited mucosal contact (Phillips 1980).

Osmotic Diarrheas. These are caused by the presence in the intestinal lumen of osmotically active solutes that are poorly absorbed by the intestinal mucosa. Acute osmotic diarrheas are exemplified by the ingestion of magnesium sulfate, lactulose, or magnesium hydroxide as laxatives. Chronic osmotic diarrheas occur in patients with the postgastrectomy dumping syndrome upon ingestion of a hyperosmolar feeding, or in patients with oligosaccharidase deficiencies following consumption of indigestible disaccharides, such as lactose, maltose, or sucrose. Osmotic diarrheas characteristically disappear when oral feedings are discontinued and are not likely to be associated with damage to the small intestinal mucosa.

Secretory Diarrheas. These are the result of an active process in the intestinal epithelium stimulated by the presence of a toxin, chemical, or nutritional product in the intestinal lumen. Some of these agents, such as heat-labile enterotoxin of *Escherichia coli* and cholera enterotoxin, stimulate adenylate cyclase and increase mucosal concentrations of cyclic adenosine 5′-monophosphate (cAMP). This agent causes luminal accumulation of water and electrolytes by both inhibition of neutral NaCl absorption and stimulation of active Cl^- secretion, the former action occurring presumably at villous epithelial membranes, and the latter at epithelial crypt cells. Cytological damage does not occur, and the absorption of glucose at villous epithelial brush borders remains normal. Other toxins, such as the heat-stable enterotoxin of *E. coli*, induce guanylate cyclase activity and cause increases of mucosal guanosine 5′-monophosphate (GMP) and secretory diarrhea, although the mechanism of GMP action has not as yet been elucidated. Vasoactive intestinal polypeptide and prostaglandins also increase adenylate cyclase activity in intestinal epithelium. Prostaglandin release has been shown to be at least a partial mediator of secretory diarrhea caused by certain laxative agents, such as ricinoleic acid (castor oil), senna, and dioctyl sodium sulfosuccinate (Buebler and Juan 1979), and of the diarrhea caused by dihydroxy bile acids and fatty acids.

Acute secretory diarrheas thus may be caused by bacterial exotoxins, certain laxatives, and viruses. Chronic secretory diarrheas occur, as we have seen, in the colon due to malabsorption of bile acids and the hydroxylation of unabsorbed fatty acids in patients with steatorrhea. Increased secretion of hormones may cause chronic secretory diarrhea through a variety of mechanisms. In the so-called pancreatic cholera (Verner-Morrison) syndrome, secretion of vasoactive intestinal polypeptide and prostaglandins by islet-cell-derived tumor tissue is believed to be responsible. Patients with medullary carcinoma of the thyroid show increased circulating levels of prostaglandins and calcitonin, and the diarrhea of the carcinoid tumor syndrome is believed to result from increased secretion of serotonin (5-hydroxytryptamine), which leads to a secretory diarrhea unrelated to cyclic AMP release.

Secretory diarrheas, unlike osmotic diarrheas, are generally not relieved by fasting. Some, like those due to cholera and *E. coli* enterotoxins, are unassociated with damage to the intestinal epithelium. On the other hand, structural lesions are usually found in secretory diarrheas due to invasive bacteria, viruses, and dihydroxy bile acids.

Exudative Diarrheas. These are always associated with mucosal damage, which leads to an outpouring of mucus, blood, and plasma proteins, and to a net accumulation of electrolytes and water. The diarrheas of salmonellosis, radiation enteritis, and chronic ulcerative colitis have been shown to be associated with increased prostaglandin release. Salmonellosis, shigellosis, and *E. histolytica* infections produce acute exudative diarrheas in the small intestine and colon, while chronic ulcerative colitis, radiation enteritis, and large bowel cancers may produce chronic exudative diarrheal states.

Limited Mucosal Contact Diarrheas. These refer to those conditions in which contact of chyme with absorbing epithelium is inadequate. Such diarrheas are always chronic in nature and result from inadequate mucosal surface, as in extensive epithelial damage (Crohn disease, radiation enteritis), extensive small intestinal resections, or small intestinal bypasses (high intestinal fistulas). Such diarrheas also occur in patients with disordered intestinal motility and inadequate mixing of chyme, like those with intestinal pseudo-obstruction, diabetic enteropathy or scleroderma. This latter type of limited mucosal contact diarrhea is usually also complicated by steatorrhea resulting from bacterial overgrowth and reduced luminal concentrations of conjugated bile acids.

BACTERIAL DIARRHEAS (TABLE 16-1)

The intestinal effects of bacterial infections are due either to the production of diarrheal toxins, to penetration of the intestinal epithelium by the infectious agent, or to both mechanisms operating simultaneously. Bacterial toxins are classified as enterotoxins (or exotoxins) if they are secreted into culture media by intact organisms, or endotoxins if they are released only after lysis of the bacteria. Diarrheas caused by bacterial toxins are primarily enterotoxigenic. Enterotoxins are highly soluble in water, usually antigenic, and usually polypeptides (Grady and Keusch 1971). By and large, purely enterotoxigenic organisms cause diarrheal states, while penetrant organisms cause dysentery.

Cholera

This condition is the prototype of acute, self-limited, enterotoxigenic secretory diarrheas. The causative agent, *Vibrio cholerae*, produces an enterotoxin (mol wt 84,000) which binds to epithelial receptors and stimulates the adenylate cyclase-cAMP system which, in turn, blocks the absorp-

Table 16–1. Classification of Infectious Diarrheas

Agent	*Type of Disease*	*Location*	*Mechanism*	*WBC in stool*	*Vectors*
Vibrio cholerae	toxigenic	small intestine	adenylate cyclase	no	water
E. coli	heat-labile toxin	small intestine	adherence factor Adenylate cyclase	no	fecal-oral
	heat-stable toxin	small intestine	guanylate cyclase	no	fecal-oral
Invasive	penetrates mucosa	ileum-colon	? prostaglandins	yes	food borne
Enteropathic	mucosal adherence	small intestine	disrupts brush borders	no	fecal-oral
Salmonella	invasive	ileum-colon	prostaglandins	yes	food borne
Shigella	enterotoxic invasive	ileum-colon	? adenylate cyclase ? prostaglandins	yes	fecal-oral
Campylobacter fetus	invasive, enterotoxic	small intestine, colon	?	yes	food, pets
V. parahemolyticus	invasive	small intestine	?	yes	fish, crustaceans
Yersinia enterocolitica	invasive, enterotoxic	ileum-colon	?	yes	food, pets
Clostridium perfringens	enterotoxic	small intestine	? adenylate cyclase	no	food borne
Staphylococcus aureus	preformed enterotoxin	small intestine	? adenylate cyclase	no	food borne
Cl. difficile	adherence; toxin	colon	exudative disease	yes	altered flora
Norwalklike virus	invasive	? small intestine	villous atrophy	no	? fecal
Rotavirus	invasive	duodenum	villous atrophy	no	fecal; ? oral
Giardia lamblia	adherence	small intestine	villous atrophy	no	water borne
E. histolytica	invasive	colon	invasive, exudative	yes	water, food

tion of NaCl and stimulates the active secretion of Cl^-, resulting in copious watery diarrhea. While cholera toxin reduces intestinal motility and causes dilatation of mucosal capillaries, it does not damage the epithelial cell in any recognizable way. The capillary dilatation is probably the result of increased tissue permeability, a state which cholera toxin has been shown to produce in tissues other than the intestinal mucosa. Both vibrios and enterotoxin are destroyed by gastric acidity, and their activity is enhanced by alkalinization of gastric juice.

Cholera enterotoxin has been isolated in two antigenically identical forms, an active variety called choleragen, and a nontoxic type known as choleragenoid. The active subunit of choleragen has been shown to behave as an enzyme that catalyzes the hydrolysis of nicotinamide adenine dinucleotide to adenine diphosphate- (ADP)-ribose. The ADP-ribose transfers to the guanadino moiety of arginine subunits contained in acceptor proteins on epithelial membranes. This protein normally regulates the activity of adenylate cyclase, but ADP-ribosylation leads to increased stability of this catalytic complex, induces increased activity of adenylate cyclase, and results in increased production of cyclic AMP (Moss and Vaughn 1977). The enterotoxin of *E. coli* appears to operate in the same fashion as choleragen, although its activity is much less (Gill and Richardson 1980).

The action of cholera enterotoxin on epithelial cells appears to be permanent and is terminated only when the cell has completed its normal life cycle. The bacterial infection, however, appears to be terminated by the elaboration of secretory IgA and by the appearance of circulating vibriocidal antibodies, the latter probably being more effective than the former. Killed cholera vaccines are of little value in promoting lasting resistance to infection, and the presence of antibodies to choleragen does not seem to prevent disease, although it may reduce the severity of individual attacks.

Clinical cholera appears to result from the ingestion of bacteria rather than toxin (Banwell and Sherr 1973). Bacteria adhere to epithelial surfaces throughout the small intestine and commence shortly to produce toxin. The resultant diarrhea is of sudden onset and is profuse, frequently accompanied by rapid dehydration, acidosis, and shock.

Treatment. Treatment consists primarily of rapid replacement of fluid and electrolytes. When diarrhea is copious, patients may require as much as 1 liter of fluid per hour. Oral fluid replacement may be very effective if glucose is contained in the medium. A balanced fluid contains sodium 110, potassium 25, chloride 87, and bicarbonate 48 (mEq per liter) and glucose 100 mmole per liter. For more seriously ill patients, initial fluid replacement should be by the intravenous route. The use of tetracycline as an antibacterial agent appears to shorten the duration of the diarrhea.

Transmission. Cholera occurs in areas where sanitation is poor, but the reservoir is not known. The possibility that virulent *V. cholera* (biotype El

Tor) may live for extended periods in brackish marshes and then infect shellfish is strongly supported by an outbreak which occurred in coastal Louisiana, involving an organism similar to one found five years before (Blake et al 1980). Positive cultures were found in crabs and in the waters themselves. Moderate cooking did not apparently destroy the organisms, which seem to have an affinity for adherence to chitinous structures. It is currently recommended that shellfish from suspect areas be boiled before eating for at least 15 minutes. The disease usually occurs in epidemics but does not appear to be particularly seasonal. Human carriers have been identified occasionally, although their small numbers could hardly account for the spread of the disease.

Escherichia-coli-Induced Diarrheas

These diseases are caused by three different classes of bacteria: enterotoxigenic, invasive, and enteropathogenic.

Enterotoxigenic E. coli. These produce either a heat-labile or a heat-stable enterotoxin. Some strains produce both types. The heat-labile toxin is similar to choleragen in molecular weight and in metabolic effects. Heat-stable enterotoxin, on the other hand, is a low molecular weight protein which stimulates watery diarrhea by activation of the guanylate cyclase–cyclic GMP system (Edelman and Levine 1980). Strains of toxigenic *E. coli* producing heat-stable enterotoxin are more common than those producing the heat-labile form.

As is the case with cholera, the diarrhea produced by enterotoxigenic *E. coli* is watery, copious, and nondysenteric. It is rarely as severe, however, as cholera. These organisms are prominent causes of the diarrhea of travelers and, especially in areas with poor sanitation, are major causes of infantile diarrheas as well. One study has shown that even gastroenterologists, when traveling in areas with marginal sanitary facilities, are not in the least immune to the rigors of diarrhea induced by enterotoxigenic *E. coli* (Merson et al 1976). Proliferation of these organisms in the gut depends upon their carrying one or more adherence factors (pilae) capable of binding to epithelial receptors. In the absence of adherence factors, *E. coli* are not pathogenic.

Invasive E. coli. These are typified by their ability to intrude into epithelial cells of the ileum and colon, and to produce a dysenteric disorder similar to shigellosis. In contrast to toxigenic *E. coli* infections, disease from invasive varieties is usually food borne rather than water borne and is rarely a problem among infants. These organisms do not appear to produce enterotoxins.

Enteropathogenic E. coli. These are not invasive, and may produce a toxin which is distinct from the two forms produced by enterotoxigenic varieties.

This toxin has not been fully characterized but appears to be able to produce a severe secretory diarrhea. In some studies enteropathogenic strains have been shown to be responsible for more cases of childhood diarrhea than either *Shigella* or *Salmonella*.

Ulshen and Rollo (1980) have described a variety of enteropathogenic *E. coli* in humans which is neither toxigenic nor invasive, but appears to be able to adhere to intestinal epithelium and to disrupt microvilli, with consequent reduction of brush border enzymes. The mechanism of the watery diarrhea is not clear.

Treatment. Treatment of diarrheas caused by *E. coli* does not require antibiotics and is usually quite well accomplished by the oral use of balanced glucose-electrolyte solutions. Bismuth subsalicylate has been shown to be helpful in controlling diarrhea, probably by the adsorption of enterotoxins (DuPont et al 1977). Opiates generally relieve the cramps and diarrhea but may prolong the infection. There is also evidence that the incidence of *E. coli*-induced diarrhea among travelers in endemic areas can be significantly reduced by the administration of prophylactic doses of doxycycline, which is a form of tetracycline distinguished by a long half-life and excretion into the intestinal lumen (Sack et al 1979). It is not clear that this form of prophylaxis should be used widely, since it may encourage the emergence of resistant strains of *E. coli*. Travelers to endemic areas should be advised to become fastidious in their eating and sanitary habits.

Salmonellosis

This infection is primarily acquired through the ingestion of contaminated foods, and all of the 1,500 serotypes of *S. enteritides* produce diarrhea through invasion of the intestinal lamina propria and the release of prostaglandins. At least one strain has also been shown to produce an enterotoxin. *S. typhi* is heavily invasive, and is capable of producing severe ileocolitis with hemorrhage.

No specific treatment is required for *S. enteritides* infections, except for management of the occasionally encountered carrier. Typhoid fever responds well to chloramphenicol, ampicillin, or trimethoprim-sulfamethoxazole.

Shigellosis

Infection with *Shigella* is spread by person-to-person contact, largely through the fecal-oral route. It is one of the major causes of diarrheal epidemics among both adults and children, and though some species produce enterotoxins, the major effects are the result of deep invasion of the mucosa. *Shigella dysenteriae I* enterotoxin has been shown to be capable of activating mucosal adenylate cyclase in the presence of substrate (ATP) excess (Charney et al 1976).

Campylobacter fetus

This organism, which was known earlier as *Vibrio fetus*, has become an increasingly recognized major cause of acute gastroenteritis, among both adults and children. This microaerophilic organism is invasive and grows especially well in stool. The subspecies *jejuni* of *V. fetus* causes an acute ulcerative colitis and a secretory diarrhea in humans (Blaser et al 1979; Loss et al 1980). The colitis may appear segmental on endoscopy. Abdominal pain, fever, and dehydration are common. Stools often contain neutrophils and red blood cells. Invasion is marked by the presence of *C. fetus* in blood at times, and by rising antibody titers. The disease is often food borne and may also be transmitted from reservoirs in animals. Clinical symptoms are often severe but not as explosive as those of cholera, and treatment with erythromycin is often beneficial.

Vibrio parahemolyticus

This and other marine vibrios are noncholeragenic, and some tend to cause diarrhea due to mucosal invasion. Outbreaks are usually the result of ingesting contaminated raw fish or crustaceans. They have been most prevalent in the Orient, but are recognized increasingly in the West.

Yersinia enterocolitica

Subtypes 3 and 9, and *Y. pseudotuberculosis* are also most probably transmitted to humans in infected foods, as well as from sick pets. Those organisms are both invasive and enterotoxigenic. *Y. enterocolitica* produces fever, diarrhea, and abdominal pain (Leino and Kalliomäki 1974). Erythema nodosum, monoarticular arthritis, and mesenteric adenitis are often associated with *Y. pseudotuberculosis* infections, and occasionally lead to the mistaken diagnoses of acute appendicitis, inflammatory bowel disease, or rheumatic fever. The diagnosis is usually confirmed by rising agglutination titers, and treatment with tetracyclines or sulfonamides is generally effective.

Clostridium perfringens (C. welchii)

This organism is the major cause of gas gangrene infections in skin and other tissues and is also probably the "prime cause of food-borne diarrhea of documented origin" (Grady and Keusch 1971). Five types are recognized, the most common etiological variety in human disease being type A, a heat-resistant, spore-forming species, producing a heat-sensitive enterotoxin. The disorder itself causes diarrhea and abdominal pain, and is usually self-limited. Type C *C. perfringens* causes a severe necrotizing jejunitis, characterized by the onset of bloody diarrhea and the presence of intramural gas collections in the bowel wall. This variety is rare in most parts of the world, but travelers to New Guinea should be warned against participating, orally at least, in New Guinean pig feasts. The precious meat, given as a sign of friendship to neighbors and visitors, is cooked well before the feast and then laid upon the ground for hours to cool. The ground itself is well supplied with *C. perfringens*, and organisms quickly contaminate the meat, and eventually the jejunum of susceptible consumers.

Staphylococcus aureus

This organism produces a tasteless, heat-stable enterotoxin which is capable in itself of causing severe outbreaks of diarrheal food poisoning. Its victims are usually incapacitated for two to three days by diarrhea and vomiting and, while the disease itself is almost invariably nonfatal, patients frequently state that they wish it were otherwise. Like most types of food poisoning, *S. aureus* gastroenteritis is the direct result of careless storage of cooked foods. Rapid, sustained chilling is essential for all foods that are prepared for consumption without recooking at a later time.

Clostridium difficile and Pseudomembranous Enterocolitis

A relatively uncommon disorder prior to the introduction of broad-spectrum antibiotics in the fifth and sixth decades of this century, pseudomembranous enterocolitis is characterized early by the occurrence of discrete exudative lesions on the mucosa of the colon and small bowel. These lesions eventually coalesce into a contiguous process, and the exudate takes the form of a "pseudomembrane" covering the mucosa. The membrane is initially quite adherent to the bowel surface, but later loosens and may slough spontaneously. The underlying mucosa is hyperemic, edematous, and often extremely friable. The pseudomembrane itself is composed of shed epithelium, pus cells, and mucin (Bartlett and Gorbach 1977). Fever, exudative diarrhea, and dehydration are the major symptoms of the disease, although the diarrhea itself may at times be mild. The enterocolitis develops rapidly, may become fulminant, and without treatment, mortality rates as great as 80 percent have been reported.

Prior to 1950, pseudomembranous enterocolitis was reported primarily in patients who were recuperating from gastrointestinal surgery and occasionally in newborns, or adults with uremia, cardiovascular disease, or obstructing colonic neoplasms. Intestinal ischemia or changes in bowel flora were felt to be possible causes. Since 1950, the majority of cases have been associated with the administration of broad-spectrum antibiotics, initially tetracycline and ampicillin, and more recently, lincomycin and clindomycin. For a time the use of fecal enemas from healthy donors was suggested as a means of restoring normal bowel flora. While these were found to be effective occasionally, their use never became popular with patients or nursing personnel. Supportive therapy and discontinuation of antibiotics appeared to be most reliable, and a few reports suggested that glucocorticoids were also of value. For a time *Staphylococcus aureus* was felt to be the causative agent, and this may occasionally still be true. However, most patients with true pseudomembranous colitis did not have this organism in their stools.

One good result of the original postantibiotic epidemic was discontinuation of the willy-nilly prescription of prophylactic antibiotics for patients about to undergo almost any form of surgery. The disease almost disappeared entirely, although it was recognized that many patients receiving broad-spectrum antibiotics would also develop transitory diarrhea. However, the development of internal prosthetic appliances, such as artificial joints and blood vessels, led to a renewed interest in the use of prophylactic antibiotics, especially those effective against anaerobic organisms. The synthesis of lincomycin and clindomycin, both with a broad range of effectiveness against anaerobes, occurred at about the same time, and they were used increasingly in preoperative patients. Suddenly, a new form of pseudomembranous enterocolitis, now called clindomycin colitis, appeared on the roll call of iatrogenic disease. Tedesco (1976) demonstrated that as many as half of the patients receiving clindomycin developed diarrhea, and that a considerable percentage of these also developed pseudomembranous disease. In some, diarrhea did not develop until after the antibiotic was discontinued. Sigmoidoscopic findings in patients with antibiotic diarrhea ranged all the way from a normal mucosa to erythema, ulcerative proctitis, and well-developed pseudomembranous disease. Pseudomembranous enterocolitis was thus found to be the most advanced stage of antibiotic colitis.

Two bacterial observations in laboratory animals eventually implicated *Clostridium difficile* as the causative organism of pseudomembranous enterocolitis in essentially all patients, and as a factor associated with antibiotic diarrhea in around 20 percent of patients. This bacterium, a fastidious anaerobe, was cultured from animals who developed hemorrhagic typhlitis (cecitis) after receiving clindamycin, and that disease could also be produced by introducing pure cultures of *C. difficile* into the colons of untreated animals (Bartlett 1980). The same bacterium was eventually cultured from stools of patients with pseudomembranous colitis, and stool supernatants were found to contain an enterotoxin cytopathic to cultured human amniotic cells. This enterotoxin was neutralized by gas gangrene antitoxin and is now believed to be solely responsible for the fully developed clinical picture of pseudomembranous colitis.

C. difficile is susceptible to vancomycin, an antibiotic which is poorly absorbed after oral administration. It is only indicated in patients whose stool contains the cytotoxic enterotoxin, and it must be given for extended periods of time, since the disease may relapse if normal bacterial flora have not been fully restored (George et al 1979). Oral metronidazole or bacitracin may also be helpful at times (George et al 1980). The milder disease usually subsides spontaneously after clindomycin is discontinued. Cholestyramine has also been found to be useful in some patients with pseudomembranous colitis, probably by binding the enterotoxin (Burbige and Milligan 1975). Prostaglandin-induced cytoprotection has been determined to prevent clindamycin colitis in laboratory animals (Robert et al 1980) and may eventually be useful in humans.

Viral Diarrheas

Norwalklike viruses, variously identified as Hawaii, Montgomery County, and Ditchling agents, have been identified as the cause of a 24- to 48-hour gastroenteritis among adults and older children in a number of epidemics (Schreiber et al 1977). These viruses are not infectious to laboratory animals, and patients infected with one of the agents do not develop immunity to the others, and may indeed develop reinfections with the original agent. A small intestinal lesion is produced, including villous shortening, hyperplasia of crypt cells, decrease in microvilli, and cellular infiltrates in the lamina propria, resembling the changes of tropical sprue. Patients show transitory decreases in fat and xylose absorption, but no activation of adenylate cyclase. The virus itself is probably an RNA type agent, consisting of unenveloped 27-nm particles. It is recognized with difficulty by immune electron microscopy (Blacklow and Cukor 1981).

Rota (reolike) viruses have been determined to be the major causes of infantile diarrhea, and also may cause disease in adults coming into contact with infected infants (Wenman et al 1979). The 70-nm, double-shelled viruses consist of 11 segments of double-stranded RNA and cause diarrhea and abdominal cramps lasting five to eight days. Over half of infected infants also develop fever, lymphadenopathy, and dehydration. The affected small intestinal mucosa shows atrophic changes and, unlike the case with Norwalklike infections, particles can be found in the cisternae of the endoplasmic reticulum and in nuclear membranes. The diagnosis can also be confirmed by counter immunoelectrophoresis with immune guinea pig serum. A high rate of previous infection, but not necessarily of active disease, is indicated by the fact that antibodies to reolike viruses have been found in up to 90 percent of infants tested up to two years of age. Active disease is most common in the fall and winter months, and infants infected prior to two months of age appear to develop only mild symptoms, if any. This protection is not related to breast feeding. There appear to be two serotypes of rotavirus, and no cross-immunity has been demonstrated.

Protozoan Diarrheas

Giardia lamblia infection of the small intestine is one of the most common causes of acute diarrhea in adults and children. The pathogenesis of the disease has been discussed in Chapter 15. Suffice it to say that giardiasis should be considered as a possible cause of acute diarrhea in patients with sustained symptoms, particularly if they have recently traveled to endemic areas or have been on camping trips where they may have ingested water from contaminated lakes or streams. Diagnosis is established by finding *Giardia* cysts in stool or in duodenal aspirates; the organism may also be detected by microscopic examination of a length of cotton tape which has been swallowed and passed into the duodenum for a few hours. While *Giardia* produce an atrophic lesion in the small intestine, the mechanism of diarrhea is not presently established. In most cases, it appears to be secretory in nature. Treatment with quinacrine hydrochloride (100 mg three times daily for 10 days) or with metronidazole (250 mg three times daily for 7 days) is usually very effective (Stevens 1980).

Entamoeba histolytica infection remains a troublesome, though uncommon, cause of acute and chronic colitis in the Western world, and a very common problem elsewhere (Pittman 1980). The disease is spread from person to person by fecal contamination of water supplies, similar to giardiasis, although there are no known alternate hosts of amebiasis. Only amebic cysts are infectious to others, and only trophozoites cause active disease.

Acute amebic colitis may resemble ulcerative proctitis, shigellosis, or *Campylobacter* colitis on proctoscopic examination, since the lesion may present with diffuse hyperemia, friability, and ulceration of the mucosa. Careful examination of the bloody exudate for the trophozoites of *E. histolytica* will generally substantiate the diagnosis. Barium enema will occasionally show acute ulcerative lesions, especially in the cecum, and may also show areas of skip involvement similar to the picture found at times in patients with Crohn disease of the colon. Rarely, patients will present with a picture of toxic megacolon. Because of the numerous possible causes of acute hemorrhagic proctitis, there is some sense in examining all patients with acute disease for amebiasis, including the use of mucosal biopsy.

Once the diagnosis of amebic colitis is made, it is usually wise to perform an isotopic scan of the liver as well, in search of a possible amebic abscess of that organ. While hepatic abscesses are uncommon, the possibly serious consequences of this complication justify the search, even when no suggestive symptoms are present.

Metronidazole is probably the most effective treatment for colonic and hepatic amebiasis. The recommended dosage is 750 mg three times daily for

10 days, followed by careful stool examination to make certain that the infection has been completely eliminated. Since the danger of reinfection in areas with poor sanitation is great, attention should also be given to improving sewage facilities as well.

Factitial Diarrhea

Drugs that are intended for occasional use as laxatives can cause chronic diarrhea when taken continuously. Such a habit can produce profound discomfort for both the patient and associates, and deep problems for the physician who is called upon to treat the disorder at a time when the patient, for personal reasons, will not divulge the fact of surreptitious ingestion. Although the psychodynamic mechanisms which lead to factitial diarrhea are frequently murky, the problem itself is quite common. In one study of 27 subjects with chronic sustained diarrhea of obscure cause, nine patients, all of them women, were found to be ingesting diarrheal agents surreptitiously (laxatives in seven, diuretics in two) (Read et al 1980).

Factitial diarrhea often presents as an osmotic diarrhea, with stool weight returning to normal (less than 225 g per day) on fasting; but this is certainly not always the case. Hospitalization does not tend to change the course of the disorder, because patients frequently bring their cathartics with them. Physicians must have a high index of suspicion regarding the possibility of factitial diarrhea, especially when the patient has had previous stool and X ray studies which were normal, the diarrhea is chronic, weight loss has not been excessive, and the patient is a woman.

Demonstration of the laxative agent is simple at times, difficult at others. The presence of phenolphthalein in diarrheal stool is easily demonstrated by the development of a reddish pink color upon the addition of alkalis. Magnesium salts produce an "osmolar gap" in chemical measurements of stool electrolytes. Normally, the concentration of sodium in stool water is around 40, and of potassium around 90 mEq per liter. The osmolality of stool water is about 350 mOsm per kg, the 60 mOsm increase over plasma osmolality being due largely to the bacterial content of stool. Any major increases in stool osmolality beyond this figure should, in the absence of disaccharidase deficiency, lead to the suspicion of surreptitious ingestion of unabsorbable laxative agents. The ingestion of cascara as a laxative agent is often confirmed by finding a brownish black pigmentation of the rectal mucosa on protoscopy. When suspicion remains high and the diagnosis of factitial diarrhea can still not be confirmed, it may be justifiable to search the patient's belongings in hospital. This should not be done, however, without obtaining immediate prior permission from the patient to do so.

Treatment should be undertaken with great care. To confront the patient with the knowledge of surreptitious ingestion is a very poor practice, in the sense that "confrontation" implies revelation of wrongdoing. It is far wiser merely to inform the patient that the ingestion is known, that this is the cause of the diarrhea, and that improvement will follow its cessation. Physicians should indicate a willingness to discuss the matter in a friendly fashion, and to obtain psychiatric help, if the patient is willing. It is usually not a good idea to reveal the diagnosis to family members without the clear permission of the patient, since nothing must be done to alter the position of the patient in the family setting.

Radiation Enterocolitis

X ray and radium therapy are commonly employed in the management of intra-abdominal and pelvic cancers. An unfortunate feature of this treatment is the almost obligatory presence of portions of the gastrointestinal tract in the radiation pathway. Serious chronic tissue injury may result, even though the therapist attempts to avoid overexposure of any one intestinal segment by changing the position of the patient from treatment to treatment. The stomach is relatively resistant to chronic radiation disease, the rectum and colon are somewhat less so, and the small intestine is the most sensitive of all. Since most intensive radiation therapy is administered for pelvic carcinomas, the lower small intestine, colon, and rectum are the commonest disease sites. Age does not appear to correlate with the incidence of chronic radiation enteritis, and while one study showed an increased incidence among patients with hypertension, diabetes, and arteriosclerosis (DeCosse et al 1969), this association could not be confirmed in another series (LoIudice et al 1977). Both studies agree, however, that previous abdominal surgery, especially appendectomy and hysterectomy, significantly increases the risk of chronic enteritis from subsequent radiotherapy. This is believed to be the result of postoperative adhesions which confine loops of bowel to one portion of the abdomen or pelvis, and thereby increase the chances of radiation exposure to a single area of intestine, despite changes in the position of the patient. The overall incidence of chronic radiation enterocolitis ranges between 2 and 10 percent of patients at risk, and does not appear to be dose related in the therapeutic range.

Nature of the Injury. Exposure of the intestine to radiation leads to suppression of epithelial regeneration, mucosal infiltration, and, eventually, ulceration. This acute lesion is reversible and disappears completely within 12 days after the exposure ceases (Trier and Browning 1966). Chronic changes appear in weeks, months, or even years after exposure, and are characterized by swelling and proliferation of the endothelium of small blood vessels and infiltration with subintimal foamy histiocytes. This endarteritis leads to fibrinoid necrosis of the vessel wall, thrombosis, and eventually chronic ischemia of the bowel. Ischemia may be associated with ulceration, hemorrhagic necrosis, fibrosis, strictures, and eventually fistulas or free perforations (Warren and Friedman 1942). Acute radiation presents a troublesome, though transitory problem. It is the chronic disease which causes the major difficulty.

Type of Disease. In a personally studied series consisting largely of patients treated for gynecological tumors, radiation proctitis, including rectal ulcers and strictures, was the most common lesion. Rectovaginal fistulas occurred in nearly 30 percent of patients, enteritis in 25 percent, and colitis in 17 percent. Malignant change induced by the radiation appeared in only one patient (1 percent).

Symptoms. Acute radiation enteritis presents most commonly with abdominal cramps and diarrhea. Tenesmus is an important symptom in patients with proctitis, and mild to moderate hemorrhage may be encountered at times.

In the chronic disease, symptoms depend on the bowel segment(s) involved. Diarrhea, abdominal cramps, malabsorption, and loss of weight are common symptoms in patients with small intestinal disease. Strictures may lead to bacterial overgrowth and partial or complete obstruction of the intestine. A sudden increase in diarrhea and malabsorption suggests the occurrence of an enteroenteric or enterocolic fistula. In the colon, chronic diarrhea may occur with extensive, nonobstructing disease; constipation is the major complaint of patients with colonic strictures. Recurrent hemorrhage may be seen in either type. Chronic radiation proctitis is associated with tenesmus and bleeding. If a rectal ulceration is present, pain may be a major complaint. Upon deep penetration, ulcerations may lead to the formation of rectovaginal fistulas.

Treatment. The acute disease usually responds well to antidiarrheal agents (opium, loperamide, diphenoxylate) or to bulking agents (psyllium), and to reduced frequency or dosage of radiation treatments. The chronic disease may be responsive to glucocorticoids, especially if medication is administered locally for rectal ulcerations or proctitis. Symptomatic therapy is also helpful. However, for major complications, such as intestinal obstruction, recurrent hemorrhage, fistulas, and nonhealing ulcers, surgery is generally indicated. While surgery usually involves bowel resection, there is good evidence that a temporary deviating colostomy may be followed by slow healing of proctosigmoiditis and rectal ulcers, and occasionally of rectovaginal fistulas. Postoperative morbidity and mortality may be high because of poor healing, but parenteral hyperalimentation can often accelerate healing by improvement of nutrition.

CONSTIPATIVE DISORDERS

It is the purpose of this section to focus on those disorders of colonic motility which are associated with constipation; organic disorders, such as intestinal obstruction, cancer of the large bowel, strictures, and distal colitis are intentionally excluded because they are considered elsewhere in this volume or because their mechanisms are self-obvious. It should also be made clear that despite all appearances to the contrary, diarrhea and constipation are not physiologic opposites. It is almost certain that diarrhea results either from luminal or mucosal events, and that motility changes, if important at all, are only secondary contributory factors. Binder (1980) cites evidence which tends to dispel the notion that even opiates, long and successfully used in the management of diarrheal disorders, work their magic solely by increasing muscular tone. An endogenous opioid, metenkephalin, has been found to increase active intestinal absorption of sodium and chloride, and exogenous opiates may well behave in the same fashion. On the other hand, constipation is believed to result almost entirely from motility disorders in the colon; it is unassociated with alterations in mucosal physiology.

Definition

In a physiologic sense, one can do worse than define constipation as the passage of less than 3 bowel movements per week, when diet is randomly selected. Ninety-nine percent of normal subjects have between 3 and 21 motions weekly (Martelli et al 1978). When healthy subjects ingest small radioopaque markers, continue to eat a normal diet, and submit to daily abdominal radiographs, the markers have been entirely expelled by the eighth day in everyone, and the rapidity of expulsion does not correlate with the frequency of bowel movements. Corazziari et al (1975) suggest that the normal total gastrointestinal transit time measured by this technique should not exceed 96 hours. Thus, at the outset, we find that a universally acceptable definition of constipation has not as yet been devised.

We must also consider the individual views of laymen in our definition, since constipation is often in the eye of the beholder. Some people inflict much anxiety on themselves and their families by insisting upon having one or two large, satisfying bowel movements daily, and by considering themselves and others to be constipated, and indeed in need of laxatives, if nature delivers anything less. Others, whose bowels may move less than once weekly, frequently give the matter no thought at all and often appear to be none the worse for it. Physicians must learn to recognize these extremes of bowel behavior, to reassure patients with what has been called "imaginary" constipation, and to avoid becoming overly alarmed themselves when they encounter truly constipated patients who are not obviously concerned about their condition.

Constipative disorders encountered in medical practice fall into two general categories, those in which the rectum is full or partially full of unimpacted stool, and those in which the rectum is essentially empty. The radiological counterparts of these categories have been defined by Corraziari et al, who described three groups of patients with nonorganic constipation of the basis of the transit of swallowed radiopaque markers; patients with left colonic slowing, patients with rectal slowing, and an intermediate group with slowing in both areas. They did not find any evidence of functional constipation due to slowing of right colonic motility, although others have documented such cases.

Aspects of Colonic Motility

The two basic aspects of colonic motility are the electrical rhythm and the muscular response. While electrical activity appears to pace muscular contractions, it most often occurs without producing corresponding muscular responses. The latter, however, do not occur without electrical stimuli.

Electrical activity in the colon is discontinuous and occurs in two slow-frequency ranges, the more common appearing at 6 to 11 cycles per minute, the less common at 2 to 4 cycles. The oscillatory rates of the higher frequency slow waves remain essentially the same throughout the upper colon and sigmoid but decrease in a gradual gradient from the lower sigmoid to the rectum. The absence of a steep gradient in these waves throughout most of the colon suggests an environment which affords slow propulsion of intestinal contents in that portion of the bowel, while the steeper gradient from lower sigmoid to rectum suggests a more propulsive environment. Low-frequency (3 cycles per minute) slow waves are present throughout the colon, but especially in the cecum and lower rectum, and do not exhibit an oscillatory gradient (Taylor et al 1975). These waves appear to be associated with nonpropulsive colonic contractions which would facitate absorption in the right colon and continence in the rectosigmoid. Muscular contraction is signaled by the appearance of electrical spike potentials on depolarizing slow waves, the rate of the slow waves thus controlling the rate of muscular contractions. Spike potentials occur only in depolarizing smooth muscle, but their source is not known. Migrating spike bursts of higher frequency slow waves suggest peristaltic activity (Christensen et al 1974), while the spike bursts on 3-cycle slow waves suggest the appearance of spastic contractions of circular muscle, which inhibit propulsive activity. In the cat, about two-thirds of migrating spike potentials progress distally, while the remainder move in an oral direction. The "pacemaker" for this activity appears to reside in the transverse colon.

Defecation is transiently stimulated by distention of the rectum, the distention producing a decrease in pressure in the upper portion of the anal canal (rectoanal inhibitory reflex). Pressure in the lower anal canal is under voluntary control and tends to rise if the rectoanal/ inhibitory reflex occurs at an inopportune time, and to fall with actual defecation. At rest, pressures in the upper anal canal are higher (average 54 cm water) than in the lower anal canal (average 35 cm water) (Martelli et al 1978). In general the more the rectum is distended, the longer is the relaxation time in the upper canal, and the lower is the pressure at maximum relaxation.

The Irritable Bowel Syndrome

This is believed to be a pure disorder of intestinal motility, in which increased contractility of both muscular coats is the basic defect. Irritable bowel syndrome (IBS), which is far and away the most common cause of visits by patients to gastroenterologists, usually commences early in life, and rarely starts after the age of 35 years. Switz (1976) estimates that 19 percent of visits to gastroenterologists are for "functional" disorders, prime among which is IBS.

Occurrence of IBS is very high in Europe and North America, and probably also in other Western cultures. The disorder is more commonly seen in women and is frequent in childhood. In primitive cultures, IBS is almost unknown, and while this fact has been attributed to the use of a high residue diet in these societies (Trowell 1974), the point is far from proved. Thompson and Heaton (1980) report that nearly 14 percent of young and elderly healthy adults experience IBS symptoms frequently.

Symptoms are almost invariably attributable to disorders of intestinal motility: constipation associated with scybalous stools and frequently increased expulsion of thin or thick mucus; borborygmi indicating increased small intestinal activity; a form of low-volume diarrhea, generally associated with mucus; pain almost anywhere in the abdomen, but most commonly in the lower left quadrant; bloating; tenesmus; and a frequent feeling of incomplete evacuation of the bowels. Symptoms may occur at any time, least commonly at night, and most frequently after meals, through initiation of the gastrocolic reflex. At times pain is referred into the left chest or substernal area, where it may resemble angina pectoris (Dworken et al 1952). Nausea is a common symptom, but vomiting and loss of weight are rare. Gross blood in the stool is noted only if hemorrhoids or anal fissures are associated. Fever never appears with IBS. Symptoms are often episodic, and many patients note that they frequently exacerbate during or following periods of emotional or physical stress.

Pathogenesis. Esler and Goulston (1973) documented a widely held belief that patients with IBS display a much higher degree of neuroticism than do controls, but there is still some uncertainty whether the psychological elements precede or follow the disease. Mendeloff et al (1970) showed that patients with IBS have experienced a significantly higher incidence of life stresses than have healthy subjects. Other medical writing from the time of the Civil War onward has commented on the high association between emotional and physical stress and IBS (Drossman et al 1977). But numerous patients with this disorder have not experienced unusual stresses and cannot be classified as psychoneurotic. In fact, Almy et al (1949) demonstrated that even healthy subjects, when subjected to stressful interviews, may develop spastic sigmoidal contractions demonstrable both by balloon kymography and by direct sigmoidoscopic observation.

In recent years, smooth muscular myoelectric abnormalities have been found among IBS patients. Ritchie (1973) has shown that patients demonstrate more frequent painful, spontaneous sigmoidal contractions, have greater sensitivity of the rectal mucosa to painful stimuli, and perceive pain more quickly upon distention of the rectum than do normal subjects. Numerous other studies have also shown increased colonic activity. Snape et al (1977) have shown that patients with IBS also have increased three cycle per second myoelectric activity in the basal state, and increased spastic contraction after receiving gastrin or cholecystokinin when compared with normal subjects. However, Latimer et al (1981) were unable to find any significant differences in colonic slow wave activity between patients with IBS, psychoneurotic patients without IBS, and normal controls. Sullivan et al (1978) found that the spike burst activity and contraction responses to a meal are delayed, but prolonged, in patients with IBS, and that colonic propulsion of contents is delayed. Finally, Martelli et al (1978b) have detected a group of patients with chronic constipation in whom the rectoanal inhibitory reflex was present, although reduced in magnitude, suggesting a mild form of anal "achalasia," and possibly representing another myoelectrical abnormality which could be associated with IBS. One may conclude from these observations that, while stress and anxiety may indeed stimulate symptoms in patients with IBS, the syndrome itself is probably engendered by an underlying myoelectrical disorder.

Diagnosis. Diagnosis should be made on the basis of a characteristic history and suggestive physical findings followed by exclusion of other diseases which may present with somewhat similar manifestations. Physical findings in IBS commonly include slight abdominal distention, increased bowel sounds, and localized tenderness, especially in the lower left quadrant of the abdomen. A tender loop of spastic intestine may be palpable. Patients also frequently have scars from previous operations, especially pelvic procedures in women, appendectomies, and cholecystectomies. It is my impression that many of these operations had been performed for symptoms that were due to previous attacks of IBS, since the same symptoms often recur following the procedure.

Rectal examination commonly reveals tightness of the anal sphincter, and sigmoidoscopy shows moderate to marked spasm of the rectum and sigmoid without significant mucosal abnormalities. Passage of the sigmoidoscope commonly reproduces the patient's symptoms. Stool specimens are guaiac negative. A barium enema should always be performed to rule out disorders, such as diverticulitis or cancer of the colon; it may occasionally reveal increased colonic haustrations, which are occasionally seen in IBS. Laboratory abnormalities are unassociated with IBS.

Management. In my experience, management requires clear understanding on the part of patients that they do indeed have colonic problems which are identifiable by an overabundance of segmental spasms, particularly in the left colon. The disease is neither imagined nor self-induced and, while those afflicted with it are probably always susceptible to recurrences, much can be done to reduce the severity of symptoms. This simple reassurance is often the most important element of therapy.

The importance of emotional and physical stress factors promoting exacerbations of IBS must also be emphasized. Adequate time must be made available to discuss a patient's personal problems. These are almost always of an intimate nature, but it is most uncommon for patients to be unwilling to discuss them. One must ask about relationships with spouse, children, and other family members, about sexual fulfillment, about problems with finances or in the workplace, and about lifetime goals. For it is within these areas that most of our personal problems lie; patients with IBS rarely, if ever, find that symptoms flare when pondering such global problems as Soviet imperialism, freeing of hostages in Iran, or world overpopulation. Physical stress must also be evaluated, since many patients lead a fairly disorganized life, attempt to do too much for too many people, and leave little time for sleep or leisure pursuits. When discussing these life stresses, it is important to explain to patients that while these are important factors in their illness, they are not the root cause of the problem.

Dietary restrictions appear to play no part whatsoever in exacerbations of IBS, and should not play a large part in therapy. This observation does not imply, however, that patients should not be allowed to use their own judgment in choosing food; they should merely be encouraged to select a well-balanced diet, with considerable variety. The intentional emphasis on high residue foods, such as bran, may be helpful, but may also aggravate bloating and cramps in some patients. Although never actually measured, the ingestion of three proper meals daily appears to benefit many patients, especially those whose habits had been unordered previously. Regular brisk physical exercise also seems to be helpful.

Over the years, antispasmodic medications have been administered to many patients with IBS. Results have been mixed even though Sullivan et al (1978) have shown that anticholinergic agents tend to reduce spike potentials and intraluminal pressure in the sigmoid colon. In a critical review of the numerous studies on anticholinergic medications in IBS, Ivey (1975) concludes that they may be of occasional value. Much of the same opinion attends the evaluation of bulking agents, such as bran and psyllium products, both of which have been shown to reduce intraluminal pressure and to increase the colonic motility index, but have received a mixed reception from patients.

When applied to patients with IBS, these therapeutic principles result in clearly beneficial responses about two-thirds of the time. Although newer techniques involving the use of biofeedback and conditioning have also been suggested, they do not appear to offer better results. Physicians must be prepared to experience therapeutic failures, but must persist in their efforts because beneficial responses often come only after long trials of therapy. They must also reject any thought about removing asymptomatic stony gall bladders or innocent uterine fibroids, since such surgical measures invariably fail to quell the colonic problem.

Hirschsprung Disease

While the genesis of constipation in IBS is related to increased myoelectrical potentials in the sigmoid colon, the cause of Hirschsprung disease is the absence of myenteric plexi in varying lengths of rectum and colon. The problem is congenital and appears to result from the failure of neurons to migrate distally in the intestine during the fifth to twelfth weeks of embryonic development (Okamoto and Veda 1967). Neuroblasts appear to emerge from the vagus into the esophagus and proceed caudally. Submucous plexi are formed by migration of myenteric neurons. While the length of aganglionic bowel differs from patient to patient, the pathologic process is always contigous from the point of origin to the distal-most rectum and is never spotty. The disease is much more common in boys and frequently occurs in families. In around 10 percent of cases long segments of colon, at times even the entire organ, may be involved.

Just as in achalasia of the esophagus, the aganglionic segment in Hirschsprung disease is spastic, and fails to undergo reciprocal relaxation when the proximal ganglionated segment is distended. Severe, unrelenting constipation is the result in those patients whose involved segment of rectum is greater than 6 cm in length. Newborns with Hirschsprung disease may develop intestinal obstruction, abdominal distention, vomiting and severe enterocolitis. The clinical picture in affected children is characterized by loss of weight, underdevelopment, and a distended abdomen. On the other hand, patients with shorter segments of disease may have only minimal trouble with chronic constipation.

Diagnosis. This disorder is suspected as the cause of constipation commencing in infancy or childhood. Characteristically, the rectum is free of stool on examination, and a barium enema often reveals a partially distensible, spastic rectum. In neglected cases or in long-segment diseases, megacolon proximal to the involved area may be marked. The diagnosis is confirmed by detection of the absence of ganglia on deep rectal mucosal biopsy. Myenteric plexi in dilated portions of the colon are disorganized, while nonmyelinated nerve fibers in the submucosa and muscularis of spastic segments are enlarged and do not ontor muscle fibers (Smith 1967). Just as it may produce a lesion resembling achalasia of the esophagus, Chagas disease may also be associated with findings suggesting Hirschsprung disease.

Treatment. Treatment of symptomatic Hirschsprung disease is solely surgical, the object being to remove all or almost all of the aganglionic bowel. In infants with advanced intestinal obstruction and in children with massive megacolon, preliminary decompression of the colon by a cecostomy or ascending colon colostomy is often necessary. Swenson (1950) advocated resection of the entire aganglionic segment down to the mucocutaneous junction, a "pullthrough" of the upper normal bowel, and anastomosis of this to the anal margin. Duhamel (1956) elected to retain the posterior wall of the lower rectum as a partially retentive pouch, and to anastomose the ganglionated upper portion of the colon anteriorly to the mucocutaneous junction and posteriorly to the retained lower rectum. Both procedures are quite successful in correcting the physiological defect. Martelli et al (1978b) have found that simple posterior anorectal myectomy is effective in patients with short-segment Hirschsprung disease.

Idiopathic Constipation

This disorder probably includes a number of etiological agents and has been variously named as simple constipation, habit constipation, and hypotonic constipation. It should be distinguished from those types of constipation in which the ability to defecate is reduced by paralysis or weakness of the diaphragm or abdominal musculature and by injuries or disease of the lower spinal cord. It is probable that idiopathic constipation can be induced by habitual rejection of normal urges to defecate, a problem which is commonly seen in children, or by a lack of adequate toilet facilities among large families living in crowded quarters. Diets that are low in fiber have also been implicated as a cause of constipation in Western societies, and it has been clearly shown that lack of stool bulk greatly increases colonic transit times (Parks 1974). A token of the importance of these social elements is the fact that idiopathic constipation is almost never seen among people living in societies where diets high in fiber are universal and where defecation may be looked upon as acceptable almost anywhere at almost any time.

Diagnosis. Stool remains in the colon for longer than normal periods of time in patients with idiopathic constipation and is, accordingly, drier and firmer than normal in most cases. Transit time is increased, stool weight is decreased, and absorption of sodium and water is greater than in nonconstipated persons (Devroede and Soffié 1973). The rectum almost invariably contains large amounts of stool, indeed at times immediately after defecation. The anal sphincter may be more relaxed than normal, spastic, or normal in tone, and the rectoanal inhibitory reflux may also be variable. Sigmoidoscopy and barium enema are normal, although the latter may show some degree of elongation of the colon and some increase in colonic width.

Balloon motility studies tend to show decreased contractions; no systematic study of myoelectric activity has been reported.

Treatment. There appears to be general agreement at present that the most effective treatment of idiopathic constipation involves efforts to increase stool bulk by increasing dietary fiber, especially through the use of bran and fibrous fruit and vegetables, and by adding bulking agents, such as psyllium or methlycellulose. Osmotic laxatives, such as magnesium hydroxide, may be needed at the start of therapy, but can generally be discontinued once a high bulk diet has been established. The regular use of laxatives that stimulate peristaltic activity should be discouraged, because they tend to develop dependence and may also lead to a spastic form of constipation.

Complications of Chronic Constipation

Aside from the intestinal obstruction of Hirschsprung disease, the complications of constipation are not life threatening but do constitute a major cause of disability and suffering. These include anorectal disorders and fecal impactions. Very little research has been devoted to the cause of these disorders, and many gastroenterologists devote little effort to their treatment. Though common, they are not fashionable—few wish to be known among their colleagues as "hemorrhoid" specialists. However, patients do not realize that anorectal disorders are considered to be déclassé, and persist in asking for therapeutic advice. Since the traditional advice given to patients with anorectal disorders by internists is to consult a surgeon, and since surgeons tend to prefer surgical methods of treatment over other approaches, it is the purpose of this section to suggest that anorectal disorders can often be treated quite well by nonsurgeons and that recurrences can frequently be prevented by following simple therapeutic measures.

Hemorrhoids. These have been for many years rather pompously attributed to upright posture, as though they were some sort of penalty to be paid for being virtuous. A brief medical experience in less developed societies, however, shows clearly by the absence of anorectal disorders that uprightness has very little if anything to do with these diseases. Burkitt (1975) considers hemorrhoids to be one of several "pressure" diseases, which also include diverticulosis of the colon, hiatal hernias, and varicose veins and attributes them to idiopathic constipation arising from a low-residue diet, prolonged straining at stool and extended periods of cogitation on the Western-style commode. His theory makes good sense but has not been clearly proved to be correct.

Venous supply to the anorectal area is very rich, and can be roughly grouped into two major complexes, the internal hemorrhoidal and the external hemorrhoidal networks. While these channels anastomose freely, most drainage from the external system is into the vena cava by way of the iliac veins, while drainage from the internal hemorrhoidal system is into the portal system through the inferior mesenteric vein. This richly anastomotic network thus provides an excellent collateral route for return of portal blood to the systemic circulation in patients with portal hypertension and accounts for the common presence of distended anorectal veins (hemorrhoids) in such patients.

Clinically, one sees patients with internal or external hemorrhoids, or both. External hemorrhoids are covered with skin, and rarely rupture. They tend, rather, to develop thrombotic clots, followed by phlebitis. The clots are probably caused by venous stasis resulting from spasm of the anal sphincters. The resulting inflammation is acutely painful and is greatly aggravated by defecation. Internal hemorrhoids, on the other hand, are covered with mucosa and rarely thrombose. With time they tend to enlarge, and to prolapse through the anal sphincter with defecation or spontaneously. They often rupture, and may bleed slightly or heavily. Very often, patients will note fresh blood on the toilet tissue, and a tendency for pure blood to spurt from the anal canal upon straining to defecate.

Treatment of internal hemorrhoids involves the use of bulking agents to soften and enlarge stools. Local applications of heat tend to relax anal sphincters, and suppositories containing aluminum paste and cocoa butter are emollient and slightly astringent. Patients must be carefully instructed in the use of suppositories. Although physicians may think it fatuous to suggest that suppositories should be unwrapped before insertion into the anal canal, they must also remember that even fairly sophisticated patients may not be aware of this. The importance of full insertion should also be mentioned, since suppositories will not remain in the anal canal and must, therefore, be pushed inward until they are felt to rise into the rectum. Local treatment with daily warm baths and suppositories for a period of two weeks usually stops bleeding, while the use of bulking agents reduces prolapse. A diet high in fiber should be followed permanently. Surgical removal of hemorrhoids is indicated only when these simpler efforts fail to control symptoms or to prevent prompt relapses. Freezing of hemorrhoids with a probe cooled by liquid nitrogen or ligation or hemorrhoids with rubber bands have been shown to be less painful than extirpative surgery and to require less convalescence.

External hemorrhoids are best managed by bulking agents, and careful attention to anal hygiene. Small flannel pads soaked in witch hazel are often useful as astringent cleansing agents. Painful thrombosed hemorrhoids can be immediately relieved by local anesthesia, followed by incision of the hemorrhoid and removal of the contained thrombus.

One must be cautioned, prior to attributing rectal bleeding to hemorrhoids, that a complete sigmoidoscopy should also be done to exclude other disorders, especially cancer of the colon, colonic polyps, and colitis, which may also cause this symptom. I am most happy about making the diagnosis when an actual hemorrhoidal bleeding point can be demonstrated on anoscopy, and when stool taken from above the site is negative for occult blood. If any doubt remains after endoscopy, a barium enema should always be performed.

Anal fissures. These are painful inflammatory tears in the anal mucosa overlying the internal anal sphincter. Nothmann and Schuster (1974) have shown that the rectoanal inhibitory reflex response to rectal distention reveals normal relaxation of the upper anal canal in patients with anal fissures, but that a much stronger than normal contraction appears after this relaxation response. This abnormality tends to disappear with healing and may well be a result of the fissure rather than a cause. A history of constipation and straining at stool is common among these patients.

Treatment is similar to that for internal hemorrhoids, except that suppositories containing small amounts of hydrocortisone may speed healing. Where these measures are not effective, surgical excision of the fissure is usually indicated, although some success has attached to doing partial myotomies of the internal sphincter. Perianal abscesses and fistulas may occur as a complication of untreated and inflamed anal fissures.

Rectal Prolapse. This is a very troublesome disorder associated with diminished sensitivity to rectal distention, decreased contractility of the pelvic muscles involved in defecation, diminished muscular tone, and reduced sphincteric tone in response to distention of the anal canal (Schuster 1975). In a form of intussusception, small or large portions of the rectum and sigmoid protrude through the anal canal; patients are often incontinent of stool and frequently complain of bleeding and discharge from the prolapsed tissue. The disorder may occur in infants, where it has been attributed to the lack of proper angulation at the anorectal junction, a problem which cures itself with growth. Rectal prolapse becomes a major problem, however, among the elderly, and the only effective long-term therapy involves an abdominal surgical procedure in which the rectum is first mobilized and then sutured to the sacrum.

Pruritus Ani. This is probably not a complication of constipation but is often associated with it. It may result from poor anal hygiene, from the presence of slight anal incontinence in persons with internal hemorrhoids or fissures, from sweating and maceration of tissues in the perianal area, or from specific infections, as with pinworms or cutaneous fungi. Most patients respond well to scrupulous cleansing with witch hazel or other lotions, and occasionally to low-strength glucocorticoid creams. If pinworms or mycotic infections are demonstrated, they, of course, should be treated specifically.

HISTORICAL DIGRESSION

Proper names referred to in this chapter without citation include: Carlos CHAGAS (1879–1934), Brazilian bacteriologist, Rio de Janeiro, described diseases due to *Trypanosoma cruzi* in 1916; Theodor ESCHERICH (1857–1911), Austrian pediatrician, Graz and Vienna, enteric bacteria named in his honor by Castellani and Chalmers, 1919; Harald HIRSCHSPRUNG (1830–1916), Danish physician, Copenhagen, described congenital megacolon in 1886; Daniel Elmer SALMON (1850–1914), American pathologist and veterinarian, Washington, D.C., organisms named in his honor, 1900; Kiyoshi SHIGA (1870–1957), Japanese bacteriologist, Tokyo, organisms named in his honor, 1919; William Henry WELCH (1850–1934), American pathologist, Baltimore, described vector of gas gangrene with H.F. Nuttall in 1892; and Alexandre Émile Jean YERSIN (1863–1943), Swiss bacteriologist working in Vietnam.

SELECTED REFERENCES

Almy TP, Kern Jr F, Tulin M. Alterations in colonic function in man under stress. II. Experimental production of sigmoid spasm in healthy persons. Gastroenterology 12:425–36, 1949.

Banwell G, Sherr H. Effect of bacterial enterotoxins on the gastrointestinal tract. Gastroenterology 65:467–97, 1973.

Bartlett JG. Postantibiotic diarrhea. Pract Gastroent 4:23–27, 1980.

Bartlett JG, Gorbach SL. Pseudomembranous enterocolotis (antibiotic-related colitis). Adv Int Med 22:455–76, 1977.

Binder HJ. Net fluid and electrolyte secretion: the pathophysiologic basis of diarrhea. Viewpoints Dig Dis 12:1–6, (Mar.) 1980.

Blacklow NR, Cukor G. Viral gastroenteritis, N Engl J Med 304:397–406, 1981.

Blake PA, Allegra DT, Snyder JD, et al. Cholera, a possible endemic focus in the United States. New Engl J Med 302:305–9, 1980.

Blaser MJ, Berkowitz ID, LaForce FM, et al. Campylobacter enteritis: clinical and epidemiological features. Ann Int Med 91:179–85, 1979.

Buebler E, Juan H. Effect of ricinoleic acid and other laxatives on net water flux and prostaglandin E release by the rat colon. J Pharmacol 31:681–85, 1979.

Burbige EJ, Milligan FD. Pseudomembranous colitis. Association with antibiotics and therapy with cholestyramine. JAMA 231:1157–58, 1975.

Burkitt DP. Dietary fibre and "pressure diseases." J R Coll Physicians Lond 9:138–47, 1975.

Charney AN, Gots RE, Formal SB, et al. Activation of intestinal mucosal adenylate cyclase by *Shigella dysenteriae* I enterotoxin. Gastroenterology 70:1085–90, 1976.

Christensen J, Anuras S, Hauser RL. Migrating spike bursts and electrical slow waves in the cat colon: effect of sectioning. Gastroenterology 66:240–47, 1974.

Corazziari E, Dani S, Pozzessere C, et al. Colonic segmental transit time in non-organic constipation. In: Vantrappen G, ed. Proceedings of the Fifth International Symposium on Gastrointestinal Motility. Herentals, Belgium: Typoff-Press, 1975:425–28.

DeCosse JJ, Rhodes RS, Wentz WB, et al. The natural history and management of radiation induced injury of the gastrointestinal tract. Ann Surg 170:369–84, 1969.

Devroede G, Soffié M. Colonic absorption in idiopathic constipation. Gastroenterology 64:552–61, 1973.

Drossman DA, Powell DW, Sessions JT, Jr. The irritable bowel syndrome. Gastroenterology 73:811–22, 1977.

Duhamel B. Une nouvelle opération pour le mégacolon congénital: l'abaissement rétrorectal et trans-anal du colon, et son application possible au traitement de quelques autres malformations. Presse Med 64:2249–50, 1956.

Dworken HJ, Biel FJ, Machella TE. Supradiaphragmatic reference of pain from the colon. Gastroenterology 22:222–31, 1952.

Edelman R, Levine MM. Acute diarrheal infections in infants. II. Bacterial and viral causes. Hosp Pract 15:97–104, 1980.

Esler MD, Goulston KJ. Levels of anxiety in colonic disorders. New Engl J Med 288:16–20, 1973.

George WL, Rolfe RD, Finegold SM. Treatment and prevention of antimicrobial agent-induced colitis and diarrhea. Gastroenterology 79:366–72, 1980.

George WL, Volpicelli NA, Stiner DN, et al. Relapse of pseudomembranous colitis after vancomycin therapy. New Engl J Med 301:414–15, 1979.

Gill DM, Richardson SH. Adenosine diphosphate—ribosylation of adenylate cyclase catalyzed by heat-labile enterotoxin of *Escherichia coli:* comparison with cholera toxin. J Infect Dis 141:64–70, 1980.

Grady GF, Keusch GT. Pathogenesis of bacterial diarrheas. New Engl J Med 285:831–41, 891–900, 1971.

Ivey KJ. Are anticholinergics of use in the irritable bowel syndrome? Gastroenterology 68:1300–7, 1975.

Latimer P, Sarna S, Campbell D et al: Colonic motor and myoelectrical activity: a comparative study of normal subjects, psychoneurotic patients, and patients with irritable bowel syndrome. Gastroenterology 80:893–901, 1981.

Leino R, Kalliomäki JL. Yersiniosis as an internal disease. Ann Intern Med 81:458–61, 1974.

LoIudice T, Baxter D, Balint J. Effects of abdominal surgery on the development of radiation enteropathy. Gastroenterology 73:1093–97, 1977.

Loss Jr RW, Mangla JC, Pereira M. *Campylobacter* colitis presenting as inflammatory bowel disease with segmental colonic ulcerations. Gastroenterology 79:138–40, 1980.
Martelli H, Devroede G, Arhan P, et al. Some parameters of large bowel motility in normal man. Gastroenterology 75:612–18, 1978.
Martelli H, Devroede G, Arhan P, et al. Mechanisms of idiopathic constipation: outlet obstruction. Gastroenterology 75:623–31, 1978.
Mendeloff AI, Monk M, Siegel CI, et al. Illness experience and life stresses in patients with irritable colon and with ulcerative colitis. An epidemiological study of ulcerative colitis and regional enteritis in Baltimore, 1960–1964. New Engl J Med 282:14–17, 1970.
Merson MH, Morris GK, Sack DA, et al. Travelers' diarrhea and toxigenic *Escherichia coli.* New Engl J Med 292:933–36, 1975.
Moss J, Vaughn M. Mechanism of action of choleragen. Evidence of ADP-ribosyl transferase activity with arginine as an acceptor. J Biol Chem 252:2455–57, 1977.
Nothmann BJ, Schuster MM. Internal anal sphincter derangement with anal fissure. Gastroenterology 67:216–20, 1974.
Okamoto E, Veda T. Embryogenesis of intramural ganglia of the gut and its relation to Hirschsprung's disease. J Pediat Surg 2:437–43, 1967.
Parks TG. The effects of low and high residue diets on the rate of transit and composition of faeces. In: Daniel EE, ed. Proceedings of the Fourth International Symposium on Gastrointestinal Motility. Vancouver: Mitchell Press, 1974:369–79.
Phillips SF. Evaluation of patients with chronic diarrhea. Pract Gastroent 4: 13–19, 1980.
Pittman FE. Intestinal amebiasis. Pract Gastroent 4:33–39, 1980.
Read NW, Krejs GJ, Read MG, et al. Chronic diarrhea of unknown origin. Gastroenterology 78:264–71, 1980.
Ritchie J. Pain from distention of the pelvic colon by inflating a balloon in the irritable colon syndrome. Gut 14:125–32, 1973.
Robert A, Nezamis JE, Lancaster C, et al. Prevention through cytoprotection of clindamycin-induced colitis in hamsters with 16,16-dimethyl PGE_2. Gastroenterology 78:1245, 1980.
Sack RB, Froelich JL, Zulich AW, et al. Prophylactic doxycycline for travelers' diarrhea. Results of a prospective double-blind study of Peace Corps volunteers in Morocco. Gastroenterology 76:1368–73, 1979.
Schreiber DS, Trier JS, Blacklow NR. Recent advances in viral gastroenteritis. Gastroenterology 73:174–83, 1977.
Schuster MM. The riddle of the sphincters. Gastroenterology 69:249–62, 1975.
Smith B. Myenteric plexus in Hirschsprung's disease. Gut 8:308–12, 1967.
Snape WJ, Jr, Carlson GM, Matarazzo SA. Evidence that abnormal myoelectrical activity produces colonic motor dysfunction in the irritable bowel syndrome. Gastroenterology 72:383–87, 1977.

Stevens DP. Giardiasis. Clinical presentation, diagnosis and treatment. Pract Gastroent 4:23–28, 1980.

Sullivan MA, Cohen S, Snape WJ, Jr. Colonic myoelectrical activity in the irritable bowel syndrome: Effect of eating and anticholinergics. New Engl J Med 298:878–83, 1978.

Swenson O. A new surgical treatment for Hirschsprung's disease. Surgery 28:371–83, 1950.

Switz DM. What the gastroenterologist does all day. A survey of a state society's practice. Gastroenterology 70:1048–50, 1976.

Taylor I, Duthie HL, Smallwood R, et al. Human large bowel myoelectrical activity. In: Vantrappen G, ed. Proceedings of the Fifth International Symposium on Gastrointestinal Motility. Belgium: Typoff-Press, Herentals, 1975:429–33.

Tedesco FJ. Clindamycin-associated colitis. Am J Dig Dis 21:26–31, 1976.

Thompson WG, Heaton KW. Functional bowel disorders in apparently healthy people. Gastroenterology 79:283–88, 1980.

Trier JS, Browning TH: Morphologic response of the mucosa of human small intestine to x-ray exposure. J Clin Invest 45:194–204, 1966.

Trowell H. Fibre and irritable bowels. Br Med J 3:44, 1974.

Ulshen MH, Rollo JL. Pathogenesis of *Escherichia coli* gastroenteritis in man —another mechanism. New Engl J Med 302:99–191, 1980.

Warren S, Friedman NB. Pathology and pathologic diagnosis of radiation lesions in the gastro-intestinal tract. Am J Pathol 18:499–514, 1942.

Wenman WM, Hinde D, Feltham S, et al. Rotavirus infection in adults. Results of a prospective family study. New Engl J Med 301:303–6, 1979.

DISCUSSION QUESTION

A 102-member symphony orchestra from a large industrial city in the northern United States is preparing to embark on a concert tour of New Orleans, Mexico, and Central America for three weeks. All members will lodge in the same hotels in each city, but aside from the 15 concerts, several receptions, and a number of master classes, they will be left to their own devices much of the time. As the orchestra physician, you are asked to provide instructions for preventing enteric infections and to supply yourself with symptomatic and therapeutic medications. Describe what your instructions would be, what diagnostic equipment you would need to have available, and what medications you would carry.

CHAPTER 17

Inflammatory Bowel Disease

How to delineate the pathophysiology of two idiopathic diseases usually distinct, but at times indistinguishable from one another, and about which so much is known and so much is dubitable? Their very names, Crohn disease and chronic ulcerative colitis, evoke clear images in the minds of physicians who are alive to these disorders, but students must be understandably dismayed when they learn that the term *Crohn disease* includes much more than the "regional ileitis" which Crohn, Ginzburg, and Oppenheimer described in 1932, and that *ulcerative colitis*, in most cases, presents to the percipient sigmoidoscopist with an erythematous, edematous, excessively friable mucosa, that is not ulcerated! The answers lie in the fact that Crohn disease is a term of convenience used to describe a disorder associated with dense lymphocytic infiltration of the entire thickness of the affected bowel, blockage and dilatation of lymphatics, thickening of the mesentery and hyperplasia of regional lymph nodes, and often granuloma formation, similar to the lesions identified in the original patients, but capable of much more widespread intestinal distribution than was originally thought to be the case; and that colitis may indeed ulcerate but is now recognizable and treatable long before gross ulcerations occur.

Each disease, it is generally agreed, may be caused by more than a single agent, mediators which may be transmissible, especially in cases of Crohn disease, but are currently unknown. The inflammatory reactions and the clinical pictures are clearly distinguishable from one another at each end of a spectrum, but in the middle of the scale, ah, that is where nature confuses and distinction may present a problem. This, plus the fact that both diseases progress slowly and may first be diagnosed in early stages before completely manifesting themselves, led Schacter and Kirsner (1975) in attempting to establish definitions of these two diseases to caution that "all patients with inflammatory bowel disease should be reviewed periodically — to monitor diagnostic accuracy and to facilitate diagnostic revision where appropriate."

One may conclude that in most instances Crohn disease and chronic ulcerative colitis can be clearly recognizable for what they are. Thus, when the inflammatory process involves one or more lengthy segments of small intestine, whether or not the right side of the colon is also diseased, the process is clearly that of Crohn disease. When the process occupies the rectum and progresses proximally into short or long segments of the colon in one continuous segment of involvement, while sparing all or a part of the right colon and all of the small intestine, it is almost certainly ulcerative colitis. Distinction is blurred primarily in those patients with inflammatory disease of the entire colon and rectum and in a few patients with distal colonic disease alone. Fortunately for diagnostic accuracy, this group makes up no more than 10 to 15 percent of all patients with chronic inflammatory bowel disease.

INCIDENCE AND DISTRIBUTION

The incidence of Crohn disease, especially those cases with more extensive involvement of the intestine than the terminal ileum alone, appears to be increasing in the United States and western Europe, while the incidence of ulcerative colitis is remaining stationary or declining somewhat. Because both diseases are essentially incurable and not highly lethal, the prevalence rates are high. Miller et al (1974) noted a threefold increase in hospital admission rates for patients with Crohn disease in the United Kingdom from 1958 to 1971, and estimate an annual incidence of between 3.0 and 5.0 new cases per 100,000 population per year. Most investigators agree that the greatest incidence of new cases occurs in the second to fourth decades of life, especially between ages 10 and 20, and Gryboski and Spiro (1978) note that the number of children and adolescents seen at one hospital during 1955 to 1965 exceeded the entire patient population with newly diagnosed Crohn disease seen during the previous decade. Where data are available, the prevalence rates of Crohn disease appear to vary from a low of 12 to 15 cases per 100,000 in Israel to a high of 75 cases in Malmo (Rozen et al 1979). In many societies, especially in underdeveloped parts of the world, Crohn disease is essentially nonexistent.

The average annual incidence rate for chronic ulcerative colitis is also variable in different parts of the world, ranging from a low of 3.6 cases per 100,000 in Tel Aviv to a high of 7.3 in Copenhagen (Gilat et al 1974). Prevalence ranges from 37 to 87 cases per 100,000. Peak incidence rates appear to occur in the third decade, and most studies also show a smaller peak in the sixth decade. The cause of this secondary peak is not clear. It may be due to the appearance with aging of a lesion similar to that of ulcerative colitis but resulting from a different cause, such as ischemia. As with Crohn disease, ulcerative colitis is almost unknown in emergent societies.

In addition to geographical differences in the occurence of these diseases, there are also curious racial distinctions. The frequency of Crohn disease particularly, but also ulcerative colitis, is severalfold greater among

Jews of European extraction than it is among non-Jews and among Jews of African or Oriental descent. Both diseases are quite rare among Orientals, but are not infrequent among American blacks. There is also a distinct familial tendency for Crohn disease, Gryboski and Spiro noting a 22 percent association among first- and second-degree relatives. No clear inheritance has been detected, but the disease occurs commonly among twins, even in one instance in a pair of twins who had been separated shortly after birth, raised in geographically distinct communities, and who had seen each other rarely during childhood and adolescence. Where the disease is present on both sides of a family, the chances for occurrence among offspring are quite likely. Two studies, however, show no distinct HLA profile among patients with Crohn disease (Delpre et al 1980; Eade et al 1980). Familial tendencies also exist for chronic ulcerative colitis, but they do not appear to be as striking as they are in Crohn disease, although Delpre et al did show an association of HLA-BW 35 in over half of 60 Israelis with colitis, and of AW 24 in half of 22 patients with early onset colitis, and in nearly 44 percent of patients with moderate or severe disease. This association did not appear to be related to the ethnic origin of patients. Many studies have shown an almost equal sexual incidence of Crohn disease and a moderate predominance of ulcerative colitis among women and girls.

THE LESIONS

Crohn Disease

While any segment of the alimentary tract may be involved with Crohn disease, including the stomach and esophagus, inflammation is most common in the lowermost portions of the ileum, the cecum, and the ascending colon. Frequently, two or more segments of bowel (skip lesions) are involved simultaneously, separated by lengths of normal intestine. Diseased segments may be as short as a centimeter or two, and as long as a meter or more. With time, the disease may appear in originally spared areas, even though the involved tissue has been already removed surgically.

Gross Appearance. Crohn disease appears to be essentially the same sort of process in both the small intestine and the colon. The bowel wall is thickened in all layers, with a commensurate decrease in the intestinal lumen and increase in intestinal rigidity (Figure 17–1). The serosal surface of the intestine is often partially enveloped by fat and may be hyperemic, edematous, and granular. This chronic visceral peritonitis gives a plastic quality to the surface of the inflamed segment which allows it to adhere to adjoining loops of normal bowel and to other viscera in the neighborhood. This adhesive quality of the peritoneum in Crohn disease leads to spreading

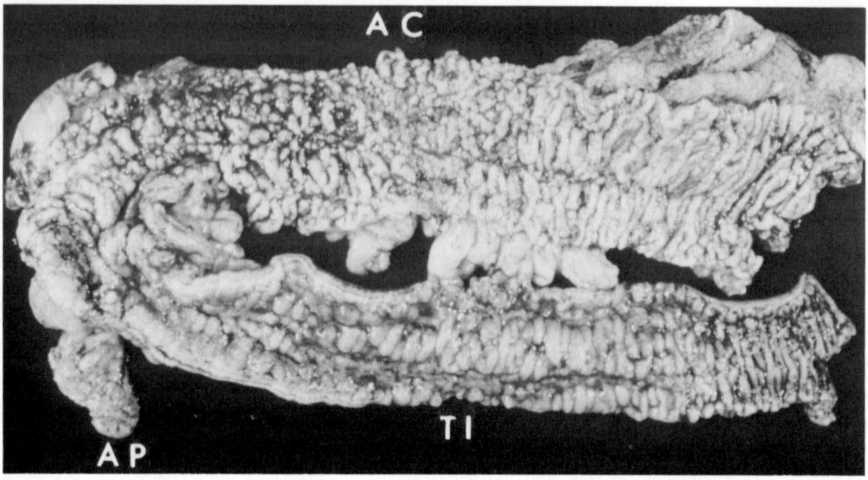

Figure 17–1. Crohn disease. In this ileocolectomy specimen, the terminal ileum (TI) and ascending colon (AC) show a polypoid, cobble-stoned mucosal surface associated with deep longitudinal and transverse ulcerations. The terminal ileum just proximal to the ileocecal valve shows fibrous thickening of the wall and narrowing of the lumen. The appendix (AP) is also involved in the disease process.

of the inflammatory process and to fistulas between diseased and normal bowel or other tissues, such as the urinary bladder, the vagina, and the pelvic wall.

The mucosa in Crohn disease is thickened and nodular; hyperemia and friability are rare. With increased mucosal thickening, the epithelium may burst, producing long, deep fissures in the bowel wall, or large ulcerations. Acute hemorrhage may occur if these fissures or ulcers rupture into an artery or vein. Especially in the colon and rectum, this nodular process may be patchy, with areas of involvement being a few centimeters in diameter and the intervening mucosa appearing normal. This asymmetry of the Crohn lesion serves to distinguish it on both sigmoidoscopy and barium enema from the lesion of ulcerative colitis.

Inflammatory complications in the anal area are common in patients with Crohn disease, especially when portions of the colon are involved. These consist of marked inflammation and hypertrophy of anal papillae, anal fissures, and fistulas, and perianal abscesses. Indeed, cases have been encountered in which only the anal canal is involved with the Crohn process, and the occurrence of these complications, especially among children, should alert physicians to the possibility of this disease. Marked fibrotic strictures of the anus may occur when deep fissures heal.

The mesentery in diseased areas is also thickened and heavily laden with fat. Mesenteric lymph nodes are firm and greatly swollen. As is also the case in the bowel itself, the transition from diseased to normal mesentery is quite abrupt.

Microscopic Appearance. The lesion of Crohn disease demonstrates that the transmural thickening is the result of a dense infiltration of all layers of the bowel by lymphocytes and plasma cells, and of secondary obstruction of lymphatics by the inflammatory process (Figure 17-2). Lymphocytes contain prominent nucleoli; plasma cells are often hypertrophied, and mast cells may be increased. The infiltrate is usually greatest in the lamina propria, and as these accumulations increase in density, ulcerations are formed by disruption of the epithelium. Occasionally, abscesses may be seen in the crypts of Lieberkuhn, but these are not nearly as prominent as in ulcerative colitis. Fissures may penetrate from the epithelial ulcers into or through the bowel wall.

Much attention has been given to the fact that well over half of resected bowel segments in Crohn disease contain well-developed, noncaseating granulomas, whose presence almost completely distinguish the lesion

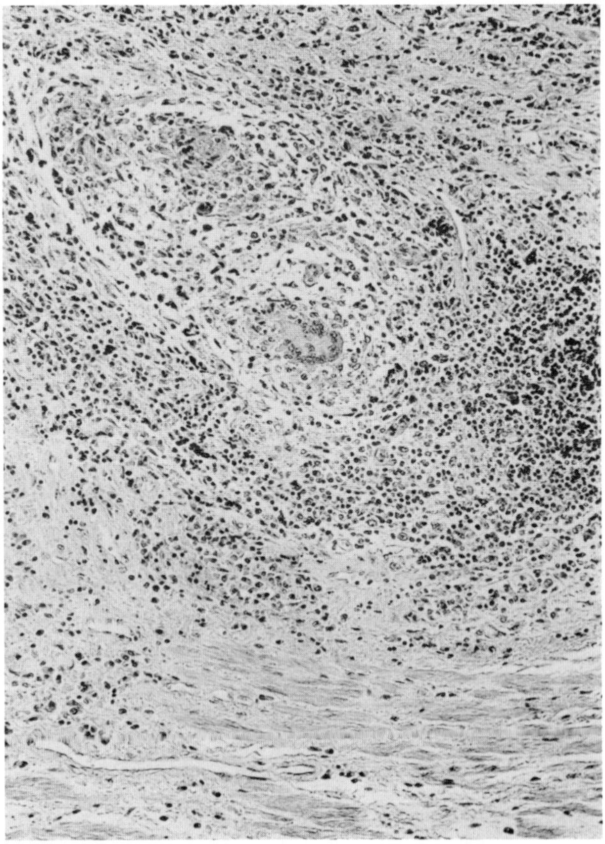

Figure 17-2. Crohn disease. The presence of noncaseating sarcoidlike granulomatous inflammation consisting of multinucleated giant cells, epithelioid cells, plasma cells, and lymphocytes in the submucosa of the small intestine is diagnostic for this disease. Original magnification x120.

from that of ulcerative colitis. These granulomas consist of giant cells and epithelioid cells and resemble those seen in sarcoidosis. They are also frequently present in regional lymph nodes, along with large lymphocytes. The presence of granulomas suggests a tissue response to antigen-antibody complexes, just as the prevalence of lymphocytes and plasma cells suggests a mighty immunological reaction.

Ulcerative Colitis

Cross Appearance. When viewing the lesion of active ulcerative colitis at surgery or through the sigmoidoscope, one is most impressed with the active bleeding tendency of the mucosa, a tendency which is either present initially or can be elicited with very gentle rubbing by a cotton pledget. This process is known as "friability." In nonbleeding areas, the mucosa is hyperemic and edematous. In the rectum, one is unable to see the prominent tracery of submucosal veins that is normally present. The surface of the mucosa is also granular and has lost its usually glistening appearance. Rectal valves, which are usually sharp and pliant, become thickened, blunted, narrower, and more rigid. The inflammatory process is pervasive and not patchy, and it almost invariably commences at the mucocutaneous junction of the anal canal. The proximal extent of the lesion is variable; it may be confined to the rectum alone (ulcerative proctitis), it may extend as far as the cecum, or it may stop at any level of the colon. But regardless of the extent of the disease, the process is always contiguous; skip lesions do not occur, and the rectum is always involved. Ulcerations are very common, although they are not invariable, and their size varies from tiny to very large (Figure 17–3). The disease involves the mucosa primarily and is transmural in only the most

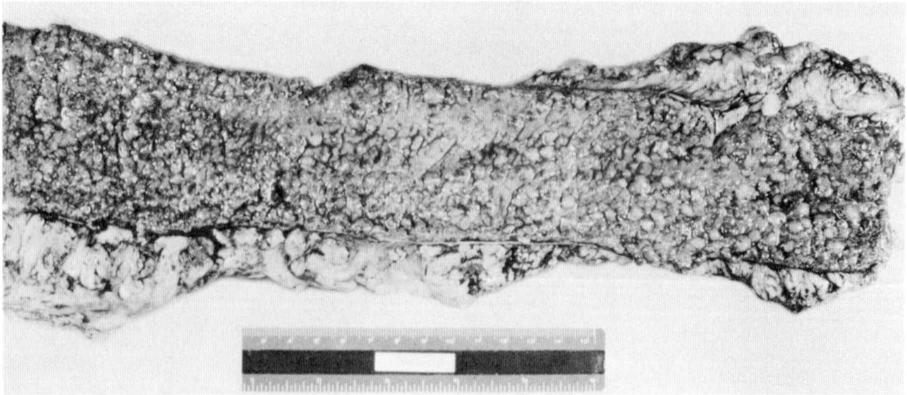

Figure 17–3. Chronic ulcerative colitis, showing diffuse mucosal ulcerations, mucosal bleeding, and multiple polypoid nodules (pseudopolyps).

severe cases. The bowel wall is not thickened as it is in Crohn disease, and, while the colon may be narrowed and haustrations destroyed by scarring, the marked luminal constriction so common in Crohn disease is not seen.

Severe perianal disease and anal strictures are most uncommon in patients with chronic ulcerative colitis, although hemorrhoids are fairly frequent. The presence of anal fistulas, abscesses, or deep fissures in patients with inflammatory proctitis is most suggestive of Crohn disease.

Microscopic Appearance. The earliest lesion of chronic ulcerative colitis is best seen by examining grossly normal-appearing bowel immediately proximal to the inflammatory area (Lumb 1961). This lesion consists of nuclear degeneration and cytoplasmic vacuoles in columnar epithelium at the base of mucosal crypts plus plugging of the crypt lumina by "polymorphonuclear leukocytes with a surrounding mild degree of capillary dilatation and infiltration of the lamina propria with lymphocytes." These *crypt abscesses* are almost diagnostic of ulcerative colitis. Goblet cells are reduced in number. Ulcerations develop when tissue lymphocytes break through the epithelial membrane and coalesce as adjacent crypts become involved. The disease is primarily confined to the mucosa, although submucosal vessels may also be dilated (Figure 17–4). In patients with advanced disease (toxic megacolon), the inflammatory process does indeed extend into the submucosa and muscularis, and spontaneous perforations of the colon may actually occur.

ETIOLOGICAL COGITATIONS

While various viruses, cell-wall defective bacteria, and autoimmunity have all been implicated in the pathogenesis of chronic inflammatory bowel diseases, no single agent has been found to be responsible for either Crohn disease or ulcerative colitis. The probability today is that these cytopathic agents "are at least as likely to be present as superinfections rather than as etiologic agents" (Gitnick 1980), and that both diseases are the result of adverse immunological reactions to tissues altered by a variety of possible exogenous agents. Let us examine some of the evidence.

Crohn Disease. Proportional studies of the lymphocyte population in inflammatory tissue indicates that there is a relative decrease in IgA-containing cells, and a relative increase in cells containing IgG and IgM (Kraft 1978). Cultures of these lymphocytes show that the proportion of B-cells is increased, null cells decreased, and T-cells about the same as normal. But Britton et al (1978) have shown that a large proportion of these T-cells, at least in regional lymph nodes of Crohn disease specimens, have receptors which are capable of binding with the Fc portion of IgG and of lysing target cells coated with antibody, and can thus be classified as "killer" T-cells. There is also some evidence that circulating lymphocytes show increased

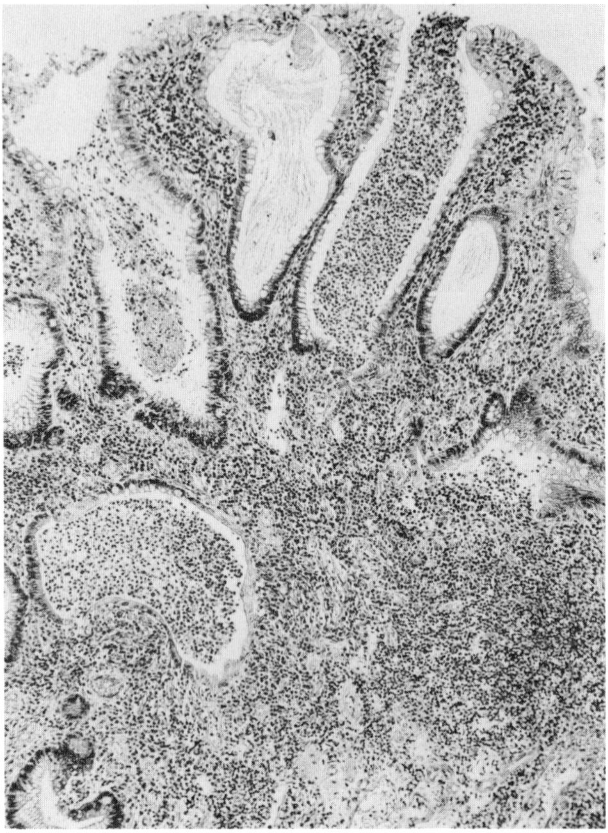

Figure 17–4. Chronic ulcerative colitis, during the active phase. Crypt abscesses, hyperemia, and lymphocytic infiltration are prominent. Crypt abscesses are colonic glands filled with neutrophils. The lining cells undergo degeneration and necrosis leading to ruture of the glands and mucosal ulceration. Original magnification x80.

proportions of killer cells, but how these cells are generated is not clear. It is postulated that some foreign agent, a virus, a cell-wall defective bacteria, or a chemical constituent in intestinal contents, somehow modifies tissue cell receptors and causes these cells to be perceived as foreign by the patient's own lymphocytes. This alteration in perception probably involves a change in the major histocompatibility complex, and invokes proliferation of lymphocytes, especially of T-cells and plasma cells, coating of the altered antigen by cellular antibodies, and subsequent lysis by killer cells. Such a process could easily be self-perpetuating, even if all grossly diseased tissue has been removed, since sensitized cells may remain after surgery. Beginning with Mitchell and Rees (1970), a number of investigators have shown that filtrates of Crohn disease tissue may indeed cause granulomatous inflammatory reactions in certain laboratory animals, but not all have been able to substantiate this reaction. It is possible that Crohn disease may be caused at times by a transmissible agent and at other times by nontransmissible factors. Certainly, no single agent has come to the fore; this has led Mayberry et al (1980) to proclaim that if there is a single agent, it "is either very unusual, particularly difficult to culture, or does not exist!"

Ulcerative Colitis

It is now felt that altered immunogenicity is also the most likely cause of ulcerative colitis. The route to this conclusion has been circuitous primarily because, for so very long, this disease had been felt by so many to have a basically psychogenic origin. This thinking was a classic example of putting the cart in front of the horse. Many patients with active ulcerative colitis are indeed querulous, sullen, anxious, and depressed, but who would not be equally ill-humored when assaulted by a prolonged disorder causing continuous tenesmus, rectal bleeding, abdominal cramps, and malaise, and for which the results of treatment are unpredictable? My own faith in the psychogenic theory was lost when, as a young practitioner, I began to note how pleasant and "normal" patients with ulcerative colitis become when their disease is treated successfully. A recent study by Alpers et al (1980) confirms the fact that psychiatric disease is not more prevalent in colitis patients than it is in matched controls, although it appears to be an increased problem among patients with Crohn disease.

Credit for suggesting the existence of altered immunity in patients with ulcerative colitis should go to Broberger and Perlmann (1959), who showed that the number of ulcerative colitic patients who demonstrated circulating antibodies to colonic epithelial cells was much greater than the number of controls with the same antibody, and that differences were highly significant. While these observations have been amply confirmed by others, most investigators feel that the demonstrated antibodies and the associated cytotoxic lymphocytes in colitis lesions are secondary to a more basic mechanism. Two contemporary studies have succeeded in producing the histologic and gross lesions of ulcerative colitis in laboratory animals by the use of dinitrochlorobenzene (DNCB), a contact agent producing T-cell-mediated delayed hypersensitivity. In the one (Rabin and Rogers 1978), rabbits were skin sensitized to DNCB and, 10 days later, challenged by rectal instillations of a weak solution of the same agent. Within 2 days, typical colitic lesions appeared, complete with crypt abscesses, epithelial disarray, capillary dilatation, and ulcerations. The lesions heals within a bit more than a month, provided that no further DNCB is given, and continue when the challenge is administered repeatedly. Colitic animals also develop periportal hepatic infiltrates, a lesion commonly encountered in human colitis, and eventually develop delayed tissue immunity to colon antigens as well. This latter phenomenon was demonstrated by the observation of inflammatory reactions to extracts of rabbit colon injected intracutaneously in colitic animals. The authors conclude that chronic colitis could theoretically result from the presence in the colon of any antigen to which the subject has been previously sensitized, and would continue as long as the antigen remained. Humoral immunity appears to have little if any role in the cause of ulcerative colitis, since the presence of, or the administration of, colonic antibodies does not cause colitis in either humans or laboratory animals.

The other study (Askenase et al 1978) is even more exciting, since DNCB was shown to cause colitis in guinea pigs by repeated intrarectal instillations without previous cutaneous sensitization. Some of these animals, however, did not develop the systemic sensitization found in the first study. Streilein (1978) points out that the number of antigens that are potentially able to cause this colitic reaction is legion and suggests that T-lymphocytes can perceive self-tissues as foreign and initiate an immune reaction, once "the host's own major histocompatibility complex cell surface determinants — have been modified by virus or reactive small molecules."

Many questions remain to be answered. What are the causative antigens? How can they be eliminated? Why do some colons respond to the antigens while other do not? Is it possible that responsivity is evanescent, being greater at times of stress and less during repose? But, while searching for the answers to these and other related questions, physicians can be fairly well assured that at least some of the pathophysiology of chronic ulcerative colitis is now clarified.

SYMPTOMS AND SIGNS

Crohn Disease

Normal physiology is subverted in diverse ways by Crohn disease — inflammation, obstruction, decreased absorptive surface, fissurization of the intestinal wall, and fistulization to the skin or to neighboring viscera. Symptoms depend on the site of the intestinal involvement and on the extent and chronicity of the inflammation.

Acute Crohn disease commonly causes fever, especially if an abscess has formed in or around a diseased segment. Since the terminal ileum and cecum are frequent early sites of the disease, patients may complain of midabdominal pain that shifts to the lower right quadrant when the parietal peritoneum becomes involved, a picture that may be virtually indistinguishable from that of acute appendicitis. On examination, lower right quadrant tenderness and occasionally muscular rigidity are present, and a small mass may be palpable. Moderate leukocytosis is also found. Preexisting diarrhea and loss of weight suggest Crohn disease rather than appendicitis, but these symptoms may be absent. If the diagnosis of acute Crohn disease is made at surgery, it is usually best to leave the appendix alone, for fear of later fistulization and to submit the patient to a trial of medical therapy.

Obstructive symptoms, consisting of abdominal cramps and distention, particularly after meals, are a result of narrowing of the intestinal lumen by the inflammatory process. This leads to loss of weight, which may often be profound, and to failure of growth and development in children and adolescents. Complete small intestinal obstruction is a recognized complication of chronic Crohn disease and is usually due to marked diminution of the lumen by inflammatory infiltrates and scarring, or to kinking of a normal segment of bowel caught in the inflammatory process extending from an adjacent diseased segment.

Diarrhea is a common symptom of Crohn disease and may be caused by a variety of mechanisms, several of which may coexist in a single patient. Malabsorption of bile salts in the terminal ileum and their bacterial deconjugation in the upper colon is probably the major cause of diarrhea. Decrease in the bile salt pool by this mechanism leads to fat malabsorption in the jejunum by reduction of conjugated jejunal bile acid levels below the critical micellar concentration. The resultant fat malabsorption causes unsaturated fatty acids to enter the colon where they are converted to dihydroxy fatty acids by bacterial action, damage colonic mucosa, and increase colonic secretion. This chronic decrease in bile acid pool also leads to the augmented incidence of cholelithiasis among patients with Crohn disease. In patients with colonic inflammation, diarrhea also results from the inability of the colon to absorb water and electrolytes. When Crohn disease causes strictures in the upper small intestine, bacterial overgrowth occurs and contributes to steatorrhea by deconjugation of bile acids and by leading to villous atrophy. Thus, Crohn disease is a major cause of bile acid and fatty acid diarrhea and of small intestinal panmalabsorption.

Fistulas between loops of bowel may lead to diarrhea by bypassing large segments of intestine. The development of a fistula between intestine and urinary bladder is heralded by the appearance of air and particulate matter in the urine, while other fistulas may lead to the passage of stool through the vagina or into the perineal area.

Bleeding in a chronic form, with resultant iron deficiency, is common among patients with Crohn disease; gross continued bleeding is not. This element often serves to distinguish the disorder from ulcerative colitis, in which gross bleeding is almost always found. Massive acute hemorrhage does occasionally occur in Crohn disease, when intestinal fissures or indolent ulcers erode into large submucosal vessels.

Anal and perianal disorders are common in patients with Crohn disease and also serve to distinguish that disorder from ulcerative colitis. Indolent anal fissures, perianal abscesses, and anal fistulas are hallmarks of Crohn disease and may be the sole or initial lesion. Spontaneous perianal lesions, especially in a child, should prompt radiological studies of the intestine in search of other inflammatory lesions and should be biopsied to determine if granulomatous inflammation is present. The lesion may at times be difficult to distinguish from that of lymphogranuloma venereum, but the relative rarity of the latter disorder makes this an uncommon problem.

The variety and indolence of Crohn disease symptoms accounts, at least in part, for the delay between their onset and the time of diagnosis. In the National (U.S.) Cooperative Crohn's Disease Study of 1,084 patients, the average interval from onset of symptoms to diagnosis was about 35 months (Mekhjian et al 1979). Major symptoms in 569 randomized patients included diarrhea in 92 percent, abdominal pain in 95 percent, loss of weight in 85 percent, fever in 56 percent, lower gastrointestinal bleeding in 41 percent, and perianal disease in 36 percent. Arthritis was present in 19 percent and cutaneous disorders in 5 percent of patients. Thirty-one percent of patients had involvement of the small intestine only, and in nearly half of these that involvement was confined to the terminal ileum. The colon and small intestine were involved simultaneously in 58 percent of patients, and the colon alone in 11 percent. Twenty-two percent of patients had involvement of the colon, terminal ileum, and proximal small bowel, and 6 percent had disease of the entire colon, including the rectum.

Ulcerative Colitis

The pathology of ulcerative colitis delineates the symptoms it produces, their type and severity being proportional to the amount of colon affected by the disease. Passage of blood, either alone or mixed with stool, is a major complaint in almost every case. When inflammation is confined to the rectum and sigmoid colon, passage of blood may be the only symptom. Bowel movements may be formed and no more frequent than usual, although occasionally the edema and spasm of the rectosigmoid acts as a partial obstruction and the patient may actually be constipated. In these cases, large amounts of stool may accumulate in the right and transverse colon. Diarrhea becomes increasingly likely as greater amounts of the colon are involved, as do fever and other complications of colitis, such as hypoalbuminemia and edema as a result of protein loss into the lumen of the colon. Iron deficiency anemia is a common complication of sustained ulcerative colitis.

Frank colonic hemorrhage is occasionally seen in severe ulcerative colitis and may not be responsive to blood replacement and medical therapy. With deep extension of the inflammatory process into the submucosa and muscularis, the colon may dilate markedly, producing the condition called *toxic megacolon*. Patients with this complication are often febrile, dehydrated, hypokalemic, and hypotensive and run a great risk of spontaneous perforation of the colon. Although toxic megacolon may occur in patients with Crohn disease of the colon and in some patients with colitis due to *Entameba histolytica* infection, its occurrence is most common among patients with ulcerative colitis.

Examination of patients with mild colitis may reveal no external abnormalities or may reveal tenderness in the lower abdomen. A distended, tympanitic abdomen, especially when bowel sounds are decreased or absent, raises the suspicion of toxic megacolon. Proctosigmoidoscopy will invariably substantiate the diagnosis by revealing the almost pathognomonic signs of edema and friability of the rectal and sigmoidal mucosa, with or lacking visible ulcerations. Although this examination confirms the diagnosis, it may mislead physicians in appraising the severity of the disease, for colitis is commonly much more severe in areas beyond the reach of the sigmoidoscope than it is in the rectum.

RADIOLOGICAL DIAGNOSIS OF INFLAMMATORY BOWEL DISEASE

All patients suspected of having Crohn disease or ulcerative colitis should have barium contrast studies of the intestinal tract performed, unless they are too ill, liable to bowel perforation, or possibly suffering from intestinal obstruction. In these patients, one commences by taking plain films of the abdomen in anteroposterior and lateral projections. Such films may reveal evidence of megacolon, small bowel obstruction or, by examination of the colonic gas pattern, mucosal changes suggesting inflammatory disease.

Barium contrast studies of the colon should be done with less than the usual amount of preparation if patients are having profuse diarrhea or are partially obstructed. Mild cleansing enemas, or no preparation at all, often permit an adequate examination. The administration of strong laxatives should be postponed until the patient has begun to improve during treatment.

In Crohn disease, areas of inflamed portions of the colon show a nodular, irregular mucosal pattern after evacuation of the barium, transverse and longitudinal ulcerations, asymmetric involvement with one wall being more ulcerated than the opposite side, and frequently no involvement of the rectum (Marshak and Lindner 1976). Skip lesions, intramural abscesses, strictures, and fistulas may also be found. In early cases, numerous tiny ulcers may also be seen (Figure 17-5). The presence of skip lesions and the absence of rectal disease support a diagnosis of Crohn colitis, but with total involvement of the colon, distinction between Crohn and ulcerative colitis may be extremely difficult, especially if the entire small intestine is normal.

In ulcerative colitis, although the disease can be invariably diagnosed by proctosigmoidoscopy, the extent and severity is best estimated by the degree of abnormality found on barium enema. In patients with early colitis or ulcerative proctitis, the barium enema may be normal, although often the rectal lumen can be seen to be displaced anteriorly from the sacrum on lateral projections. Fine serrations along the margins of the barium column represent either small ulcerations or increased collections of mucus. Frank

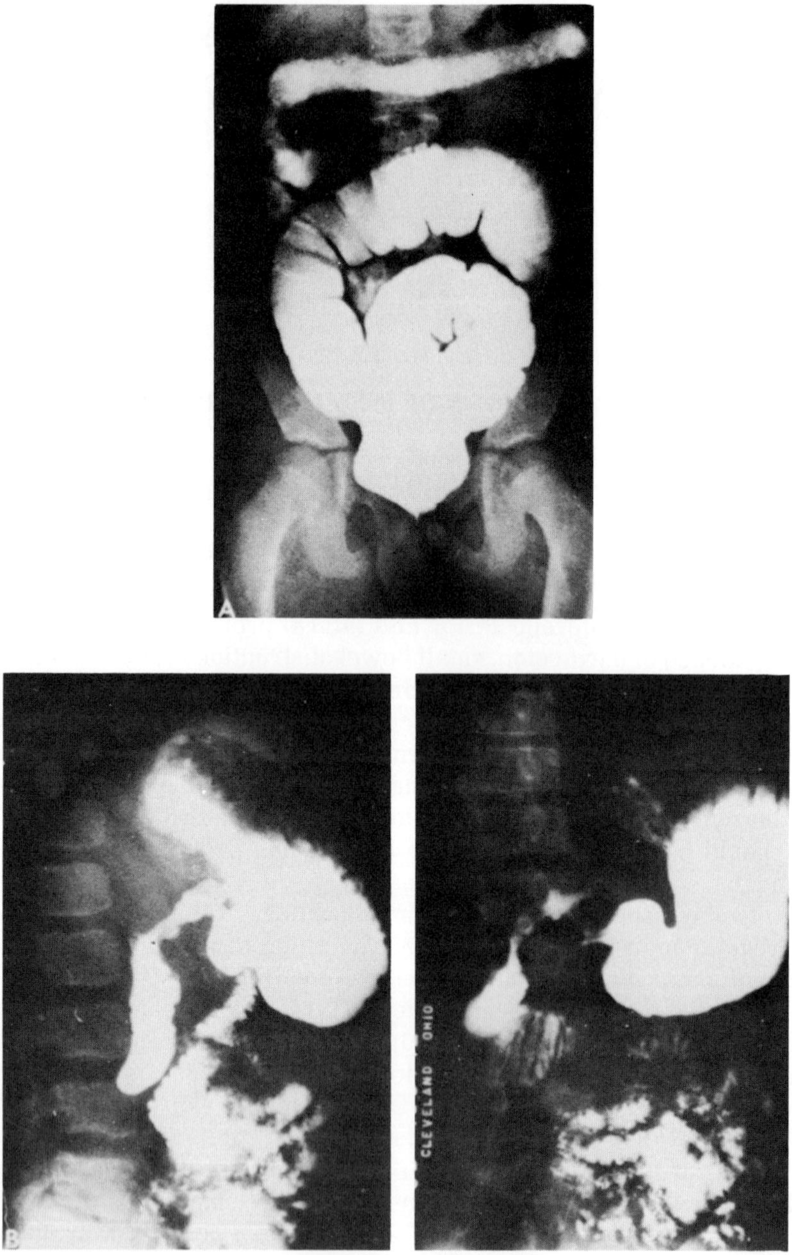

Figure 17-5. Upper and lower bowel X rays in a patient with Crohn disease, showing simultaneous multiple areas of involvement. *A*, barium enema shows extensive disease of the entire colon above the sigmoid. Note the nodular character of the mucosal pattern and the loss of haustrations. *B*, a short segment of disease is also present in the postbulbar area of the duodenum.

ulcerations and pseudopolyps are seen in patients with more severe disease (Figure 17–6). Loss of haustrations, shortening of the colon, and stricture formation represent scarring in the submucosa and muscularis in chronic cases (Figure 17–7). The process always involves the distal colon, though it may be more severe proximally, and the disease is always contiguous, without skip areas.

Crohn disease of the small intestine may occur at any level, from distal stomach to terminal ileum, and has been occasionally reported to occur in the esophagus. Marshak and Lindner (1976) describe nonstenotic and stenotic phases of the Crohn lesion. Early on, there is thickening and flattening of the valvulae conniventes, folds become rigid, and affected areas of intestine lose their normal pliability. The lumens of adjacent loops of intestine become separated as the intestinal wall thickens from inflammation. The mucosa may appear cobblestoned and ulcerated (Figure 17–8). In some areas, all mucosal pattern is lost, save for occasional nodules, and the bowel segment appears sausagelike. In the stenotic stage, the intestinal lumen becomes narrowed and the bowel loops more rigid. Stenotic areas may be quite short or quite extensive. Normal bowel proximal to a stenotic segment may become distended. Numerous stenotic segments may be present along the course of the intestine. Fistulas may also be demonstrable between adjacent loops of bowel, and diseased loops of bowel may be shown at fluoroscopy to be adherent to one another. At times, stenosis may be so marked that only a thin trickle of barium can pass through the diseased segment, giving rise to the characteristic "string sign" of Crohn disease.

NONINTESTINAL MANIFESTATIONS OF INFLAMMATORY BOWEL DISEASE

A number of nonintestinal disorders may accompany inflammatory bowel disease and should be readily recognized by experienced physicians. They are often concomitants of active bowel disease and present no diagnostic problems when patients also have significant intestinal complaints. However, since they may at times be the sole symptoms of inflammatory bowel disease, delay in recognition of the association of the extraintestinal manifestation with possible bowel disease may lead to an unfortunate delay in coming to the proper diagnosis. By and large, these complications occur in both Crohn disease and ulcerative colitis, and most are felt to be immunogenic (altered immunity, circulating antigen-antibody complexes) in origin, although it is not clear why they occur in some patients more than others. Their incidence does not necessarily correlate with the severity of the underlying inflammatory bowel disease. The nonintestinal complications of cutaneous lesions, ocular inflammations, arthritis, and hepatitis occurred either singly or in various combinations among 137 of 569 patients (24 per-

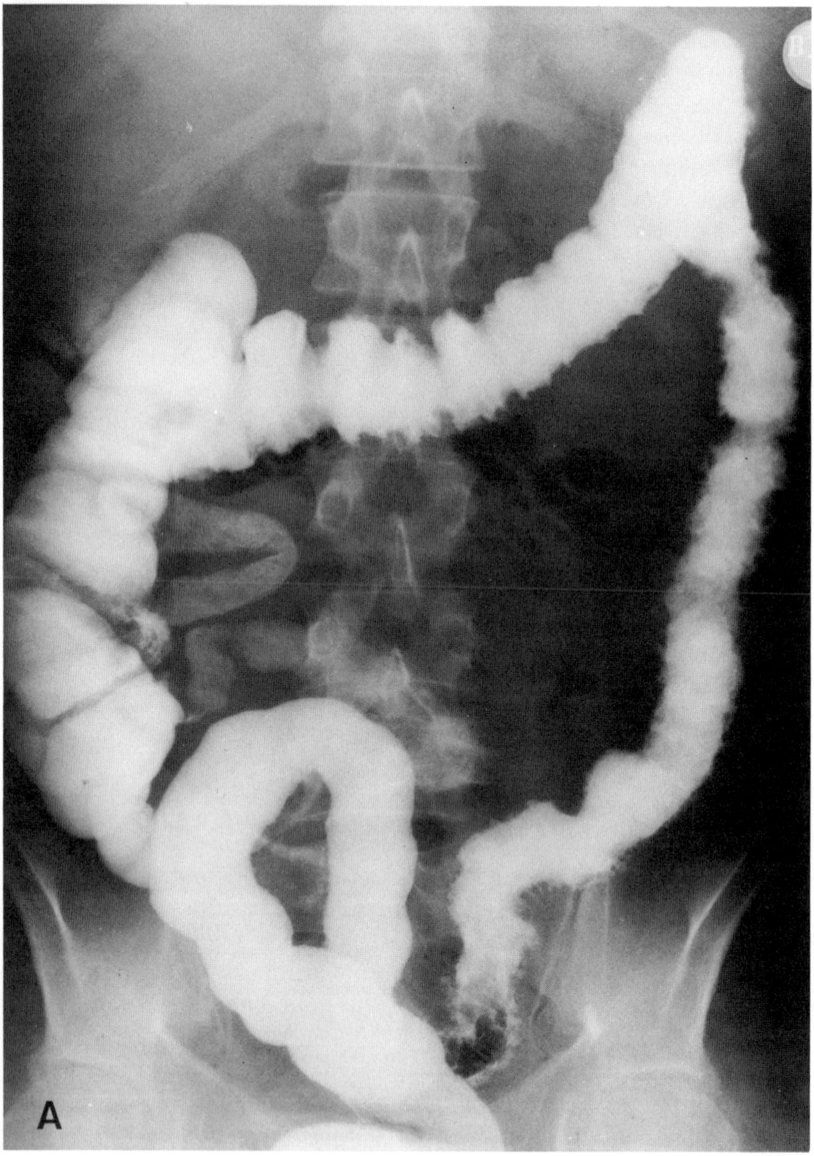

Figure 17-6. Active ulcerative colitis of the entire colon distal to the hepatic flexure. *A*, shows numerous ulcerations in the colon and loss of normal haustral features in the involved portions. *B*, shows diffuse ulcerations in the region of the splenic flexure, and *C* shows extremely deep sigmoidal ulcerations.

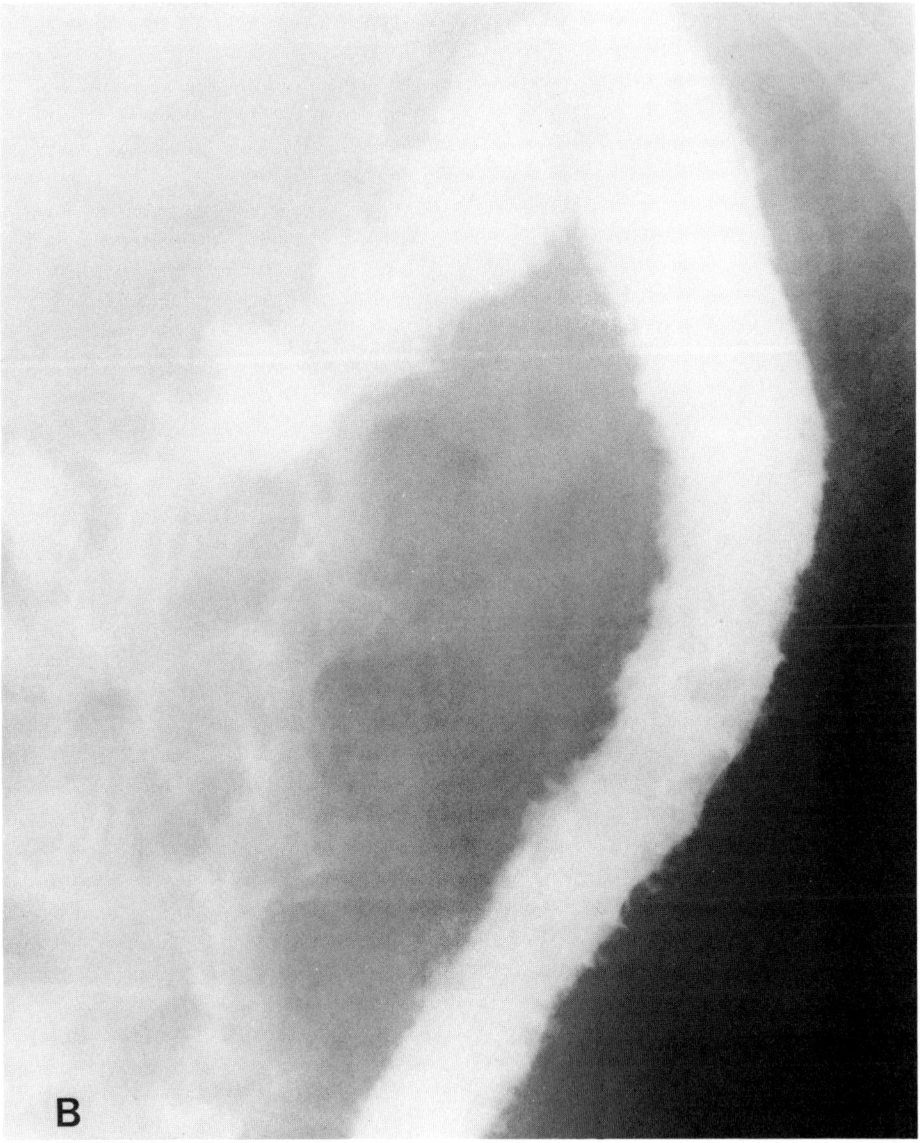

Figure 17-6B.

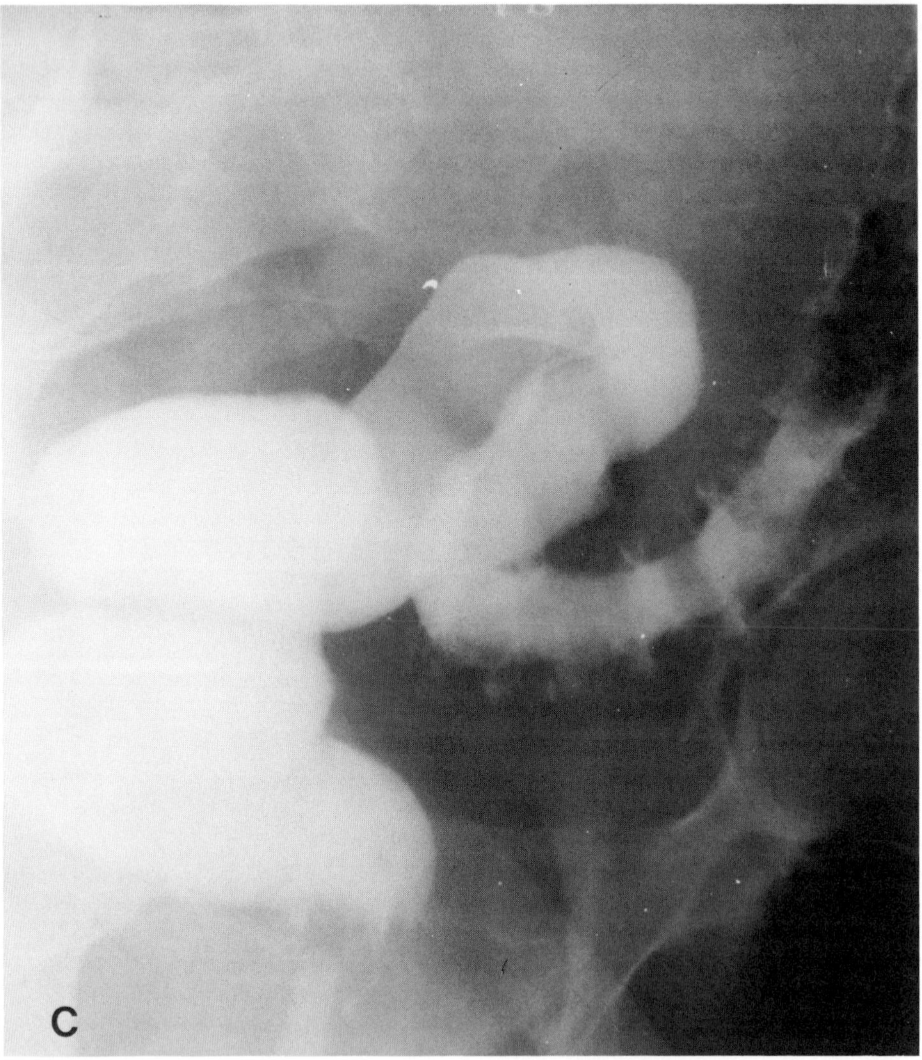

Figure 17–6C.

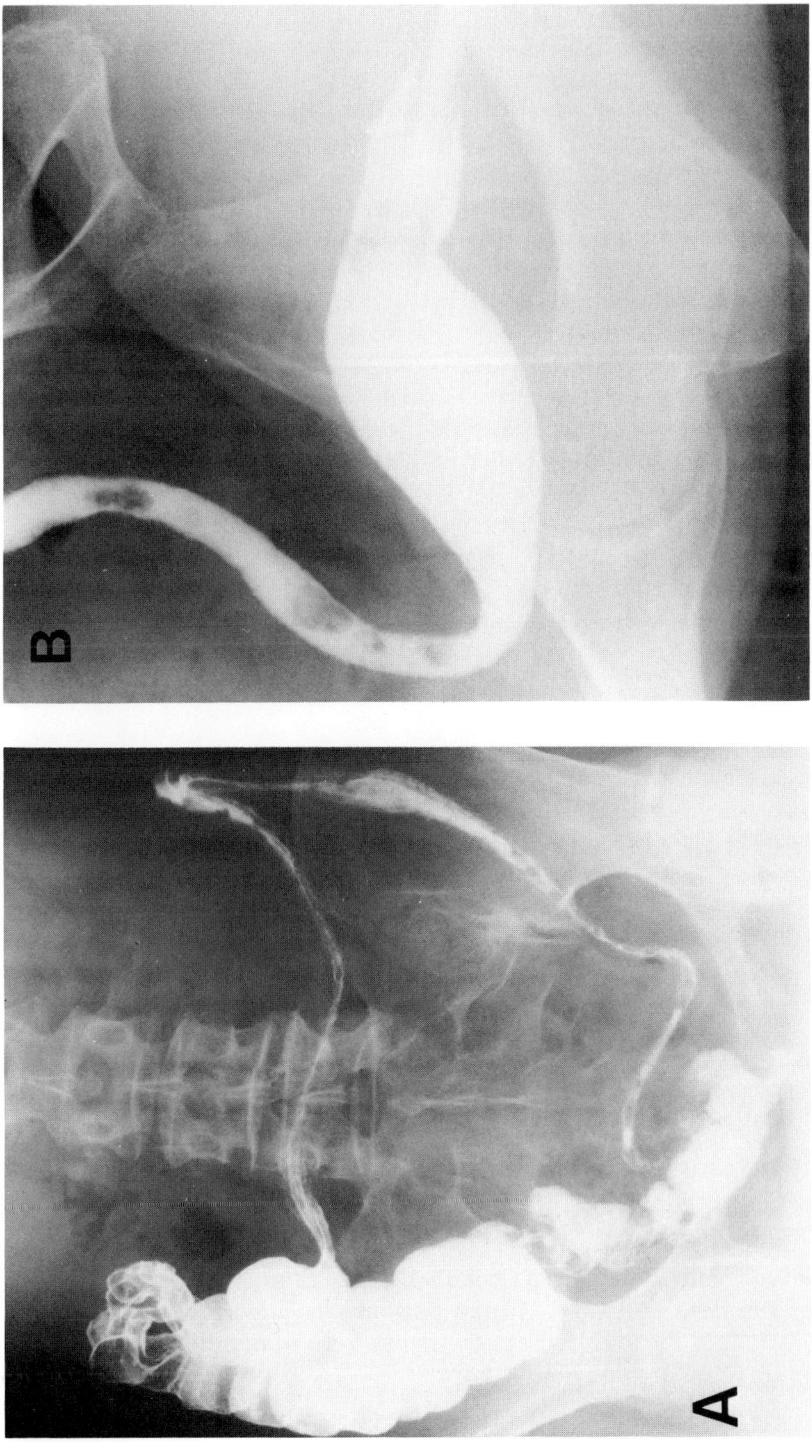

Figure 17–7. Chronic ulcerative colitis with stricture formation and pseudopolyposis. *A*, shows that the process is continuous from rectum to hepatic flexure. *B*, demonstrates marked narrowing of rectum and sigmoid; opacities in the sigmoid are pseudopolyps.

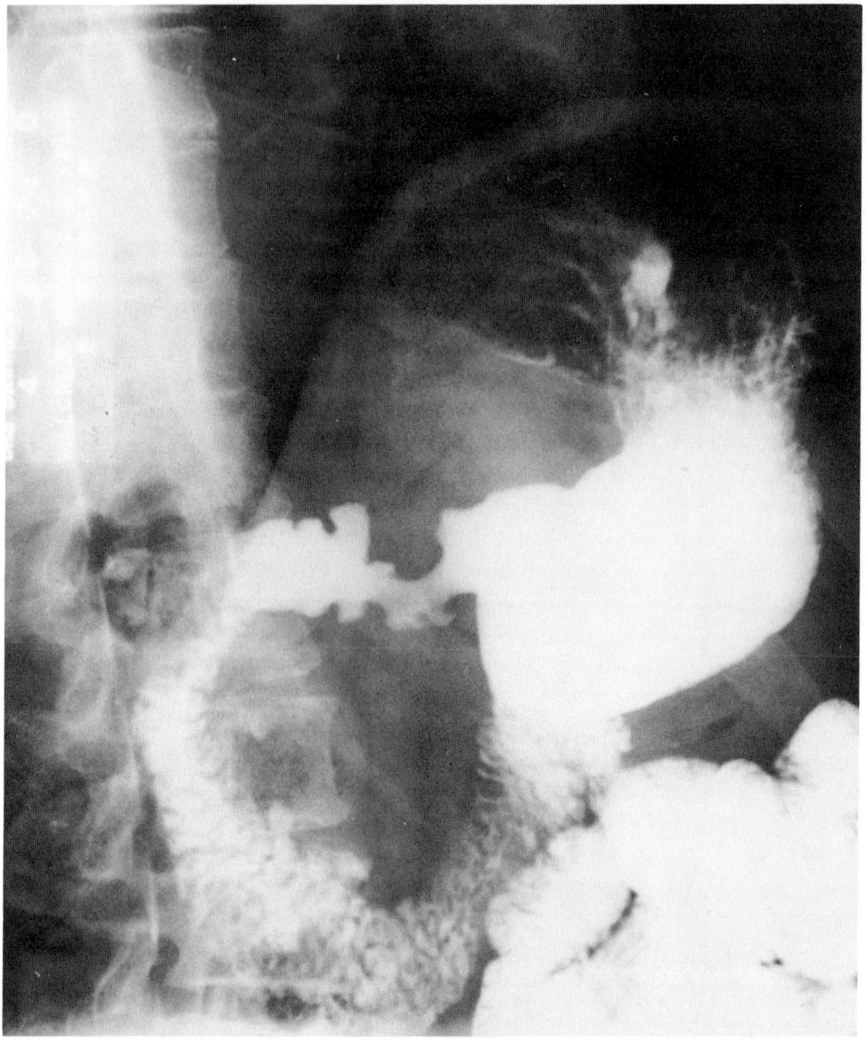

Figure 17–8. Crohn disease of the antrum of the stomach. Note the marked narrowing and deep ulcerations in the antrum. This lesion caused gastric outlet obstruction and was originally felt to be a malignant neoplasm of the stomach.

cent) in the National Cooperative Crohn's Disease Study (Rankin et al 1979). Analysis of the data collected on 624 patients by Edwards and Truelove (1964) suggests that these complications occur with something less than half this frequency in ulcerative colitis.

Fever

Fever may be the sole or principal manifestation of inflammatory bowel disease, especially in children. Its presence correlates fairly well with the severity of the underlying disease, and it occurs in about 40 percent of patients with ulcerative colitis and 60 percent of those with Crohn disease. Where fever occurs as the sole manifestation of bowel disease, the underlying diagnosis can be quite obscure and may be confused with an occult infection, rheumatic fever, collagen disease, or tuberculosis. Proctosigmoidoscopy and intestinal radiography will often be diagnostic and should be performed in all patients with fevers of uncertain etiology.

Cutaneous Complications

Cutaneous complications include erythema nodosum and pyoderma gangrenosum (Figure 17–9). Erythema nodosum is a mild, though painful, manifestation consisting of single or multiple, discrete, raised, tender pinkish red nodules, usually on the anterior aspect of the legs or thighs, and occasionally on the upper arms. Individual lesions range in diameter from less

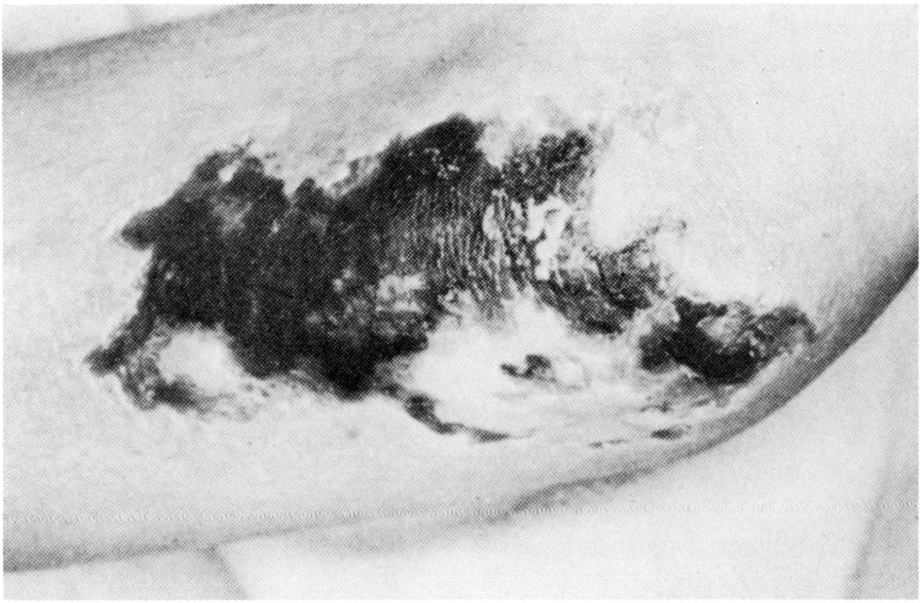

Figure 17–9. Pyoderma gangrenosum in a patient with active chronic ulcerative colitis. This large lesion on the elbow healed promptly and completely following a total proctocolectomy. Courtesy of Dr. Ralph DePalma.

than one to several centimeters, and are indistinguishable from those which occur spontaneously or in association with tuberculosis, sarcoidosis, or with other infections. The lesion is an inflammation of the microvasculature without vascular necrosis and may be the result of deposition of circulating immune complexes. Erythema nodosum appears in slightly over 2 percent of patients with ulcerative colitis and shows a striking predominance among women (Edwards and Truelove 1964), and in about 5 percent of patients with Crohn disease. The lesions are usually very responsive to therapy with glucocorticoids.

Pyoderma gangrenosum is a much more grave disorder, manifested by necrosis and sloughing of small or large areas of skin in any portion of the body. The resulting ulcerations may require skin grafting for treatment, although the early lesions are responsive to large doses of glucocorticoids. Occasionally, progress of the pyoderma can be halted only by surgical removal of diseased bowel. Lesions usually commence as small boils that grow quickly and rapidly become necrotic; no bacteria are found in the exudate and polymorphonuclear leukocytes are present only in small numbers. This serious complication affects less than 1 percent of patients with inflammatory bowel disease.

Occasionally patients with Crohn disease involving the anus have indolent ulcerations of the perianal skin, and these may spread to involve the buttocks as well. Resultant ulcerations are painful and can usually be distinguished from pyoderma by the presence of a heavy lymphoid infiltrate with granulomas in the ulcer base or in the surrounding skin.

Arthritis

Both forms of inflammatory bowel disease may be associated with what has been termed a *nondestructive oligoarticular arthritis*, usually in large joints and serologically distinct from rheumatoid arthritis. Affected joints are associated with swelling, redness, limitation of motion, and occasionally, sterile effusions. Multiple joint involvement is generally asymmetrical, striking, for example, the hip on one side of the body, and the wrist on the other. This acute, nondeforming type of arthritis usually parallels the acute activity of the bowel inflammation and occurs in approximately 6 percent of patients with ulcerative colitis and around 15 percent of patients with active Crohn disease. The lesions usually respond promptly and well to therapy with glucocorticoids.

Chronic arthritis in the form of spondylitis and inflammation of the sacroiliac joints is less common than acute arthritis, but is deforming and progressive, even at times when the underlying bowel disease is under control. There is a very high association of this complication among patients of HLA type B27, especially among whites, and the arthritis may progress to the point of severe ankylosis of joints. Just as is the case with psoriatic arthritides, the association of B27 antigen extends only to those patients with chronic spondylitis, and not those with acute arthritis. Apparently, a variety of diseases, including inflammatory bowel disease, may light up a susceptibility to anklyosing spondylitis and sacroilitus, while not being the proximate cause of the complication. Around 2 percent of patients with inflammatory bowel disease develop chronic arthritides.

Ocular Lesions

Ocular lesions, most commonly conjunctivitis or iritis, occur in something less than 10 percent of patients with ulcerative colitis and 5 percent with Crohn disease. Here again, there is an increased association with HLA type B27, and ocular disease is commonly found in association with arthritis and erythema nodosum. Although corneal ulcers may also appear, the lesions in the eyes are rarely destructive.

I have also seen patchy retinal necrosis in two patients with inflammatory bowel disease, one with Crohn disease and one with ulcerative colitis. In both patients, the lesion was associated with activity of the inflammatory disease, and in both the residual visual defect is permanent, though not disabling.

Liver and Biliary Tract Involvement

This is common in patients with inflammatory bowel disease. The changes are often insidious and may result in cirrhosis of the liver. Liver biopsy may reveal fairly severe changes at a time when hepatic function tests are normal, and the changes may not be related to the severity of the bowel disease. The initial lesion appears to be a spreading type of cholangitis, starting in portal areas. Fatty degeneration of hepatocytes may also be present. Dordal et al (1967) found abnormal liver biopsies in 103 patients with inflammatory bowel disease, in whom the indications for biopsy were variable. Twenty patients had cirrhosis of the liver, and 13 of these were of the "portal-biliary type." Pericholangitis was present in 33 biopsies, 22 showed fatty changes, and 22 others showed nonspecific abnormalities. Mistilis et al (1965) performed 49 liver biopsies in 441 patients with ulcerative colitis because of abnormal physical findings and liver function tests and demonstrated periocholangitis in 24, chronic hepatitis in 8, and cirrhosis in 3. Serum alkaline phosphatase; asparate aminotransferase, and bilirubin levels are the best indicators of hepatobiliary disorders in inflammatory bowel disease. Over 7 percent of patients with ulcerative colitis in the Edwards-Truelove series showed transient or chronic hepatitis, compared with 5 percent of Crohn disease patients in the study of Mekhijian et al.

The best etiological bet for the hepatobiliary complications is the transfer of lymphocytes with altered immunity and destructive capacity from diseased bowel to the liver. It is in this connection that the observation of periportal infiltrates in the livers of rabbits made colitic by DNCB sensitization by Rabin and Rogers (1978), quoted earlier, are so fascinating. Other possibilities, such as transmission of bacteria to the liver from diseased bowel, malnutrition, and toxic reactions to therapeutic agents have been rather well ruled out by appropriate studies. There is no evidence for an increase of HBsAg positivity among inflammatory bowel disease patients.

Sclerosing cholangitis is another curious disorder which may rarely complicate the course of inflammatory bowel diseases. In patients with this disorder, the bile duct system in and outside of the liver, and even the gall bladder, may become the site of a fibrosing inflammatory process associated with generalized or segmental obstruction of the ductal system. Cholestasis is the earliest lesion seen in the liver biopsy, but as it progresses, peribiliary infiltrates, fibrosis of intrahepatic bile ducts, and eventually, nodular biliary cirrhosis may appear. Up to one-third of patients with sclerosing cholangitis have chronic ulcerative colitis (Thorpe et al 1967), and the course is usually quite prolonged. While portal hypertension and bleeding esophageal varices may develop in time, hepatic function may remain normal for many years. Glucocorticoids appear to relieve the jaundice and pruritus commonly associated with the disorder and may also arrest the progress of the disease, which is not related to the activity of the intestinal inflammation.

Several cases of *biliary ductal carcinoma* have also been reported in patients with chronic ulcerative colitis. Some of these patients have also had a prolonged previous history of sclerosing choledochitis, but others have not.

The incidence of cholesterol gallstones is moderately increased among patients with Crohn disease of the lower small intestine, and this is almost certainly a result of reductions in the bile acid pool due to decreased enterohepatic uptake. Chronic fat malabsorption and deficiency of fat-soluble vitamins may also result from a reduced bile acid pool.

Anemia

In patients with inflammatory bowel disease, anemia is almost always the result of acute and chronic blood loss. Ulceration and friability of the mucosa leads to chronic bleeding in patients with ulcerative colitis, while friability and fissurization are probably responsible for the chronic iron deficiency in Crohn disease. Megaloblastic anemias, resulting from malabsorption of vitamin B_{12} and folic acid are also seen. Over 40 percent of patients with Crohn disease have occult intestinal bleeding, and many of these develop mild to marked iron deficiency, while almost all patients with active ulcerative colitis develop at least a degree of iron lack, with a reduction of hemoglobin levels to 9 to 12 g per dl. In the Edwards-Truelove series, 20 percent of patients had severe anemia (hemoglobin less than 9 g), while about 3.5 percent had massive colonic hemorrhages.

Failure of Growth and Development

Failure of growth and development is a serious complication of chronic inflammatory bowel disease and, especially in children with Crohn disease, may be the only symptom. If development is delayed long enough, throughout the major growing years, permanent short stature and absence of secondary sexual characteristics may result. The causes for this are manifold and are primarily nutritional. They include inadequate food intake, loss of protein into the gut lumen, fever, low-grade and chronic intestinal obstruction, and especially in patients with Crohn disease, malabsorption of fat and protein. Furthermore, the use of antianabolic drugs, such as glucocorticoids, may benefit the primary disease considerably but can also serve to aggravate the growth failure. Their detrimental effects can, however, be limited by administering them on an alternate day rather than a daily basis.

Growth hormone levels are normal in developmental failure due to chronic inflammatory bowel disease; no other endocrine deficiencies have been noted, and end organ responsiveness to hormonal stimulation also appears to be intact (Kirschner et al 1978). Negative nitrogen balance, decreased intake of calories, enteric loss of protein, and hypoalbuminemia are common. Growth retardation and delayed sexual development occur in approximately 20 percent of children and adolescents with active Crohn disease and in a somewhat smaller percentage of children with ulcerative colitis.

The effects of growth failure are often devastating to both patients and parents, and physicians must remain alert to detecting this complication in its early, and potentially reversible, stages. Comparison of bone age, determined by radiological study, with the patient's chronological age usually serves to reveal the extent of the growth gap. Many authors have defined growth failure as a height of less than the third percentile for a given age, but the complication can be more clearly diagnosed when several measurements of height are recorded over a period of five or six months.

Once the diagnosis of growth failure is made, special attention should be given to nutritional supplementation, preferably with oral solutions rich in protein. Short periods of parenteral hyperalimentation may also be helpful. But, if these measures are not permanently successful, prompt consideration should be given to surgical removal of diseased bowel. Such therapy is often justifiable in children at a much less extensive stage of disease than it is in adults, because once the growth and development years (up to age 14 in girls and age 16 in boys) have passed, no amount of later nutrition can remedy the problem. The observed growth spurt after successful extirpation is justification enough for the surgical decision.

Urinary Tract Disorders

Confined primarily to Crohn disease, these include ureteral calculi, hydronephrosis, and renal failure. In regard to ureteral calculi, Chadwick et al (1973) showed that patients with ileal resections and ileal dysfunction excreted three to five times more urinary oxalate than did controls, and that this was due to increased absorption of oxalate from the intestinal tract. Dobbins and Binder (1977) showed that hyperoxaluria occurs only in patients with ileal disease or resection in whom the colon was intact, and that it was worsened by accompanying steatorrhea. Patients with ileostomies do not have hyperoxaluria. Reduction of the fat content of the diet reduces the absorption of oxalate. In experimental animals, bile acid perfusion has been shown to increase the absorption of oxalate by the colon.

One may conclude from these studies that hyperoxaluria in patients with Crohn disease is the result of increased colonic absorption of oxalate, and that this results from both decreased luminal calcium, which normally forms poorly absorbable calcium oxalate in the intestinal lumen, and from damage to the colonic mucosa by poorly absorbed bile acids. Steatorrhea is important because the increased presence of free fatty acids in the intestinal lumen leads to the formation of calcium soaps and makes less calcium available for combination with oxalic acid. Where ureteral calculi of calcium oxalate are a problem in patients with any sort of steatorrhea, but especially in patients with Crohn disease, a low-fat diet supplemented with calcium is often beneficial. Oxalates should also be restricted in the diet, but they cannot be totally excluded.

Hydronephrosis in patients with Crohn disease usually results from obstruction of the ureteral-vesical junction by the inflammatory bowel mass. It is a frequent complication of this disease, and involves the right ureter more commonly than the left. Ureteral obstruction occurs in up to 10 percent of patients with Crohn disease and may precede the formation of an ileovesical fistula. Its frequency justifies performing radiological studies of the urinary tract in all patients, especially since many with ureteral obstruction present no urinary tract signs or symptoms. In my experience, the obstructive uropathy may occasionally be relieved with glucocorticoid therapy, although resection of diseased bowel is more lastingly effective. In addition to infection of the upper urinary tract, patients with hydronephrosis also show an increased tendency to develop ureteral calculi, usually not of the oxalate variety. Uric acid calculi are fairly frequent in patients with severe chronic diarrhea, and a tendency to form them can often be controlled by the use of allopurinol.

Renal failure is a fortunately rare complication of Crohn disease, and usually follows recurrent attacks of obstructive uropathy, ureteral calculi, and ascending urinary tract infections. This complication can be best avoided by efforts to maintain adequate urine flow by controlling diarrhea, by meticulous attention to possible urinary tract infections, and by measures directed at relieving urinary tract obstruction and formation of calculi.

THE COURSE OF INFLAMMATORY BOWEL DISEASE

The foregoing discussion implicitly suggests a notable feature of both Crohn disease and chronic ulcerative colitis—each tends to be a chronic condition, capable of recurring after healing, and occasionally involving more bowel during recurrences than in initial attacks. Eighty percent of patients who had undergone a single attack of ulcerative colitis in the Edwards-Truelove series suffered a second attack during the first year, and each of the 19 patients who had been followed for at least 17 years had had second attacks. Chronic, continuous disability is even more of a problem for patients with untreated Crohn disease than it is for those with ulcerative colitis.

Crohn Disease

Crohn disease tends to cause chronic, continuing symptoms in all patients, unless the inflammatory reaction is responsive to therapy. These symptoms are generally either obstructive or diarrheal in nature, and at times both. Malnutrition, the result of caloric deprivation, malabsorption, or chronic obstruction generally occurs in patients with more advanced disease. Although occasional patients can outlive their disease to the extent that therapy can be discontinued without return of symptoms, most patients who respond well to medical therapy require continuing treatment, even though therapeutic agents can often be decreased in quantity. In certain patients with less extensive disease, diarrhea may become so much a part of life that it may be considered by them to be a nearly normal characteristic.

There tends to be some difference in the manner with which Crohn disease presents itself, depending on the portion of bowel involved by the process. Thus, patients with duodenal disease commonly present with vomiting and gastric outlet obstruction. In patients with disease of the upper and middle small intestine, diarrhea, weight loss, cramps, and fever are common complaints. Patients with terminal ileal disease tend to have obstructive symptoms of abdominal bloating, cramps, and vomiting, with or without diarrhea. Diarrhea, cramps, gross bleeding, and anorectal complications are common among patients with colonic disease. One study (Willwerth et al

1971) noted that Crohn disease of the colon alone appears to be more common in women, to present at an earlier age, and to be less commonly treated surgically than disease confined to the small intestine alone or to the ileum and colon simultaneously.

Exacerbations may occur at times of emotional or physical stress, but often enough there is no clear precipitating factor. Radiological changes may improve with therapy, but they rarely disappear without surgery. Untreated internal or external fistulas almost never heal without treatment. While it is uncommon for Crohn disease to involve more areas of the intestine in patients who have not undergone surgery, there is a great and devilish tendency for it to recur following surgical extirpation of all initially diseased bowel. Mekhjian et al (1979) noted a recurrence rate of approximately 75 percent in 15 years among patients with Crohn disease who had previously been subjected to an operation at which all diseased bowel was removed. Recurrences were most common between 5 and 10 years after the initial operation. Approximately 90 percent of their patients had had at least one operation during the course of 30 years of disease. Intestinal obstruction and failure of medical therapy appear to be the major causes of primary and secondary operations, with perianal and fistulous complications also being major indications. Because of the great percentage of postsurgical relapses, physicians can never be free to assure patients that their disease is permanently cured.

While the morbidity from Crohn disease is extremely high, the mortality rate is extremely low, especially when one considers the depredations and possible complications of the disease. Farmer et al (1975) noted a 7 percent mortality among 252 patients with ileocolitis followed for four years, a 5 percent mortality among 166 patients with Crohn colitis alone, and a 4 percent mortality among 178 patients with small intestinal disease only. During a 10-year period, Gryboski and Spiro noted no mortality among 86 children with Crohn disease, 52 percent of whom had ileocolitis, 19 percent terminal ileitis, 20 percent more extensive small bowel disease, and 9 percent colitis alone. These low mortality figures indicate that supportive care, surgery, and the use of various anti-inflammatory agents are effective in maintaining life, if not always removing all symptoms.

Ulcerative Colitis

Ulcerative colitis is a disease of considerable variability, depending both on the percentage of colon and rectum involved in the process and on the nature of the inflammatory process. In the Edwards-Truelove series, 26 percent of patients had involvement of only rectum and sigmoid colon at the initial attack; 24 percent, of the entire colon; and 50 percent, of "substantial" amounts of the colon. Eight percent of patients, usually with total colitis, had fulminant first attacks with toxic megacolon, 66 percent developed the chronic intermittent type of disease with healing followed by recurrence, 7 percent had chronic continuous disease, and 19 percent had only a single attack during the follow-up period. The extent of colonic involvement increased in 13 percent of patients at risk during subsequent attacks of colitis. Mortality statistics for ulcerative colitis are very murky, because they are continually changing for the better. The advent of glucocorticoids followed by improvement in surgical techniques and a far better understanding of when to resort to surgery have led to a reduction in mortality rates from a peak of 25 percent prior to 1950 to less than 2 to 3 percent today when management is placed in the hands of experienced and competent physicians. The major unsolved problems affecting mortality from ulcerative colitis today are the means for detection of colonic cancer in patients with long-term disease and the identification of the "precancer lesion."

COLONIC CANCER IN INFLAMMATORY BOWEL DISEASE

Colonic cancer is an undoubted complication of both chronic ulcerative colitis and Crohn disease of the colon. If it occurs at all, colonic cancer is most likely to arise late in the course of chronic colitis, appearing ironically at a time when the underlying inflammatory disease may be causing few if any symptoms. It is, in a way, the final affront to patients who have long suffered from the indignities and depredations of an onerous disease.

Ulcerative Colitis

Persons at greatest risk for developing cancer of the colon engrafted on chronic ulcerative colitis are those whose disease has existed continuously for a decade or more, usually in a smoldering form, and in whom colonic involvement is extensive. The neoplastic lesions are often multifocal and tend to be highly anaplastic. When compared to conventional colonic cancers, malignant lesions in patients with chronic ulcerative colitis appear in a far younger age group and are considerably more likely to appear in the upper colon than in the sigmoid. The proportion of rectal lesions in conventional cancer is similar to that in ulcerative colitis.

The symptoms of colonic cancer are often distressingly misleading at the outset, since they completely mimic the rectal bleeding, mucus secretion, and obstructive symptoms so typical of a mild attack of colitis. At times, patients may note no new symptoms whatsoever. The only way to diagnose colonic cancer at an early and curable stage is to perform sigmoidoscopies on patients with chronic active colitis at least annually, especially after seven to eight years of continuous disease, and to biopsy any areas which look suspicious. Annual X ray examination of the colon, with particular emphasis on the appearance of new strictures or mucosal irregularities, is also advised by many gastroenterologists, but the cautious patient often becomes fearful of repeated barium enemas and may reject this recommendation. The advent of suitable instruments has led to the suggestion that biannual colonoscopies with biopsies should alternate with biannual proctoscopy and rectal biopsy (Nugent et al 1979) in all colitic patients after five years of disease, but here again the patient's reluctance to undergo the procedure may be difficult to overcome. At the very least, patients should clearly be told of the risk of cancer, of the means available for early detection, and thence be allowed to make up their own minds. A few investigators have advocated "prophylactic" total proctocolectomies for all patients, regardless of symptoms, who have had chronic ulcerative colitis for over a decade. Fortunately, this opinion is not widely held and not widely prescribed.

In the Edwards-Truelove series there was an overall incidence of 22 patients (3.5 percent) who developed carcinoma of the colon; an incidence of 0.5 percent would have been anticipated in a matched general population. The incidence of cancer was nearly 18 percent among patients with both involvement of the entire colon and chronic continuing symptoms, and 10 percent among those with subtotal colitis and continuing symptoms. The cumulative annual risk of colonic cancer was 0.5 percent during the first 7 years of disease, 1.0 percent during the next 7 years, and 4.5 percent from the 15th through 19th years. After the 20th year, the incidence of cancer rose to over 12 percent, but the number of patients in this category was small. Greenstein et al (1979) discovered 26 colonic cancers among 267 colitic patients seen during a period of 17 years; the incidence was 13 percent among patients with total involvement of the colon, and 5 percent among those with "left-sided" colitis. They estimated a 34 percent cancer risk at 30 years, and a 64 percent risk after 40 years of disease. Sackett and Whelan (1980) have suggested that the results of this investigation cannot be generalized to other groups because of sampling bias and qualifications for admission to the study. Despite this, the data show beyond a doubt that cancer risk is indeed great among patients with chronic continuing colitis.

Precancer. Is it possible to more clearly select patients at greatest risk for developing cancer of the colon? The answer is both yes and no: yes, because a dysplastic lesion, indicating a tendency toward definite malignant change, has been identified and described by Morson and Pang (1967); no, because pathologists still differ about the gradations of these dysplastic changes and may have difficulty distinguishing them from the hyperplastic mucosal changes accompanying an acute exacerbation of colitis. Riddell (1976) describes both macroscopic and microscopic changes suggesting precancer. Grossly, lesions may appear to be either flat, looking thicker and more opaque than the usual mucosa of chronic colitis, or villous, being velvety and slightly raised. Microscopically, dysplastic lesions show adenomatous and basal cell changes commonly, and "in situ anaplasia," clear cell change and pancellular change infrequently. Adenomatous changes consist of branching of mucosal crypts, progressively decreased numbers of goblet cells, hyperchromatic nuclei, and occasionally villous transformation of the mucosa. Basal cell changes consist of proliferation and stratification of basal cells, narrowing of crypts, total loss of goblet cells, and mucosal thickening. In situ anaplasia occurs only in flat mucosa and consists of either total absence of crypts with replacement by undifferentiated cells or a continuing persistence of degenerating crypts. Clear cell change consists of enlargement of epithelial cells, with elongated and hyperchromatic nuclei, and loss of the tendency of nuclei to be aligned at the base of mucosal cells. Pancellular changes include clear cell changes plus abnormalities of Paneth, argentaffin, and goblet cells. Paneth cells appear at places other than their normal location at the base of crypts; goblet cells appear to be distended, with nuclei at the luminal border instead of at the base; argentaffin cells become hyperplastic and may surround the mucosal crypt.

That the association of dysplasia with cancer is high is indicated by the fact that Riddell was able to demonstrate dysplastic mucosal changes at a distance from the actual cancer in 65 of 80 colitic colons removed for carcinoma. But the findings also show that cancer may exist without dysplasia, and there is certainly evidence that dysplasia may exist without cancer. In reviewing the incidence of precancer in a collected series of 453 colectomies, Dobbins (1977) reports that mucosal dysplasia (precancer) was found in 88 percent of the colons containing cancers and in 13 percent of colons without cancer. He concludes that precancer alone is not a very precise indication of malignancy, that it develops in 19 percent of patients having ulcerative colitis for 10 years or more, and that its absence is no indication that cancer may be excluded. On the basis of our current knowledge, it is probably best to recommend against colectomy if dysplasia, particularly if it is mild, is demonstrated on only one set of sigmoidoscopic or colonoscopic biopsies. However, if it can be shown to persist or to worsen on at least two sets of biopsies taken one year or more apart, colonic resection is probably indicated.

Crohn Disease

The association of cancer of the colon with chronic Crohn colitis has been indicated in a number of studies, and there is general agreement that the risk is increased over normal. However, the risk does not appear to be as great in Crohn disease as it is in ulcerative colitis, and this may be due to the fact that more patients with the former condition have undergone extirpative surgery. The increased amount of colonic surgery in Crohn disease may reflect the fact that permanent ileostomy is not commonly necessary since, in most cases, severe inflammation tends to avoid the rectum and lower sigmoid colon. In ulcerative colitis, however, definitive surgery always requires total colectomy and permanent ileostomy. At all accounts, Weedon et al (1973) noted the incidence of eight colonic cancers among 499 patients with Crohn colitis observed for a total of over 7,000 patient years, an incidence which is quite a bit greater than would be expected in a matched general population. Data on the occurrence of dysplasia in this condition are not presently available.

THERAPEUTIC APPROACHES IN PATIENTS WITH INFLAMMATORY BOWEL DISEASE

Any physician who endeavors to treat patients with inflammatory bowel disease must be reminded of five very important facts: (1) There is no specific therapy for either of these disorders at present, even though a great deal can be done to ameliorate them. (2) Therapy must be continuous, often extending over many years, and, in the case of a true clinical remission, prophylactic management is often beneficial, especially among patients with ulcerative colitis. (3) Permanent cures with medical management alone do occur in both diseases, but are uncommon. (4) Since surgery is not infrequently indicated, physicians must acquaint themselves with the procedures available, discuss them in detail with surgeons of their choice before and during the operation, and be prepared to reassume the care of the patient afterwards. (5) Patients must be informed of both the chronic nature of their illness and the quintessential importance of their willingness to cooperate with the recommended treatment. One does not then undertake the care of such patients lightly. There are many triumphs and many disappointments to be enjoyed and weathered. Physicians must be ready to delight in the former and to comfort and reassure in the latter. In few other disorders is proper therapy so dependent upon knowledge of the patient and the patient's world. So much for the grave caveats; now, on to the specifics.

Glucocorticoids

Adrenocorticotrophic hormone (ACTH), cortisone, prednisone, prednisolone, and dexamethasone were first used in the treatment of ulcerative colitis at midcentury, and somewhat later became fashionable in the treatment of Crohn disease as well. The results in many cases were truly outstanding, and numerous case reports and controlled studies quickly attested to their value, especially in the control of acute flares of illness. Edwards and Truelove ascribed largely to glucocorticoids the fact that the mortality rate in the first attack among untreated patients with ulcerative colitis was 27 percent (6 of 22 cases), compared with approximately 7 percent (7 of 102 cases) among treated patients. Similarly, the National Cooperative Crohn's Disease Study showed that prednisone induced at least a transient remission in 78 percent of actively symptomatic patients during a 17-week study, and that 60 percent maintained this remission. A comparable group of patients on a dummy preparation showed 49 percent developing a transient remission, and 30 percent maintaining it. These effects of prednisone were significant among patients with small bowel disease alone or with simultaneous small bowel and colonic disease, but not in patients with colonic Crohn disease alone (Summers et al 1979). The results in patients with colonic disease alone are debatable, for the groups were small and there is considerable anecdotal evidence suggesting that glucocorticoids are beneficial.

As can be seen from these results, total elation about the benefits of glucocorticoids was rather quickly replaced with hopeful circumspection when it became clear that not all patients responded to these drugs. Furthermore, the advent of intolerable side effects tends to limit the continuous use of glucocorticoids, especially in high doses. Nevertheless they continue to be a major and most powerful therapeutic tool. ACTH and cortisone were quickly discarded for routine use because both tend to cause greater degrees of sodium retention than do the other glucocorticoids, and the former drug must be administered parenterally. Most physicians today rely primarily upon prednisone and prednisolone because of their lower cost and relatively milder side effects.

Dosage Schedule. Glucocorticoids are usually commenced at relatively high doses (up to 60 mg prednisone daily) and diminished shortly after maximum symptomatic benefits are obtained. In patients with ulcerative colitis, symptomatic improvement in bleeding, bowel frequency, and malaise and reduction of nonintestinal symptoms and fever commonly occurs well before any mucosal improvement can be demonstrated by proctosigmoidoscopy. It is for this reason that dosage should be reduced slowly and cautiously. Usually the dose of prednisone can be reduced to 30 mg daily in two to three weeks, to 20 mg in six to eight weeks, and to alternate-day dosage thereafter (commencing with 40 mg every second day). The use of alternate-day therapy has been shown to be accompanied by a distinct reduction of side effects, especially of growth failure in children, along with fairly good maintenance of therapeutic benefits. Further reductions in dosage should be governed by improvements in the mucosal lesions, which should be appraised proctoscopically at each visit.

Rectal Administration. Rectal administration of glucocorticoids by retention enema is a practical and useful measure in the treatment of Crohn disease and ulcerative colitis confined to the rectum or sigmoid colon. The response is often quite prompt, and the incidence of side effects is reduced by the lessened systemic absorption of the drug. In practice, nightly retention enemas containing 100 mg of hydrocortisone or 40 mg of methyl prednisolone in 60 to 90 ml of water can be continued for extended periods of time and repeated with beneficial responses if the disease recurs.

Side Effects. Side effects of glucocorticoids are common and range from slight to nearly disabling. Most patients promptly feel an early sense of well-being and euphoria. Rarely does the latter effect become a serious problem, but insomnia, which is a mild manifestation of this feeling, is a frequent complication. Periodic drenching sweats and occasional cramping in the thighs and legs may also occur. Many patients gain weight from increased appetite, and most also experience small ecchymoses on the extremities. These particular complications of glucocorticoid therapy are usually quite tolerable.

For many patients, facial rounding, cutaneos striae, acne, or hirsutism limit the tolerance for prednisone. Occasionally, these cosmetic complications can be reduced by resorting to the use of lower doses or to alternate-day therapy. For the physician, the dangers of osteoporosis and growth failure loom as more significant complications of long-term therapy with glucocorticoids. It is for this reason that other means have been sought to allow a decrease of adrenocorticosteroids in those patients in whom high dosage levels are required for sustained control of symptoms.

Sulfasalazine

Sulfasalazine (SAS) is a curious combination of sulfapyridine and 5-aminosalicylic acid. It was originally devised in the 1940s as a compound which had a special "affinity" for connective tissue and might therefore be useful in the treatment of rheumatoid arthritis and ulcerative colitis, both of which were felt to be connective tissue diseases. SAS has indeed been found to be effective in the treatment of colitis, although its mechanism of action is still not clear, and the incidence of side effects is fairly high, though often dose related. Claims for its efficacy have ranged from as high as 90 percent improvement in patients with ulcerative colitis (Svartz 1954) to something like 65 percent improvement in controlled studies. In Crohn disease, the National Study has also shown that SAS is significantly better than a dummy preparation, especially in patients whose involvement is confined to the colon. Of equal interest is the fact that the continuing use of SAS has been shown to be of significant benefit in reducing the recurrence rate of ulcerative colitis among patients in the healed stage of disease (Dissanayake and Truelove 1973), and many patients with healed colitis are now being carried on maintenance doses.

After oral administration, a small portion of SAS is absorbed in the small intestine and excreted, essentially unchanged, into the urine or the biliary tract. In this form it appears to have little or no therapeutic activity (Das et al 1979). In the lowermost small intestine and colon, SAS is hydrolyzed, presumably by bacterial action, into 5-aminosalicylic acid (5-ASA) and sulfapyridine. The latter constituent is believed to have no therapeutic effect, while the 5-ASA has been shown to be a strong inhibitor of prostaglandin synthetase activity and to be capable of reducing the high levels of PGE_2 which are usually found in the colonic mucosa of patients with active colitis (Sharon et al 1978). 5-ASA alone, given as a rectal retention enema, has moderate effect in reducing inflammation in patients with active colitis.

Therapeutic dosage of SAS averages between 4.0 to 6.0 g per day, given in divided amounts after meals and at bedtime. The side effects of nausea and headache can often be relieved by a transient reduction of dosage, or by administering the medication in enteric-coated tablets. Patients with deficiencies of glucose-6-phosphate dehydrogenase should probably not be given the drug at all, since it may provoke a variable degree of hemolysis. All patients should be observed for evidence of leukopenia, especially during the first few weeks of treatment, and SAS should be discontinued if the white blood count falls below 4,500 per cu mm.

Immunosuppressive Agents

These have been used with varying success in the treatment of inflammatory bowel diseases, and their efficacy is still somewhat uncertain. *Azathioprine* was first lauded highly in the management of patients with Crohn disease, but the National Study showed it to be ineffectual when given alone. and also demonstrated a 5 percent incidence of complicating pancreatitis. Presently, the drug might be useful in allowing physicians to reduce the dosage of glucocorticoids in those patients whose disease is controlled by the latter drugs, but only at the expense of intolerable side effects. *6-Mercaptopurine*, the metabolite of azathioprine, has been used in an extended study of patients with Crohn disease (Present et al 1980) and has been fairly well shown to allow for reduction or discontinuation of glucocorticoids in 75 percent of patients and for healing of fistulas in 31 percent, all without excessive toxicity. The response to this drug is slow, averaging greater than three months. It seems to be most beneficial among patients with Crohn disease involving the colon. The use of *metronidazole*, which is both an antibiotic and an immunosuppressive agent, has also been associated with the healing of fistulas in some patients. At present, such agents must be considered to be third-line drugs for the treatment of inflammatory bowel diseases, coming after both glucocorticoids and sulfasalazine. The possibility that they may lead to mutagenesis and oncogenesis has not be excluded.

Supportive Therapy

Supportive therapy may be crucial to the severely ill patient with inflammatory bowel disease. Such treatment is largely parenteral and consists of electrolytes, blood, albumin, and iron lost as a result of the disease itself and nutriment that often cannot be provided as effectively by oral feeding. Central venous hyperalimentation has indeed been lifesaving in many patients with marked caloric deprivation. By this mechanism, patients can be provided with over 3,000 kcal of balanced nutrition per day. The resultant bowel rest may allow for some healing of the inflammatory disease in a significant percentage of patients, although this has been questioned. At the very least, the nutritional complications of severe inflammatory bowel disease can be overcome with this highly valuable therapeutic technique, and it can be continued for extended period of time without serious difficulty. In fact, a small, but significant, number of patients with extensive small intestinal Crohn disease are now being maintained by permanent home hyperalimentation, which has proved to be a practical, but costly, form of therapy (Rault and Scribner 1977).

Emotional Support

Emotional support must be a continuing form of treatment during both relapses and remissions of illness. Although most evidence indicates that psychic stress is either a precipitating or concomitant factor, rather than an etiological agent, in inflammatory bowel disease, its effects can be exceedingly deleterious. So too is the awareness by patients of the fact that they are different from others, and have a disease which is somehow more loathsome than others. Reassurance and understanding are essential. Anything more than superficial psychotherapy, however, should not be employed in the acutely ill patient, lest the underlying disease be aggravated further. Physicians must be both therapists and counselors and must be able to anticipate the concerns of patients. Other patients may also be helpful counselors, but they must be selected carefully, for fear that what they have to say may actually heighten a patient's anxiety. Physicians must also learn that patients may wish to seek medical guidance elsewhere, especially when therapeutic progress has been slow or when surgery has been recommended. They should be encouraged to seek such help whenever they become plaintive, but such advice should be given in an amicable fashion to avoid evoking a feeling of abandonment. The management of patients with inflammatory bowel disease is indeed quite a trick!

Surgical Management

Surgical management becomes a consideration in patients with ulcerative colitis when the acute threats of colonic perforation or hemorrhage, and the more chronic problems of continuing disability, growth failure, anemia, threat of cancer, or failure to respond to more conservative therapy outweigh the disadvantages of total proctocolectomy and permanent ileostomy. In acutely ill patients, such as those with toxic megacolon unresponsive to large doses of glucocorticoids for two or three days, many internists dally too long before advising colectomy and increase the risk of complications. In patients with chronic problems, the seed of surgical intervention should be planted in a patient's mind well before the actual recommendation is made. This suggestion should be reserved only for those symptomatic patients with subtotal or greater involvement of the colon. It is hardly ever necessary for patients with chronic proctosigmoiditis. Approximately 15 percent of all patients with ulcerative colitis will eventually require a total colectomy. Experience has shown that anything less than a total resection of the lower bowel is unlikely to be successful in eliminating the disease, since colitis is likely to exacerbate in portions of the colon which appear at surgery to be grossly normal.

In Crohn disease, surgery is required much more commonly than it is in patients with ulcerative colitis. Approximately two-thirds or more of patients will require at least one such definitive procedure. The indications for surgery vary somewhat with the location of the disease. Thus, Farmer et al (1976) found that patients with disease in both the ileum and colon were operated upon mainly for internal fistulas and abscesses (44 percent), intestinal obstruction (35 percent), and perianal disease (12 percent), while patients with small intestinal disease only required surgery mainly for intestinal abscess and fistula (23 percent). Where the disease was confined to the colon, 26 percent were operated upon for failure to respond to medical therapy, 23 percent for internal fistula and abscess, 23 percent for toxic megacolon, and 19 percent for anorectal disease.

In the National Cooperative Crohn's Disease Study, the probability of surgery was 78 percent after 20 years of disease, the time from onset to first operation being shortest in patients with involvement of the small bowel and colon, longer for patients with small intestinal disease only, and longest in those with colitis only (Mekhjian et al 1979). It is estimated that about three-quarters of these patients will require a second operation within 15 years of the first. It is findings such as these which give rise to the conclusion that no patient, once having had Crohn disease, can ever be said to be completely free of the risk of recurrence. Surgery in Crohn disease consists of sleeve resections of diseased bowel with primary end-to-end intestinal anastomosis, except in cases of distal colonic disease, where total or subtotal proctocolectomies, often with colostomy or ileostomy, are necessary. The patient who has had a total colectomy for ulcerative colitis is considerably better off than the patient whose colectomy was performed for Crohn disease, since the danger of any significant recurrence is almost negligible in the former case, and moderate in the latter.

Ileostomy

Life with a permanent ileostomy is certainly no bed of roses for the patient, but it is invariably far more comfortable than was the disease for which it was performed. Despite this, patients must contend with a major change in their own bodily image and must be guided carefully through this period by their medical counselors. No physician should recommend total colectomy for a patient without having the knowledge of ileostomy care and the willingness to manage the adjustment process. The construction of ileostomies today involves the eversion of the protruding intestinal segment upon itself, with the formation of a mucosal covered stump which is unlikely to become strictured. Ileostomy appliances can now be tailored to the configuration of the abdominal wall and of the stoma itself, so that leakage and irritation of the skin can be prevented. Sealing material made of karaya gum is also a useful means of preventing leakage. Disposable appliances have also made cleaning a much less odious process than formerly. Fellow patients and enterostomal therapists may also provide useful guidance, so long as they do not criticize the surgeon or the technique which was employed. "Ostomy clubs" have been useful in forming purchasing cooperatives for the procurement of ileostomy equipment. Although life with an ileostomy is not without its trials and cares, better surgical techniques, better appliances, effective counseling services, and greater popular understanding have greatly reduced its problems to the point where no patients with a healthy ileostomy need feel any physical limitations whatsoever.

Recently, some surgeons have begun to construct a continent ileostomy for patients with colectomies for ulcerative colitis. This involves forming an intra-abdominal pouch from the lower 25 to 40 cm of ileum, which is in turn attached to the abdominal wall by way of a distal ileal stump. These pouches need be emptied with a plastic tube a few times a day, do not discharge continuously, and avoid the use of external appliances. They have not been perfected, however, and for the time being do not appear to be likely replacements for conventional ileostomies.

SELECTED REFERENCES

Alpers DH, Norland CC, Stillings WA, et al. Increased prevalence of psychiatric disease in Crohn's disease but not ulcerative colitis. Gastroenterology 78:1131, 1980.

Askenase PW, Boone WT, Binder HJ. Colonic basophil hypersensitivity. J Immunol 120:198–201, 1978.

Britton S, Eklund AE, Bird AG. Appearance of killer (K) cells in the mesenteric lymph nodes in Crohn's disease. Gastroenterology 75:218–220, 1980.

Broberger O, Perlmann P. Autoantibodies in human ulcerative colitis. J Exp Med 110:657–74, 1959.

Chadwick VS, Modha K, Dowling RH. Mechanism for hyperoxaluria in patients with ileal dysfunction. N Engl J Med 289:172–76, 1973.

Crohn BB, Ginzburg L, Oppenheimer GD. Regional ileitis: pathologic and clinical entity. JAMA 99:1323–29, 1932.

Das KM, Chowdhury JR, Zapp B, et al. Small bowel absorption of sulfasalazine and its hepatic metabolism in human beings, cats and rats. Gastroenterology 77:280–84, 1979.

Delpre G, Kadish U, Gazit E, et al. HLA antigens in ulcerative colitis and Crohn's disease in Israel. Gastroenterology 78:1452–57, 1980.

Dissanayake AS, Truelove SC. A controlled therapeutic trial of long term maintenance treatment of ulcerative colitis with sulphasalazine (salazopyrin). Gut 14:923–26, 1973.

Dobbins JW, Binder HJ. Importance of the colon in enteric hyperoxaluria. N Engl J Med 296:298–301, 1977.

Dobbins WO, III. Current status of the precancer lesion in ulcerative colitis. Gastroenterology 73:1431–33, 1977.

Dordal E, Glagov S, Kirsner JB. Hepatic lesions in chronic inflammatory bowel disease. I. Clinical correlations with liver biopsy diagnoses in 103 patients. Gastroenterology 52:239–53, 1967.

Eade OE, Moulton C, MacPherson BR, et al. Discordant HLA haplotype segregation in familial Crohn's disease. Gastroenterology 79:271–75, 1980.

Edwards FC, Truelove SC. The course and prognosis of ulcerative colitis. Gut 4:299–315, 1963; Gut 5:1–22, 1964.

Farmer RG, Hawk WA, Turnbull RB, Jr. Clinical pattern in Crohn's disease: a statistical study of 615 cases. Gastroenterology 68:627–35, 1975.

Farmer RG, Hawk WA, Turnbull RB, Jr. Indications for surgery in Crohn's disease: analysis of 500 cases. Gastroenterology 71:245–250, 1976.

Gilat T, Ribak J, Benaroya Y, et al. Ulcerative colitis in the Jewish population of Tel Aviv-Yafo. Epidemiologic and clinical aspects. Gastroenterology 66:335–42, 1974.

Gitnick GL. Etiology of inflammatory bowel diseases: are we making progress? Gastroenterology 78:1090–92, 1980.

Greenstein AJ, Sachar DB, Smith H, et al. Cancer in universal and left-sided ulcerative colitis: factors determining risk. Gastroenterology 77:290–94, 1979.

Gryboski JD, Spiro HM. Prognosis in children with Crohn's disease. Gastroenterology 74:807–17, 1978.

Kirschner BS, Voinchet O, Rosenberg IH. Growth retardation in inflammatory bowel disease. Gastroenterology 75:504–11, 1978.

Kraft SC. The regional lymphocytes in regional enteritis. Gastroenterology 75:319–21, 1978.

Lumb G. Pathology of ulcerative colitis. Gastroenterology 40:290–98, 1961.

Marshak RH, Lindner AE. Radiology of the small intestine, 2nd ed. Philadelphia: WB Saunders, 1976:179–300.

Mayberry JF, Rhodes J, Heatley RV. Infections which cause ileocolic disease in animals: are they relevant to Crohn's disease? Gastroenterology 78: 1080–84, 1980.

Mekhjian HS, Switz DM, Melnyk CS, et al. Clinical features and natural history of Crohn's disease. Gastroenterology 77:898–906, 1979.

Mekjian HS, Switz DM, Watts HD, et al. National cooperative Crohn's disease study: factors determining recurrence of Crohn's disease after surgery. Gastroenterology 77:907–13, 1979.

Miller DS, Keighley AC, Langman MJS. Changing patterns in epidemiology of Crohn's disease. Lancet 2:691–93, 1974.

Mistilis SP, Skyring AP, Goulston AJM. Pericholangitis and ulcerative colitis. Ann Intern Med 63:1–26, 1965.

Mitchell DN, Rees RJW. Agent transmissible from Crohn's disease tissue. Lancet 2:168–71, 1970.

Morson BC, Pang LSC. Rectal biopsy as an aid to cancer control in ulcerative colitis. Gut 8:423–34, 1967.

Nugent FW, Haggitt RC, Colcher H, et al. Malignant potential of chronic ulcerative colitis. Gastroenterology 76:1–5, 1979.

Present DH, Korelitz BI, Wisch N, et al. Treatment of Crohn's disease with 6-mercaptopurine. A long-term, randomized, double blind study. N Engl Med 302:981–87, 1980.

Rabin BS, Rogers SJ. A cell-mediated immune model of inflammatory bowel disease in the rabbit. Gastroenterology 75:29–33, 1978.

Rankin GB, Watts HD, Melnyk CS, et al. National cooperative Crohn's disease study: extra-intestinal manifestations and perianal complications. Gastroenterology 77:914–20, 1979.

Rault RMJ, Scribner BH. Treatment of Crohn's disease with home parenteral nutrition. Gastroenterology 72:1249–52, 1977.

Riddell RH. The precarcinomatous phase of ulcerative colitis. In: Morson BC, ed. Pathology of the gastrointestinal tract. Berlin: Springer-Verlag, 1976:179–220.

Rozen P, Zonis J, Yekutiel P, et al. Crohn's disease in the Jewish population of Tel Aviv-Yafo. Epidemiologic and clinical aspects. Gastroenterology 76:25–30, 1979.

Sackett DL, Whelan G. Cancer risk in ulcerative colitis: scientific requirements for the study of prognosis. Gastroenterology 78:1632–35, 1980.

Schachter H, Kirsner JB. Definitions of inflammatory bowel disease of unknown etiology. Gastroenterology 68:591–600, 1975.

Sharon P, Ligumsky M, Rachmilewitz D, et al. Role of prostaglandins in ulcerative colitis. Enhanced production during active disease and inhibition by sulfasalazine. Gastroenterology 75:638–40, 1978.

Streilein JW. Inflammatory bowel disease: T lymphocytes may be the culprits. Gastroenterology 75:150–52, 1978.

Summers RW, Switz DM, Sessions JT, et al. National cooperative Crohn's disease study: results of drug treatment. Gastroenterology 77:847–69, 1979.

Svartz N. The treatment of ulcerative colitis. Gastroenterology 26:26–28, 1954.

Thorpe MEC, Scheuer PJ, Sherlock S: Primary sclerosing cholangitis, the biliary tree, and ulcerative colitis. Gut 8:435–448, 1967.

Weedon DD, Shorter RG, Ilstrup DM, et al. Crohn's disease and cancer. N Engl J Med 289:1099–1103, 1973.
Willwerth B, DeCosse JJ, Dworken HJ, et al. Natural history of regional enterocolitis. Arch Surg 103:315–19, 1971.

CLINICAL CONFERENCE 10

A 15-year-old boy was brought to a physician by his parents because of failure to grow and loss of 17 pounds in weight during the previous two years. He felt well except for mild weakness, and he attributed his loss of weight both to a lack of appetite and to early satiety. About six weeks before his visit to the doctor he had begun to have two or three loose stools per day, usually without cramps or tenesmus, although there would at times be slight soreness in the lower abdomen. His stools contained neither gross blood nor particles of food, and no obvious change in odor was noted. In the previous week stools had become more normal, with only one movement per day. He had occasional chilly sensations without obvious fever, and there was no evidence of rash, arthralgia, sore throat, swollen ankles, or ocular difficulty. He did note occasional rectal pain when his bowels were loose.

History was not remarkable. The patient was an extremely good student and bright for his age. His parents and brother were all rather short in stature, but in good health. Their concern was not that the patient was short, but that he had stopped growing at an early age and that the onset of puberty had been delayed.

On examination the patient weighed 41 kg and stood 60.25 (274 cm) inches tall. He appeared slightly pale, and his temperature was 37.2°C orally. The entire physical examination was normal, except for the presence of a slightly tender loop of bowel in the right lower quadrant of the abdomen and a 3-mm raised, red, tender area just anterior and to the right of the anal orifice. His testes were small and there was very scant pubic hair. His voice was high pitched. A small amount of stool obtained on rectal examination was negative to guaiac testing.

Urinalysis showed a specific gravity of 1.016 and only a few white blood cells per hpf in the sediment. Red blood count was 5.15 million, hematocrit 39 percent, hemoglobulin 11.5 g. White blood count was 10,400 with 63 percent segmented neutrophils. An upper gastrointestinal and small bowel series was obtained (Figure 17–10). A tuberculin tine test was administered during the examination and was negative.

Over the next few days, the rectal pain increased greatly, and one week after his first visit he returned to his physician. Examination at that time revealed a large, tender, swollen perirectal mass measuring about 5 cm in diameter located where the tender spot had been seen a week before. The center of the mass was fluctuant, and the tightly drawn skin was quite red at

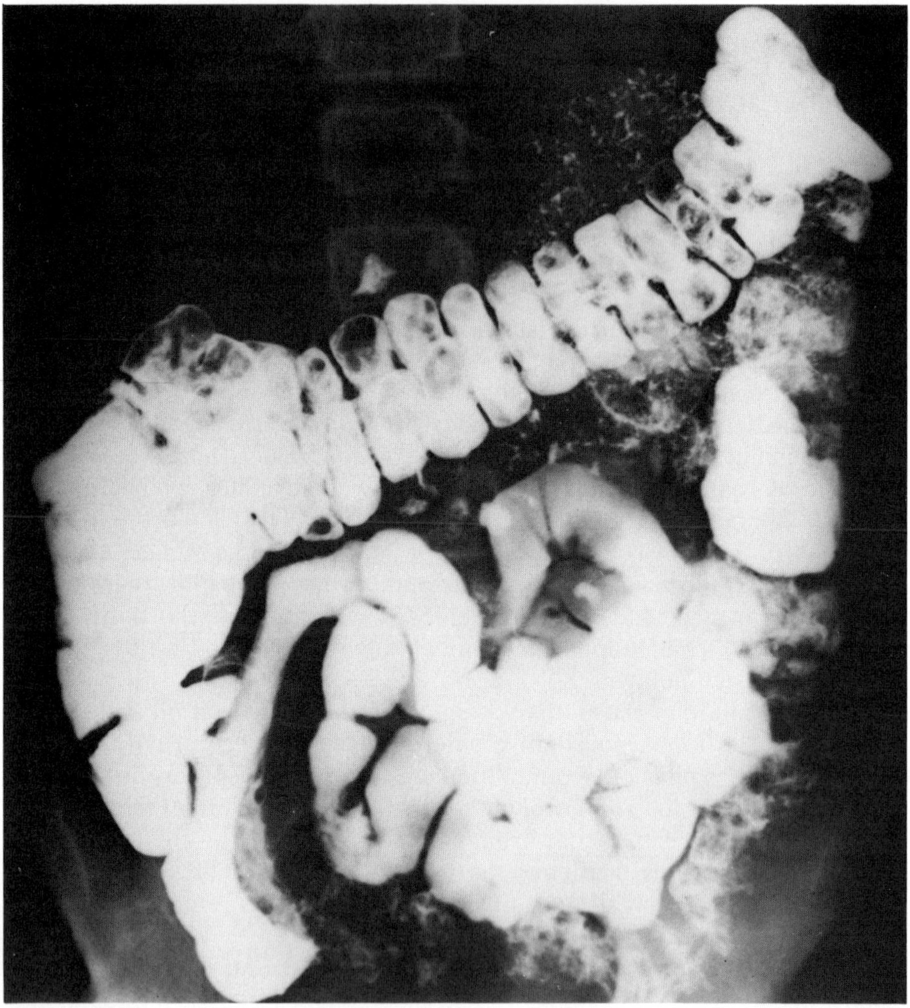

Figure 17–10. *A*, small bowel series, Clinical Conference 10. *B*, spot films of ileocecal area.

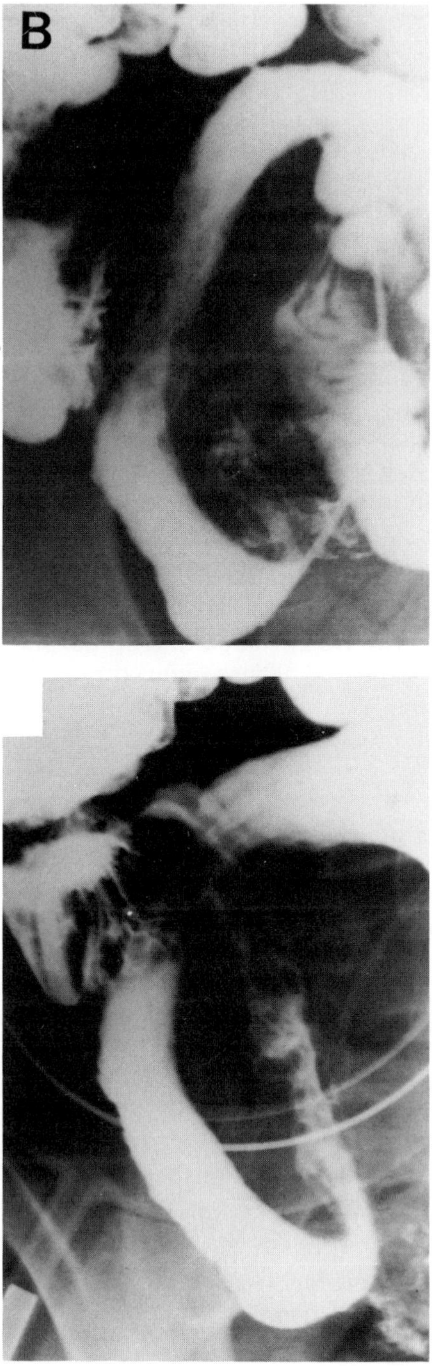

Figure 17–10B.

this point. Incision of this area produced about 25 ml of thick pus and was accompanied by great relief of pain.

The patient was placed on a regimen of hot sitz baths and given medication for his primary disease. He began to feel quite well in a few days but still did not gain weight. In about two weeks he began noting slight nausea after meals and slight epigastric pain late in the evening. The latter was usually relieved quickly by taking Tums. The abscess site continued to drain, although the volume of exudate gradually decreased. On the 24th day following the incision he awakened nauseated in the morning, and shortly thereafter he vomited a large amount of coffee-grounds material. In the next few minutes he felt an urge to defecate, passed a large tarry stool, and promptly fainted.

He was immediately hospitalized, and his vital signs on admission showed a blood pressure of 155/68, pulse 108 and bounding, respirations 24, and temperature 36.6°C. He complained of great thirst. Upon his sitting erect, his blood pressure dropped to 96/64, he felt quite faint and began to perspire profusely. The remainder of a quick physical examination was not remarkable, the site of the abscess showing little exudate and no evidence of healing. Shortly after the examination he passed another tarry stool, and his pulse rate rose to 126. His hematocrit at that time was 32 percent.

Response to therapy was prompt, and on the sixth hospital day his intestinal X rays were repeated. These showed changes as demonstrated on the previous study but also showed "persistent rather marked constriction of the apex of the duodenal bulb, without demonstration of an actual crater."

1. List all possible disease processes in this patient and your reasons for selecting them. Which one(s) would you consider most likely?
2. What complications have already occurred?
3. What medication would you have employed after drainage of the abscess? After the hemorrhage?
4. What definitive therapy is indicated for long-term management?

CLINICAL CONFERENCE 11

A 33-year-old man was hospitalized three weeks after the onset of a migratory type of polyarthritis, which began in the left knee and eventually involved the right ankle, left elbow, and left shoulder. As the joints became involved, they exhibited moderate swelling and slight redness. Movement was quite painful, and the discomfort did not tend to subside during the day. There was some benefit from aspirin, although the relief was never complete. There was no history of chills, fever, or rash.

The patient had never noted any previous episodes of arthritis but had been afflicted with chronic diarrhea since the age of 21. His stools were generally watery and often numbered as many as 8 to 10 per day. There was occasional gross bleeding with his bowel movements. For the previous 12 years he had taken no medication for the diarrhea, save for a few doses of paregoric. One year before this admission there was marked aggravation of the diarrhea associated with rather high fever and considerable gross blood in his stools. The symptoms became progressively severe for several weeks, during which time he also lost weight for the first time. He was eventually hospitalized in another city, required several blood transfusions, and improved while being treated with adrenocorticosteroids.

Following that hospitalization he continued to receive glucocorticoids and sulfasalazine. He gradually regained weight and strength, and within three months was able to return to his work as a college teacher. During the ensuing six months his physician gradually decreased the prednisone to a dose of 15 mg per day. His arthritic symptoms recurred about two weeks after the dose of prednisone had been reduced to 15 mg.

The patient's past health had been excellent, and there was no family history of a similar disorder in either of his parents or his sister. He was married and had two children, both of whom were in good health. During the four years prior to his hospitalization he had been under marked emotional stress as a result of difficulties with his wife. Much of their disagreement concerned his career. His wife felt that the patient could accomplish a great deal more and be better off financially were he able to obtain a responsible job in industry. Whenever he and his wife discussed this subject, his diarrhea became much more severe. He did not admit to being particularly tense otherwise, and stated that he had in the past been quite happy at home and at school and had rarely encountered any major personal problems.

On examination the patient was a well-developed, well-nourished man, weighing 63.2 kg. He appeared to be quite relaxed, but complained of pain on movement of his left arm and right ankle. Blood pressure was 120/80, pulse 96 and regular, respirations 12, and temperature 36.0°C. The positive findings on examination included rather marked swelling and tenderness in the right ankle, left wrist, and left knee. The skin over these joints was slightly reddened. Abdominal examination was normal, save for slight tenderness to pressure in the right lower quadrant where a sausage-shaped loop of bowel was palpable. Sigmoidoscopy to a distance of 15 cm showed normal rectal architecture and a healed anal fissure. The mucosa of the rectum was diffusely granular, moderately edematous, and slightly friable. There was no evidence of ulceration. Two small polypoid lesions measuring 2 mm in diameter were seen at a 15-cm depth.

Urine examination was normal except for four to five white blood cells per hpf. BUN was 16 mg per dl, fasting glucose, 115 mg; alkaline phosphatase, 210 IU. Latex fixation and antinuclear tests were negative. Hematocrit was 37 percent; white blood count, 14,100, differential: neotrophils, 81; lymphocytes, 14; and monocytes, 5 percent. Sedimentation rate was 30 mm per hour, prothrombin 80 percent of normal. Guaiac testing on four stools, all of which were quite watery, varied from negative to 4 plus. A representative film from his barium enema examination is reproduced in Figure 17–11.

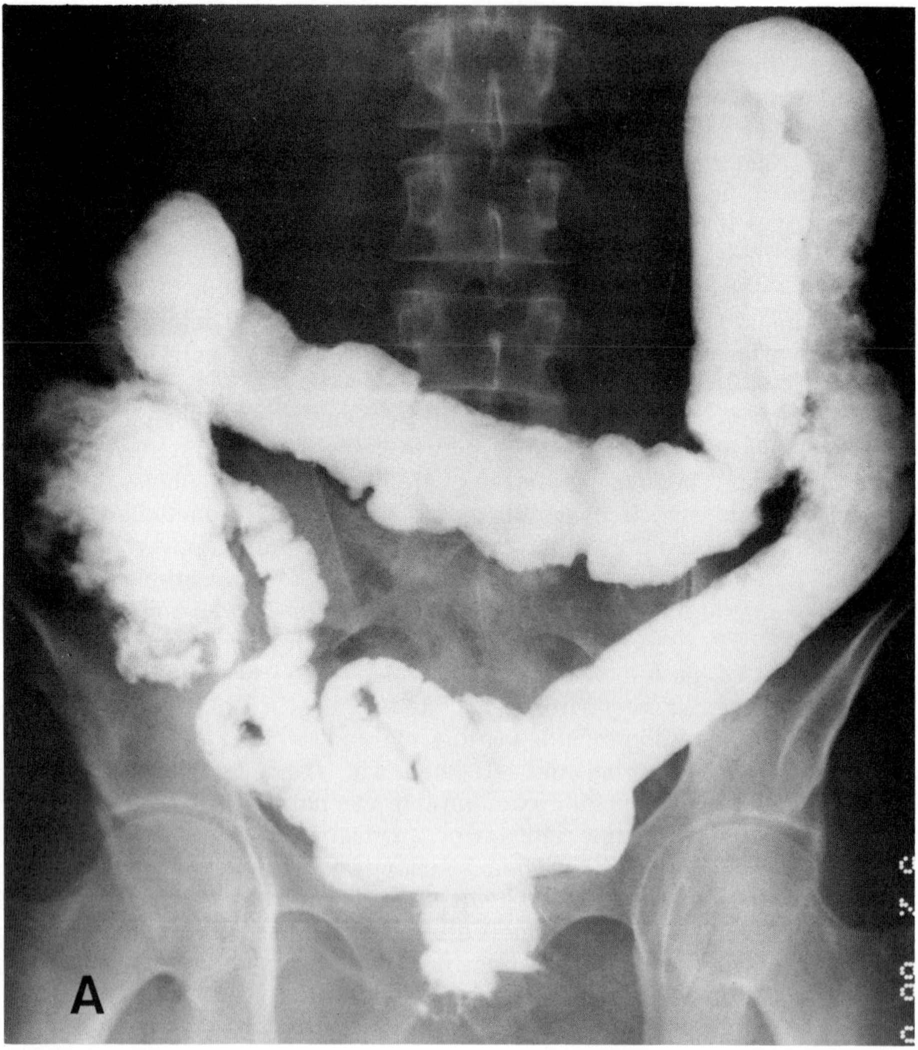

Figure 17–11. *A*, barium enema, Clinical Conference 11. Spot films (*B*) of splenic flexure and (*C*) of cecum.

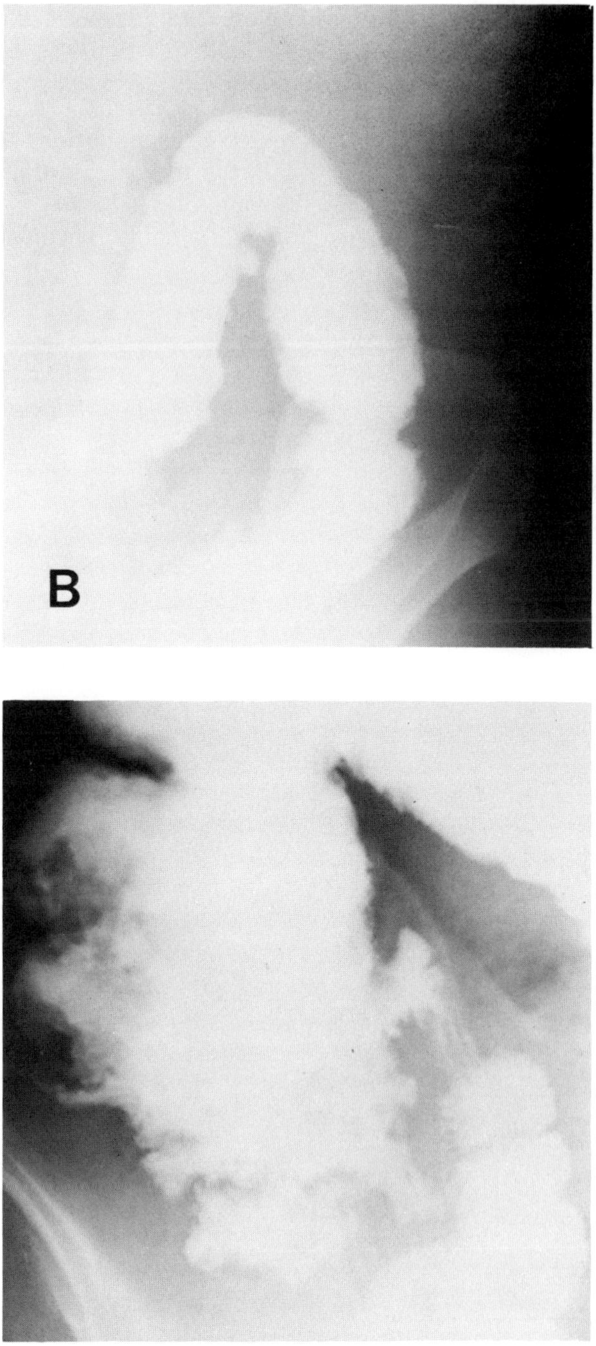

Figure 17–11B.

1. What disease processes would have to be considered in this patient, and which appears to you to be the most probable diagnosis? Using the case history, laboratory findings, and X ray as a guide, select those aspects that tend to support your conclusion.
2. What complications have already occurred in this patient, and what might you expect as possible complications in the future?
3. If a colonic biopsy were available for examination, what would you expect it to show microscopically?
4. At this stage, what types of therapy could be considered? Which would you choose and why?

CHAPTER 18

Mesenteric Vascular and Angiodysplastic Disorders

We have already seen that the macrocirculation to the stomach and intestine is provided by three large branches of the abdominal aorta: the celiac axis, the superior mesenteric artery, and the inferior mesenteric artery. The microcirculation is equally important in maintaining the integrity of the intestine and in providing energy for the three major elements of intestinal function, the absorption of nutrients, their conveyance from the intestine, and the mixing and propulsion of intestinal contents. The microcirculation is a complex apparatus that has its own autoregulatory mechanisms and is responsive as well to extrinsic hormonal and neural stimuli. Its physiologic responses vary from segment to segment in a fashion that allows each region of the intestine to subserve its own distinctive functions. A detailed review of this topic has been written by Lanciault and Jacobson (1976).

THE INTESTINAL MICROCIRCULATION

Circulation to the intestinal wall may be divided into two distinct components, that which supplies the intestinal villi and that supplying the mucosal crypts and the submucosa. Blood flow through both of these vascular components is controlled by two features, the arteriolar musculature and the precapillary sphincters. At any one time, some precapillary sphincters are open (about 20 percent) while others are closed, so that cellular demand for oxygen is not continuous. Arteriolar muscle is responsive to local vasoactive substances and to neurotransmitters. Cholecystokinin, secretin, serotonin, and β-adrenergic agonists appear to increase mucosal blood flow, while α-adrenergic agonists and angiotensin II constrict the vasculature. The relative physiologic importance of these agents has not been conclusively determined. Vasodilatation appears to be mediated by accumulation of cyclic adenosine 5′-monophosphate (cAMP) which stimulates adenosine triphosphatase (ATPase) activity and releases enough energy to decrease cellular calcium. Hypoxia also causes vasodilatation but appears to operate through another mechanism.

Precapillary sphincters are responsive to changes in tissue pressures of O_2, CO_2, and unspecified metabolites. Depression of tissue O_2 by arteriolar constriction causes more precapillary sphincters to open so that a greater proportion of oxygen than usual is removed from that blood which continues to flow through the arteriolar system. This compensatory form of autoregulation is more active in the villous circulation than it is in the submucosal component and appears to differ quantitatively from one portion of the intestine to another.

Countercurrent Exchange in Villi

Villous circulation is provided by an ascending artery and a descending vein connected by a hairpin turn at the villous tip. Circulation proceeds in opposite directions in the two vessels, and especially at the base of the villus, they are separated by only a thin layer of stroma which appears to act as a semipermeable membrane. This membrane allows for the diffusion of solutes from one vessel to the other without passage through the capillary bed, providing a countercurrent exchange mechanism. Oxygen, for example, has been shown to diffuse from artery to vein, especially at villous bases where A-V oxygen differences are greatest. This "shunt" of oxygen is aggravated by hypotension and may explain why mucosal necrosis commences at the tips of villi during episodes of ischemia. During absorption of fat, venous lipid levels are initially higher than arterial, and lipids may thus diffuse to the arterial side and act as a brake to further absorption. The existence of a countercurrent mechanism may also explain why the absorption of sodium at villous tips is four times greater than at villous bases, and why this gradient is increased by the presence of glucose in the surrounding medium. Such a mechanism also explains the fact that the passive absorption of water is greatest at villous tips, where the concentrations of sodium and other absorbed solutes is likely to be greatest.

PATHOPHYSIOLOGY OF MESENTERIC AND ANGIODYSPLASTIC VASCULAR DISORDERS

Among a series of 100 patients with primary mesenteric ischemia, Williams and Wittenberg (1973) found that 64 patients suffered extensive disease, usually in the distribution of the superior mesenteric artery, while 36 suffered from milder segmental disease, usually in the distribution of the inferior mesenteric artery. Mortality among patients with extensive disease was 84 percent; that among patients with segmental disease, 33 percent. Sixty-six percent of patients with extensive disease showed no evidence of vascular occlusion, 28 percent had arterial occlusions, and 3 percent showed venous occlusions. All but two of the patients with segmental disease had nonocclusive ischemic colitis. The proportion of patients with nonocclusive disease varies considerably from one series to another but makes a significant contribution in each, reflecting the importance of low flow states in the pathogenesis of intestinal ischemia and infarction. The incidence of thromboembolic mesenteric arterial and venous disease is significantly increased in women taking oral contraceptives, especially following elective surgery (Vessey et al 1970).

Occlusive mesenteric arterial disease results both from obstruction by arteriosclerotic thrombi and by emboli. Since thrombi develop slowly, and since collateralization is considerable among organs supplied by the mesenteric arteries, significant ischemic necrosis does not usually develop from thrombosis of only a single large mesenteric vessel. Sudden occlusion, however, by a dissecting aortic aneurysm may cause rapid ischemic necrosis of bowel. Embolic obstructions appear most commonly in patients with atrial fibrillation, rheumatic heart disease, mural thrombi, or prosthetic heart valves. The superior mesenteric artery and its branches are more commonly involved by emboli than either the celiac axis or the inferior mesenteric artery because it arises at a more acute angle than the other vessels and is thus in the main line of blood flow. Sudden embolization of a mesenteric vessel is likely to cause immediate distal vasoconstriction and ischemia. Extensive small or large vessel occlusions may also complicate diffuse forms of vasculitis, such as that occurring with rheumatoid arthritis, periarteritis, and lupus erythematosus.

Occlusive mesenteric venous disease is much less common than arterial disease, and usually complicates hypercoagulable hematologic states, such as polycythemia vera. Venous mesenteric occlusions have also been described in patients with cirrhosis of the liver and with vasculoinvasive abdominal neoplasms.

Nonocclusive mesenteric arterial disease is most often encountered in older patients with low flow states, including congestive heart failure, excessive diuresis, sustained hypotension, extensive burns, or endotoxic shock. Reduced blood flow leads to release of α-adrenergic agents, vasospasm, and feedback responses in aid of maintaining cerebral circulation. The prior use of digitalis glycosides appears to aggravate the tendency to bowel ischemia by causing spasm of arterioles and precapillary sphincters. Nonocclusive mesenteric infarction usually occurs in patients over age 60 who also have considerable evidence of arteriosclerosis. Thus, while thrombosis itself does not have a role in nonocclusive ischemia, it is quite likely that loss of vascular elasticity does play an important part.

Another element which doubtless contributes to nonocclusive vascular ischemia, especially in the colon, has been described by Binns and Isaacson (1978). They have shown that long colic arteries undergo marked increases of tortuosity with aging, and that this change is unrelated to arteriosclerosis. It is believed that increased tortuosity causes increased flow resistance and increased susceptibility to ischemia whenever blood flow is reduced.

Angiodysplastic lesions of the gastrointestinal mucosa are common causes of alimentary bleeding, and may occur in the stomach, small intestine, or colon. Individual lesions consist of thin-walled capillary or venous telangiectases which eventually enlarge enough to behave functionally as arteriovenous fistulas (Figure 18–1). The hemorrhagic telangiectases described by Rendu (1896), Osler (1901), and Weber (1907), and those described by von Willebrand (1931), are hereditary in origin, while the increasingly recognized venous dysplasia of the right colon has been ascribed solely to aging by Boley et al (1977). Acquired angiodysplasia results from irradiation in some cases, while numerous others are found curiously associated with aortic valvular stenosis.

The lesions of hereditary hemorrhagic telangiectasia may occur in the mucosa of the nose, mouth and alimentary tract, the skin, and the liver. Col-

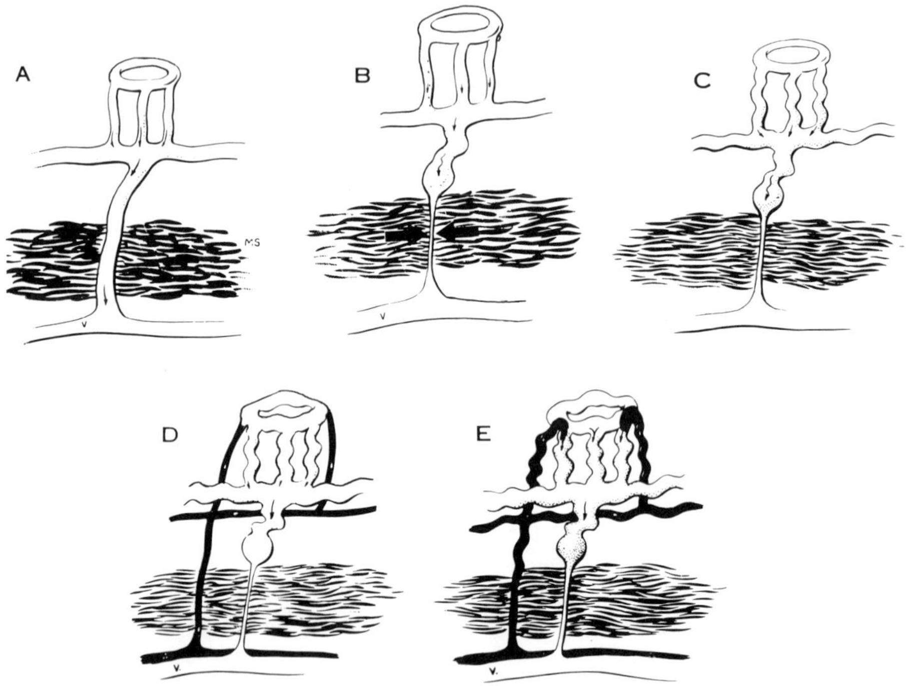

Figure 18–1. Diagrammatic illustration of proposed concept of the development of cecal vascular ectasias. *A*, normal state of vein perforating muscular layers. *B*, with muscular contraction or increased intraluminal pressure, the vein is partially obstructed. *C*, after repeated episodes over many years the submucosal vein becomes dilated and tortuous. *D*, later the veins and venules draining into the abnormal submucosal vein become similarly involved. *E*, ultimately the capillary rings become dilated, the precapillary sphincter becomes incompetent, and a small arteriovenous communication is present through the estasia. From Boley SJ. Reprinted by permission of the publisher from Gastroenterology 72:650–68, 1977. Copyright 1977 by The American Gastroenterological Association.

lectively they may produce enough arteriovenous shunting of blood to cause cardiac enlargement and heart failure. The lesions of von Willebrand disease may appear anywhere in the alimentary tract and usually do not involve the mouth and skin (Ahr et al 1977). A similar distribution has been noted with the angiodysplasia of aortic stenosis (Weaver et al 1979). Lesions similar to the vascular ectasias of the aging right colon have also been described in the left colon and in the stomach. Bleeding from any area of vascular dysplasia has been presumed to result from progressive distention of venous and capillary walls. Because precapillary sphincters have been gradually dilated by the dysplastic process, bleeding is primarily arterial in nature and often extremely heavy. This bleeding tendency is greatly aggravated in patients with hereditary or acquired von Willebrand disease owing to deficient platelet function.

PATHOLOGY

Pathologic changes related to intestinal ischemia are the same in both colon and small intestine, and the lesions from arterial and venous ischemia are indistinguishable from one another. Mucosal necrosis is followed by hemorrhage and nodular swelling of the submucosa, and then by deep ulcerations which may heal rapidly in reversible cases. It is these ulcerations which are responsible for the "thumbprint" pattern noted at times in patients with ischemic segmental colitis. In the small intestine, necrosis is noted earliest at the tips of villi and later extends to involve the entire mucosa. The base of mucosal ulcers is laden with granulation tissue and fibroblasts and, most characteristically, macrophages containing hemosiderin. These latter cells are not found in ulcerative colitis and Crohn disease and serve to distinguish them pathologically from ischemic disease. In specimens showing transmural necrosis, bacterial colonization is also frequently found.

SYMPTOMS AND SIGNS OF MESENTERIC ISCHEMIA AND NECROSIS

Although abdominal pain is the prime symptom of mesenteric vascular insufficiency, it is often nondescript and occasionally mild enough in the patient seriously ill with a low flow state so as to attract little clinical attention. In patients with recurrent ischemia alone, pain is usually brought on by eating (*abdominal angina*), and may lead to decreased food intake and loss of weight. Chronic ischemia can also cause mucosal atrophy and malabsorption. Bowel infarction is usually a catastrophic episode causing pain, ileus, sweating, and intestinal hemorrhage from necrosis and ulceration of the bowel mucosa. Peritonitis occurs from transmural infarction and perforation of the bowel, and is commonly associated with sepsis.

Examination of the patient with abdominal angina frequently shows no abnormality whatsoever, although at times a loud systolic bruit may be audible on auscultation of the upper abdomen. In a large number of patients, the relief or prevention of postprandial pain by the use of 0.32 mg nitroglycerine sublingually is of diagnostic value. In patients with ischemic necrosis of the bowel, abdominal distention and hypomotility are common findings. Peritoneal signs are elicited if transmural necrosis is present, and fever usually accompanies these. Stools are usually grossly bloody in patients with ischemic necrosis, but they may only reveal occult blood early on. Proctoscopy in the presence of distal colonic mucosal necrosis commonly reveals a normal appearance of the distal few centimeters of rectum, with edema and dusky cyanosis of the infarcted area above. The distal rectum is often spared because it receives arterial blood by way of the iliac vasculature.

DIAGNOSIS

The diagnosis of mesenteric ischemic necrosis is suspected from the history and examination, and from the detection of ileus on plain films of the abdomen. In patients with colonic infarctions, examination of the air-filled splenic flexure and descending colon may reveal mucosal irregularities suggesting edema and ulceration. If the patient's general condition is good, despite the passage of bloody stools intermittently, a barium enema may be performed. The presence of distinct mucosal irregularities suggesting "thumbprints" is nearly diagnostic of segmental colonic infarction, especially if the disease is confined to a single segment of bowel (Figure 18–2).

Mesenteric angiography should be performed as soon as possible in all patients felt to have extensive ischemic necrosis of the bowel. This is the only technique which will clearly demonstrate the presence of vascular occlusion, and it must be done promptly in order to allow surgical intervention prior to the development of irreversible ischemic necrosis. Angiography in patients with nonocclusive extensive infarction may demonstrate the presence of diffuse spasm of the mesenteric vasculature. In patients suspected of having intestinal angina, angiography may be performed at a more leisurely pace and will provide diagnostic information. Patients with angiodysplasias can also be diagnosed often by this technique, and actual extravastion of dye into the lumen of the colon may be demonstrable at times.

TREATMENT OF MESENTERIC VASCULAR DISEASES

In patients with extensive disease, following stabilization and arteriography, therapy should depend upon the radiographic and clinical findings. There is some evidence that patients with nonocclusive ischemia may bene-

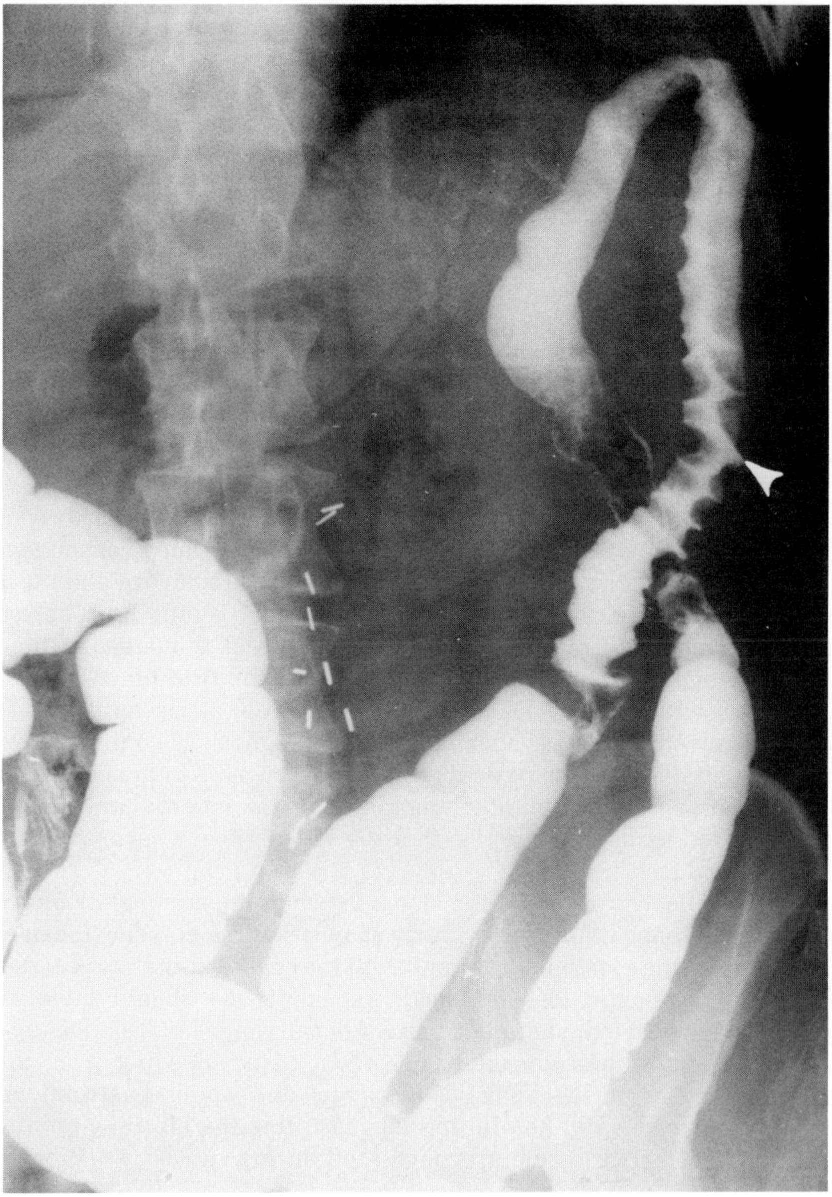

Figure 18–2. Arterial infarction of the splenic flexure of the colon. Arrow points to typical "thumbprint" lesions caused by edema and ulceration of mucosa following segmental infarction. Patient recovered spontaneously after a short period of colonic hemorrhage.

fit from the perfusion of vasodilating substances into the superior mesenteric artery after performing angiograms. Papaverine has been used with some success in these patients, and glucagon and phenoxybenzamine have also been found to be beneficial at times. The disadvantage of papaverine is that as systemic levels of the drug increase, mesenteric blood flow may be further compromised by systemic hypotension. Prostaglandin E_1 has been proposed to be the ideal mesenteric vasodilator, but experience with this drug is still too limited to make any judgments. While giving vasodilator agents, it is probably also advisable to explore patients with extensive nonocclusive vascular disease surgically in order to determine whether any irreversible ischemic necrosis has occurred, and to remove such areas. All patients with extensive occlusive vascular disease must be operated on as soon as a degree of circulatory stability has been achieved.

Wide clinical experience has shown that patients with segmental vascular infarctions do not require surgery initially unless signs of transmural necrosis have occurred. Mucosal infarctions, especially in the colon where collateral circulation between the superior and inferior mesenteric systems is fairly rich, heal within a short time and cause no serious consequences. Occasionally, where the infarction has involved the submucosa and the muscularis, stenotic strictures may appear. These can usually be repaired at leisure. The important element of therapy is to treat the cause of the low flow state which caused the segmental infarct in the first place.

Patients with intestinal angina due to stenosis of mesenteric vessels also require elective surgery shortly after the diagnosis is confirmed by angiography. Left alone, these patients commonly progress to the point of complete occlusion and to bowel infarction. Patients taking oral contraceptives should be asked to discontinue this therapy at least two weeks prior to any surgical procedures.

Angiodysplastic lesions of the stomach, small intestine, and colon also require surgery once it has been clearly shown that the ectasias themselves are the cause of the bleeding. It is important to remember in these cases that not all angiodysplastic lesions bleed, and that one should have clear evidence that they are the actual source of hemorrhage before advising surgery. In patients who have not been shown to be bleeding from angiodysplasia during arteriography, colonoscopy and upper gastrointestinal endoscopy are frequently helpful in demonstrating the bleeding points. At times, such lesions can be electrocoagulated during endoscopy (Weaver et al 1979).

SELECTED REFERENCES

Ahr JD, Rickles FR, Hoyer, et al. Von Willebrand's disease and hemorrhagic telangiectasia. Association of two complex disorders of hemostasis resulting in life-threatening hemorrhage. Am J Med 62:452–58, 1977.

Binns JC, Isaacson P. Age-related changes in the colonic blood supply: their relevance to ischemic colitis. Gut 19:384–90, 1978.
Boley SJ, Sammartano R, Adams A, et al. On the nature and etiology of vascular ectasias of the colon: degenerative lesions of aging. Gastroenterology 72:650–60, 1977.
Lanciault G, Jacobson ED. The gastrointestinal circulation. Gastroenterenterology 71:851–73, 1976.
Osler W. A family form of recurring epistaxis, associated with multiple telangiectases of the skin and mucous membranes. Bull Hopkins Hosp 12:333–37, 1901.
Rendu M. Epistaxis répétés chez un sujet porteur de petits angiomes cutanés et muquez. Bull Soc Med Hop Paris 13:731–33, 1896.
Vessey MP, Doll R, Fairbairn AS, et al. Postoperative thromboembolism and the use of oral contraceptives. Br Med J 3:123–26, 1970.
von Willebrand EA. Über hereditäre pseudohämophilie. Acta Med Scand 76:521–50, 1931.
Weaver GA, Alpern HD, Davis JS, et al. Gastrointestinal angiodysplasia associated with aortic valve disease: part of a spectrum of angiodysplasia of the gut. Gastroenterology 77:1–11, 1979.
Weber FP. Multiple hereditary developmental angiomata (telangiectasia) of the skin and mucous membranes associated with recurring haemorrhages. Lancet 2:160–62, 1907.
Williams LF, Jr, Wittenberg J. Vascular insufficiency of the intestine. Separating fact from fad and fiction. Viewpoints Dig Dis 5:1–4 (March), 1973.

DISCUSSION QUESTION

A 64-year-old man complains of having had postprandial midabdominal pain for the previous three months. He also has had foul-smelling stools and has lost 10 percent of his previous weight in that period. Describe and give reasons for studies that would show whether this patient suffers from mesenteric ischemia.

CHAPTER 19

Diverticular Diseases of the Colon and Lower Small Intestine

This chapter is concerned with the pathogenesis and management of the diseases of those blind pouches of the lower intestine called diverticula. Diverticula may be congenital or acquired. They may also be classified as true diverticula if they contain in their wall each layer of the bowel, or false diverticula if their walls consist only of mucosa and submucosa which has partially or completely penetrated the muscularis. The appendix, Meckel diverticula, and solitary diverticula of the right colon are congenital true diverticula, the appendix being a normal anatomical structure while the others are anomalies. Zenker and jejunal diverticula are examples of acquired false diverticula, the former being a prominent cause of dysphagia and aspiration pneumonitis in older patients, particularly men, while the latter when multiple are an uncommon cause of malabsorption of fat and macrocytosis, due to colonization by bacteria and resultant intraluminal deconjugation of bile acids and consumption of vitamin B_{12}. By these classifications, the ubiquitous disorder known as diverticulosis of the colon is also a collection of acquired false diverticula.

DIVERTICULOSIS OF THE COLON

It has often been stated about colonic diverticulosis that the disorder is almost solely encountered among persons living in Western industrialized societies, was almost unknown prior to the turn of the twentieth century, and almost invariably increases in incidence with aging. There has been enough support for these facts during the past decade to consider them to be axiomatic (Connell 1977; Almy and Howell 1980). The estimated frequency of diverticulosis among urban populations in western Europe and North America ranges from an incidence of 10 percent among persons over age 40 to nearly 50 percent among healthy individuals over age 70. In emergent agrarian populations, on the other hand, the incidence of colonic diverticulosis approaches zero, regardless of age (Painter and Burkitt 1971). Among patients aged 65 or more in the United States, the frequency of hospitalization for colonic diverticular disease is more than two and one-half times the percentage of this age group in the entire hospitalized population (Commission on Professional and Hospital Activities 1977).

How does one explain these facts? Current wisdom attributes great importance to dietary factors. Painter and Burkitt point out that in underdeveloped agrarian societies the diet consists of large amounts of whole grain, little meat, and almost no processed food. The result of this diet is bulky and heavy stools, rapid intestinal transit, low intracolonic pressures, and infrequent diverticulosis. Urbanized populations consume primarily milled flour, processed foods, considerable meat, and refined sugars. Such a diet results in small and hard stools, slowed intestinal transit, increased intracolonic pressures and, in time, a high incidence and prevalance of diverticulosis. These impressions have been supported by observations that patients with diverticulosis of the colon do indeed have considerable increases of intracolonic pressures over normal (Arfwiddson 1964), and that the addition of dietary fiber to patients reduces both the intestinal transit time and the luminal colonic pressures. Furthermore, there is increasing evidence that dietary changes over a period of years may be associated with moderate increases in the incidence of diverticulosis among populations which had been formerly free of that disorder. Segal et al (1977) have demonstrated the emergence of diverticulosis among South African blacks in the years following their removal to an urban setting from the countryside, and Stemmerman and Yatani (1973) have shown a similar effect among Japanese immigrants to Hawaii. Although each of these observations strengthens the dietary hypothesis, final confirmation in animal models or in prospective studies is not at hand.

Pathogenesis

Diverticulosis of the colon probably results from a combination of two contributory factors, decreased integrity or tensile strength of the musculature of the colon, and increased intraluminal pressure. The relative importance of each of these factors in any one case of diverticulosis probably has a direct bearing on the size, location, and configuration of individual diverticula, and perhaps also on the total number of diverticula and the likelihood for certain complications to occur.

Decreased Integrity of the Colonic Musculature. The circular musculature of the colon is not a seamless homogeneous layer. It is rather a closely knit lattice of muscle fibers supported by connective tissue and penetrated at regular intervals by nutrient arteries extending from the serosa to the mucosa. With aging, it has been demonstrated that the synthesis of type III collagen, which is essential for the normal tensile strength of intestinal tissue, is decreased (Prockop et al 1979). The rate of synthesis and degradation, and the quality of collagen, also decreases with aging. These physiologic phenomena might explain both why the incidence of diverticulosis increases with aging, and why colonic diverticulosis tends to be more extensive throughout the colon among the elderly than it is in younger individuals. It is an impression also that diverticula tend to be larger among the elderly, and that the diverticular necks leading from the intestinal lumen into the pouch of herniated mucosa tend to be of greater diameter, perhaps again as a result of reduced tensile strength of the collagen. Many older patients with diverticulosis show little or no evidence of increased intracolonic pressure, suggesting again that the connective tissue defect is probably of major importance in the etiology of this type of the disease.

In some patients with genetic and acquired connective tissue disorders, an increased incidence of colonic diverticulosis has been described. Beighton et al (1969) describe colonic diverticulosis as one of the digestive complications found among patients with the Ehlers-Danlos syndrome, a congenital disorder of connective tissue. And among patients with scleroderma involving the large intestine, there is also a significant incidence of diverticulosis. Diverticula in this disorder tend to have large stomas and a decreased likelihood of becoming obstructed. The increased stomal size is probably a direct result of reduced muscular tensile strength occasioned by the fibrotic infiltration characteristic of the disease.

Increased Intraluminal Pressure. While diverticula resulting primarily from connective tissue and muscular weaknesses tend to be large and more disseminated throughout the colon, those caused mainly by increased intraluminal pressure tend to congregate at points where intraluminal pressures are likely to be greatest. They are also likely to be smaller in size and to have narrower necks. In these patients, there is a tendency for an associated hypertrophy of the colonic muscular layer to be present. This muscular hypertrophy in the sigmoid colon has been noted to occur in some patients without diverticulosis and has been considered by Arfwiddson (1964) and others to be a prediverticular condition. That pressure-related diverticula tend to occur in the sigmoid and descending colons primarily has been attributed to the fact that these segments of the colon, being smaller in diameter than the more proximal segments, react to a given strength of muscular contraction with proportionately greater increments of intraluminal pressure (Almy 1965). Painter et al (1965) attribute the genesis of pressure-induced diverticula to the increased tension and resulting "blow-out" of mucosa caused in the colonic haustrum located between two successive segments of spastic circular muscle (Figure 19–1).

Reference has already been made to the moderating effect which dietary fiber has on intracolonic pressure. There is also some feeling that patients with a long history of irritable colon syndrome are at greater risk than others for developing diverticulosis. In support of this contention is the

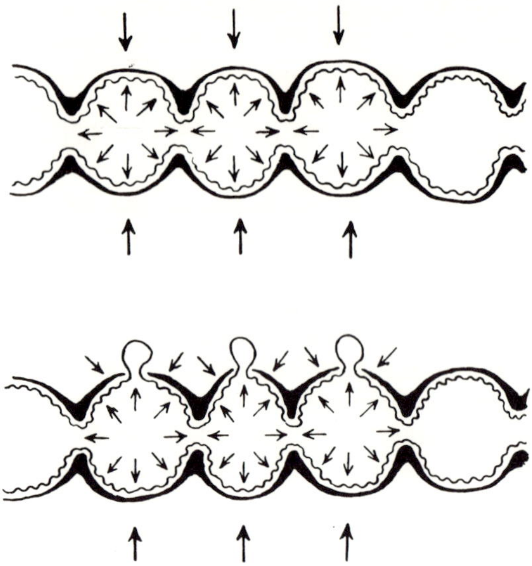

Figure 19-1. Diagram to show how segmentation produces the pulsion force that distends colonic diverticula, and probably causes the initial mucosal herniation. From Painter NS, Truelove SC, Adran GM, et al. Gastroenterology 49:169–77, 1965. © 1965 The William & Wilkins Co., Baltimore.

fact that some patients with sigmoid diverticulosis show physiologic responses similar to those of patients with irritable bowels. Among these are increased pressure responses in the sigmoid to eating and increased motor responses to cholecystokinin. However, most patients with new symptoms related to diverticular disease have no preceding history of irritable bowel symptoms, and many patients with irritable bowel symptoms of long duration do not appear to develop diverticulosis.

Symptoms and Signs

Many patients with diverticulosis of the colon experience no symptoms whatsoever. When present, symptoms are the result of motility disturbances, acute or chronic inflammation of clustered or single diverticula, and bleeding, either singly or in varying combinations.

Most commonly, the complaints of patients with diverticulosis resemble those of patients with the irritable bowel syndrome, and include abdominal distention, cramping pain, tenesmus, diarrhea, or constipation. Signs of inflammation are absent, and the complaints are probably the result of muscular irritability alone. The bowel is often tender to palpation, particularly in the lower left quadrant of the abdomen. While the rectum is usually normal on sigmoidoscopy, considerable spasm of the sigmoid is commonly found. In fact, introduction of the instrument into the upper rectum or lower sigmoid is often impossible because of muscular spasm and pain, often with reproduction of the patient's spontaneous symptoms. While the symptoms are often severe, this type of diverticular disease should not be confused with actual diverticulitis.

True diverticulitis is much less common than the muscular irritability syndrome, and probably results from diverticular obstruction by feces and mucus, mucosal edema and inflammation, followed by microperforations into the submucosa, muscularis, and surrounding tissues. In these patients, signs of localized peritonitis, fever, and leukocytosis are usually present. Walled-off and free peritoneal perforations may occur, the latter leading at times to generalized peritonitis with free air in the peritoneal cavity. While most instances of diverticulitis occur in the left colon and sigmoid amid clustered diverticula, large single diverticula of the right colon may occasionally become obstructed and inflamed. A walled-off perforation may lead to the development of a pelvic abscess, and deep penetrations of the inflammatory process may lead to the formation of fistulas into organs adjacent to the rectosigmoid, such as the urinary bladder or the vagina. Some patients indeed may be unaware of having chronic diverticulitis until they note the passage of gas or particulate fecal matter in the urine.

Colonic hemorrhage is an increasingly recognized complication of diverticulosis and tends to occur as frequently from right-sided as from left-sided diverticula. The hemorrhage may be profuse, and the responsible diverticulum is commonly not inflamed. The liability of hemorrhage is doubtless related to the fact that diverticula penetrate the colonic muscularis through the interstices of mural arteries, and that the arteries are consequently closely apposed to them. As the diverticulum increases in size, the artery becomes more liable to pressure necrosis and to hemorrhage.

Diagnosis

The diagnosis of diverticular disease is suspected from history and physical findings. The condition can usually be quickly distinguished from colonic cancer by the results of a barium enema examination (Figure 19–2). In cases of free perforation, the diagnosis is confirmed at surgery. Where colonic hemorrhage is the major symptom of diverticular disease, efforts should be made initially to achieve circulatory stabilization, to rule out coagulapathies, and then to proceed as quickly as possible to selective angiography of the mesenteric vasculature. Where arteriocapillary hemorrhage is active enough, the exact site of bleeding can be nicely demonstrated by this technique and the catheter may be left in place for therapy with vasospastic agents (Figure 19–3). The use of vasopressin for this purpose

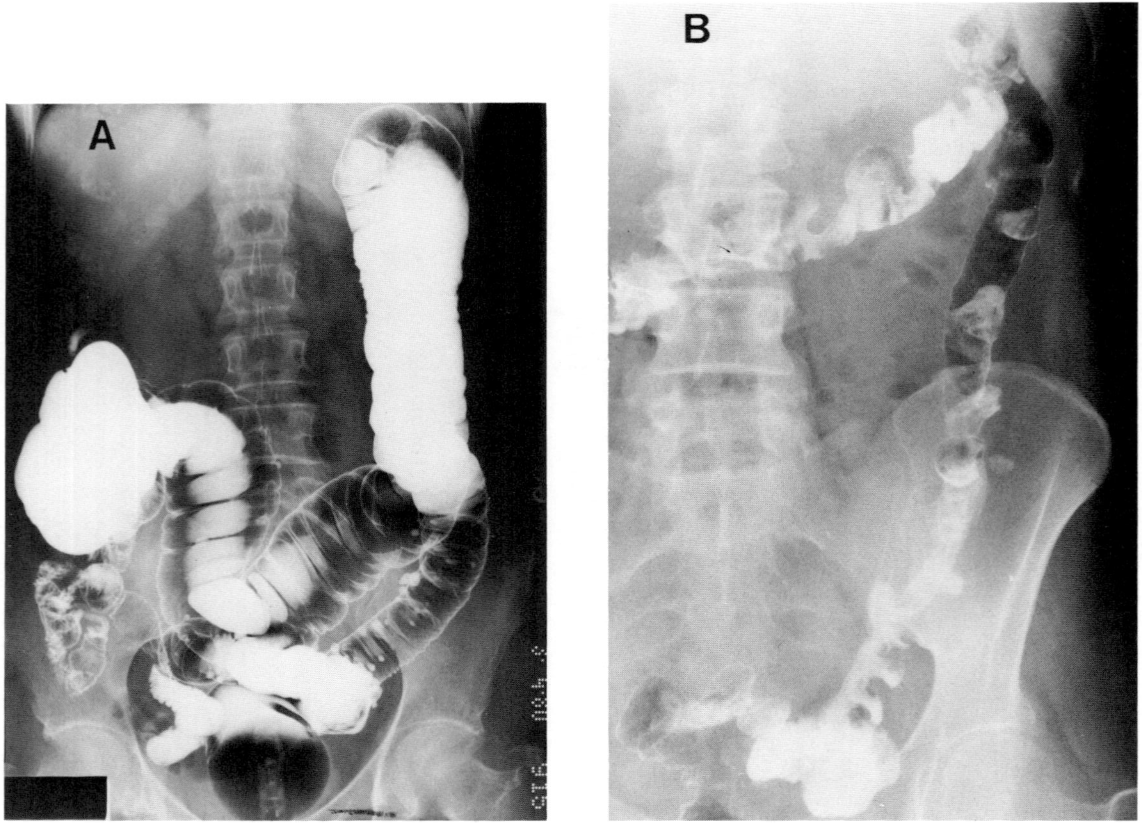

Figure 19–2. Barium enemas in two patients with diverticulosis of the colon. *A*, shows typical, small narrow-mouthed diverticula in the sigmoid and transverse colon characteristic of pulsion diverticulosis. *B*, shows numerous large diverticula with characteristic wide mouth, observed frequently in patients with progressive systemic sclerosis (scleroderma). Courtesy of Dr. Renatl Duchesneau.

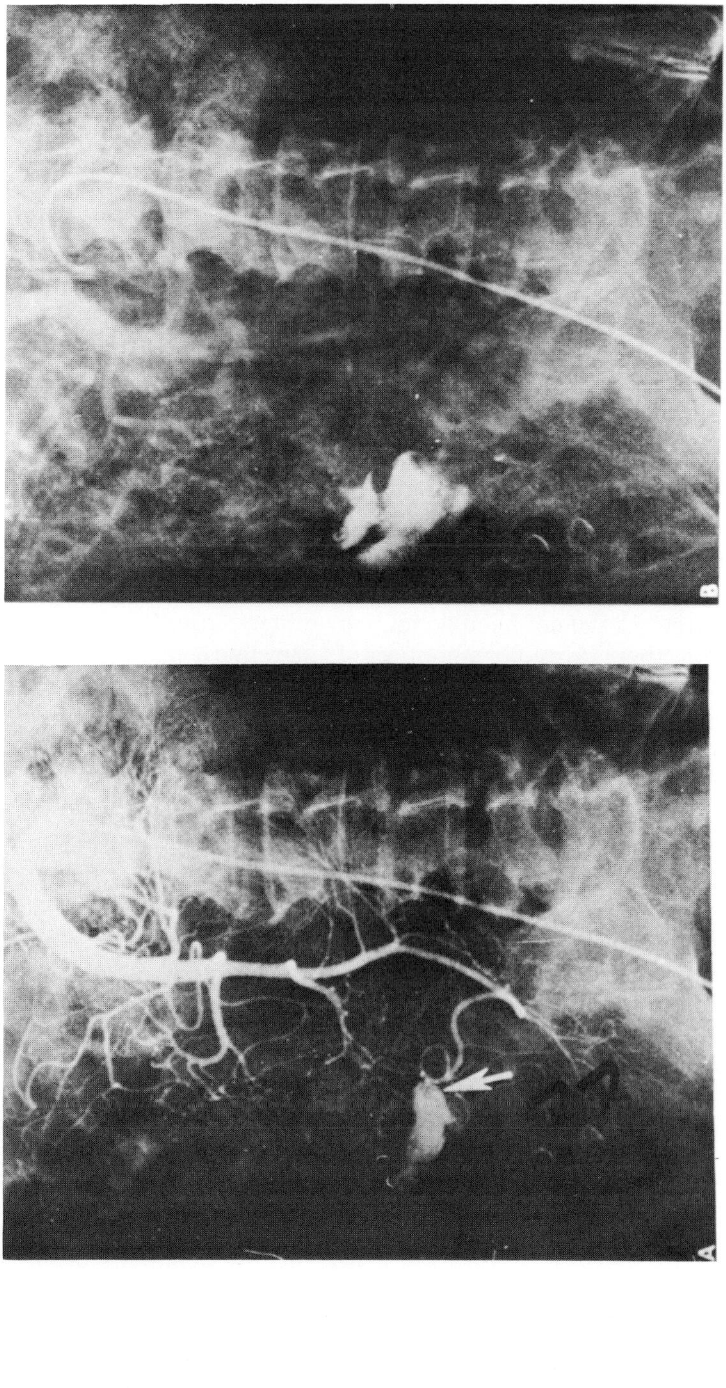

Figure 19–3. Massive hemorrhage from a diverticulum of the ascending colon in a sixty-five-year-old man. *A*, superior mesenteric arteriogram shows extravasation of contrast material from a branch of the ileocolic artery (arrow) into the ascending colon. *B*, during the later phase of the superior mesenteric arteriogram, extravasation persists, and it has assumed the circular appearance that is representative of diverticular hemorrhage due to accumulation of contrast material within the confines of the diverticulum. From Athanasoulis CA, Baum S, Rosch J, et al. Am J Surg 129:212–16, 1975. Reprinted by permission.

has been quite effective (Athanasoulis 1980), and the incidence of recurrent hemorrhage is quite low. When a bleeding site is not demonstrable and vascular ectasias are not found, patients with recent colonic hemorrhage should be given barium enemas. This procedure will detect the presence of diverticula, although it will not indicate the exact source of bleeding.

Treatment

The clear message of the observations of Burkitt and Painter (1971) is that the heavy moist stool of the country-dwelling African native is to be strongly preferred to the hard compact stool of the urbanized Westerner. Where this hypothesis has been tested by increasing dietary fiber with supplemental bran in patients with symptomatic diverticular disease, the results do indicate considerable benefit (Brodribb and Humphreys 1976; Taylor and Duthie 1976). Some patients experience initial troublesome bloating from this regimen, but these side effects tend to disappear within a short time, and associated diverticular symptoms of cramping, tenesmus, diarrhea, and constipation usually moderate considerably. Where spasm is clearly associated with symptomatic diverticulosis or diverticulitis, some of us like to administer antispasmodic agents (such as dicyclomine, 10–20 mg qid before meals and at bedtime) as well, although careful, controlled studies of their effects have not been done. In practice, patients are asked to increase gradually their daily consumption of bran to 18 to 20 g per day. Where this is not possible, equally good effects have been reported from the use of methylcellulose or psyllium hydrophylic mucilloid as bulking agents. This treatment has also been found to be effective in patients with single attacks of diverticular bleeding.

In cases of acute diverticulitis, most physicians prescribe antibiotics (ampicillin, tetracycline) for short periods of time, even though their efficacy has not been clearly documented and causative bacterial agents may not have been isolated. Patients with acute flares of diverticulitis should be fed only clear liquid diets for the first few days, until the course of their disease has been clearly shown to be improving. The efficacy of this "medical" approach to the treatment of diverticulitis has been documented in a study by Larson et al (1976).

Surgery should be reserved for patients with recurrent diverticular hemorrhage, recurrent uncomplicated diverticulitis, or acute perforations or fistulization. In all of these situations, the disease is clearly severe enough to demand extirpation of the involved bowel segment. Surgical intervention is particularly important for those patients with isolated recurrent attacks of diverticulitis, the objective being the avoidance of serious complications like abscess or perforation which usually demand more than one surgical procedure, including a temporary deviating colostomy.

MECKEL DIVERTICULA

While single antimesenteric diverticula of the lower ileum were described occasionally during the seventeenth and eighteenth centuries, Johann Friedrich Meckel the Younger was the first anatomist to attribute their origin to incomplete closure of the vitelline or omphaloenteric duct, which connects the intestine to the embryonic yolk sac. His description first appeared in 1808, and later observers noted a number of other anomalies of the vitelline duct, including fistulas between the lower small intestine and the navel, cords connecting the intestine to the abdominal wall, and enterocysts attached by a cord to the umbilicus, the lower small intestine, or both. Gastric mucosa was found in some Meckel diverticula in the late nineteenth century, but the first description of an ileal peptic ulcer due to diverticular secretion of hydrochloric acid was not published until 1913.

Pathogenesis

Meckel diverticula are single wide-mouthed pouches of varying length attached to the antimesenteric border of the ileum about 40 cm from the ileocecal valve in children and 50 cm in adults (Figure 19–4). The vitelline duct

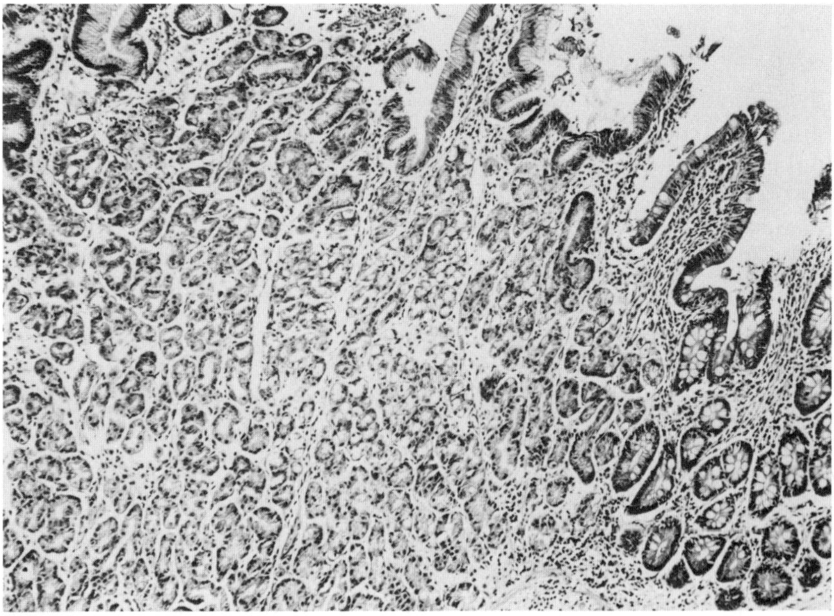

Figure 19–4. Meckel diverticulum in a patient with lower right quadrant pain and gastrointestinal hemorrhage. The mucosa is lined by gastric glands on the left and intestinal glands on the right. Original magnification x80.

usually disappears completely during the eighth week of embryonic life, and the reason for its persistence in patients with Meckel diverticula is not known. Associated anomalies are uncommon. Approximately 2 percent of newborn infants are believed to have Meckel diverticula, and they are three times more common in men than in women. Nearly half of Meckel diverticula contain aberrent gastric mucosal glands; some contain pancreatic glands and intestinal mucosa as well. Apparently, the stem cell endoderm of the diverticulum is capable of developing in a variety of directions.

Probably no more than 5 to 10 percent of Meckel diverticula ever become sympotomatic, and these symptoms may be related to ileal peptic ulcers caused by the action of gastric secretions on ileal mucosa, to intestinal obstruction caused by volvulus of bowel around the vitelline duct remnant or by intussusception of the diverticulum into the ileum, or to diverticulitis and occasionally perforation of the diverticulum from obstruction. The incidence of hemorrhage from ileal ulcers appears to be higher in children, and diverticulitis and intestinal obstruction predominate in adults. While nearly half of pathogenic Meckel diverticula become symptomatic by the age of two years, Söderlund (1959) reported that nearly 20 percent of patients were older than age 16 when their first symptoms appeared.

Symptoms

Volvulus or intussusception of a Meckel diverticulum causes abdominal distention, pain, vomiting, and the inability to pass flatus so typical of an intestinal obstruction. The presence of fever and leukocytosis suggest intestinal necrosis or diverticulitis. A mass is frequently palpable in the lower right abdominal quadrant or just below the umbilicus. Ileal peptic ulcerations cause major lower bowel hemorrhage, typified by the passage of bright or dark red stools without melena. There is usually no pain associated with the ulcerations themselves, unless they have perforated into the peritoneal cavity.

Diagnosis

Meckel diverticula should be prominently considered as the cause of lower small intestinal obstructions in infants and children. Where gastrointestinal hemorrhage is the major symptom, it should be kept in mind that melena is usually absent in patients with massive lower intestinal bleeding, and that the level of blood urea nitrogen usually does not show as great an increase as would be expected from a hemorrhage of similar volume from an upper gastrointestinal site. This distinction appears to arise from the fact that the shedding of blood into the lowermost small intestine does not lead to the proteolysis and massive absorption of protein nitrogen which occurs when blood is introduced into the upper small intestine and digested in the lumen.

Blood loss from the ileal ulcerations caused by acid-secreting Meckel diverticula may be intermittent or chronic. Small intestinal X rays demonstrate only a small proportion of these diverticula. Superior mesenteric arterial angiography will show extravasation of the contrast medium into the small intestine if the study is performed while bleeding is active, but will be normal if the bleeding is slight or has discontinued. In instances where the ileal ulcerations are not bleeding actively, and where the diverticulum contains gastric mucosa, some diagnostic success has been achieved with radioisotopic scanning (Kilpatrick and Aseron 1972). ^{99m}Tc sodium pertechnetate has an affinity for oxyntic cells, presumably because it is metabolized similarly to chloride and iodide. After blockage of thyroid uptake with iodine, the intravenously administered isotope concentrates in gastric mucosa and, if they are present, in the oxyntic cells of Meckel diverticula. The specificity of this test is rather good, but its sensitivity is only fair. When scanning is negative in cases where the clinical suspicion of a Meckel diverticulum is high, exploratory laparatomy is frequently the most advisable clinical option.

Treatment

In patients with symptomatic Meckel diverticula, whether the symptoms are related to intestinal obstruction, diverticulitis, or hemorrhage, the only acceptable treatment is surgical excision. Surgical management generally involves a sleeve resection of the ileal segment containing the diverticulum, with a primary anastomoses of the transected ends of the bowel. There is some dispute regarding the advisability of removal of asymptomatic Meckel diverticula found incidentally during surgery for other conditions. In these cases, there is evidence that the diverticula should not be removed, since the complications of the excision are likely to be greater than the benefit of the procedure (Soltero and Bill 1976).

APPENDICITIS

Because appendicitis is a most common cause of localized peritonitis in humans, and since its diagnosis presents a continuing clinical challenge, the pathophysiology of this potentially serious disorder should be clearly understood by all clinicians. The usual evolution of appendicitis illustrates very nicely the distinction between visceral and parietal peritonitis, and its recognition in early stages can prevent the serious complications of appendiceal abscess and generalized peritonitis.

The exact cause of suppurative appendicitis is not clear in all cases, but stasis of luminal flow is believed to be a major contributory factor. Actual obstruction of the narrow appendiceal lumen by feces or mucus is found in well over half the cases of acute inflammation, and other cases have been associated with the accumulation of large amounts of stool in the cecum and right side of the colon. It is possible that strictures and primary motility disturbances of the appendix play an etiologic role in still other instances. Stasis, according to this theory, permits an accumulation of enteric organisms in the appendiceal lumen. These, in turn, lead to epithelial disruption and mural inflammation. Once established, inflammation progresses rapidly through the thin wall of the appendix, and leads directly to visceral peritonitis, necrosis, and finally, to perforation.

Epidemiology

Appendicitis is largely a disease of youth, the mean age of 19.8 years in a series of 192 patients described by Law et al (1976) being typical of most other studies. However, the range of ages in this series, from 2.5 months to 68 years, strongly suggests that appendicitis must always be considered as a cause of abdominal pain in any patients, age notwithstanding, who do not bear an operative scar attesting to a previous appendectomy. Among the elderly, appendicitis is a particularly treacherous disease, because the symptoms are often mild and atypical, and because the likelihood of perforation is increased (Bradley 1959). Reduced arterial blood flow with aging is believed to be responsible for the increased risk of perforation.

Symptoms and Signs

Sir Zachary Cope (1968) has stressed that the earliest symptoms of acute appendicitis may be so mild that they are likely to be minimized by the patient, and frequently not fully appreciated by the medical advisor. To a large extent, symptoms are related to the anatomical position of the appendix. Pain and physical findings are most striking when the organ lies in one of its usual positions, alongside or just below the cecum, and they are least intense when the appendix lies low in the true pelvis or behind the cecum or terminal ileum. In other words, when the inflamed appendix is overlain by normal bowel or by pelvic organs, the onset of parietal peritonitis and sharp pain may be delayed, even though the danger of appendiceal rupture and abscess is not reduced.

The initial pain of appendicitis is usually midabdominal or epigastric. It is commonly followed by nausea, occasionally with vomiting, and is then succeeded by local tenderness in the lower right quadrant of the abdomen, often by slight fever and almost invariably by leukocytosis. The initial pain is visceral and results from transmural inflammation and edema of the organ. Pain becomes sharply perceived by the patient when the parietal peritoneum in the lower right quadrant becomes involved in the inflammatory process and somatic nerve pathways are stimulated. This shift of pain from a vaguely perceived visceral discomfort to a sharply perceived somatic distress is typical of the progress of appendicitis when the organ occupies one of its usual positions. While having visceral pain, patients often bend forward and may pace the floor; when pain becomes somatic, they prefer to lie quietly.

Examination of the abdomen before the onset of parietal peritonitis reveals tenderness deep in the lower right quadrant, usually without rigidity of the overlying abdominal musculature. Muscular spasms occur when localized parietal peritonitis develops. Tenderness can often be detected high on the right side during rectal examinations, especially if the appendix points into the true pelvis. The white blood count is usually elevated, averaging between 13,000 and 15,000 per cu mm, and temperature may be elevated about one degree or more in over a third of patients. Higher elevations of temperature are associated with appendiceal abscess and free perforations.

Patients with retrocecal or pelvis appendicitis and older patients frequently complain less of pain and show less evidence of muscular spasm on abdominal examination. Sometimes only vague abdominal discomfort and tenderness and slight leukocytosis are the only findings. Extension and outward rotation of the right thigh may aggravate abdominal pain in patients with inflammation of a retrocecal appendix (psoas sign).

Diagnosis

The diagnosis of appendicitis can be made with relative certainty only after pelvic inflammatory disease, tubal pregnancy, rupture of an ovarian follicle, and upper urinary tract infections have been ruled out by appropriate examinations. A plain film of the abdomen is also useful in ruling out the possibility of intestinal obstruction. Acute mesenteric adenitis and acute Crohn disease of the terminal ileum may closely simulate the symptoms of appendicitis. The former can be diagnosed occasionally by the simultaneous presence of upper respiratory symptoms and a nearly normal white blood count, while the latter is frequently suggested by a history of diarrhea for days or weeks before the acute attack. Symptoms and signs of Meckel diverticulitis are indistinguishable from those of acute appendicitis.

Even though appendicitis should be suspected in all patients with signs of inflammation and localized peritonitis who do not bear the telltale scar of previous appendectomy, it should not be considered when abdominal pain and tenderness are unaccompanied by muscular spasm, fever, or leukocytosis. Many patients with the irritable bowel syndrome have lost their appendices unnecessarily because their physicians did not appreciate this point.

Treatment

Although single attacks of appendicitis may subside spontaneously, appendectomy is the only acceptable form of treatment. The danger of rupture followed by peritonitis far outweighs the risk of surgery, even in those patients in whom the preoperative diagnosis is not crystal clear. In most carefully monitored series of appendectomies done for presumed acute inflammation, approximately 10 to 15 percent reveal either no evidence of any pathology or the presence of nonappendiceal disease. Because of the uncertainties of diagnosis, there is certainly no shame attached to removing a normal appendix occasionally. The greater shame comes from allowing a perforation to occur while debating whether to operate.

HISTORICAL DIGRESSION

Names mentioned in this chapter without further reference include: Henri Alexander DANLOS (1844–1912), French physician, Paris; Edward EHLERS (1863–1937), Danish dermatologist, Copenhagen, described hyperelasticity of skin in 1901; Johann Friedrich MECKEL, Jr. (1781–1833). German anatomist and surgeon, Halle, described congenital ileal diverticulum, 1809.

SELECTED REFERENCES

Almy TP. Diverticular disease of the colon–the new look. Gastroenterology 49:109–12, 1965.

Almy TP, Howell DA. Diverticular disease of the colon. N Engl J Med 302: 324–31, 1980.

Arfwidsson F. Pathogenesis of multiple diverticula of the sigmoid colon in diverticular disease. Acta Chir Scand (Suppl):342, 1964.

Athanasoulis CA. Therapeutic applications of angiography. N Engl J Med 302:1117–25, 1980.

Beighton PH, Murdoch JL, Votteler T. Gastrointestinal complications of the Ehlers-Danlos syndrome. Gut 10: 1004–8, 1969.

Bradley RL. Appendicitis in the aged. Gastroenterology 33:925–28, 1959.

Brodribb AJM, Humphreys DM. Diverticular disease: three studies. Br Med J 1:988–90, 1976.

Commission on Professional and Hospital Activities. Hospital Mortality, PAS Hospitals, 1974–75. Ann Arbor, 1977.

Connell AM. Pathogenesis of diverticular disease of the colon. Adv Int Med 22:377–95, 1977.

Cope Z. The early diagnosis of the acute abdomen, 13th ed. London: Oxford University Press, 1968:47–60.

Kilpatrick ZM, Aseron CA, Jr. Radioistope detection of Meckel's diverticulum causing acute rectal hemorrhage. N Engl J Med 287:653–54, 1972.

Larson DM, Masters SS, Spiro HM. Medical and surgical therapy in diverticular disease. A comparative study. Gastroenterology 71:737–37, 1976.

Law D, Law R, Eiseman B. The continuing challenge of acute and perforated appendicitis. Am J Surg 131:533–35, 1976.

Painter NS, Burkitt DP. Diverticular disease of the colon: a deficiency disease of Western civilization. Br Med J 2:450–54, 1971.

Painter NS, Truelove SC, Ardran GM, et al. Segmentation and the localization of intraluminal pressures in the human colon, with special reference to the pathogenesis of colonic diverticula. Gastroenterology 49: 169–77, 1965.

Prockop DJ, Kivirikko KI, Tuderman L, et al. The biosynthesis of collagen and its disorders. N Engl J Med 301:13–23, 77–85, 1979.

Segal I, Solomon A, Hunt JA. Emergence of diverticular disease in the urban South African black. Gastroenterology 72:215–19, 1977.

Söderlund S. Meckel's diverticulum. A clinical and histologic study. Acta Chir Scand (Supp):248, 1959.

Soltero MJ, Bill AH. The natural history of Meckel's diverticulum and its relation to incidental removal. AM J Surg 132:168–73, 1976.

Stemmerman GN, Yatani R. Diverticulosis and polyps of the large intestine: a necropsy study of Hawaii Japanese. Cancer 31:1260–70, 1973.

Taylor I, Duthie HL. Bran tablets and diverticular disease. Br Med J 1:988–90, 1976.

CLINICAL CONFERENCE 12

A 63-year-old man was hospitalized with lower midabdominal cramps, diarrhea, tenesmus, loss of weight, and urinary frequency for three weeks. He had been well previously, except for constipation requiring occasional laxatives for 20 years. He had initially consulted his physician for 10 days before hospitalization and was placed on paregoric for diarrhea. This medication relieved diarrhea somewhat but did not affect the cramps or tenesmus. He ascribed his loss of five pounds to the fact that eating tended to aggravate the lower abdominal pain.

Physical examination showed a well-developed man whose oral mucosa was somewhat dehydrated. Vital signs showed blood pressure

152/76, pulse 94, respirations 16, and temperature 38.4°C. Abnormal findings consisted of moderate tenderness in the left lower quadrant of the abdomen, slight muscular rigidity in this area, and a palpable, slightly movable, sausage-shaped mass, measuring 20 cm at its widest diameter parallel to the left pelvic brim. Bowel sounds were normal, save for one rush that was associated with a complaint of cramping pain. Rectal examination showed early symmetrical enlargement of the prostate and produced a small amount of soft brown stool that was 2-plus positive to guaiac. Sigmoidoscopy was performed to a depth of 22 cm and could not be continued because of marked sigmoidal spasm associated with dusky reddening of the mucosa without friability. The rectum and lower sigmoid were normal. A barium enema showed moderately extensive diverticulosis of the colon, with an area of clustered diverticula in the midsigmoid. The colonic lumen was narrow in this area, and it was difficult initially to force barium through it. In one spot the radiologist thought he might have seen penetration of a thin stream of barium into a lateral colonic mass. Hematocrit was 46 percent, white cell count 13,600, with 78 percent polymorphonuclear leukocytes. Urinalysis showed 20 to 30 white blood cells per high-power field and a few red blood cells but was otherwise normal. Serum electrolytes were normal.

1. Define the probable pathophysiology of this disorder, considering alternate possibilities for symptoms as well.
2. What therapeutic mechanisms are available to you? What alternatives should be used in the event that primary therapy is not effective?

CHAPTER 20

Polyps and Cancer of the Colon

COLONIC POLYPS AND POLYPOSIS SYNDROMES

Any mucosal protuberance which juts into the lumen of the intestine may justifiably be called a polyp. There is a considerable variety of types of polyp which are of clinical importance. The most important of these types are the inflammatory, the hamartomatous, the metaplastic, and the adenomatous. Of these, only adenomatous polyps are true neoplasms, and thus are of the greatest clinical interest because of the frequency with which they undergo malignant change.

Colonic polyps of any type may occur singly or in small numbers, or may appear in multitudes. Only the latter situation is designated as "polyposis." Morson and Dawson (1979) describe the following colonic polyposis syndromes: inflammatory polyposis (as may occur in ulcerative colitis, Crohn disease, or lymphoid hyperplasia); hamartomatous polyposis (as in juvenile polyposis, the Cronkhite-Canada syndrome, or the Peutz-Jeghers syndrome); metaplastic polyposis; and adenomatosis (as in familial polyposis of the colon, Gardner syndrome, or Turcot syndrome). Most polyposis syndromes are heredible, familial polyposis, Gardner syndrome, and Peutz-Jeghers syndrome as dominant traits, and Turcot syndrome and juvenile polyposis as recessives. Sex-linkage does not occur. There appears to be no genetic mechanism involved in the Cronkhite-Canada syndrome. While inheritance is clear in most types of polyposis, the disorders are not congenital, and may not appear in persons at risk until after the first or second decades of life.

Nonneoplastic Polyps

Inflammatory Polyps (Figure 20–1). These lesions are commonly seen as areas of inflamed and swollen colonic mucosa between open or epithelialized ulcerations in patients with Crohn disease of the colon or ulcerative colitis. They have also been called pseudopolyps to distinguish them from adenomata. They have no known malignant potential and frequently disappear when the colitis heals. Inflammatory polyps and adenomatous polyps

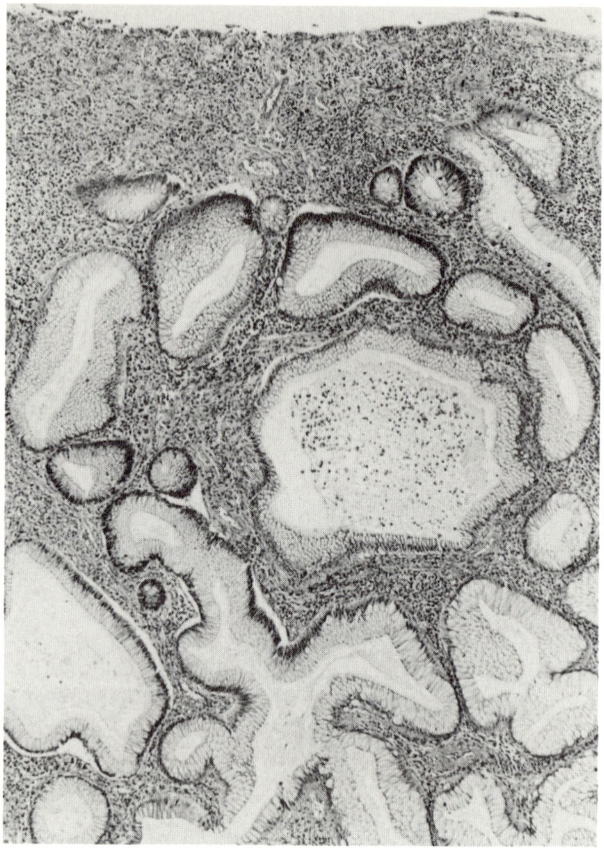

Figure 20-1. Inflammatory colonic polyp. Note that the mucosa is ulcerated, the colonic glands are cystically dilated, and there is chronic inflammatory infiltrate in the lamina propria. Original magnification x50.

may coexist in the same colon and may be difficult to distinguish from one another by gross examination. The symptoms and treatment of inflammatory polyps are not different from those of the underlying inflammatory bowel disease. Their presence does, however, emphasize the severity of the inflammatory process.

Hamartomatous Polyps (Figure 20-2). Hamartomas are abnormal combinations of tissues which normally appear in the bowel. While strands of muscle are commonly found to be coursing throughout a hamartomatous polyp in an irregular fashion, epithelial cytology is normal (Enterline 1976). The population of goblet cells is normal, nuclear crowding and hyperchromasia are absent, nuclei are located at the base of the epithelial cell and no atypia of nuclei or layering of epithelial cells is found.

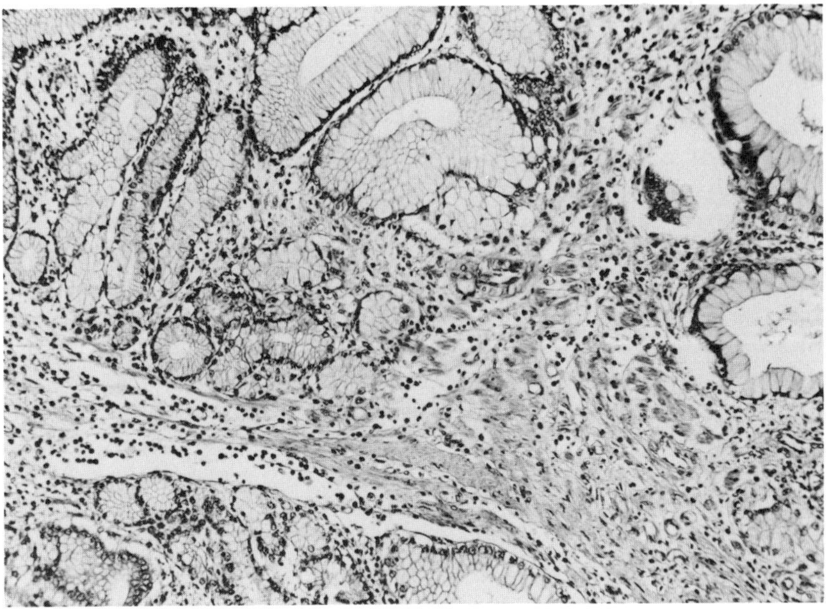

Figure 20–2. Hamartomatous polyp in Peutz-Jeghers syndrome. Proliferating colonic glands, some of which are dilated, are intermingled with smooth muscle cells. Original magnification x100.

In the syndrome described by Peutz (1921) and Jeghers (1949), numerous hamartomatous polyps are found throughout the stomach and intestines, but they predominate in the small bowel. Spots of mucocutaneous melanin pigmentation, particularly in the mouth, lips, and face, are characteristic of this syndrome. The polyps themselves vary considerably in size, and their enlargement has been attributed to hyperplasia of the muscularis mucosae.

The symptoms of Peutz-Jeghers syndrome consist primarily of vomiting, abdominal pain, and bloating, relating to varible degrees of intestinal obstruction caused by the polyposis. In milder attacks, the symptoms disappear spontaneously, while severe attacks of complete intestinal obstruction may very possibly require surgical repair. The obstructive symptoms result from the effects of peristaltic traction on the larger polyps which leads, over a period of time, to the development of mucosal pedicles or stalks. Eventually, this repeated peristaltic tugging causes intussusception of the intestine, with a large polyp acting as the leading edge of the intussusceptum. Occasional polyps may ulcerate and bleed; they rarely if ever undergo malignant changes. Treatment is directed only at the complications, usually intestinal obstruction or hemorrhage, of the Peutz-Jeghers syndrome. Prophylactic surgery is useless, because the occurrence of these complications is not predictable, and because polyps may develop at a later date in segments of bowel found to be free of disease at the time of the initial study (Schwabe and Lewin 1980).

The Cronkhite-Canada syndrome (Cronkhite and Canada 1955) is a rare disorder consisting of hamartomatous sessile polyposis largely in the stomach and colon, and occasionally in the small intestine, associated with brown macular cutaneous lesions on the face and upper trunk in many patients, atrophy of the fingernails, loss of hair, iron-deficiency anemia, anorexia, loss of weight, protein-losing enteropathy, and occasional steatorrhea. The average age of onset is about 60 years. Colonic mucosal lesions show both atrophy of the epithelium and tortuosity and cyst formation of glands. The gastric mucosa may show proliferation of epithelial cells above the foveolar neck, suggestive of the changes seen in the Menetrier-Hurst syndrome, a disorder which is also associated with loss of serum protein through the intestinal or gastric mucosa (Enterline 1976). Secondary mucosal inflammation may be found in patients with the Cronkhite-Canada syndrome, and the disease itself may be partially responsive to glucocorticoids and parenteral hyperalimentation.

Metaplastic Polyps (Figure 20–3). These lesions are benign mucosal elevations which may appear in any portion of the colon but tend to congregate

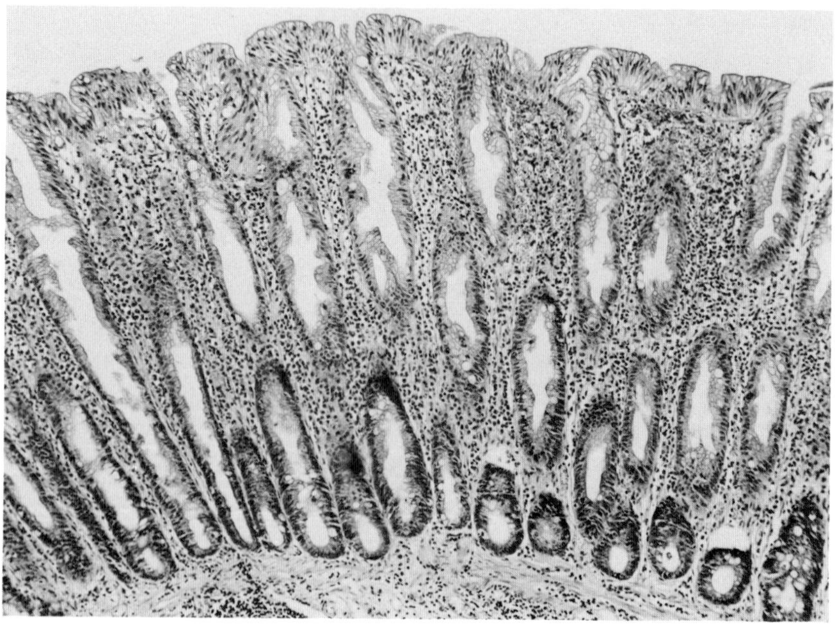

Figure 20–3. Metaplastic colonic polyp. Stellate-shaped colonic glands are lined by a single layer of tall columnar cells without any nuclear atypia. Original magnification x80.

primarily in the rectum. The incidence of metaplastic polyps increases with age and approaches 75 percent in persons over age 55. They are rarely greater than 0.5 cm in diameter, and they rarely become symptomatic. They tend to be sessile and of paler shade than normal mucosa. On microscopy, metaplastic polyps show reduced migration rates of colonic epithelial crypt cells when compared to normal epithelium. Cytological characteristics are otherwise normal, and cellular atypia is never seen.

Neoplastic (Adenomatous) Polyps

Single or Random Adenomata. Adenomatous polyps of the colon are extremely common with aging. They are quite variable in size and configuration, ranging from sessile to pedunculated, and from a few millimeters in diameter to several centimeters. Grossly, adenomatous polyps are bright to deep red and mild to moderately friable to gentle touching. They are readily distinguishable from metaplastic polyps by their size and color. Microscopy reveals their true neoplastic nature by showing hyperchromasia, enlargement, and crowding of nuclei (Figure 20-4). The production of mucin is usually reduced in adenomatous mucosa, and the mucus itself is believed to be

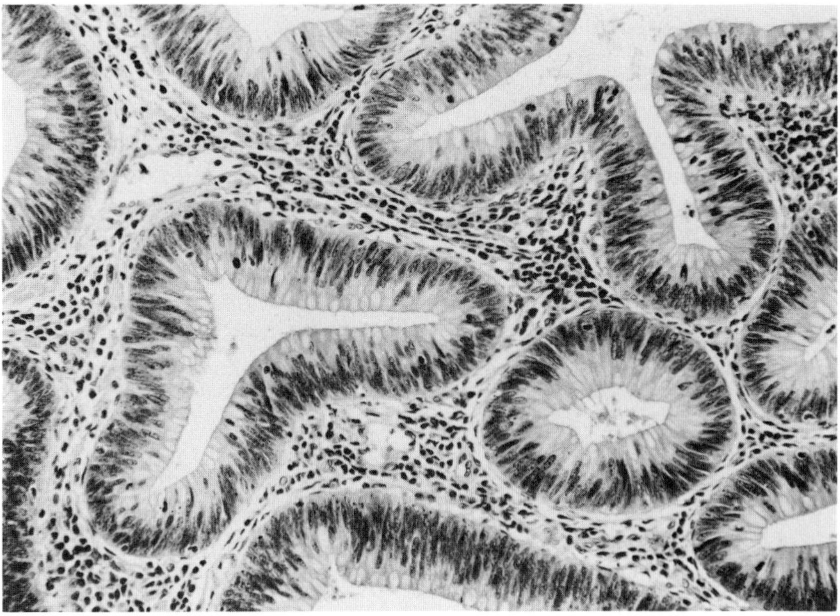

Figure 20-4. Adenomatous polyp of colon. The glands are lined by columnar cells with pseudostratified nuclear arrangement, minimal nuclear atypia, and abundant mitotic figures. Original magnification x200.

abnormal. Paneth cells appear throughout adenomatous polyps rather than being located only in the bases of mucosal crypts, as in normal mucosa. Epithelial cell division is also abnormal in these lesions (Bottomley and Cooper 1973). Tritiated thymidine studies have shown that DNA synthesis may occur in epithelial cells at any level on an adenomatous polyp, rather than being suppressed in the middle of colonic crypts as in normal tissue. Clearly, normal growth regulation has been lost in adenomatous tissue.

Classification. Neoplastic polyps are of three types: (1) tubular adenomata, consisting of branching epithelial tubules surrounded by lamina propria (Figure 20–5); (2) villous adenomata (Figure 20–6), which are long, frondlike processes of lamina propria covered by crowded neoplastic epithelium; and (3) tubulovillous adenomata (Figure 20–7), which contain features of both of the other types (Morson and Sobin 1976). While any type of

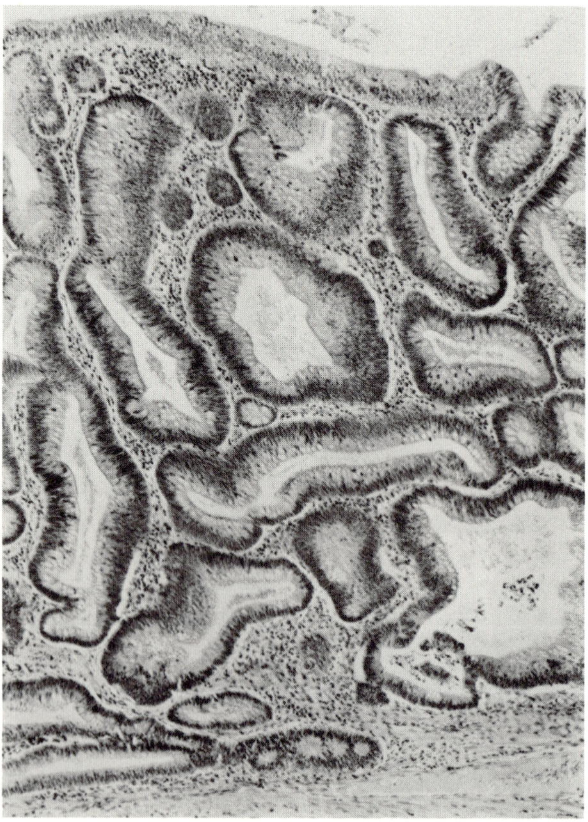

Figure 20–5. Tubular adenoma of the colon. The glands have a tubular or dilated appearance and show evidence of branching. Original magnification x68.

neoplastic polyp may show areas of nuclear atypia (less basal polarity, and more irregularity in shape and size than usual), carcinoma in situ (atypia plus distorted glandular growth pattern without invasion beyond gland sites) (Figure 20-8), or intramucosal carcinoma (carcinoma in situ plus a desmoplastic reaction and cell clusters outside of gland, but not deep to the muscularis mucosae), villous adenomata are usually considered to have a greater potential for malignant change than tubular adenomata. Despite this, many observations support the notion that any neoplastic polyp should be considered to be a potentially malignant lesion.

The close relationship of colonic adenomata to cancer of the colon is supported by many observations (Winawer et al 1976). While these observations are quite disparate, they collectively build a strong case of circumstantial evidence supporting the adenoma-cancer connection. (1) Colonic adenomata tend to appear at an earlier average age (fifth decade and beyond) than do colonic cancers (sixth decade and beyond), thus suggesting the effect of time in promoting the conversion of neoplasia to anaplasia. (2) The predominant sites of adenomata and cancers in the colon (sigmoid and rectum, cecum and ascending colon) are similar. (3) It is common to discover satellite adenomatous polyps in the immediate neighborhood of established colonic cancers. (4) Patients with adenomatous polyps have an increased risk for developing cancer of the colon at a later date. (5) There is a

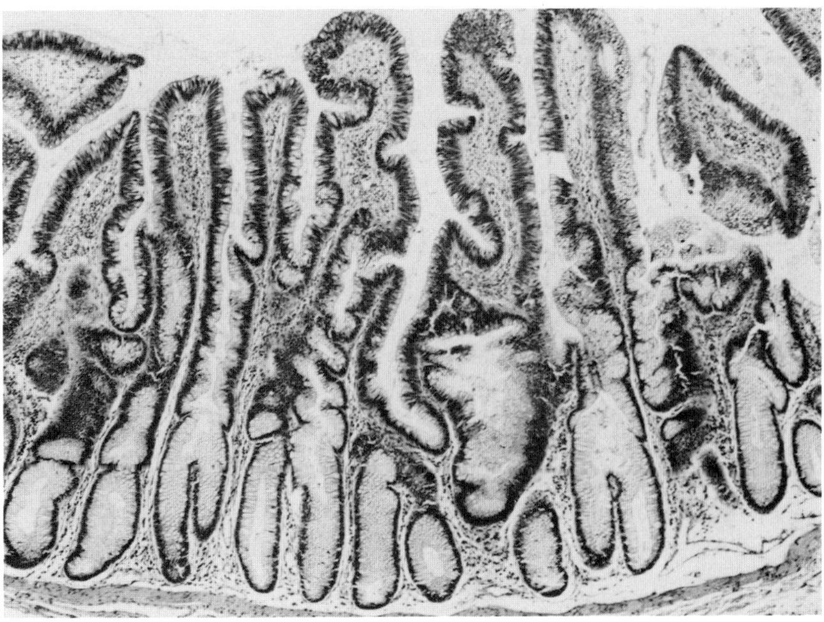

Figure 20-6. Villous adenoma of the colon. Papillary fronds projecting from the base of the lamina propria are characteristic of this lesion. Original magnification x50.

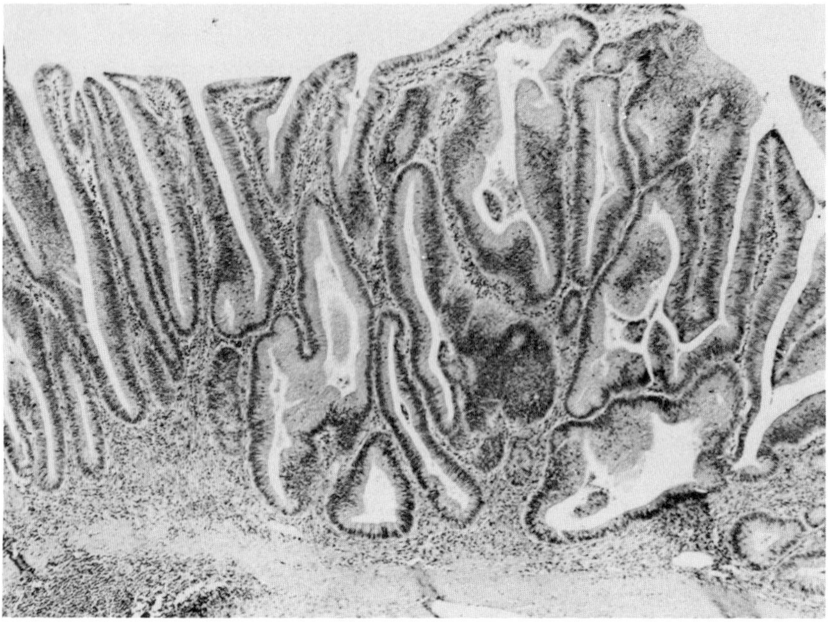

Figure 20–7. Tubulovillous adenoma of the colon. There is a mixture of tubular glands (*right*) and villous growth (*left*). Original magnification x50.

significant incidence of nuclear atypia, carcinoma in situ, and intramucosal cancer in rectal (7 percent) and sigmoidal (12 percent) adenomata. (6) The incidence of carcinoma is proportional to the size of polyps, occurring rarely in adenomata less than 1.0 cm in diameter and commonly (25 to 45 percent) in polyps greater than 2.0 cm in diameter (7) Larger adenomata tend to be more villous and thus more premalignant in character. (8) Satellite adenomata in the immediate vicinity of established colonic cancers show a greater incidence of dysplasia and nuclear atypia than do adenomata in other locations. (9) There are few if any reliable reports of actual small carcinomas of the colon starting in any setting other than in an adenoma. (10) Careful, repeated sigmoidoscopic screening in over 18,000 subjects followed for up to 25 years, with removal of all polyps, resulted in less than one-sixth of the number of rectosigmoid cancers being discovered during the same period of time in a similar, but unscreened, population (Gilbertsen 1974).

Surveillance for Adenomatous Polyps. The American Cancer Society recommends that all asymptomatic adults of age 50 years or over should have a sigmoidoscopy performed to screen for adenomatous polyps and cancer (Eddy et al 1980). Following two negative examinations one year apart, repeat sigmoidoscopies need not be performed more often than every three to five years, except among persons at higher than usual risk for co-

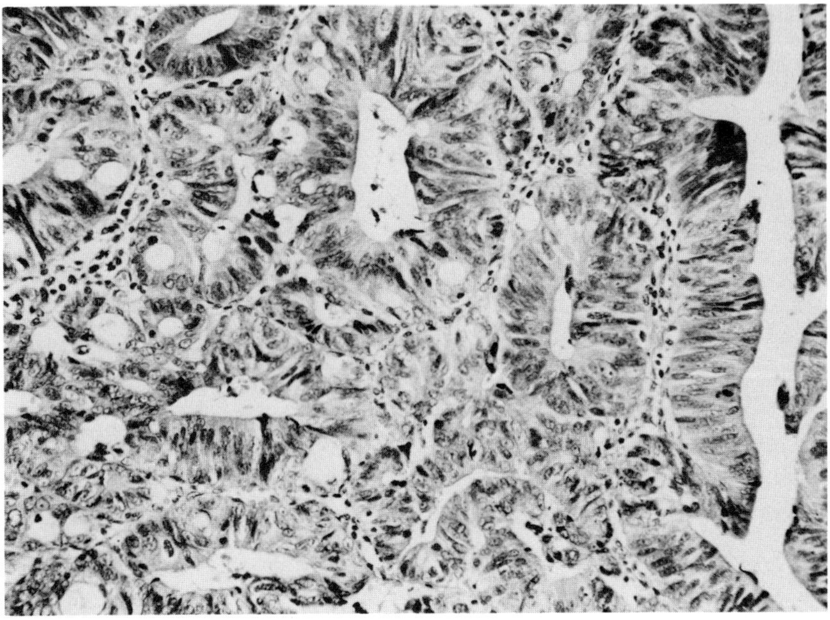

Figure 20-8. Carcinoma in situ in an adenomatous polyp. The glands are closely packed, and adjacent strands of mucosa are closely packed against one another. In addition there is a greater degree of nuclear atypia than there is in simple adenomas (see Figure 20-4). Original magnification x200.

lonic cancer. This latter group consists of patients who have had previous polyps or cancer or who have a family history of these diseases, and patients with chronic ulcerative colitis. These recommendations are based on the known slow rate of growth of polyps, and the observation that in Gilbertsen's study no cancers were detected within seven years after a negative sigmoidoscopy.

A digital rectal examination and a stool guaiac slide test series is recommended annually, the latter to rule out the likelihood of bowel cancer above the rectum. The guaiac test series consists of two separate stool smears obtained on each of three successive days; the total cost to patients should be no more than five dollars. Five percent of subjects with at least one positive stool guaiac test have been found to have bowel cancer, and cellular atypia has been found in 3 percent. Benign neoplasms or nonneoplastic polyps have been found in 25 percent of patients with positive stool guaiac tests.

In practice, the discovery of a stool positive for occult blood should be followed by a proctosigmoidoscopy and an air-contrast barium enema examination (Figure 20-9). Detection of a malignant-appearing lesion, or a very large sessile polyp, should be followed by prompt surgical removal, while discovery of a pedunculated polyp should be followed by colonoscopy and

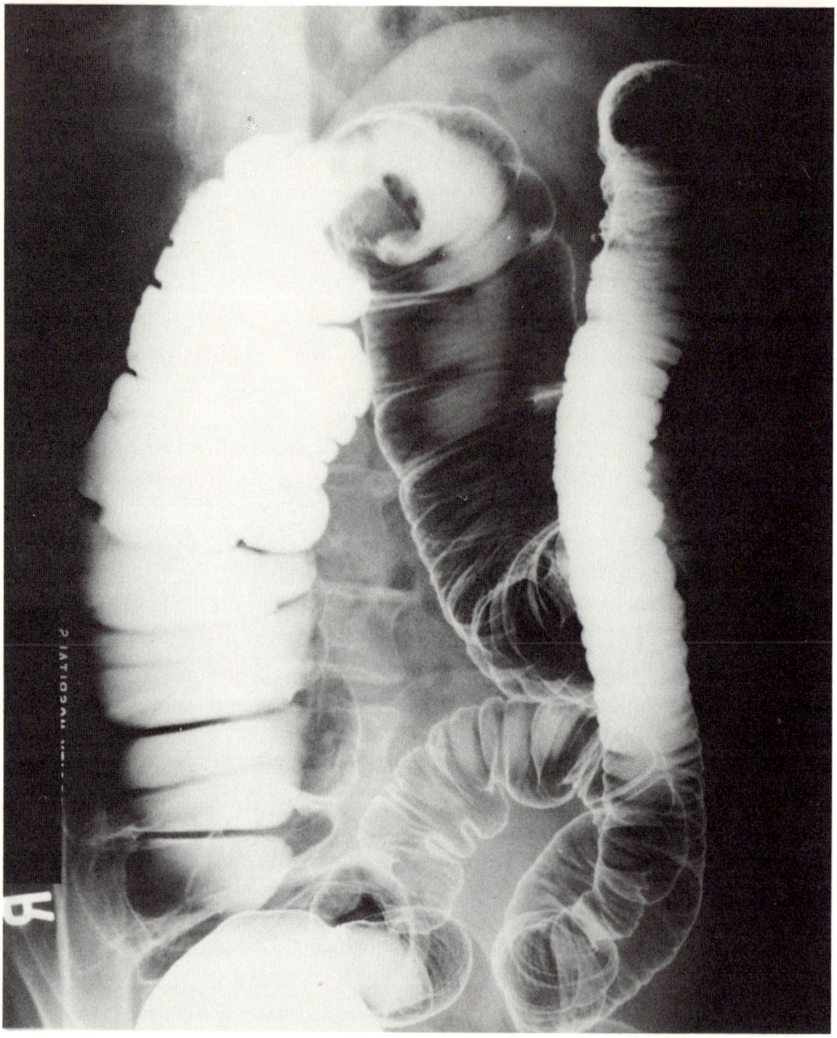

Figure 20-9. Barium enema showing a large polypoid lesion in the hepatic flexure of the colon. This proved to be a benign villous adenoma at surgery.

endoscopic polypectomy. If the barium enema is negative, and if no other sites of possible bleeding are detected by radiologic study of the upper gastrointestinal tract and small intestine, a diagnostic colonoscopy should be performed, since flat cecal carcinomas and small polyps may occasionally be missed by X ray studies. If this study is negative and if occult bleeding appears to be continuing, it may be possible to detect the level at which the bleeding originates by passage of a long intestinal tube with regular monitoring of the guaiac reaction of aspirated intestinal contents as passage continues. When material positive for occult blood is aspirated, further progress of the tube should be halted, and angiographic, followed by barium contrast, studies performed with special attention given to the area of bowel in the neighborhood of the tip of the tube.

Symptoms. Symptoms of adenomatous polyps relate almost exclusively to minor gross or occult bleeding. Occasionally, larger pedunculated polyps may become the vanguard of a colonic intussusception and lead to intermittent abdominal cramps. Large villous adenomata may cause a profound, watery secretory diarrhea, hypokalemia, and hypovolemia (Babior 1966).

Diagnosis. Diagnosis of adenomatous polyps of the colon is by barium enema and endoscopy. Because of their vascularity, adenomatous polyps almost invariably appear to be both hyperemic and friable when seen through the colonoscope and are readily distinguished from normal or metaplastic mucosa. It is usually not possible to distinguish small villous adenomata from tubular forms.

Treatment. Treatment is by surgical removal, preferably by snaring and cautery through the colonoscope. Larger pedunculated polyps, over 2.0 to 3.0 cm in diameter, may have to be removed piecemeal by this technique, and sessile polyps over 5.0 to 10 mm in diameter cannot be properly snared without running the risk of colonic perforation. These should probably be removed surgically, after biopsy. Smaller sessile polyps can be successfully fulgurated through the colonoscope, since the risk of cancer in such small lesions is very slight indeed.

Adenomatous Polyposis. This condition occurs in three hereditary syndromes, two of which, familial polyposis of the colon and Gardner-Richards syndrome (1953), are transmitted as autosomal dominant traits. The third disorder involving adenomatous polyposis, the Turcot-Despres-St. Pierre syndrome (Turcot et al 1959), is an exceedingly rare autosomal recessive characteristic. In each of these syndromes, the risk of malignant degeneration of the colonic polyps is very great, and continuous regular surveillance is essential.

Familial polyposis of the colon was probably first described in 1847 by Couvisant (Lynch et al 1979), and consists of literally myriads (up to 5,000 or more) of colonic adenomata of varying size. The disorder is not congenital, and the average age at diagnosis is in the late third or early fourth decade. Within 25 years of diagnosis, colonic cancer will have developed in nearly half of unoperated patients, and within 35 years, in all. While the polyposis is confined to the colon in almost every case, there have been a few reports of simultaneous adenomatous polyps occurring also in the stomach and small bowel.

In Gardner syndrome (Gardner and Richards 1953) colonic adenomatosis is associated with benign bony tumors (osteomas), soft-tissue tumors (fibromas, lipomas) and, frequently, dentigerous cysts and unerupted or supernumerary teeth. These latter phenomena often precede the development of polyposis. Malignant degeneration of small and large intestinal polyps is common.

Turcot syndrome (Turcot et al 1959) consits of adenomatous polyps of the colon associated with malignant tumors of neural origin, especially medulloblastomata or glioblastomata of the brain or spinal cord.

Diagnosis. The diagnosis of adenomatous polyposis syndromes depends on awareness of the family history of the disease and careful observation of the asymptomatic children of patients. Regular checking of stools for occult blood and sigmoidoscopy should commence about age 10 years and continue until at least age 40. The chances are good that an offspring who has not developed adenomatous polyposis by the end of the fourth decade of life has not inherited the responsible genome.

Treatment. Treatment of adenomatous polyposis requires colectomy if more than 100 polyps are found, or if careful and frequent observation is not feasible. Subtotal colectomy with ileoproctostomy reduces the risk of colonic cancer considerably, but requires a lifetime of at least semiannual sigmoidoscopy plus complete fulguration of any polyps seen. While total colectomy requires a permanent abdominal or perineal ileostomy, recent experiences with the continent ileostomy (Beart et al 1979), and with ileoperineal pull-through procedures, including construction of a perineal ileal reservoïr, offer some hope for reducing the discomfort of patients to a satisfactory minimum. It must be remembered that patients with adenomatous polyposis are still at some risk after colectomy for developing small intestinal and gastric polyps. Because of this, periodic stool guaiac testing must be continued for an indefinite period.

CANCER OF THE COLON

Colonic and rectal adenocarcinoma is second in incidence only to bronchogenic carcinoma among all internal maglignancies seen in the United States and western Europe. The American Cancer Society estimates an occurrence of nearly 115,000 new cases of this disease, and 53,000 deaths from it, during 1980 in the United States alone. Among women, the incidence of colonic cancer is somewhat higher than it is among men, and the incidence of rectal cancer is somewhat lower. Incidence rates continue to show various geographical differences. They are very low in Mexico, Central America, and Thailand, moderate in Japan, Poland, and Finland, high in the United States, France, and England, and very high in Scotland, New Zealand, and Chile. While it is difficult to draw any hard and fast conclusions from these figures as they stand, studies on persons who have migrated from low-incidence to high-incidence areas provide a clue that suggests that environment is probably stronger than heredity in rectocolonic cancer, a conclusion opposite to those relating to polyposis. Migrants from Japan to Hawaii have been shown to develop bowel cancer at a greater rate than do their countrymen who chose not to emigrate (Haenszel et al 1973). Similar results have been reported among migrants from Poland and Norway to the United States.

The Role of Diet in the Etiology of Colonic Cancer

Several lines of reasoning have involved the type of dietary intake to the genesis of large bowel cancer. First is the fact that the diets of migrants to the United States contain considerably more fat and meat protein than did their premigratory diets. Second is the fact that stools of American vegetarians, who have a significantly lower average incidence of colonic carcinoma than do nonvegetarians, contain considerably lower levels of fecal sterols and bile acids than do controls (Reddy and Wynder 1973). Both sterols and secondary bile acids have chemical structures similar to known experimental chemical colonic carcinogens (LaMont and O'Gorman 1978). Third is the observation that fecal bile acids can be converted to weak carcinogens by bacteria from human stool. However, no known carcinogen has been found in the stools of human colonic cancer victims to date.

Fecal flora are altered when dietary fat is increased. This is signaled particularly by a marked increase in the amount of *Bacterioides* found. This organism produces increased levels of 7-α-dehydroxylase, the enzyme which converts primary to secondary bile acids, and there is evidence that dehydroxylation is an early step in the conversion of bile acids to carcinogens (Goldin and Gorbach 1978). Wynder et al (1977) have shown that bile acids are more extensively degraded in the stools of persons on conventional diets than they are in the stools of vegetarians. Bacterial flora have also been implicated in the production of other enzymes, β-glucuronidase, β-glucosidases, aryl nitroreductase, and azoreductase, which are capable of converting drugs, chemicals, and food colorings into potential carcinogens. The possible importance of bacteria in the sequence of diet-bile acid-carcinogen-cancer development is underscored by observations that germ-free animals are moderately well protected against experimental (dimethylhydrazine) cancers, regardless of the diet they ingest.

A model of colon cancer has been developed in rats by feeding dimethylhydrazine. This alkylating agent leads to the methylation of epithelial DNA and permanently alters its structure. Its administration is followed by increasing cellular proliferation, altered mitotic activity, and the appearance of atypia and dysplasia. Tumor yield with this agent is increased by feeding a diet high in fat (LaMont and O'Gorman 1978).

Pathology

The lion's share of colonic adenocarcinomata are very well or moderately well differentiated, and nonmucinous. Most are exophytic, rather than flat and scirrhous. They tend also to be quite vascular and friable. In time, they involve all or almost all of the colonic wall and become obstructive, especially when located at sites distal to the hepatic flexure.

For some years surgical specimens of colorectal carcinomas have been classified prognostically by the degree of mural involvement as well as by cell type, in a system originally defined by Cuthbert Dukes and colleagues at St. Marks Hospital, London (1948). In the Dukes classification, a type A cancer involves the colonic wall into but not through the circular muscle layer; type B lesions (Figure 20–10) penetrate deep to the muscularis but do not involve regional lymph nodes; type C lesions are those associated with lymph node metastases. Dukes also recognized a fourth stage of colonic carcinoma in which distant metastases are already present at the time of surgery. This has been called type D by others. Morson and Dawson (1979) estimate that nearly 50 percent of colonic carcinomas are at stage C at the time of surgery, and that only one-third of patients having such lesions survive for five years.

Beart et al (1978) point out that the Dukes classification has become clumsy. It has been modified so much over the years, by Dukes and by others, that it has lost its credibility as an internationally accepted system.

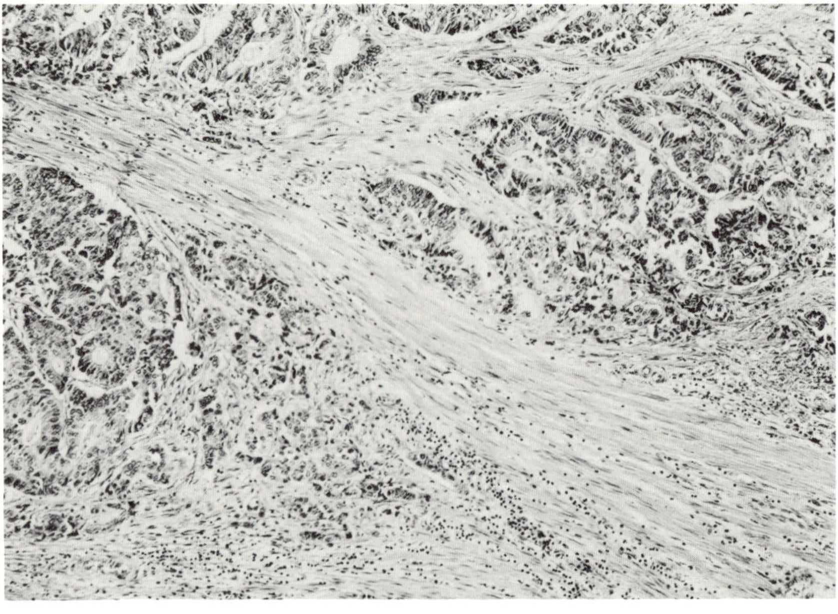

Figure 20–10. Adenocarcinoma of the colon extending into the muscularis (Dukes B, or T2, NO, MO lesion). Original magnification x80.

Each time it is employed, it must be qualified by reference to the modification being used (Roseman and Straus 1980). Furthermore, the advent of chemotherapeutic measures for cancer of the colon makes a more precise system mandatory, if small changes in prognosis are to be measured. Beart et al advocate the use of a system based on the estimation of the local penetration of the tumor (T), the degree of regional lymph node involvement (N), and the presence or absence of distant metastases (M). They suggest that use of this TNM classification (Table 20–1) will allow for more precise comparisons among different groups of patients, and for more accurate prediction of survival rates.

Symptoms and Diagnosis

The aim of the surveillance procedures outlined earlier in the discussion of colonic adenomata is to detect malignant or premalignant lesions before they become symptomatic, through the use of regular rectal examinations, stool tests for occult bleeding, and proctosigmoidoscopy. Failing detection in the presymptomatic phase, physicians and patients alike must be alert to the onset of new symptoms ranging from a simple change in bowel habits, to gross bleeding at stool, recurrent abdominal cramping, and a slowly developing iron-deficiency anemia. While these suggestions are easy to make, it is important to observe that they are frequently difficult to apply, primarily because the symptoms of bowel cancer are often so mild and so insidious. This is especially true among elderly patients, among patients with a previous history of hemorrhoids or the irritable bowel syndrome, and among those patients who tend to procrastinate before consulting a physician. Indeed, medical advisors themselves occasionally fail to initiate diagnostic studies promptly, being lulled often by the minor nature of their patient's complaints. The diagnosis of colonic cancer depends largely on endoscopic and radiologic confirmation, as described for colonic polyps.

Treatment

Surgical resection is the only satisfactory definitive treatment for colorectal carcinomas. Even when distant metastases to the liver or lungs are known to be present, there is merit in removing the primary tumor, both to prevent later obstruction of the colon and hemorrhage and to reduce the tumor burden prior to chemotherapy. The presence of a large rectal cancer usually requires proctocolectomy with permanent descending colostomy, but smaller exophytic rectal tumors may be successfully managed at times with extensive fulguration followed by radiation therapy.

Chemotherapy for metastatic disease has been used with slight success. Adriamycin and 5-fluorouracil have been employed most frequently, and some studies have added radiation therapy to either or both of these

Table 20-1. TNM Classification and Staging of Carcinoma of Colon

T: Primary tumors

TO:	no tumor clinically demonstrable
T1:	clinically benign lesion or confined to mucosa or submucosa
T2:	involvement of muscular wall or serosa, no extension beyond
T3:	involvement of all layers of colon with extension to immediately adjacent structures and organs and no fistula present
T4:	fistula present with any of the above degrees of tumor penetration
T5:	T3 or T4 with direct extension beyond immediately adjacent organs
TX:	depth of penetration not specified

N: Regional lymph node involvement

NO:	nodes not believed involved
N1:	nodes believed involved—distal to origins of the ileocolic, right colic, middle colic, and inferior mesenteric arteries
NX:	nodes not assessed or involvement not recorded

M: Distant metastasis

MX:	not assessed
MO:	no known distant metastasis
M1:	distant metastasis present

5.0 Stage Grouping

Stage 0:	
TIS NO MO	carcinoma in situ as demonstrated by histologic examination of tissue—biopsy or other
Stage I:	
Stage IA:	
TO,1 NO MO TO,1 NX MO	tumor confined to mucosa or submucosa with no demonstrable metastasis to regional lymph nodes and no evidence of distant metastasis
Stage IB:	
T2 NO MO T2 NX MO	tumor involves muscularis but has not extended beyond serosa with no demonstrable metastasis to regional lymph nodes and no evidence of distant metastasis
Stage II:	
T3-5 NO MO T3-5 NX MO	a tumor that has extended beyond the bowel wall or serosa with no demonstrable metastasis to regional lymph nodes and no evidence of distant metastasis
Stage III:	
Any T N1 MO	any degree of penetration of bowel or rectal wall by tumor, with metastasis to regional lymph nodes but no evidence of distant metastasis
Stage IV:	
Any T Any N M1	any degree of penetration of bowel or rectal wall by tumor with or without metastasis to regional lymph nodes and with evidence of distant metastasis

This material was taken from page 80 of the *Manual for Staging of Cancer 1977*, which was prepared by the American Joint Committee for Cancer Staging and End-Results Reporting. It was reprinted in Beart, RW, Jr, van Heerden JA, Beahrs RW. Surg. Gynec. Obst. 146:257–59. Reprinted by permission.

agents. While some prolongation of useful life may be obtained with these measures, the outlook for patients with metastatic disease is still grim. The greatest benefit from chemotherapy today seems to be in improving the prognosis for those patients with extensive mural lesions (Dukes B; T2, NO, MO), or with regional but not distant metastases (Dukes C; AnyT, Nl, MO).

Follow-up of all patients who have been successfully operated on for rectocolonic cancer should consist of endoscopic evaluation of the anastomosis at 6 and 12 months, then annually thereafter for up to five years. Recurrent tumor is most likely to occur at the point of previous surgery. Following this period, guaiac testing of two stools per day for three days should probably be done semiannually.

Measurement of serum levels of carcinoembryonic antigen may also be useful in detecting recurrent disease. If the levels of this antigen were known to have been normal or only slightly elevated following surgery, a later significant rise is strongly suggestive of recurrent cancer, provided that the patient does not also have ulcerative colitis, cirrhosis of the liver, or chronic pancreatitis, and is not a heavy smoker. Because of its poor specificity, this test has not been widely used.

SELECTED REFERENCES

Babior BM. Villous adenoma of the colon. Study of a patient with severe fluid and electrolyte disturbances. Am J Med 41:615–21, 1966.

Beart RW, Jr, Beahrs OH, Kelly KA, et al. The continent ileostomy. A viable alternative. Mayo Clin Proc 54:643–45, 1979.

Beart RW, Jr, van Heerden JA, Beahrs OH. Evolution in the pathologic staging of carcinoma of the colon. Surg Gynec Obst 146:257–59, 1978.

Bottomley JP, Cooper EH. Cell proliferation in colonic mucosa and carcinoma of the colon. Proc R Soc Med 66:1183–84, 1973.

Cronkhite LW, Jr, Canada WJ. Generalized gastrointestinal polyposis: an unusual syndrome of polyposis, pigmentation, alopecia, and onychotrophia. N Engl J Med 252:1011–15, 1955.

Dukes CE, Bussey HJR, Lamb GW. The examination and classification of operation specimens of intestinal cancer. Bull Int Assoc Med Mus 28: 55–65, 1948.

Eddy D, ed. Guidelines for the cancer-related checkup. Recommendations and rationale. Ca 30:208–15, 1980.

Enterline HT. Polyps and cancer of the large bowel. In: Morson BC, ed. Pathology of the gastro-intestinal tract. Berlin: Springer-Verlag, 1976: 97–141.

Gardner EJ, Richards RC. Multiple cutaneous and subcutaneous lesions occurring simultaneously with hereditary polyposis and osteomatosis. Am J Hum Genet 5:139–47, 1953.

Gilbertsen VA. Proctosigmoidoscopy and polypectomy in reducing the incidence of rectal cancer. Cancer 34:936–39, 1974.

Goldin B, Gorbach SL. Colon cancer connection: beef, bran, bile and bacteria. Viewpoints Dig Dis 10:1–4 (May), 1978.

Haenszel W, Berg JW, Sezi M, et al. Large bowel cancer in Hawaiian Japanese. J Natl Cancer Inst 51:1765–69, 1973.

Jeghers H, McKusick VA, Katz KH. Generalized intestinal polyposis and melanin spots of the oral mucosa, lips and digits: a syndrome of diagnostic significance. N Engl J Med 241:993–1005, 1031–36, 1949.

LaMont JT, O'Gorman TA. Experimental colon cancer. Gastroenterology 75:1157–69, 1978.

Lynch HT, Lynch PM, Albano WA, et al. Hereditary cancer: ascertainment and management. Ca 29:216–32, 1979.

Morson BC, Dawson IMP. Gastrointestinal pathology, 2nd ed. Oxford: Blackwell Scientific Publications, 1979:607–48.

Morson BC, Sobin LH. Histological typing of tumours. In: International histological classification of tumours, No. 15. Geneva: World Health Organization, 1976.

Peutz JLA. On a very remarkable case of familial polyposis of the mucous membrane of the intestinal tract and the nasopharynx accompanied by a peculiar pigmentation of the skin and mucous membranes (Dutch). Nedrl Maandschr v Geneesk 10:134–46, 1921.

Reddy BS, Wynder EL. Large bowel carcinogenesis: fecal constituents of populations with diverse incidence rates of colon cancer. J Natl Cancer Inst 50:1437–42, 1973.

Roseman DL, Straus AK. Staging of carcinoma of the colon and rectum. Surg Gynecol Obstet 151:93–95, 1980.

Schwabe AD, Lewin KJ. Gastrointestinal polyposis syndromes. Viewpoints Dig Dis 12:1–4 (January), 1980.

Turcot J, Despres JP, St. Pierre F. Malignant tumors of the central nervous system associated with familial polyposis of the colon: report of two cases. Dis Colon Rectum 2:465–68, 1959.

Winawer SJ, Sherlock P, Schottenfeld D, et al. Screening for colon cancer. Gastroenterology 70:783–89, 1976.

Wynder EL, Reddy BS, McCoy GD, et al. Diet and cancer of the digestive tract. Adv Int Med 22:397–419, 1977.

CLINICAL CONFERENCE 13

Part 1

A 70-year-old woman sought treatment at a hospital emergency room for moderately severe substernal pain radiating into the left shoulder and upper back. The pain had lasted steadily for eight hours and was associated with shortness of breath. There was no sweating, nausea, or vomiting. During the previous year she had experienced increasingly frequent episodes of substernal pressure, dyspnea, and weakness on exertion, the pressure readily disappearing at rest. She also volunteered that for several months she had become quite dizzy on standing quickly. There was no cough, orthopnea, or swelling of the ankles. Weight, appetite, and digestion were unchanged. Bowel movements were regular, and stool was always normal in color.

Her past medical history was not remarkable. She had had a hysterectomy performed at age 47, and a hemorrhoidectomy one year later. Four years prior to admission she was told by a physician that her examination was completely normal, save for a serum cholesterol "over 300." Since that time she had decreased the amount of fat in her diet, and had lost a few pounds in weight. There was no family history of cancer, hypertension, or anemia. Her father had died after a heart attack at age 72. Patient was a homemaker, with no known exposures to possibly toxic chemicals.

On examination, she was a pale, well-oriented woman lying comfortably in bed. Her temperature was 37.2°C, blood pressure 100/80, pulse 80 and regular, respirations 18. Positive findings included only a few crepitant rales at the base of the left lung, left border of cardiac dullness 11 cm from the midsternal line, a grade 2 systolic murmur at the base, and slight epigastric tenderness.

Laboratory work included a urinalysis which was normal. Hematocrit was 23 percent, with small, pale red cells on smear; white blood count 5,500 with a normal differential; aspartate aminotransferase (AsAT) 10 units per ml. An electrocardiogram was interpreted as normal. The patient was hospitalized.

1. What are the probable mechanisms responsible for this patient's illness?
2. What specific diseases may be causing them?
3. What further studies would you order in this case? Why?

Part 2

On the day following admission, the electrocardiogram was unchanged. AsAT, 12 units; hematocrit 24 percent; red blood count, 3.86 million; hemoglobin, 5.8 g per dl; reticulocytes, 2.0 percent of red blood cells; and prothrombin time 11.4 seconds, control 10.4 seconds. Over the next two days, the electrocardiogram remained unchanged, and the AsAT was 12 and 18 units per ml. Serum iron was 0 μg per dl, iron-binding capacity 477. Ten successive stool specimens were positive for occult blood testing, but were tan in color.

Because of the intermittent chest pain, the patient was given 1,000 ml of whole blood on the third hospital day. Following this she felt very well and asked to be discharged. However, she agreed to have further studies performed.

4. How has this information helped you in arriving at a diagnosis? What diseases have been ruled out?
5. What further studies should be done? When? Why? What will you do if the studies are normal?
6. What criticism do you have of this patient's management thus far?

Part 3

Several more stools were positive for occult blood during the next seven days. The hematocrit rose to 34 percent after transfusion and remained at that level. The patient continued to feel well.

On the 12th hospital day, gastric analysis showed a basal acid production of 4.78 mEq in one hour, and a maximal production of 21 mEq per hour after administration of pentagastrin. The next day, a barium enema was performed and the following day an upper gastrointestinal and small intestinal series. All of these studies were technically adequate and reported as normal.

However, the day after her final X ray study, stool specimens were still strongly positive for occult blood. Accordingly, a long intestinal tube was passed into the duodenum under fluoroscopic guidance, and intestinal contents were aspirated continuously as the balloon on the end of the tube carried it through the small intestine. Aspirated samples were checked regularly for occult blood, and all were negative until 48 hours after the tube was initially placed. At that time, the tip of the tube was in the lower right quadrant of the abdomen and the aspirate was positive for occult blood for the first time (Figure 20–11). A rectal specimen of stool at the same time was also positive for occult blood.

7. How have these studies helped in arriving at a diagnosis?
8. What possible lesions could be responsible for the findings?
9. What should be done now?

CLINICAL CONFERENCE 14

A 45-year-old man consulted a gastroenterologist for diagnosis and treatment of profuse watery diarrhea and gripping abdominal pain which had become increasingly severe during the previous seven months. Though his appetite was only fair, he had lost no weight. His bowel movements, while watery and profuse, were occasionally thick but never formed during

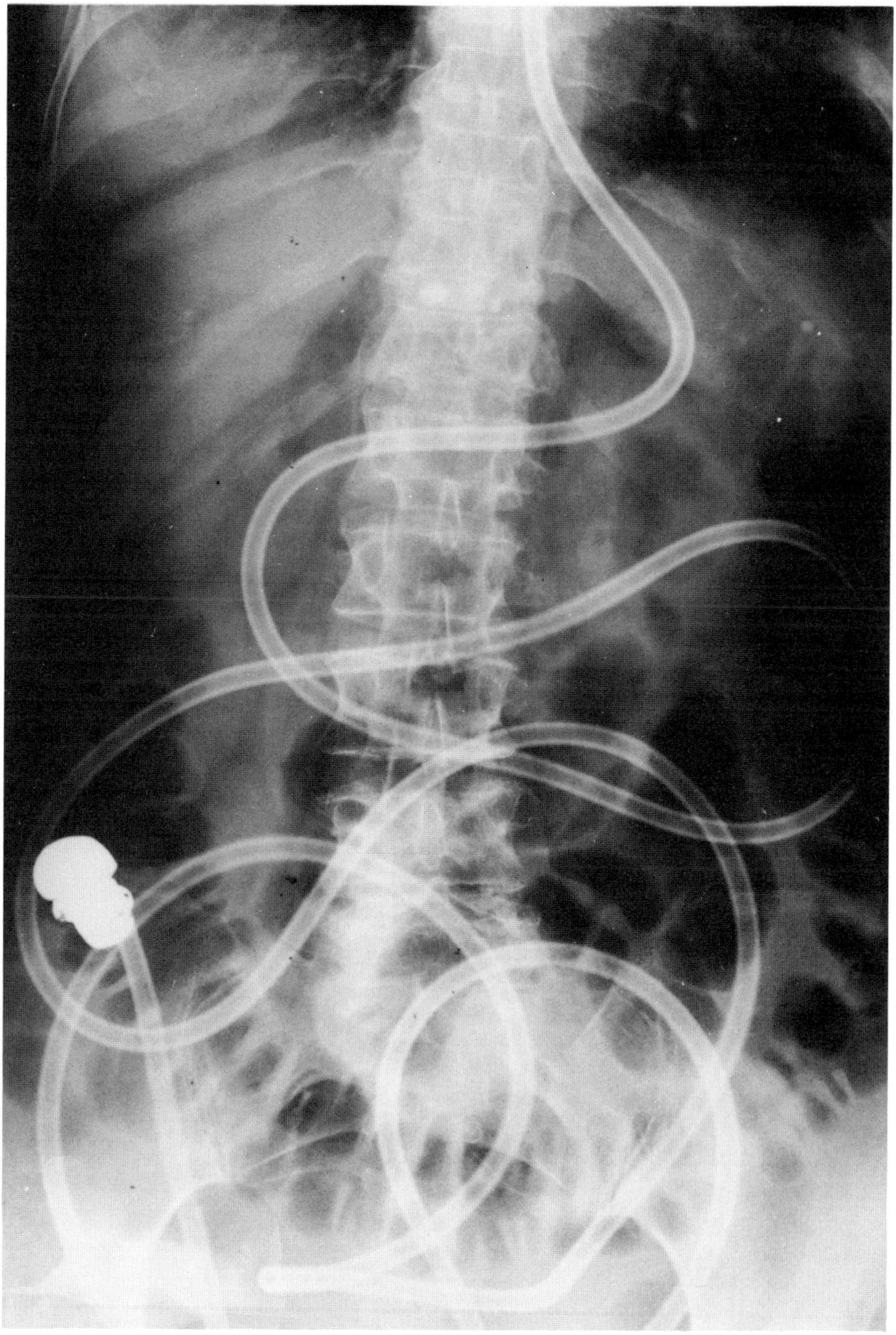

Figure 20–11. Clinical Conference 13, Part III. Plain film of the abdomen.

this illness. The gripping abdominal pain was usually temporarily relieved by a bowel movement, and the diarrhea would commonly awaken him from sleep. He denied melena and gross bleeding. Anticholinergic drugs and loperamide did not relieve the symptoms. Prior to this illness, he had normal stools with occasional constipation. He denied taking laxatives.

Patient worked as a free-lance photographer. He had graduated from college in the Midwest with a degree in journalism. He admitted to considerable aggravation and nervousness since suffering a great financial loss when his uninsured photographic equipment was stolen 10 months before. A barium enema and intravenous pyelogram were negative one month previously, and an upper gastrointestinal series, performed for forgotten reasons, had been normal two years before.

His past health had been fair. At the age of 28 he passed the first of a series of ureteral calculi, and had experienced about five similar attacks between that time and the age of 41. The stones were always associated with typical colic, and all had passed spontaneously without the need for surgery. He had become mildly diabetic at age 39, and this was well controlled with tolbutamide 0.5 g twice daily. He had suffered from transient diarrhea for one month at the age of 43, after returning from a trip to Mexico. A maternal uncle is diabetic. Two paternal first cousins have polycystic kidneys. The patient has no siblings, and his mother is alive and well at the age of 75. His father died at the age of 64, "with a large tumor in his chest." His paternal grandfather had died at age 35 "with many small tumors in his brain." The patient was married for the first time at age 39. His wife is well, and they have no children.

Physical examination revealed a blood pressure of 130/82, pulse 74 and regular, respirations 14. Aside from moderate facial acne and a late systolic murmur in the second left intercostal space along the sternal border, the physical examination was normal. Sigmoidoscopy was normal to 25 cm, and a specimen of soft, brown stool was negative for occult blood, fat, and cysts or ova. Complete blood count and urinalysis were also normal. The patient was placed on antispasmodic therapy pending review of his X rays.

Over the next several days, the diarrhea increased greatly in volume, and the patient commenced vomiting for the first time. With this, he became extremely weak and eventually unable to stand without support. He was hospitalized and found to have marked postural hypotension but an otherwise normal physical examination. Initial studies in the hospital showed a hematocrit of 48 percent, white blood count 9,000 with a normal differential smear, and a normal urinalysis save for a specific gravity of 1.028 and 2-plus albuminuria. Serum sodium was 138, potassium 3.1, chloride 106, and carbon dioxide content 18 mEq per liter. Blood pH was 7.38. Plasma glucose was 280, BUN 32, serum calcium 14.2, phosphorus 2.0 mg per dl, and the alkaline phosphatase was 46 IU per liter.

He was placed on parenteral fluid replacement and, in the first 24 hours, required 8,500 ml to maintain adequate urinary output. During this same period he passed 3,800 ml of water stool with normal osmolality. An X ray of the chest was normal. Abdominal films showed small intestinal and colonic air-filled fluid levels "suggestive of paralytic ileus or early bowel obstruction." Three days later, a bone survey showed osteoporosis of the skull and bones of the hands, and enlargement of the sella turcica with destruction of its floor. An operation was performed on the eighth hospital day.

APPENDIX:

Clinical Conference Discussions

DISCUSSION OF CLINICAL CONFERENCE 1

1. Diagnostic possibilities include weakness of lower esophageal sphincter with esophagitis and stricture.

An uncomplicated sliding hiatal hernia could not be responsible for this patient's symptoms, since dysphagia, loss of weight and regurgitation of undigested food are not symptoms of this condition. Heartburn as a symptom of mild esophagitis is commonly associated with a sliding hernia, but the patient denied ever having heartburn. In addition, there was no evidence that the recumbent position aggravated her difficulties. A larger paraesophageal hernia, which may cause obstruction of the lower esophagus, is unlikely because of the X ray findings.

Favoring the diagnosis of esophagitis and stricture secondary to lower sphincter weakness are (1) the fact that the patient had been told in the past that she had a herniation of the stomach, and (2) the identification of a cardioesophageal junction 38 cm from the incisors (normal, 40 cm) during esophagoscopy. However, the diagnosis of small hiatal hernias by X ray is frequently uncertain, and the identification of the cardioesophageal junction at esophagoscopy may be inexact. The transitional zone is not always obvious, and there may be a small amount of telescoping of the esophagus on the instrument. Hiatal hernias are commonly asymptomatic, so the existence of a small hernia does not mean that this is the cause of the symptoms, particularly if reflux is not demonstrated.

Evidence against the diagnosis of esophagitis and stricture secondary to a hernia are the absence of previous pyrosis; the difficulty from onset of swallowing both solids and liquids; the lack of a stricture on X ray; the absence of esophagitis on endoscopy; and the marked degree of esophageal dilatation.

Diffuse Esophageal Spasm

The prolonged history of pain on swallowing is compatible with this diagnosis, since this disorder causes obstruction by marked tonic esophageal spasms initiated by swallowing. Patients afflicted with diffuse esophageal spasm commonly experience equal difficulty in swallowing both liquids and solids, although they rarely lose as much weight as this patient did. The X ray and esophagoscopy, however, do not support the diagnosis. The esophagus would not be so dilated with diffuse spasm, nor would the endoscopist have encountered so much debris in the esophagus.

Scleroderma

This systemic disorder can cause severe dysphagia as a result of gradually decreasing propulsive peristalsis of the esophagus. Major aspects favoring the diagnosis are a history suggestive of Raynaud phenomenon and the patient's sex. However, Raynaud phenomenon is not uncommon, and femininity can hardly be considered a symptom of disease, so the association of these with dysphagia does not establish cause and effect.

Scleroderma does not cause the esophagus to dilate as much as this, tending rather to produce a nonperistaltic organ, which is only slightly dilated. It rarely causes the amount of pain that this woman suffered and is most commonly associated with heartburn, owing to the tendency for this disease to involve the esophagus intially at the level of the inferior sphincter. One would also expect to find other evidence of scleroderma after an eight-year period of esophageal symptoms.

Carcinoma of the Esophagus

A malignant obstruction of the esophagus could be suspected on the basis of dysphagia, loss of weight, and distress in the chest. Cancer of the esophagus may lead to dysphagia in one of two ways: by obstruction from the tumor itself or by infiltration into the muscularis with destruction of the myenteric plexi. The former mode of obstruction is unlikely in this patient because of the initial dysphagia for both liquids and solids, the absence of an obstructing lesion on X ray, and the negative mucosal findings on esophagoscopy.

Esophageal Diverticulum

This diagnosis cannot be seriously entertained here, because the only type of diverticulum that could cause this degree of obstruction is a large pulsion (Zenker) diverticulum of the cervical esophagus. This disorder would be apparent on X ray and would not cause the distal esophagus to dilate.

Achalasia of the Esophagus

If one discounts the history of Raynaud phenomenon and remains skeptical about the localization of the cardioesophageal junction, this history is completely typical of moderately severe achalasia, and the ancillary data obtained on both X ray and endoscopy are confirmatory.

In view of the patient's nativity, it would be impossible to exclude chronic Chagas disease completely, although the absence of cardiac or colonic signs or symptoms speaks strongly against the diagnosis. One might also entertain the diagnosis of an infiltrative carcinoma of the cardia or lower esophagus, since the signs and symptoms of esophageal dilatation and obstruction may be the earliest indications of this disorder.

2. Achalasia is the most likely diagnosis. Valuable information regarding the status of the lower esophageal segment and the cardia of the stomach could be obtained from further X rays, especially cinematic fluoroscopy. These procedures would be performed primarily to rule out a carcinoma of the stomach or lower esophagus. Cytologic studies would also be useful. A metacholine (Mecholyl) test would hardly be indicated, since the test is occasionally positive in patients with carcinoma, and the present X rays are otherwise diagnostic. Specific testing for *Trypanosoma cruzi* would also be useful.

3. Assuming that the additional studies outlined above confirm the diagnosis of achalasia, the only effective therapy would be to attempt to rupture the circular muscle of the inferior sphincter by forcible balloon distention or by a surgical myotomy (Heller procedure). The former procedure is less troublesome and would, in most patients, be performed first.

DISCUSSION OF CLINICAL CONFERENCE 2

Part 1

1. The history of regurgitation of acrid material without actual vomiting is suggestive of incompetence of the closing mechanism at the gastroesophageal junction. The disorder commonly causing this symptom is an incompetent lower esophageal sphincter (LES), frequently associated with a sliding (direct) hiatal hernia. The hernia is readily seen on X ray. The diagnosis of sphincter incompetence is confirmed by the fact that the patient's symptoms are aggravated by lying flat or bending over, and relieved by standing erect.

Heartburn, dysphagia, and hematemesis are not seen in patients with uncomplicated sphincter incompetence and suggest the presence of associated esophagitis. The acid-perfusion test strongly indicates esophagitis. These symptoms may also indicate the presence of an obstructing lesion.

Such complaints may suggest a paraesophageal hernia, but the X rays disprove this, and such hernias do not lead to gastroesophageal reflux. One may also entertain the possibility of achalasia, but the absence of weight loss and the failure of the X rays to demonstrate esophageal dilatation are against this.

The major differential diagnosis is between esophageal or gastric carcinoma and esophagitis. Absence of weight loss is contrary to the former diagnosis, but does not rule it out completely. The esophagoscopy confirms both the presence of a hernia (gastroesophageal junction at 36 cm) and of inflammation (friability). The biopsy (Figure 3–16) shows infiltration of round cells in mucosa and submucosa, compatible with esophagitis, and a mucosal erosion.

The findings after surgery indicate the presence of continued esophagitis and support the impression of sustained gastroesophageal reflux. They also indicate that surgical repair of hiatus hernias may not, at times, relieve reflux esophagitis—if, indeed, this is the type of operation that was performed.

2. Sphincter incompetence and hiatus hernias are managed by measures that tend to increase sphincter tone, keep the hernia from protruding into the chest, and modestly decrease gastric acidity. The first objective is approached indirectly by stimulating gastrin production through the use of cholinergic drugs and measures to alkalinize the antrum. Cholinergic drugs might be helpful by increasing pressure in the LES. Steps designed to decrease intra-abdominal pressure, such as reduction of weight or ascites and avoidance of tight corseting, tend to decrease herniation. The patient is also instructed to avoid assuming postures that aggravate the reflux, such as bending over or lying flat. To this end, he is advised to stoop rather than bend, and to raise the head of his bed 15 to 20 cm from the floor for sleeping; the use of pillows alone rarely achieves this result. Gastric acidity can be reduced by liquid antacids. Anticholinergic drugs decrease vagal stimulation of the fundic glands, but also reduce sphincter tone. It is also well for the patient to avoid foods such as alcohol and caffeine, which reduce sphincter pressure. These measures are very helpful in controlling the reflux manifestations of an incompetent lower sphincter, and are often successful in treating accompanying esophagitis.

3. Surgical repair of the hernia was doubtless attempted for the reasons outlined above. It was apparently unsuccessful, possibly because the esophagogastric sphincter remained incompetent. Despite this, a further course of intensive nonsurgical therapy is indicated in an effort to avoid another operation. If the management were unsuccessful, a fundal plication procedure should be effective.

Part 2

1. The appearance of serious dysphagia and the loss of weight suggest the possibility of an esophageal carcinoma, despite its lack of evidence on

previous examination. The X rays clearly show a stricture in the body of the esophagus, and esophagoscopy reveals an abrupt narrowing at 30 cm. The fact that no ulceration or neoplasm was seen is reassuring, although it is possible that the carcinoma was not detected because it was impossible to pass the esophagoscope beyond 32 cm. Cytologic material provides helpful information, but there is always concern about false negative reports.

The biopsies provide the most useful information. Here (Figure 3–18) one sees columnar epithelium and inflammatory cells in esophageal mucosa that is located at least 8 cm above the esophagogastric junction. This is the type of mucosa described by Barrett in patients with esophagitis and esophageal strictures. In this patient the fact that squamous epithelium was obtained four years earlier at a lower level of the esophagus argues strongly in favor of metaplasia. The proclivity of these areas to develop strictures is well known. The presence of columnar epithelium in mid esophagus does not rule out carcinoma at a lower level, but certainly can explain the patient's symptoms and findings. This patient's stricture probably arose from Barrett epithelium consequent to chronic esophagitis. Reflux from incompetence of the esophagogastric sphincter is the most likely cause of the esophagitis, although that disorder may also have been aggravated by general anesthesia and possibly by a nasogastric tube at the time of surgery.

2. In view of the diagnosis, especially with the stricture, surgery is indicated. One may try to dilate the stricture periodically with mercury-filled bougies or hard rubber dilators, but most patients with a stricture of this degree require surgery.

DISCUSSION OF CLINICAL CONFERENCE 3

1. Possible diagnoses, considering the protocol and the X rays, are: (1) a benign gastric ulcer of the lesser curve; (2) a benign gastric ulcer with malignant change; and (3) an ulceration in a malignant tumor of the stomach.

The most likely diagnosis is a benign gastric ulcer, although the answer to this cannot be conclusive on the basis of the information given. In arriving at this diagnosis, one could place great weight on the facts that: (1) the patient's pain was generally relieved by antacids; (2) his maximal acid output was quite high; (3) early in his illness the pain, loss of weight, and vomiting had improved on limited therapy for a period of nearly two years; and (4) X ray, particularly the spot films, show a deeply penetrating ulcer that, unlike an ulcerated carcinoma, goes well beyond the normal boundaries of the lesser curve of the stomach.

2. The most useful additional studies would be a gastroscopy with biopsy of the ulcer margins, and a brush cytology. Both these procedures would be performed to obtain a closer look at the lesion in order to rule out the presence of a carcinoma.

3. If the ulcer is believed to be benign, the major mechanisms of onset are probably the patient's previous anxiety regarding the loss of work and

the subsequent alcoholism. Both these factors in a patient with a large parietal cell mass can be ulcerogenic.

4. The X rays indicate that the ulcer has already penetrated well beyond the wall of the stomach into surrounding tissues. The patient's symptoms of dyspnea and weakness, as well as a very low hematocrit and serum iron, indicate that the ulcer has been causing bleeding for a long while. A massive gastric hemorrhage or a free perforation of the ulcer into the peritoneal cavity may appear as a later complication.

5. Two types of treatment are available, medical or surgical. Both are designed to reduce acid secretion, but surgery has the added advantage of removing the ulcer as well. The choice of treatment depends on the bias of the therapist. The gastroenterologist would probably elect a course of intensive medical therapy, including blood transfusions to a hematocrit of about 28, iron supplements, avoidance of alcohol, frequent antacids, and cimetidine, 300 mg qid. He would X ray the patient at three- to four-week intervals until assured that the ulcer had healed completely. If complete healing failed to occur, he would advise surgery.

The surgeon would consider the patient's age, the depth of his ulcer, the low hematocrit, and the poor chance of sustained healing of a large gastric ulcer without continuous therapy, and would probably opt for immediate surgery. The choice of operation would depend on his own experience.

This patient was operated on immediately. The additional photograph shows the gross and microscopic features of this deep, benign, gastric ulcer (Figure A-1). Note especially that the ulcer has penetrated deeply and that there is a large artery in its base. The findings indicate that the surgeon probably had the better side of the argument in this case!

DISCUSSION OF CLINICAL CONFERENCE 4

1. The history of infrequent but copious vomiting productive of gastric contents that contained food eaten as long as 12 hours previously and tasting very sour is highly suggestive of gastric retention. This impression is confirmed by the observation that vomiting relieved the distress, and that the illness was accompanied by a significant weight loss. The succussion splash, the large volume of gastric aspirate, and the massive gastric distention seen on X ray corroborate the diagnosis.

There are very few disorders that cause this degree of retention, and chronic peptic ulcer in the duodenum or lower portion of the stomach is always the most likely cause. An obstructing carcinoma of the lower stomach should also be considered, but this rarely causes so much distention and is usually associated with diminished volumes of gastric secretion. If the patient were a diabetic, the possibility of neuropathic gastric retention could also be entertained. Rarer lesions such as adult hypertrophic pyloric stenosis, malrotations and herniations of the upper small intestine, compres-

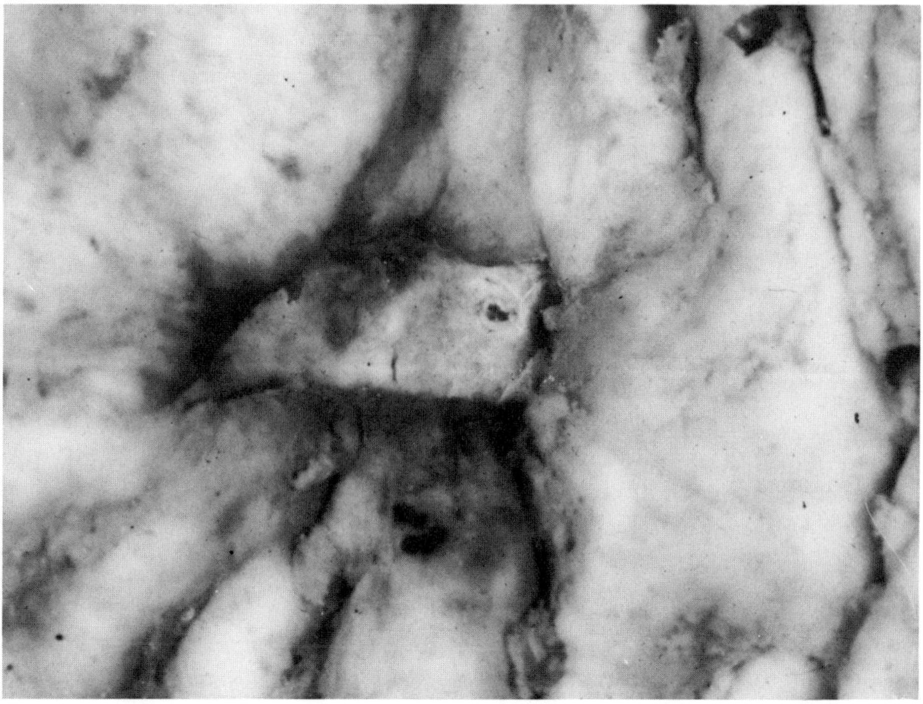

Figure A–1A. *A*, gross view of ulcer in surgical specimen, and *B*, low-power photomicrograph of ulcer. An open artery is noted in the base of this benign lesion in both pictures. Original magnification of photomicrograph x30.

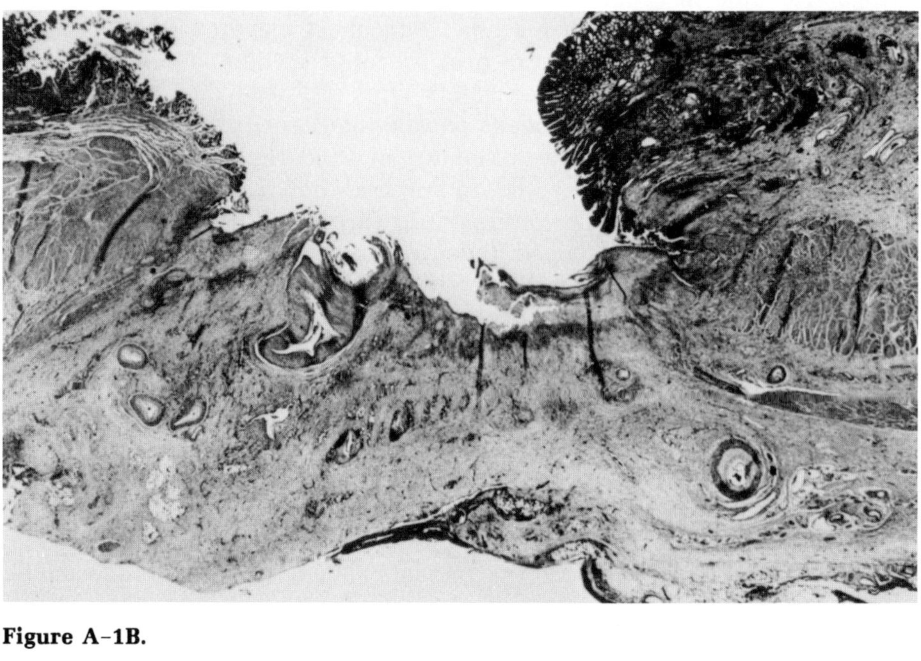

Figure A–1B.

sion of the duodenum by the superior mesenteric artery, amyloidosis of the stomach, intestinal pseudo-obstruction, and regional enteritis of the duodenum may also lead to this degree of gastric retention. But in most of these, at least some barium enters the duodenum. The episodes of epigastric distress that had troubled this patient for the previous 15 years are strongly suggestive of peptic ulcer and make this the most likely diagnosis.

2. The patient is seriously alkalotic. He is a victim of the large parietal cell mass, which is responsible for the continuous secretion of H^+ ions into the stomach, and the pyloroduodenal obstruction, which prohibits intestinal absorption of these ions. Large amounts of Cl^- and water are lost in the same way. Sodium loss is limited by aldosterome release, which also leads to kaluresis and hypokalemia. Bicarbonate is lost in the urine, which becomes alkaline. Sustained hypokalemia may lead to renal tubular damage, H^+ loss, and an acid urine. These changes are reflected by the elevated blood pH, increased CO_2 content, and decreased serum sodium and potassium. The tetany manifested by facial muscle spasm (Chvostek sign) is often seen in patients with alkalosis in the presence of normal levels of serum calcium. Decreased ionized calcium or decreased myoneural sensitivity to calcium may be responsible for the tetany of alkalosis. Alkalosis may also have been aggravated by the patient's habit of ingesting baking soda.

Losses of intracellular and extracellular water also play an important part in the clinical picture. Volume loss alone results in decreased renal blood flow, azotemia, hypotension, tachycardia, and urine of low volume and high specific gravity.

3. The patient requires early and complete gastric decompression with nasogastric tube in order to restore gastric tone and to prevent further vomiting. He should lie with his head and chest elevated to prevent reflux esophagitis and aspiration of oral secretions while on suction. Large amounts of parenteral water and electrolytes are needed to replace ionic and voluminal losses. Caloric needs can be temporarily supplied by intravenous hyperalimentation. The adequacy of fluid replacement should be monitored by recording intake and output, and daily body weight.

This treatment could be continued for three to four days, after which the patient should be endoscoped to determine whether the pylorus has become patent. If patency is demonstrated, he may be started on an acute ulcer regimen. The success of this program should be monitored by aspirating residual gastric contents each morning. If the endoscope does not pass into the duodenum after several days of suction, or if gastric retention reappears following the institution of oral feedings, the indications for surgical correction are very clear.

The choice of a surgical procedure varies with the surgeon. Most would favor an operation that removes the major stimulants to the secretion of acid (antrectomy and vagotomy) and provides an ample opening between the stomach and small intestine (gastroduodenostomy or gastrojejunostomy).

DISCUSSION OF CLINICAL CONFERENCE 5

1. Differential Diagnosis of Jaundice

First Admission. The hyperbilirubinemia is of the direct or conjugated type, as shown by the test for bilirubinuria. Hemolytic jaundice is ruled out by the conjugated type of hyperbilirubinemia, the low value for urine urobilinogen, and the normal hematocrit. The fact that the patient is 42 years old and has had no episodes of jaundice in the past, has no family history of jaundice, and was relieved of jaundice after her operation are all contrary to a diagnosis of a congenital conjugated type of hyperbilirubinemia.

The main differential diagnosis is between hepatocellular and obstructive jaundice, both of which lead to conjugated hyperbilirubinemia. Obstruction is more likely because of the rising alkaline phosphatase and the low urinary urobilinogen, associated with only slight evidence of acute hepatocellular damage (AsAT, 80 units). If hepatocellular damage were the predominant process, a more prolonged convalescence might have been expected following surgery.

Second Admission. Hyperbilirubinemia is again of the conjugated type because of bilirubinuria, and the main differential diagnosis is between hepatocellular and obstructive jaundice. Hapatocellular jaundice is more likely here, because of the marked aberrations in tests of hepatocellular function (aminotransferase, prothrombin content, and urine urobilinogen), with a relatively unaffected level of alkaline phosphatase.

2. Differential Diagnosis of Illness

First Admission. This was an acute illness, characterized by obstructive jaundice and attacks of periumbilical pain related to the ingestion of large meals. The pain later shifts to the right upper quadrant of the abdomen, radiates into the back, and is accompanied by signs of inflammation, such as fever and leukocytosis and peritoneal irritation. The obstruction clears promptly after an abdominal operation, without residual symptoms.

The differential diagnosis is between extrahepatic and intrahepatic partial biliary tract obstruction. The obstruction is considered to be partial because the patient's stools were never acholic and there was some urobilinogen in her urine. All features are compatible with a diagnosis of cholelithiasis with stones in the common bile duct, including the description of pain occurring several hours after a large meal, the relief of pain by belladonna, the signs of inflammation and peritoneal irritation, and the prompt recovery following surgery. Patient's age, sex, and obesity are also frequently associated with gallstones, but this certainly does not rule out the possibility that cholelithiasis may readily occur in thin men, young or old!

Acute pancreatitis is a less likely possibility, in view of the normal levels of serum amylase—but this, too, is not invariable. Tumors, sclerosis of the common bile duct, or carcinomas of the head of the pancreas are unlikely to be associated with the degree of acute pain experienced by this patient. These extrahepatic lesions generally produce complete biliary obstruction.

Intrahepatic partial biliary obstruction could be the result of cholestatic drugs or viral hepatitis. The latter is very unlikely, particularly in view of the extreme pain experienced by the patient and the fact that tests of hepatocellular function are not remarkably impaired. Cholestasis from chlorpromazine cannot be completely ruled out, although pain of this severity is quite uncommon. One would also not expect a drug-induced form of cholestasis to improve so promptly after surgery.

Second Admission. This illness represents an acute episode of painless hepatocelluar jaundice with rapidly deteriorating hepatic function and the appearance of hepatic coma. The picture is that of acute diffuse hepatitis with necrosis.

Possibilities include viral hepatitis, toxic hepatitis, and hepatic necrosis associated with any type of cirrhosis of the liver. The last possibility can probably be ruled out most easily, since there was no apparent disease of the liver at the time of her operation three months before. Toxic hepatitis owing to halothane anesthesia may, however, have occurred and led to this relentlessly progressive disease. The apparent absence of any symptoms during the time since her operation and the presumed fact that this was her first exposure to halothane are strong points against that possibility.

Hepatitis owing to blood transfusions remains the most likely possibility. The incubation period is typical for hepatitis virus B and the presence of HBsAg is strongly confirmatory. Type A hepatitis is much less likely for these same reasons.

3. Management of Illness

The patient has lapsed into hepatic coma and the rapid deterioration of her condition is a very poor prognostic sign. The rising urea nitrogen level confirms this prognosis.

Management of hepatic coma would consist of methods to decrease production of ammonia by the kidney and enteric bacteria (prevention of hypokalemia, use of intestinal antibiotics, catharsis to remove protein from gut, acidification of colonic contents). Circulating volume should be maintained to improve renal perfusion as much as possible. Massive doses of adrenocorticosteroids may be helpful in reducing inflammatory reaction in the liver. Trial of exchange transfusions may be indicated if donors of fresh blood are available and if other measures appear to be ineffective.

The patient did expire in hepatic coma, and a liver biopsy was then performed (Figure A–2).

DISCUSSION OF CLINICAL CONFERENCE 6

1. I.A, II.A, III.C, IV.C, V.A, VI.B, VII.C, VIII.B, IX.A, X.C.

2. This patient has symptoms and findings characteristic of both a duodenal ulcer and alcoholic disease of the liver, an association that is not uncommon in clinical practice. The response of his abdominal pain to antacids is characteristic of the ulcer syndrome, whereas the failure of response shortly before he entered the hospital indicates that a portion of the pain may be coming from another source, such as the liver. The enlarged firm liver on admission and the decreased serum albumin suggest the probability

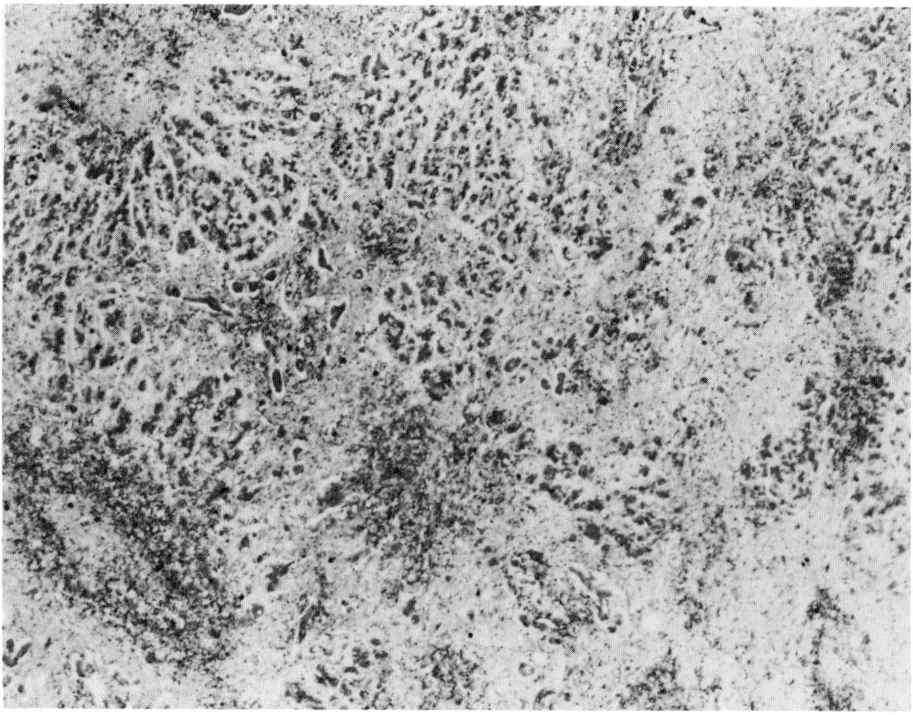

Figure A–2. Diffuse acute subtotal hepatic necrosis. Note that parenchyma is almost completely destroyed. Hemosiderin remains in the necrotic areas. Original magnification x30.

of cirrhosis. The increase in bilirubin of the unconjugated variety, the elevated levels of serum cholesterol and triglycerides, and the fall in hematocrit after admission suggest a hemolytic episode. The increased percentage of reticulocytes supports this conclusion. This picture is seen in patients with Zieve syndrome, which is occasionally associated with alcoholic cirrhosis or fatty liver.

3. The finding of shifting dullness in the abdomen signifies the presence of ascites, not great enough in amount to cause the tight distention of the abdomen necessary to produce a fluid wave. The two bits of laboratory information that suggest the reason for the ascites are the lowered serum albumin and the decreased sodium concentration and volume of the urine. Low albumin levels decrease the colloid oncotic pressure of the blood, and sodium retention increases total body water. Lowered serum albumin can be the result of either decreased production owing to liver disease or to loss of protein into the gastrointestinal tract owing to gastric rugal hypertrophy. The patient's sodium intake may have been increased by heavy consumption of liquid antacids.

4. This patient's abdominal pain, as has been indicated, is typical of ulcer distress. It is believed that it occurs when gastric and duodenal pH drops to low levels. The associated alcoholism and nervousness could be responsible for increased acid production, while the ingestion of salicylates increases the susceptibility of the gastroduodenal mucosa to injury, possibly by inhibition of tissue prostaglandins. Relief of his pain with antacids suggests the importance of a lowered luminal pH in its genesis. One might also consider the possibility of pancreatitis in this patient, since this disorder may be aggravated by factors that increase the production of acid. However, it is not usually so responsive to antacids.

5. It would be desirable to perform a liver biopsy in this patient, but it would be unreasonable and extremely dangerous! In view of the low prothrombin content and the presence of ecchymoses, which indicate an increased tendency to bleed, the procedure is absolutely contraindicated.

6. Fatty metamorphosis, cytoplasmic alcoholic hyaline, infiltration of portal areas by polymorphonuclear and mononuclear cells, and some degree of hepatocellular necrosis would certainly be anticipated. Portal fibrosis and proliferation of bile ducts with regenerating nodules would be seen if cirrhosis has actually begun.

7. The tiny positive filling defect at the apex of the duodenal bulb indicates an active duodenal ulcer. Deformity of the duodenal bulb indicates scarring from a previous ulcer or spasm associated with an active ulcer. Coarse mucosal folds throughout the stomach indicate gastric rugal hypertrophy and suggest the presence of gastritis (Menetrier disease), which may account for loss of albumin.

8. The two habits that might influence this patient's gastroduodenal and hepatic diseases are, of course, his alcoholism and the ingestion of salicylates. The ingestion of alcohol increases the secretion of acid by the stomach and may lead to mucosal damage and ulceration. The ingestion of

salicylates decreases mucosal resistance to ulcer. Nervousness can increase the secretion of acid and pepsin and also accentuate the use of alcohol.

9. Therapy should stress: (1) abstinence from alcohol because of adverse effects on liver and duodenum; (2) abstinence from aspirin; (3) frequent doses of a low sodium antacid; (4) possibly cimetidine; and (5) a well-balanced diet low in salt (1.0–1.5 g daily).

DISCUSSION OF CLINICAL CONFERENCE 7

This patient's nearly lifelong history of episodic abdominal pain, jaundice, pain in extremities, indolent cutaneous ulcers, and anemia lend strong support to a tentative diagnosis of a chronic hemolytic anemia. His race, the finding of sickle forms on blood smear, the low hematocrit, and leukocytosis support the diagnosis of sickle cell anemia. His serum bilirubin in the past has been almost solely unconjugated in type, but on this admission there is a large conjugated fraction as well, and this is confirmed by the presence of bilirubinuria. This shift to a conjugated variety of serum bilirubin indicates a clinical change from a purely hemolytic picture to an obstructive or hepatocellular form of jaundice. The elevated alkaline phosphatase suggests an obstructive disorder, and the presence of urobilinogen in his urine indicates that biliary obstruction is not complete.

The present attacks of abdominal pain are different from anything he has had in the past, so they probably do not represent sickle cell anemia crises. This impression is confirmed by the fact that his hemoglobin levels and reticulocyte counts are not different from those that he usually carries during remissions. His pain could be due to pancreatitis, a disorder that may lead to obstructive jaundice, and his serum amylase is somewhat elevated. However, it is unusual for attacks of pancreatitis to be as short and frequent as these, and amylase levels may rise in response to a variety of abdominal disorders. The possibility of intestinal infarctions owing to sickle cell disease should be considered, but the absence of abdominal distention, the presence of normal bowel sounds, the guaiac negative stool, and the onset of conjugated hyperbilirubinemia stand against it.

The plain film of his abdomen shows numerous partially calcified gallstones in the right upper abdominal quadrant. The calcification represents large deposits of pigment in the calculi, and the fact that patients with chronic hemolytic disease commonly develop gallstones, even at age 19, is well known. Although the mere presence of cholelithiasis does not mean that the gallstones themselves are responsible for his new symptoms, the symptoms themselves are quite typical of biliary spasm, and the new type of jaundice attests to the likelihood of stones in the common bile duct as well.

Treatment must be surgical because the biliary stones are symptomatic. The operation must include an exploration of the common bile duct because of the evidence of extrahepatic biliary obstruction.

The operation went smoothly, since the gall bladder was not acutely inflamed. Operative cholangiograms showed several calculi in the common bile duct, and these were also removed. Recovery was uneventful, the alkaline phosphatase fell to normal levels in 10 days, and the conjugated hyperbilirubinema disappeared in a short time.

DISCUSSION OF CLINICAL CONFERENCE 8

1. Abdominal fullness probably results from afferent loop distention after meals.

2. Loss of weight is probably related both to anorexia and absorptive disorder. Edema probably relates to protein malnutrition and malabsorption of peptides.

3. Neutral fat in untreated stool and normal intestinal mucosal pattern suggest maldigestion. The palpable bowel mass and the partially obstructed afferent loop on X ray suggest a blind-loop syndrome. The anemia is associated with an abnormal B_{12} level and Schilling test. This would account for the macrocytic anemia, but not the hypochromia. The abnormal xylose test suggests an intestinal defect, but may also result from intraluminal digestion of xylose by gut flora, a possibility which could be verified by repeating the xylose test after a short trial of antibiotics.

4. Serum iron and iron-binding capacity, repeat Schilling test, or B_{12} levels after trial of therapy with antibiotics.

5. Antibiotic treatment now would be appropriate to test hypothesis of maldigestion owing to bacterial overgrowth in an obstructed blind loop.

6. As before, patient does not have pernicious anemia because intrinsic factor did not convert Schilling test to normal. Bacterial overgrowth has now been demonstrated by aspiration of duodenum, and mucosal defect is ruled out by the normal small intestinal biopsy.

7. Antibiotics, broad spectrum.

8. Suggests another deficiency. What about serum iron?

9. Antibiotic therapy has decreased bacterial flora enough so that bile salts are no longer being deconjugated in the intestinal lumen and better mixed micelles are being formed, thus facilitating diffusion of free fatty acids and two monoglycerides across the unstirred aqueous layer bathing villous tip cells. The fact that a degree of steatorrhea persists suggests that a trial of pancreatic supplements would be in order, as might surgical correction of his obstructed afferent loop, so that food would have a better opportunity to mix with pancreatic enzymes.

10. His most recent loss of weight was the result of the disappearance of edema. Earlier, the malabsorption was responsible.

11. To repeat, blind-loop syndrome. Pancreatic insufficiency may also play a part, but it is more likely that his pancreas is normal, even though its

secretions are unable to traverse the blind loop in amounts adequate enough for complete digestion to occur.

12. B_{12} deficiency from bacterial consumption of B_{12}. Iron deficiency probably from postoperative gastritis, although one must observe stools for occult blood and perform endoscopy and lower intestinal X rays if blood loss persists.

DISCUSSION OF CLINICAL CONFERENCE 9

1. As the history unfolds, it is difficult to escape the initial impression that the patient's pain is pancreatic in origin. It is located in the midabdomen and left upper quadrant, and judging by the relief afforded by assuming a fetal position, the pain must also radiate into her back. A penetrating ulcer could cause similar symptoms, but such pain should have been at least partially relieved by food and antacids. Gall bladder disease should also be considered, but the early age of onset and the fact that no clear complications of cholecystitis have developed rules against that diagnosis.

2. If the initial impression of chronic relapsing pancreatitis is correct, her diarrhea and loss of weight could reasonably be the result of chronic pancreatic insufficiency with resultant malabsorption.

3. The regular menstrual periods, sustained fertility, and lack of anemia suggest a less than maximal degree of malabsorption. Amenorrhea and anemia are commonly seen in patients with untreated celiac sprue, and are less likely in malabsorption owing to pancreatic insufficiency. Continuing fertility is also evidence against a diagnosis of anorexia nervosa as the cause of her long-standing loss of weight and abdominal pain.

4. The glucose tolerance test shows a modestly diabetic response. Since she denies a family history of diabetes, the chances are likely that the patient is showing signs of pancreatic islet deficiency from chronic pancreatitis.

5. Large fat globules in an unacidified stool, as well as meat fibers, suggest pancreatic steatorrhea. Fat globules should not be seen in an unheated stool, although tiny scattered droplets can be seen after heating (see text).

6. Thus, one might again wish to rule out intestinal malabsorption with a xylose test and to perform a pancreatic drainage for appraisal of exocrine function.

7. Xylose test confirms the impression of normal absorption. Therefore, steatorrhea must be the result of maldigestion.

8. This question is somewhat off the main point of this case, since the patient has had no abdominal surgery aside from an appendectomy. However, had there been a history of gastric or ileal surgery, measurement of vitamin B_{12} levels and a Schilling test would be useful. Failure of an ab-

normal Schilling test to respond to intrinsic factor would implicate ileal disease and might also make one suspect bile salt deficiency as a cause of her steatorrhea.

9. No, although it does strongly implicate the pancreas.

10. A secretin test of pancreatic function.

11. Early age of onset suggests a hereditary form of pancreatitis. Hyperlipidemia, type I or type IV, should also be excluded, as should chronic cholecystitis.

12. A cholecystogram and blood lipid studies. The finding of gallstones would persuasively recommend surgery. Hyperlipemia would suggest a low fat diet.

13. See text.

14. Occasionally one sees cholesterol crystals in the bile of patients with chronic cholecystitis and no stones on cholecystography.

15. See text for answer to first question. No.

16. A family history, with pancreatic studies of blood relatives.

17. See text.

18. She has neither excessive blood loss nor folate or B_{12} malabsorption.

19. The cause of the aminoaciduria is unknown, but it is commonly seen in this patient's disorder—familial pancreatitis.

DISCUSSION OF CLINICAL CONFERENCE 10

1. Malabsorption syndromes of any type may result in growth failure, but are usually associated with abdominal complaints of bloating and distention for a much longer period of time than was the case here. Stools are usually bulky and malodorous, and unless the malabsorption results from a neoplasm such as lymphosarcoma or an infection such as tuberculosis, appetite is generally greater than normal despite loss of weight. Absence of previous respiratory infections is contrary to a diagnosis of cystic fibrosis and hypogammaglobulinemia, and the negative tine test is contrary to tuberculosis, although a state of tuberculin anergy may be present in patients with miliary disease.

Ulcerative colitis is a strong possibility, for it is often associated with growth failure and frequent stools and may be present for months or years without striking symptoms. The absence of gross blood in the stools, the perirectal abscess and, most importantly, the conclusive radiologic findings of thickening, stiffening, and loss of mucosal pattern in a long segment of terminal ileum are contrary to ulcerative colitis and point strongly to the probability that Crohn disease is the true diagnosis in this patient. The only element incompatible with this diagnosis is the massive upper gastrointestinal hemorrhage. Crohn disease may involve the stomach, but is not likely to cause bleeding of this severity. Furthermore, the second set of X rays showed a probable duodenal ulcer, which could have appeared as a result of stress from the enteritis and abscess or as a toxic response to the salicylates contained in the sulfasalazine with which the patient was originally treated.

Pituitary growth failure is most unlikely in this patient because of his gastrointestinal complaints and the absence of any signs or symptoms of other endocrine deficiency (hypothyroidism, hypoadrenalism), save for delayed onset of puberty.

2. Failure of growth and development, the perirectal abscess, and mild hypochromic anemia have already occurred. Abdominal cramps probably represent partial small intestinal obstruction. The gastrointestinal hemorrhage, probably from a duodenal ulcer, may have resulted from the patient's medication.

3. Many physicians would have used no medication at all, based on their knowledge that perirectal abscesses and fistulas rarely heal in patient's with regional enteritis without surgical extirpation of the diseased small intestine. Adrenocorticosteroids would only have aggravated the growth failure, and azathiaprine is probably too drastic a drug to use when other courses of therapy such as surgery show promise of being able to cope with the disease. In this patient sulfasalazine and oral iron were used initially, in the hope that the disease could be controlled at least temporarily, and to allow time for the patient to regain weight and strength.

The hemorrhage was treated by suspension of previous medication, a 500-ml transfusion of blood, and the administration of hourly doses of liquid antacids and milk. Bleeding stopped within 24 hours, and the patient felt well.

4. The patient's growth failure, the appearance of a duodenal ulcer, and the perirectal abscess made the indications for definitive surgery clear. The cecum and a 50-cm segment of terminal ileum were removed, and an ileoascending colostomy was formed. A duodenal ulcer was identified at surgery and treated with vagotomy and pyloroplasty. The resected ileal segment contained both normal and diseased portions (Figure A–3). No other diseased segments were identified.

The patient grew quickly after his operation. He is now in his early thirties, asymptomatic, married, 160 cm tall, and the father of two children.

DISCUSSION OF CLINICAL CONFERENCE 11

1. The most likely diagnosis in this patient is either chronic ulcerative colitis or Crohn disease. Chronic amebic colitis would be a slight possibility, although arthritis rarely occurs in association with that disorder. Chronic ulcerative colitis appears to be the most likely diagnosis, as the following tabulation suggests:

	Supports Diagnosis of Ulcerative Colitis	Supports Diagnosis of Crohn Disease
Chronic diarrhea	X	X
Migratory arthritis	X	X
Gross blood in stools	X	
Mucosal granularity	X	X
Mucosal friability	X	
Pseudopolyps	X	
Ulcerations on X ray	X	X
Precipitated by emotional stress	X	X

2. Complications that have already occurred are: malnutrition, hemorrhage, colitic arthritis, cholestasis, anal fissure, and hyperglycemia (? induced by glucocorticoids). Future possibilities are: cirrhosis of the liver, chronic iron-deficiency anemia, and carcinoma of the colon (since this disorder involves the entire colon and has lasted over 10 years).

3. At this stage, one would expect to see numerous crypt abscesses (granularity), with coalescence of some adjacent abscesses. The entire lamina propria would be infiltrated with inflammatory round cells and plasma cells (edema of mucosa). The crypts would also be shallower than normal, probably from long-continued inflammation, and the lamina propria thinned out. Small ulcers would also be seen in the colon above the rectum (X ray findings). Inflammatory exudate and some scarring would also be found in the submucosa (loss of haustrations). Mucosal capillaries would be dilated, and blood might be extravasating from them (friability). In ulcerated areas, occasional capillaries would be thrombosed.

4. A continuation of medical therapy with steroids and sulfasalazine could be considered, or colectomy could be advised. The fact that his joint symptoms had flared in a response to a dose as high as 15 mg of prednisone; that his alkaline phosphatase was high, indicating cholestasis; that he had already experienced one severe episode of colitis with hemorrhage; that his history of diarrhea has lasted over 10 years; that his family problems were unchanged; and that his fasting blood sugar was elevated (corticosteroid-induced diabetes) would all suggest colectomy. However, the patient would have to be mentally and emotionally prepared for life with an ileostomy, a responsibility that must be undertaken by the physician, using patience and sympathy.

Figure A–3. *A*, gross surgical specimen showing Crohn disease of the terminal ileum. Note normal segment of ileum proximal to the lesion, and normal cecum distally. The margins of resection were free of disease. *B*, ileal mucosa showing ulceration of the epithelium and marked infiltration of the lamina propria and submucosa with lymphocytes. Original magnification x60.

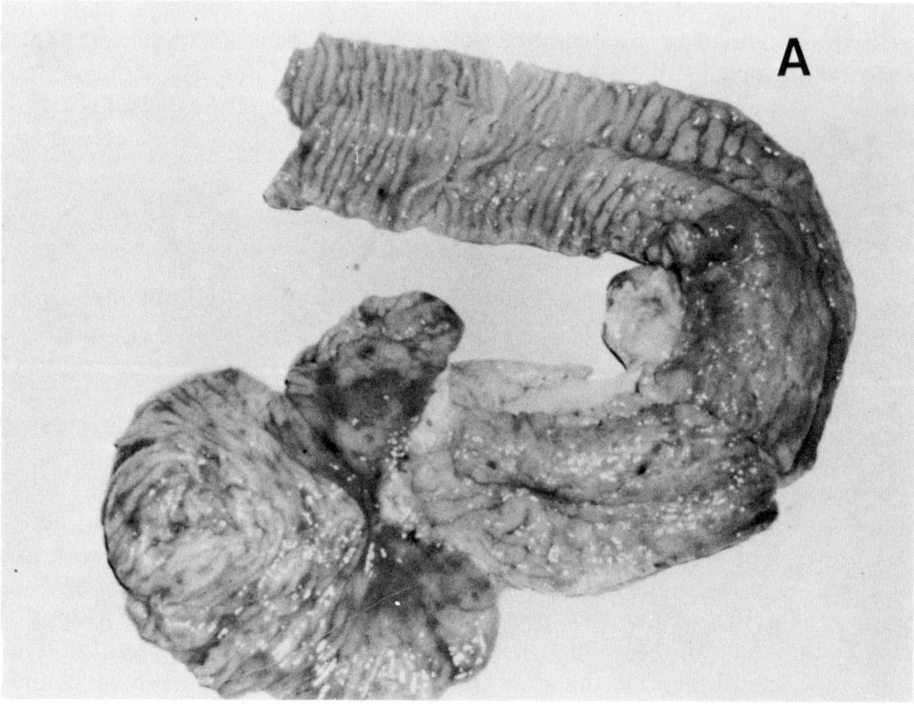
A

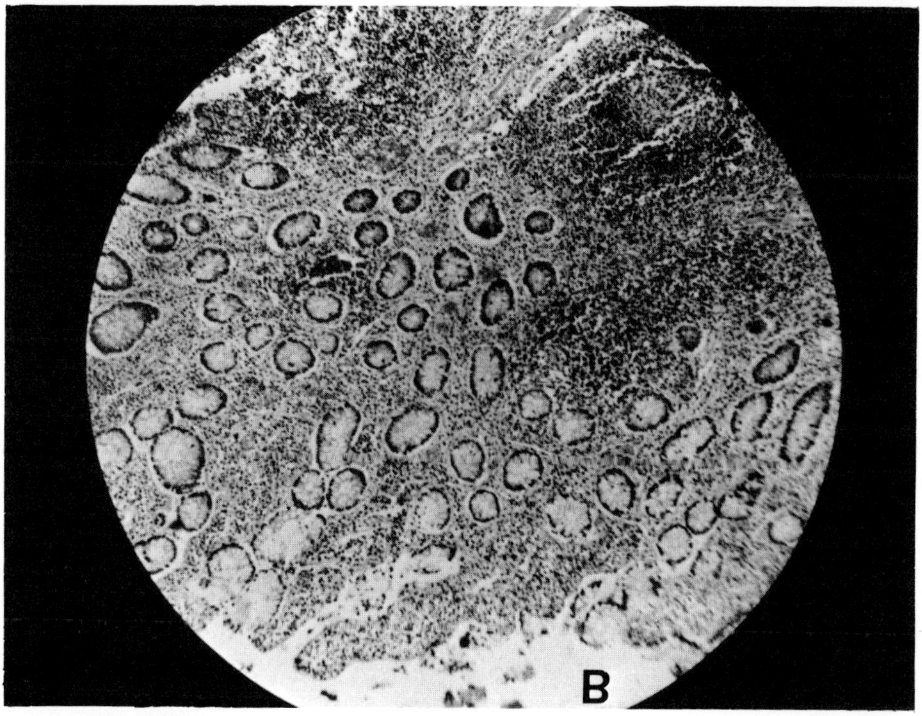
B

This patient elected to continue with prednisone treatment, since the arthritis subsided in the hospital. However, recurrent bleeding and aggravated diarrhea led him to change his mind and to undergo surgery four months later. He tolerated the operation well and has made a most satisfactory adjustment to his ileostomy.

DISCUSSION OF CLINICAL CONFERENCE 12

1. This patient has a long history of constipation, and now has symptoms of partial lower bowel obstruction (cramps aggravated by eating, diarrhea), signs of inflammation (fever, leukocytosis), and possibly localized peritonitis (left lower quadrant tenderness and muscular spasm). Peristaltic rushes with simultaneous pain support the notion of obstruction, as does the abdominal mass. The barium enema establishes a diagnosis of diverticulosis and suggests diverticulitis as well because of the clustered sigmoidal diverticula and spasm. Penetration of barium at one point beyond the confines of the bowel wall suggests the possibility of an abscess between colon and bladder. This is supported by the complaint of urinary frequency and the finding of pyuria. However, prostatic hypertrophy and urinary retention may be the cause of these abnormalities. The patient's loss of weight and the finding of occult blood in the stool should suggest that a sigmoid carcinoma may be responsible for the obstructive complaints, even though diverticulitis alone is a reasonable cause.

2. Therapeutic mechanisms for treatment of obstructive diverticulitis with possible abscess consist of relieving smooth muscle spasm, facilitating bowel movements, and combating infection. The possible complications from opiates, which stimulate smooth muscle contraction, are demonstrated by this patient's experience. Antispasmodics should be used with care, since they may lead to increasing urinary retention by relaxing the smooth muscle of the urinary bladder behind a partially obstructing enlarged prostate.

Failure of symptoms to respond to therapy within a week should lead to surgical resection of the diseased colon. Even a partial response, in which signs of infection and peritonitis subside but obstruction or occult blood persist, would be a strong indication for surgery unless another X ray examination of the colon shows enough improvement to minimize the possibility of an adenocarcinoma. A colonoscopy might also be useful in ruling out colonic cancer.

DISCUSSION OF CLINICAL CONFERENCE 13

1. One must presume at least two underlying disorders in this patient's illness: the first causing the anginal pain, the second causing her anemia. In all likelihood these disorders are interrelated, because if the chest symp-

toms are felt to be the result of myocardial ischemia or infarction, the anemia certainly contributes to the problem. The slowly progressive nature of her symptoms over the period of one year indicates that the anemia was not of sudden onset, and the normal color of her stools indicates that she at no time had a massive intestinal hemorrhage. The normal AsAT and electrocardiogram suggest that she has not had a fresh myocardial infarction.

2. The chest complaints are, in the absence of valvular heart disease, diagnostic enough of coronary arteriosclerosis to be considered pathognomonic. Although the systolic murmur may represent aortic valvular disease, it does not seem to be intense enough to suggest aortic stenosis, and we are given inadequate information regarding the character of the second sound and the presence of a systolic thrill.

The nature of the anemia is not so clear. It could certainly be the result of a slowly bleeding gastrointestinal lesion, first, because this is the commonest cause of chronic anemias among the elderly, and second, because this conference is a gastrointestinal exercise. The fact that her vital signs are normal with a hematocrit of 23 favors chronic rather than acute loss.

This patient could also have pernicious anemia, a disease that usually appears insidiously. Hemolysis is unlikely in view of the absence of jaundice, although this is not diagnostic. Aplastic and myelophthisic anemias are unlikely in view of the normal white count and differential.

If the anemia is the result of iron deficiency, we have numerous disorders to consider as the cause, ranging from chronic esophagitis to internal hemorrhoids.

3. The patient certainly requires serial cardiograms and AsAT determinations to rule on the possibility of a myocardial infarction. Red cell indices and serum iron determinations will help to decide the cause of the anemia. A gastric analysis and serum levels of vitamin B_{12} are useful in diagnosing pernicious anemia. Guaiac studies of the stool will indicate whether gastrointestinal bleeding is continuous. Finally, if the anemia is the result of loss of blood, gastrointestinal X rays may reveal the site of bleeding.

4. The information almost certainly rules out an acute myocardial infarction. The indices of the red cells, being microcytic, rule out the possibility of pernicious anemia. The serum iron studies prove the presence of iron deficiency, and the stool guaiac determinations indicate that the loss is from the gastrointestinal tract.

5. The indications for complete X rays of the gastrointestinal tract are now crystal clear, since gastrointestinal bleeding has been conclusively demonstrated. As long as the patient is free of pain and the likelihood of a myocardial infarction is minimal, the studies should be done without delay. If the X rays are normal, the temptation would be to observe the patient for a further period of time. However, this would be a mistake, since chronic gastrointestinal bleeding among the elderly is so often the result of a malignant disease. If the X rays were indeed negative, one might try to locate the point of bleeding with gastrointestinal endoscopy and intubation, then operate.

6. The point to be made by this question is the inadvisability of giving whole blood to anemic, elderly patients whose circulating blood volumes are probably normal at the time of transfusion. This may lead to volume overloads and acute left heart failure. In view of this, it would have been advisable to transfuse packed red cells rather than whole blood.

7. The patient continues to bleed and her X rays are normal. The presence of normal amounts of acid in her stomach is a further indication against pernicious anemia, but this had already been ruled out. The presence of acid certainly does not tell us that she is free of a gastric carcinoma. The absence of blood in the intestinal tract until the tip of the tube, as shown on the X rays, was in the ileocecal area is very helpful information. This almost certainly represents a bleeding lesion in that portion of the intestine. One could now perform a colonoscopy to verify the presence of a cecal lesion.

8. Several lesions could cause this type of bleeding from the ileocecal area, but first and foremost is a carcinoma of the cecum—a diagnosis that must be kept in mind even in the presence of normal X rays. Carcinoid tumors are also common in this area and may bleed slowly. Even in an elderly patient the possibility of a Meckel diverticulum must be kept in mind, although bleeding from ulcerations owing to such an anomaly is usually massive and acute.

9. Surgical exploration through a right lower quadrant incision!

This was done, and the patient was found to have two polypoid carcinomas of the cecum (Figure A–4). Nearly 30 lymph nodes were found in the surgical specimen, and none of these showed metastases, so the prognosis in this patient is quite good.

After surgery the two barium enema examinations were reviewed, and no evidence of the cecal tumors was found on the films. This illustrates the importance of persistence in discovering the cause of serious symptoms, even when commonly performed exclusion tests are negative. This case also demonstrates the well-known clinical fact that cecal carcinomas are often asymptomatic, save for bleeding.

DISCUSSION OF CLINICAL CONFERENCE 14

A patient with maturity-onset diabetes complains of relentless and progressively severe watery diarrhea for the previous seven months, unassociated with loss of weight. He also has a remote history of recurrent ureteral calculi. The diarrhea worsens rapidly after his first office visit and, when evaluated in hospital, proves to be voluminous and isosmolar in character. This is truly a secretory diarrhea of the sort associated with bacterial toxins (cholera or a toxigenic *Escherichia coli* infection, for example) or with alimentary hormonal excess of such polypeptides as gastrin or vasoactive intestinal peptide (VIP). The normal osmolality of the stools is strongly

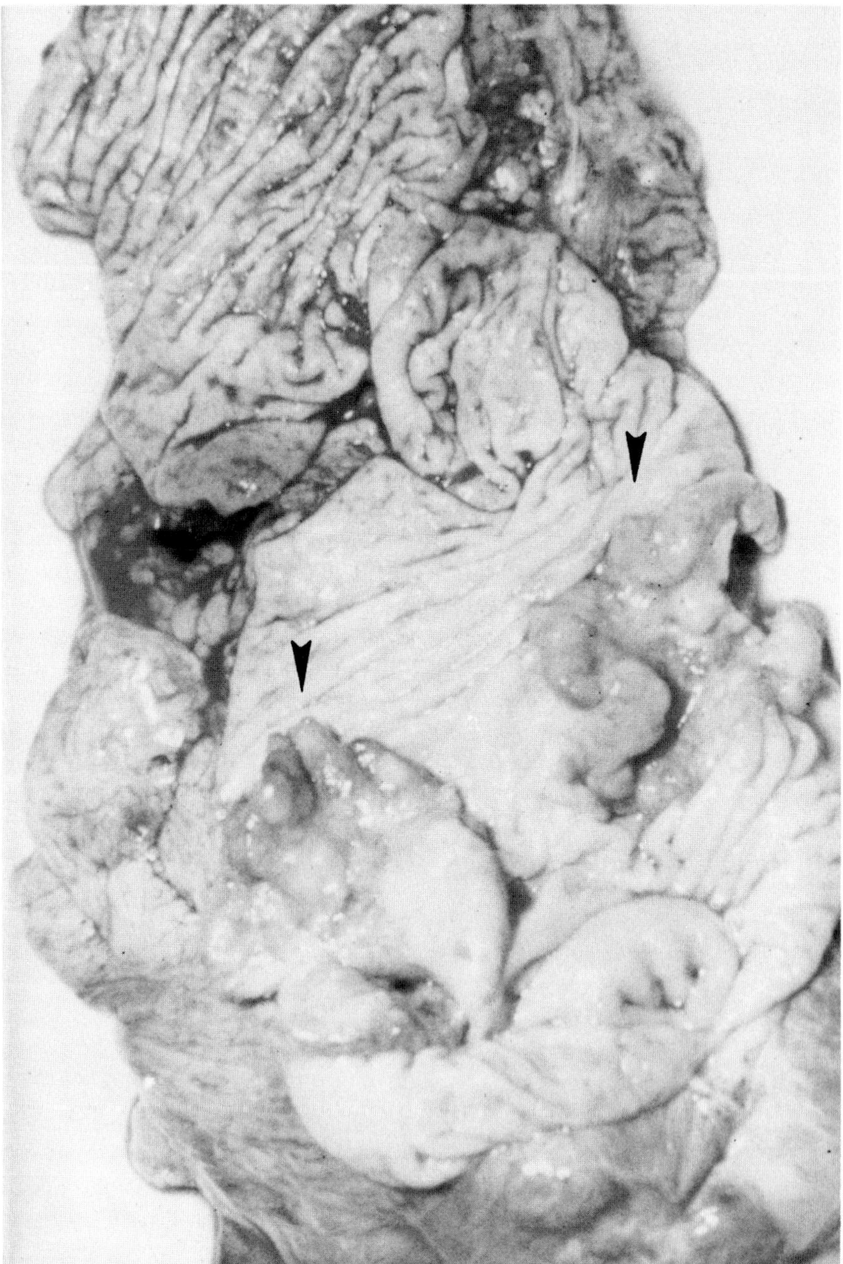

Figure A–4. Terminal ileum (*right*) and cecum. Note two polypoid carcinomas (arrows).

against the possibility that patient has been surreptitiously ingesting a poorly absorbed osmotic laxative. The prolonged history favors consideration of a hormonal cause, rather than the effects of a bacterial entertoxin. Since there is no evidence of past or present peptic ulcers, an islet-cell adenoma secreting VIP is favored over one secreting only gastrin.

Such adenomata are usually associated with adenomata in other endocrine organs, especially the parathyroids and the pituitary gland (multiple endocrine adenomatosis, type I). In this case, there is strong evidence for functioning parathyroid adenoma(s), as evidenced by the history of ureteral calculi, hypercalcemic, hyperchloremic acidosis, hypophosphatemia, elevated serum alkaline phosphatase, and the finding of scattered areas of osteoporosis. The enlarged and eroded sella turcica supports the diagnosis of a pituitary adenoma as well.

Multiple endocrine adenomatosis is inherited as an autosomal dominant with 60 to 80 percent gene penetrance (Lynch et al 1979). This patient's paternal grandfather died at an early age from an unusual malignancy, and his father also succumbed to an ill-defined cancer in the chest. Nothing further was known of his paternal relatives. This history also supports the probability that one or more of patient's adenomata may be malignant.

His plasma VIP level was greater than 400 pg per ml (normal, 43–76), and the serum gastrin was 140 pg per ml (normal, less than 100). The high levels of VIP may explain the ileus which troubled this patient, as well as being the cause of the secretory diarrhea. VIP has been shown to relax the smooth muscle of the lower esophageal sphincter, the gastric fundus, and the gall bladder, colon, and rectum (Said 1980), although the effect on ileal motility may be stimulatory. Glucagon may also be responsible for transient intestinal relaxation by inhibition of the interdigestive motor complex. Hypercalcemia may also have contributed to the ileus.

In this patient with multiple endocrine adenomatosis, it was deemed best to attack the hyperparathyroidism initially, because of the interference of sustained hypercalcemia with cardiac conduction. At surgery, adenomatous hyperplasia was found in the left superior and inferior parathyroid glands, both of which were resected. A small thyroid adenoma was also removed.

Levels of serum calcium were well controlled after surgery, and plans were then made to remove the probable pancreatic tumor. Celiac arteriography showed a tumor blush in the head of the pancreas, and also revealed a large tumor mass in the left lobe of the liver, thus indicating the probable malignant nature of the disease. Massive diarrhea persisted, and could not be controlled with prostaglandin and adenylate cyclase inhibitory agents. Surgery was undertaken primarily for tumor debulking purposes prior to the start of chemotherapy with streptozocin.

A subtotal pancreatectomy was performed. The body of the organ contained a 200-g tumor mass which, on microscopy, was composed of irregularly shaped cells with granular cytoplasm, and nuclei which were pleo-

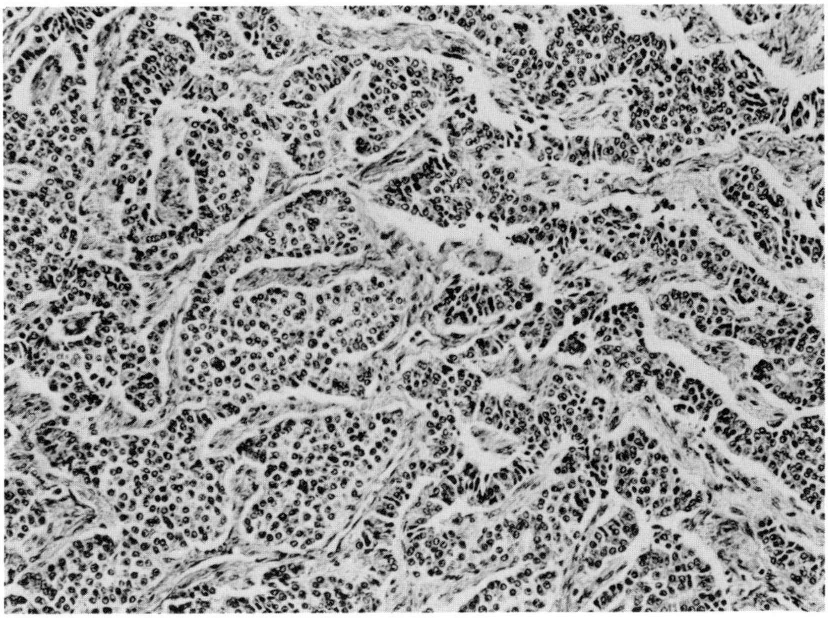

Figure A–5. Islet cell tumor of pancreas. The tumor cells are arranged in cords, ribbons, and nests. The rich vascular network is characteristic of an endocrine tumor, in this case one which secretes vasoactive intestinal polypeptide. Original magnification x150.

morphic and hyperchromatic with prominent nucleoli (Figure A-5). Several separate tumor foci in the pancreas and tissue from the hepatic mass showed the same histology.

Patient's diarrhea, consisting of up to 8 liters daily, continued after surgery. Renal damage appeared after his first treatment with streptozocin and, shortly afterward, he developed the shock lung syndrome, which could not be successfully managed. Death occurred about one month after the abdominal operation.

SELECTED REFERENCES

Lynch HT, Lynch PM, Albano WA, et al. Hereditary cancer: ascertainment and management. Ca 29:216–32, 1979.

Said SI. Vasoactive intestinal peptide (VIP): isolation, distribution, biological actions, structure-function relationships, and possible functions. In: Glass GBJ, ed. Gastrointestinal hormones. New York: Raven Press, 1980:245–74.

INDEX